This is a classic book on yoga. Practical and extensively illustrated it describes over 200 postures (āsanas and bandhas) and 14 breathing exercises (prāṇāyāmas) in detail. The 600 photographs, placed in the relevant part of the text, enable the reader to practise a posture without a teacher. There is a summary of the meaning of Yoga, and the nāḍīs, chakras and kuṇḍalinī are also considered. An Appendix directs the reader to specific exercises for a wide variety of ailments and for the serious student there is a long yoga course of over 300 weeks. B. K. S. Iyengar has been teaching yoga since 1936 and has given demonstrations throughout the world.

To. Mrs Dabir.
for Good health
[illegible]

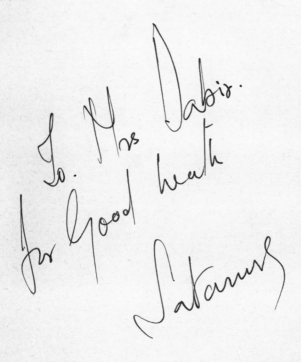

LIGHT ON YOGA

By the same author

THE CONCISE LIGHT ON YOGA
LIGHT ON PRANAYAMA

Other Yoga books

BIKRAM'S BEGINNING YOGA CLASS
YOGA AND HEALTH
YOGA FOR HEALTH AND VITALITY
YOGA SELF-TAUGHT
YOGA WEEK BY WEEK

For further information on Iyengar Yoga, the recently opened Iyengar Yoga Institute is at 223A Randolph Avenue, London W9. Phone: 01-624 3080.

Light on Yoga

Yoga Dipika

B. K. S. IYENGAR

Foreword by Yehudi Menuhin

London
UNWIN PAPERBACKS
Boston Sydney

First published in Great Britain by George Allen & Unwin 1966
Second edition 1968
Reprinted nine times
First published in Unwin Paperbacks 1976
Reprinted 1979
Re-issued 1982
Reprinted 1982
Reprinted 1984
Reprinted 1985
Reprinted 1986

Unwin® Paperbacks
40 Museum Street, London, WC1A 1LU, UK

Unwin Paperbacks
Park Lane, Hemel Hempstead, Herts HP2 4TE, UK

George Allen & Unwin Australia Pty Ltd.,
8 Napier Street, North Sydney, NSW 2060, Australia

British Library Cataloguing in Publication Data

Iyengar, B K S
Light on yoga.
1. Yoga, Hatha
I. Title
181'.45 B132.Y6

ISBN 0-04-149035-5

Printed and bound in Great Britain by
Hazell Watson & Viney Limited,
Member of the BPCC Group,
Aylesbury, Bucks

Dedicated to my Revered Gurujī

Sāmkya-yoga-Śikhāmaṇi; Veda-kesari; Vedāntavāgīśa; Nyāyāchārya; Mīmāmsa-ratna; Mīmāmsa-thīrtha

Professor, Śrīmān, T. Krishnamāchārya of Mysore (South India), India

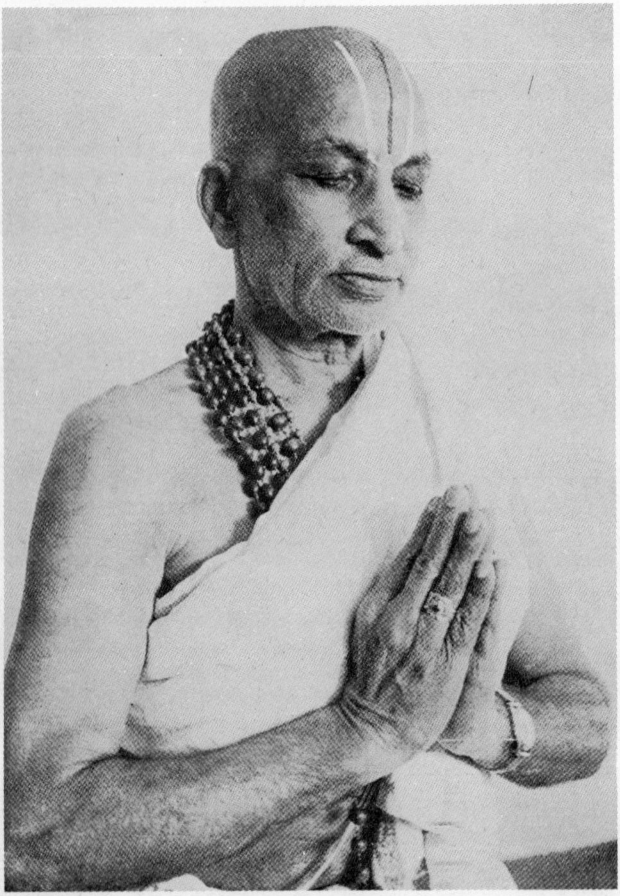

PRAYER

'I bow before the noblest of sages, Patañjali, who brought serenity of mind by his work on yoga, clarity of speech by his work on grammar and purity of body by his work on medicine.'

'I salute Ādīśvara (the Primeval Lord Śiva) who taught first the science of Haṭha Yoga – a science that stands out as a ladder for those who wish to scale the heights of Rāja Yoga.'

Foreword by Yehudi Menuhin

The practice of Yoga induces a primary sense of measure and proportion. Reduced to our own body, our first instrument, we learn to play it, drawing from it maximum resonance and harmony. With unflagging patience we refine and animate every cell as we return daily to the attack, unlocking and liberating capacities otherwise condemned to frustration and death.

Each unfulfilled area of tissue and nerve, of brain or lung, is a challenge to our will and integrity, or otherwise a source of frustration and death. Whoever has had the privilege of receiving Mr Iyengar's attention, or of witnessing the precision, refinement and beauty of his art, is introduced to that vision of perfection and innocence which is man as first created – unarmed, unashamed, son of God, lord of creation – in the Garden of Eden. The tree of knowledge has indeed yielded much fruit of great variety, sweet, poisonous, bitter, wholesome according to our use of it. But is it not more imperative than ever that we cultivate the tree, that we nourish its roots? And furthermore how dangerous is that knowledge to those who, ill at ease with themselves, would rather apply it to the manipulation of other people and things than to the improvement of their own persons.

The practice of Yoga over the past fifteen years has convinced me that most of our fundamental attitudes to life have their physical counterparts in the body. Thus comparison and criticism must begin with the alignment of our own left and right sides to a degree at which even finer adjustments are feasible: or strength of will will cause us to start by stretching the body from the toes to the top of the head in defiance of gravity. Impetus and ambition might begin with the sense of weight and speed that comes with free-swinging limbs, instead of with the control of prolonged balance on foot, feet or hands, which gives poise. Tenacity is gained by stretching in various Yoga postures for minutes at a time, while calmness comes with quiet, consistent breathing and the expansion of the lungs. Continuity and a sense of the universal come with the knowledge of the inevitable alternation of tension and relaxation in eternal rhythms of which each inhalation and exhalation constitutes one cycle, wave or vibration among the countless myriads which are the universe.

What is the alternative? Thwarted, warped people condemning the order of things, cripples criticising the upright, autocrats slumped in expectant coronary attitudes, the tragic spectacle of people working out their own imbalance and frustration on others.

Yoga, as practised by Mr Iyengar, is the dedicated votive offering of a man who brings himself to the altar, alone and clean in body and mind, focussed in attention and will, offering in simplicity and innocence not a burnt sacrifice, but simply himself raised to his own highest potential.

It is a technique ideally suited to prevent physical and mental illness and to protect the body generally, developing an inevitable sense of self-reliance and assurance. By its very nature it is inextricably associated with universal laws: for respect for life, truth, and patience are all indispensable factors in the drawing of a quiet breath, in calmness of mind and firmness of will.

In this lie the moral virtues inherent in Yoga. For these reasons it demands a complete and total effort, involving and forming the whole human being. No mechanical repetition is involved and no lip-service as in the case of good resolutions or formal prayers. By its very nature it is each time and every moment a living act.

Mr Iyengar's *Light on Yoga* will, I hope, enable many to follow his example and to become the teachers whom mankind so sorely needs. If this book will serve to spread this basic art and will ensure that it is practised at the highest level, I shall feel more than ever grateful for having shared in its presentation.

London, 1964

Preface

It is only thanks to the persistent encouragement of my devoted friends and pupils that this book is now achieved – for alone I would have repeatedly faltered not only because of my inadequate command of the English language but because I would have lost heart without their buoyant support and assurance.

Yoga is a timeless pragmatic science evolved over thousands of years dealing with the physical, moral, mental and spiritual well-being of man as a whole.

The first book to systematise this practice was the classic treatise the *Yoga Sutras* (or Aphorisms) of Patañjali dating from 200 BC. Unfortunately most of the books published on Yoga in our day have been unworthy of both the subject and its first great exponent, as they are superficial, popular and at times misleading. I have even been asked by their readers whether I can drink acid, chew glass, walk through fire, make myself invisible or perform other magical acts. Scholarly and reliable expositions of the religious and philosophical texts already exist in most languages – but the practice of an art is more difficult to communicate than a purely literary or philosophical concept.

The title of this book is *Light on Yoga* (Yoga Dīpikā in Sanskrit), as my purpose is to describe as simply as possible the āsanas (postures) and prāṇāyāmas (breathing disciplines) in the new light of our own era, its knowledge and its requirements. Instructions on āsana and prāṇāyāma are therefore given in great detail and are based on my experience for over twenty-seven years in many parts of the world. It contains the complete technique of 200 āsanas with 592 photographs from which the āsanas can be mastered: and it also covers bandha, kriyā and prāṇāyāma with a further 5 photographs.

The Western reader may be surprised at the recurring reference to the Universal Spirit, to mythology and even to philosophical and moral principles. He must not forget that in ancient times all the higher achievements of man, in knowledge, art and power, were part of religion and were assumed to belong to God and to His priestly servants on earth. The Catholic Pope is the last such embodiment of divine knowledge and power in the West. But formerly, even in the Western world, music, painting, architecture, philosophy and medicine, as well as wars, were always in the service of God. It is only very recently in India that these arts and sciences have begun to be emancipated from the Divine – but with due respect, for the emancipation of man's will, as distinct from the Divine will, we in India continue to value the purity of purpose, the humility of discipline and the selflessness that are the legacy of our long bondage to God. I consider it important as well as interesting that the reader should know the origin of āsanas, and I have, therefore, included legends handed down by practising yogis and sages.

All the ancient commentaries on yoga have stressed that it is essential to work under the direction of a GURU (Master), and although my experience proves the wisdom of this rule, I have endeavoured with all humility in this book to guide the reader – both teacher and student – to a correct and safe method of mastering these āsanas and prāṇāyāmas.

In Appendix I, I have introduced a 300 weeks' course for the intense practitioner, grouping the āsanas stage by stage according to their structure.

In Appendix II, I have arranged groups of āsanas for their therapeutic and curative value.

Study in detail the hints and cautions before attempting the āsana and prāṇāyāma techniques.

I am sincerely grateful to my esteemed friend and pupil Mr Yehudi Menuhin for his foreword and immeasurable support.

I am indebted to my pupil Mr B. I. Taraporewala for his collaboration in the preparation of this book.

I thank Messrs Allen and Unwin for their gesture in publishing this exhaustively illustrated book and presenting my work to a world-wide public.

I express my sincere gratitude to Messrs G. G. Welling of Poona (India), for their personal supervision and interest in taking innumerable photographs for me and for placing the resources of their studio at my disposal.

The author wishes to express his gratitude to Mr Gerald Yorke for the care with which he dealt with the editing of the typescript and subsequent proof correction.

B. K. S. IYENGAR

Contents

Part I
Introduction

What is Yoga?

The word Yoga is derived from the Sanskrit root yuj meaning to bind, join, attach and yoke, to direct and concentrate one's attention on, to use and apply. It also means union or communion. It is the true union of our will with the will of God. 'It thus means,' says Mahadev Desai in his introduction to the *Gita according to Gandhi*, 'the yoking of all the powers of body, mind and soul to God; it means the disciplining of the intellect, the mind, the emotions, the will, which that Yoga presupposes; it means a poise of the soul which enables one to look at life in all its aspects evenly.'

Yoga is one of the six orthodox systems of Indian philosophy. It was collated, co-ordinated and systematised by Patañjali in his classical work, the *Yoga Sutras*, which consists of 185 terse aphorisms. In Indian thought, everything is permeated by the Supreme Universal Spirit (Paramātmā or God) of which the individual human spirit (jīvātmā) is a part. The system of yoga is so called because it teaches the means by which the jīvātmā can be united to, or be in communion with the Paramātmā, and so secure liberation (mokṣa).

One who follows the path of Yoga is a yogi or yogin.

In the sixth chapter of the *Bhagavad Gītā*, which is the most important authority on Yoga philosophy, Śri Krishna explains to Arjuna the meaning of Yoga as a deliverance from contact with pain and sorrow. It is said:

'When his mind, intellect and self (ahaṁkāra) are under control, freed from restless desire, so that they rest in the spirit within, a man becomes a Yukta – one in communion with God. A lamp does not flicker in a place where no winds blow; so it is with a yogi, who controls his mind, intellect and self, being absorbed in the spirit within him. When the restlessness of the mind, intellect and self is stilled through the practice of Yoga, the yogi by the grace of the Spirit within himself finds fulfilment. Then he knows the joy eternal which is beyond the pale of the senses which his reason cannot grasp. He abides in this reality and moves not therefrom. He has found the treasure above all others. There is nothing higher than this. He who has achieved it, shall not be moved by the greatest sorrow. This is the real meaning of Yoga – a deliverance from contact with pain and sorrow.'

As a well cut diamond has many facets, each reflecting a different colour of light, so does the word yoga, each facet reflecting a different shade of meaning and revealing different aspects of the entire range of human endeavour to win inner peace and happiness.

The *Bhagavad Gītā* also gives other explanations of the term yoga and lays stress upon Karma Yoga (Yoga by action). It is said: 'Work alone is your privilege, never the fruits thereof. Never let the fruits of action be your motive; and never cease to work. Work in the name of the Lord, abandoning selfish desires. Be not affected by success or failure. This equipoise is called Yoga.'

Yoga has also been described as wisdom in work or skilful living amongst activities, harmony and moderation.

'Yoga is not for him who gorges too much, nor for him who starves himself. It is not for him who sleeps too much, nor for him who stays awake. By moderation in eating and in resting, by regulation in working and by concordance in sleeping and waking, Yoga destroys all pain and sorrow.'

The *Kaṭhopanishad* describes Yoga thus: 'When the senses are stilled, when the mind is at rest, when the intellect wavers not – then, say the wise, is reached the highest stage. This steady control of the senses and mind has been defined as Yoga. He who attains it is free from delusion.'

In the second aphorism of the first chapter of the *Yoga Sutras*, Patañjali describes Yoga as 'chitta vṛtti nirodhah'. This may be translated as the restraint (nirodhah) of mental (chitta) modifications (vṛtti) or as suppression (nirodhah) of the fluctuations (vṛtti) of consciousness (chitta). The word chitta denotes the mind in its total or collective sense as being composed of three categories: (a) mind (manas, that is, the individual mind having the power and faculty of attention, selection and rejection; it is the oscillating indecisive faculty of the mind); (b) intelligence or reason (buddhi, that is, the decisive state which determines the distinction between things) and (c) ego (ahaṁkāra, literally the I-maker, the state which ascertains that 'I know').

The word vṛtti is derived from the Sanskrit root vṛt meaning to turn, to revolve, to roll on. It thus means course of action, behaviour, mode of being, condition or mental state. Yoga is the method by which the restless mind is calmed and the energy directed into constructive channels. As a mighty river which when properly harnessed by dams and canals, creates a vast reservoir of water, prevents famine and provides abundant power for industry; so also the mind, when controlled, provides a reservoir of peace and generates abundant energy for human uplift.

The problem of controlling the mind is not capable of easy solution, as borne out by the following dialogue in the sixth chapter of the *Bhagavad Gītā*. Arjuna asks Śri Krishna:

'Krishna, you have told me of Yoga as a communion with Brahman (the Universal Spirit), which is ever one. But how can this be permanent, since the mind is so restless and inconsistent? The mind is impetuous and stubborn, strong and wilful, as difficult to harness as the wind.' Śri Krishna replies: 'Undoubtedly, the mind is restless and hard to control. But it can be trained by constant practice (abhyāsa) and by freedom from desire (vairāgya). A man who cannot control his mind will find it difficult to attain this divine communion; but the self-controlled man can attain it if he tries hard and directs his energy by the right means.'

THE STAGES OF YOGA

The right means are just as important as the end in view. Patañjali enumerates these means as the eight limbs or stages of Yoga for the quest of the soul. They are:

1. Yama (universal moral commandments); 2. Niyama (self purification by discipline); 3. Āsana (posture); 4. Prāṇāyāma (rhythmic control of the breath); 5. Pratyāhāra (withdrawal and emancipation of the mind from the domination of the senses and exterior objects); 6. Dhāraṇa (concentration); 7. Dhyāna (meditation) and 8. Samādhi (a state of super-consciousness brought about by profound meditation, in which the individual aspirant (sādhaka) becomes one with the object of his meditation – Paramātmā or the Universal Spirit).

Yama and Niyama control the yogi's passions and emotions and keep him in harmony with his fellow man. Ásanas keep the body healthy and strong and in harmony with nature. Finally, the yogi becomes free of body consciousness. He conquers the body and renders it a fit vehicle for the soul. The first three stages are the outward quests (bahiranga sādhanā).

The next two stages, Prāṇāyāma and Pratyāhāra, teach the aspirant to regulate the breathing, and thereby control the mind. This helps to free the senses from the thraldom of the objects of desire. These two stages of Yoga are known as the inner quests (antaranga sādhanā).

Dhāranā, Dhyāna and Samādhi take the yogi into the innermost recesses of his soul. The yogi does not look heavenward to find God. He knows that HE is within, being known as the Antarātmā (the Inner Self). The last three stages keep him in harmony with himself and his Maker. These stages are called antarātmā sādhanā, the quest of the soul.

By profound meditation, the knower, the knowledge and the known become one. The seer, the sight and the seen have no separate existence from each other. It is like a great musician becoming one with his instrument and the music that comes from it. Then, the yogi stands in his own nature and realises his self (Ātman), the part of the Supreme Soul within himself.

There are different paths (mārgas) by which a man travels to his Maker. The active man finds realisation through Karma Mārga, in which a man realises his own divinity through work and duty. The emotional man finds it through Bhakti Mārga, where there is realisation through devotion to and love of a personal God. The intellectual man pursues Jñāna Mārga, where realisation comes through knowledge. The meditative or reflective man follows Yoga Mārga, and realises his own divinity through control of the mind.

Happy is the man who knows how to distinguish the real from the unreal, the eternal from the transient and the good from the pleasant by his discrimination and wisdom. Twice blessed is he who knows true love and can love all God's creatures. He who works selflessly for the welfare of others with love in his heart is thrice blessed. But the man who combines within his mortal frame knowledge, love and selfless service is holy and becomes a place of pilgrimage, like the confluence of the rivers Gangā, Saraswatī and Jamunā. Those who meet him become calm and purified.

Mind is the king of the senses. One who has conquered his mind, senses, passions, thought and reason is a king among men. He is fit for Rāja Yoga, the royal union with the Universal Spirit. He has Inner Light.

He who has conquered his mind is a Rāja Yogi. The word rāja means a king. The expression Rāja Yoga implies a complete mastery of the Self. Though Patañjali explains the ways to control the mind, he nowhere states in his aphorisms that this science is Rāja Yoga, but calls it Aṣṭāṅga Yoga or the eight stages (limbs) of Yoga. As it implies complete mastery of the self one may call it the science of Rāja Yoga.

Swātmārāma, the author of the *Hatha Yoga Pradīpikā* (haṭha = force or determined effort) called the same path Haṭha Yoga because it demanded rigorous discipline.

It is generally believed that Rāja Yoga and Haṭha Yoga are entirely distinct, different and opposed to each other, that the *Yoga Sutras* of Patañjāli deal with Spiritual discipline and that the *Hatha Yoga Pradīpikā* of Swātmārāma deals solely with physical discipline. It is not so, for Haṭha Yoga and Rāja Yoga complement each other and form a single approach towards Liberation. As a mountaineer needs ladders, ropes and crampons as well as physical fitness and discipline to climb the icy peaks of the Himālayas, so does the Yoga aspirant need the knowledge and discipline of the Haṭha Yoga of Swātmārāma to reach the heights of Rāja Yoga dealt with by Patañjali.

This path of Yoga is the fountain for the other three paths. It brings calmness and tranquillity and prepares the mind for absolute unqualified self-surrender to God, in which all these four paths merge into one.

Chitta Vṛtti (*Causes for the Modification of the Mind*)

In his *Yoga Sutras* Patañjali lists five classes of chitta vṛtti which create pleasure and pain. These are:

1. Pramāṇa (a standard or ideal), by which things or values are measured by the mind or known, which men accept upon (a) direct evidence such as perception (pratyakṣa), (b) inference (anumāna) and (c) testimony or the word of an acceptable authority when the source of knowledge has been checked as reliable and trustworthy (āgama).

2. Viparyaya (a mistaken view which is observed to be such after study). A faulty medical diagnosis based on wrong hypotheses, or the formerly held theory in astronomy that the Sun rotates round the Earth, are examples of viparyaya.

3. Vikalpa (fancy or imagination, resting merely on verbal expression without any factual basis). A beggar may feel happy when he imagines himself spending millions. A rich miser, on the other hand, may starve himself in the belief that he is poor.

4. Nidrā (sleep), where there is the absence of ideas and experiences. When a man is sleeping soundly, he does not recall his name, family or status, his knowledge or wisdom, or even his own existence. When a man forgets himself in sleep, he wakes up refreshed. But, if a disturbing thought creeps into his mind when he is dropping off, he will not rest properly.

5. Smṛti (memory, the holding fast of the impressions of objects that one has experienced). There are people who live in their past experiences, even though the past is beyond recall. Their sad or happy memories keep them chained to the past and they cannot break their fetters.

Patañjali enumerates five causes of chitta vṛtti creating pain (kleśa). These are:

1. Avidyā (ignorance or nescience); (2) asmitā (the feeling of individuality which limits a person and distinguishes him from a group and which may be physical, mental, intellectual or emotional); (3) rāga

(attachment or passion); (4) dveśa (aversion or revulsion) and (5) abhiniveśa (love of or thirst for life, the instinctive clinging to worldly life and bodily enjoyment and the fear that one may be cut off from all this by death). These causes of pain remain submerged in the mind of the sādhaka (the aspirant or seeker). They are like icebergs barely showing their heads in the polar seas. So long as they are not studiously controlled and eradicated, there can be no peace. The yogi learns to forget the past and takes no thought for the morrow. He lives in the eternal present.

As a breeze ruffles the surface of a lake and distorts the images reflected therein, so also the chitta vṛtti disturb the peace of the mind. The still waters of a lake reflect the beauty around it. When the mind is still, the beauty of the Self is seen reflected in it. The yogi stills his mind by constant study and by freeing himself from desires. The eight stages of Yoga teach him the way.

Chitta Vikṣepa (Distractions and Obstacles)

The distractions and obstacles which hinder the aspirant's practice of Yoga are:

1. Vyādhi – sickness which disturbs the physical equilibrium
2. Styāna – languor or lack of mental disposition for work
3. Saṁśaya – doubt or indecision
4. Pramāda – indifference or insensibility
5. Ālasya – laziness
6. Avirati – sensuality, the rousing of desire when sensory objects possess the mind
7. Bhrānti Darśana – false or invalid knowledge, or illusion
8. Alabdha Bhūmikatva – failure to attain continuity of thought or concentration so that reality cannot be seen
9. Anavasthitattva – instability in holding on to concentration which has been attained after long practice.

There are, however, four more distractions: (1) duḥkha – pain or misery, (2) daurmansya – despair, (3) aṅgamejayatva – unsteadiness of the body and (4) śvāsa-praśvāsa – unsteady respiration.

To win a battle, a general surveys the terrain and the enemy and plans counter-measures. In a similar way the Yogi plans the conquest of the Self.

Vyādhi: It will be noticed that the very first obstacle is ill-health or sickness. To the yogi his body is the prime instrument of attainment. If his vehicle breaks down, the traveller cannot go far. If the body is broken by ill-health, the aspirant can achieve little. Physical health is important for mental development, as normally the mind functions through the nervous system. When the body is sick or the nervous system is affected, the mind becomes restless or dull and inert and concentration or meditation become impossible.

Styāna: A person suffering from languor has no goal, no path to follow and no enthusiasm. His mind and intellect become dull due to inactivity and their faculties rust. Constant flow keeps a mountain stream pure, but water in a ditch stagnates and nothing good can flourish in it. A listless person is like a living corpse for he can concentrate on nothing.

Saṁśaya: The unwise, the faithless and the doubter destroy themselves. How can they enjoy this world or the next or have any happiness? The seeker should have faith in himself and his master. He should have faith that God is ever by his side and that no evil can touch him. As faith springs up in the heart it dries out lust, ill-will, mental sloth, spiritual pride and doubt, and the heart free from these hindrances becomes serene and untroubled.

Pramāda: A person suffering from pramāda is full of self-importance, lacks any humility and believes that he alone is wise. No doubt he knows what is right or wrong, but he persists in his indifference to the right and chooses what is pleasant. To gratify his selfish passions and dreams of personal glory, he will deliberately and without scruple sacrifice everyone who stands in his way. Such a person is blind to God's glory and deaf to His words.

Ālasya: To remove the obstacle of laziness, unflagging enthusiasm (vīrya) is needed. The attitude of the aspirant is like that of a lover ever yearning to meet the beloved but never giving way to despair. Hope should be his shield and courage his sword. He should be free from hate and sorrow. With faith and enthusiasm he should overcome the inertia of the body and the mind.

Avirati: This is the tremendous craving for sensory objects after they have been consciously abandoned, which is so hard to restrain. Without being attached to the objects of sense, the yogi learns to enjoy them with the aid of the senses which are completely under his control. By the practice of pratyāhāra he wins freedom from attachment and emancipation from desire and becomes content and tranquil.

Bhrānti Darśana: A person afflicted by false knowledge suffers from delusion and believes that he alone has seen the true Light. He has a powerful intellect but lacks humility and makes a show of wisdom. By remaining in the company of great souls and through their guidance he sets his foot firmly on the right path and overcomes his weakness.

Alabdha Bhūmikatva: As a mountain climber fails to reach the summit for lack of stamina, so also a person who cannot overcome the inability to concentrate is unable to seek reality. He might have had glimpses of reality but he cannot see clearly. He is like a musician who has heard divine music in a dream, but who is unable to recall it in his waking moments and cannot repeat the dream.

Anavasthitattva: A person affected with anavasthitattva has by hard work come within sight of reality. Happy and proud of his achievements he becomes slack in his practice (sādhana). He has purity and great power of concentration and has come to the final cross-roads of his quest. Even at this last stage continuous endeavour is essential and he has to pursue the path with infinite patience and determined perseverance and must never show slackness which hampers progress on the path of God realization. He must wait until divine grace descends upon him. It has been said in the *Kaṭhopanishad:* 'The Self is not to be realised by study and instruction, nor by subtlety of intellect, nor by much learning, but only by him who longs for Him, by the one whom He chooses. Verily to such a one the Self reveals His true being.'

To overcome the obstacles and to win unalloyed happiness, Patañjali offered several remedies. The best of these is the fourfold remedy of Maitri (friendliness), Karuṇa (compassion), Muditā (delight) and Upekṣā (disregard).

Maitri is not merely friendliness, but also a feeling of oneness with the object of friendliness (ātmīyatā). A mother feels intense happiness at the success of her children because of ātmīyatā, a feeling of oneness. Patañjali recommends maitri for sukha (happiness or virtue). The yogi cultivates maitri and ātmīyatā for the good and turns enemies into friends, bearing malice towards none.

Karuṇa is not merely showing pity or compassion and shedding tears of despair at the misery (duḥkha) of others. It is compassion coupled with devoted action to relieve the misery of the afflicted. The yogi uses all his resources – physical, economic, mental or moral – to alleviate the pain and suffering of others. He shares his strength with the weak until they become strong. He shares his courage with those that are timid until they become brave by his example. He denies the maxim of the 'survival of the fittest', but makes the weak strong enough to survive. He becomes a shelter to one and all.

Muditā is a feeling of delight at the good work (punya) done by another, even though he may be a rival. Through muditā, the yogi saves himself from much heart-burning by not showing anger, hatred or jealousy for another who has reached the desired goal which he himself has failed to achieve.

Upekṣā: It is not merely a feeling of disdain or contempt for the person who has fallen into vice (apuṇya) or one of indifference or superiority towards him. It is a searching self-examination to find out how one would have behaved when faced with the same temptations. It is also an examination to see how far one is responsible for the state into which the unfortunate one has fallen and the attempt thereafter to put him on the right path. The yogi understands the faults of others by seeing and studying them first in himself. This self-study teaches him to be charitable to all.

The deeper significance of the fourfold remedy of maitri, karuṇa, muditā and upekṣā cannot be felt by an unquiet mind. My experience has led me to conclude that for an ordinary man or woman in any community of the world, the way to achieve a quiet mind is to work with determination on two of the eight stages of Yoga mentioned by Patañjali, namely, āsana and prāṇāyāma.

The mind (manas) and the breath (prāṇa) are intimately connected and the activity or the cessation of activity of one affects the other. Hence Patañjali recommended prāṇāyāma (rhythmic breath control) for achieving mental equipoise and inner peace.

Śisya and Guru (A Pupil and a Master)

The *Śiva Samhitā* divides sādhakas (pupils or aspirants) into four classes. They are (1) mṛdu (feeble), (2) madhyama (average), (3) adhimātra (superior) and (4) adhimātratama (the supreme one). The last, the highest, is alone able to cross beyond the ocean of the manifest world.

The feeble seekers are those who lack enthusiasm, criticise their teachers, are rapacious, inclined to bad action, eat much, are in the power of women, unstable, cowardly, ill, dependent, speak harshly, have weak characters and lack virility. The Guru (Teacher or Master) guides such seekers in the path of Mantra Yoga only. With much effort, the sādhaka can reach enlightenment in twelve years. (The word mantra is derived from the root 'man', meaning to think. Mantra thus means a sacred thought or prayer to be repeated with full understanding of its meaning. It takes a long time, perhaps years, for a mantra to take firm root in the mind of a feeble sādhaka and still longer for it to bear fruit.)

Of even mind, capable of bearing hardship, wishing to perfect the work, speaking gently, moderate in all circumstances, such is the average seeker. Recognising these qualities, the Guru teaches him Laya Yoga, which gives liberation. (Laya means devotion, absorption or dissolution.)

Of stable mind, capable of Laya Yoga, virile, independent, noble, merciful, forgiving, truthful, brave, young, respectful, worshipping his teacher, intent on the practice of Yoga, such is a superior seeker. He can reach enlightenment after six years of practice. The Guru instructs this forceful man in Haṭha Yoga.

Of great virility and enthusiasm, good looking, courageous, learned in scriptures, studious, sane of mind, not melancholy, keeping young, regular in food, with his senses under control, free from fear, clean, skilful, generous, helpful to all, firm, intelligent, independent, forgiving, of good character, of gentle speech and worshipping his Guru, such is a supreme seeker, fit for all forms of Yoga. He can reach enlightenment in three years.

Although the *Śiva Samhitā* and the *Haṭha Yoga Pradīpikā* mention the period of time within which success might be achieved, Patañjali nowhere lays down the time required to unite the individual soul with the Divine Universal Soul. According to him abhyāsa (constant and determined practice) and vairāgya (freedom from desires) make the mind calm and tranquil. He defines abhyāsa as effort of long duration, without interruption, performed with devotion, which creates a firm foundation.

The study of Yoga is not like work for a diploma or a university degree by someone desiring favourable results in a stipulated time.

The obstacles, trials and tribulations in the path of Yoga can be removed to a large extent with the help of a Guru. (The syllable gu means darkness and ru means light. He alone is a Guru who removes darkness and brings enlightenment.) The conception of a Guru is deep and significant. He is not an ordinary guide. He is a spiritual teacher who teaches a way of life, and not merely how to earn a livelihood. He transmits knowledge of the Spirit and one who receives such knowledge is a śiṣya, a disciple.

The relationship between a Guru and a śiṣya is a very special one, transcending that between parent and child, husband and wife or friends. A Guru is free from egotism. He devotedly leads his śiṣya towards the ultimate goal without any attraction for fame or gain. He shows the path of God and watches the progress of his disciple, guiding him along that path. He inspires confidence, devotion, discipline, deep understanding and illumination through love. With faith in his pupil. the Guru strains hard to see that he absorbs the teaching. He encourages him to ask questions and to know the truth by question and analysis.

A śiṣya should possess the necessary qualifications of higher realisation and development. He must have confidence, devotion and love for his Guru. The perfect examples of the relationship between a Guru and a śiṣya are those of Yama (the God of Death) and Nachiketā in the *Kaṭhopaniṣad* and of Śri Krishna and Arjuna in the *Bhagavad Gītā*. Nachiketā and Arjuna obtained enlightenment through their one-pointed mind, their eagerness and questioning spirit. The śiṣya should hunger for knowledge and have the spirit of humility, perseverance and tenacity of purpose. He should not go to the Guru merely out of curiosity. He should possess śraddhā (dynamic faith) and should not be discouraged if he cannot reach the goal in the time he had expected. It requires tremendous patience to calm the restless mind which is coloured by innumerable past experiences and saṁskāra (the accumulated residue of past thoughts and actions).

Merely listening to the words of the Guru does not enable the śiṣya to absorb the teaching. This is borne out by the story of Indra and Virochana. Indra, the king of Gods, and Virochana, a demon prince, went together to their spiritual preceptor Brahmā to obtain knowledge of the Supreme Self. Both stayed and listened to the same words of their Guru. Indra obtained enlightenment, whereas Virochana did not. Indra's memory was developed by his devotion to the subject taught and by the love and faith which he had for his teacher. He had a feeling of oneness with his Guru. These were the reasons for his success. Virochana's memory was developed only through his intellect. He had no devotion either for the subject taught or for his preceptor. He remained what he originally was, an intellectual giant. He returned a doubter. Indra had intellectual humility, while Virochana had intellectual pride and imagined that it was condescending on his part to go to Brahmā. The approach of Indra was devotional while that of Virochana was practical. Virochana was motivated by curiosity and wanted the practical knowledge which he believed would be useful to him later to win power.

The śiṣya should above all treasure love, moderation and humility. Love begets courage, moderation creates abundance and humility generates power. Courage without love is brutish. Abundance without moderation leads to over-indulgence and decay. Power without humility breeds arrogance and tyranny. The true śiṣya learns from his Guru about a power which will never leave him as he returns to the Primeval One, the Source of His Being.

Sādhanā (A Key to Freedom)

All the important texts on Yoga lay great emphasis on sādhanā or abhyāsa (constant practice). Sādhanā is not just a theoretical study of Yoga texts. It is a spiritual endeavour. Oil seeds must be pressed to yield oil. Wood must be heated to ignite it and bring out the hidden fire within. In the same way, the sādhaka must by constant practice light the divine flame within himself.

'The young, the old, the extremely aged, even the sick and the infirm obtain perfection in Yoga by constant practice. Success will follow him who practises, not him who practises not. Success in Yoga is not obtained by the mere theoretical reading of sacred texts. Success is not obtained by wearing the dress of a yogi or a sanyāsi (a recluse), nor by talking about it. Constant practice alone is the secret of success. Verily, there is no doubt of this.'–(*Haṭha Yoga Pradīpikā*, chapter I, verses 64–6.)

'As by learning the alphabet one can, through practice, master all the sciences, so by thoroughly practising first physical training one acquires the knowledge of Truth (Tattva Jnāna), that is the real nature of the human soul as being identical with the Supreme Spirit pervading the Universe.'–(*Gheraṇḍa Saṁhitā*, chapter I, verse 5.)

It is by the co-ordinated and concentrated efforts of his body, senses, mind, reason and Self that a man obtains the prize of inner peace and fulfils the quest of his soul to meet his Maker. The supreme adventure in a man's life is his journey back to his Creator. To reach the goal he needs well developed and co-ordinated functioning of his body, senses, mind, reason and Self. If the effort is not co-ordinated, he fails in his adventure. In the third valli (chapter) of the first part of the *Kaṭhopaniṣad*, Yama (the God of Death) explains this Yoga to the seeker Nachiketā by way of the parable of the individual in a chariot.

'Know the Ātman (Self) as the Lord in a chariot, reason as the charioteer and mind as the reins. The senses, they say, are the horses, and their objects of desire are the pastures. The Self, when united with the senses and the mind, the wise call the Enjoyer (Bhoktṛ). The undiscriminating can never rein in his mind; his senses are like the vicious horses of a charioteer. The discriminating ever controls his mind; his senses are like disciplined horses. The undiscriminating becomes unmindful, ever impure; he does not reach the goal, wandering from one body to another. The discriminating becomes mindful, ever pure; he reaches the goal and is never reborn. The man who has a discriminating charioteer to rein in his mind reaches the end of the journey–the Supreme Abode of the everlasting Spirit.'

'The senses are more powerful than the objects of desire. Greater than the senses is the mind, higher than the mind is the reason and superior to reason is He–the Spirit in all. Discipline yourself by the Self and destroy your deceptive enemy in the shape of desire.' (*Bhagavad Gītā*, chapter III, verses 42–3.)

To realise this not only constant practice is demanded but also renunciation. As regards renunciation, the question arises as to what one should renounce. The yogi does not renounce the world, for that would mean renouncing the Creator. The yogi renounces all that takes him away from the Lord. He renounces his own desires, knowing that all inspiration and right action come from the Lord. He renounces those who oppose the work of the Lord, those who spread demonic ideas and who merely talk of moral values but do not practise them.

The yogi does not renounce action. He cuts the bonds that tie himself to his actions by dedicating their fruits either to the Lord or to humanity. He believes that it is his privilege to do his duty and that he has no right to the fruits of his actions.

While others are asleep when duty calls and wake up only to claim their rights, the yogi is fully awake to his duty, but asleep over his rights. Hence it is said that in the night of all beings the disciplined and tranquil man wakes to the light.

Aṣṭāṅga Yoga – The Eight Limbs of Yoga

The *Yoga Sutra* of Patañjali is divided into four chapters or pāda. The first deals with samādhi, the second with the means (sādhanā) to achieve Yoga, the third enumerates the powers (vibhūti) that the yogi comes across in his quest, and the fourth deals with absolution (kaivalya).

Yama

The eight limbs of Yoga are described in the second chapter. The first of these is yama (ethical disciplines) – the great commandments transcending creed, country, age and time. They are: ahimsā (non-violence), satya (truth), asteya (non-stealing), brahmacharya (continence) and aparigraha (non-coveting). These commandments are the rules of morality for society and the individual, which if not obeyed bring chaos, violence, untruth, stealing, dissipation and covetousness. The roots of these evils are the emotions of greed, desire and attachment, which may be mild, medium or excessive. They only bring pain and ignorance. Patañjali strikes at the root of these evils by changing the direction of one's thinking along the five principles of yama.

Ahimsā. The word ahimsā is made up of the particle 'a' meaning 'not' and the noun himsā meaning killing or violence. It is more than a negative command not to kill, for it has a wider positive meaning, love. This love embraces all creation for we are all children of the same Father – the Lord. The yogi believes that to kill or to destroy a thing or being is to insult its Creator. Men either kill for food or to protect themselves from danger. But merely because a man is a vegetarian, it does not necessarily follow that he is non-violent by temperament or that he is a yogi, though a vegetarian diet is a necessity for the practice of yoga. Blood-thirsty tyrants may be vegetarians, but violence is a state of mind, not of diet. It resides in a man's mind and not in the instrument he holds in his hand. One can use a knife to pare fruit or to stab an enemy. The fault is not in the instrument, but in the user.

Men take to violence to protect their own interests – their own bodies, their loved ones, their property or dignity. But a man cannot rely upon himself alone to protect himself or others. The belief that he can do so is wrong. A man must rely upon God, who is the source of all strength. Then he will fear no evil.

Violence arises out of fear, weakness, ignorance or restlessness. To curb it what is most needed is freedom from fear. To gain this freedom, what is required is a change of outlook on life and reorientation of the mind. Violence is bound to decline when men learn to base their faith upon reality and investigation rather than upon ignorance and supposition.

The yogi believes that every creature has as much right to live as he has. He believes that he is born to help others and he looks upon creation with eyes of love. He knows that his life is linked inextricably with that of others and he rejoices if he can help them to be happy. He puts the happiness of others before his own and becomes a source of joy to all who meet him. As parents encourage a baby to walk the first steps, he encourages those more unfortunate than himself and makes them fit for survival.

For a wrong done by others, men demand justice; while for that done by themselves they plead mercy and forgiveness. The yogi on the other hand, believes that for a wrong done by himself, there should be justice, while for that done by another there should be forgiveness. He knows and teaches others how to live. Always striving to perfect himself, he shows them by his love and compassion how to improve themselves.

The yogi opposes the evil in the wrong-doer, but not the wrong-doer. He prescribes penance not punishment for a wrong done. Opposition to evil and love for the wrong-doer can live side by side. A drunkard's wife whilst loving him may still oppose his habit. Opposition without love leads to violence; loving the wrong-doer without opposing the evil in him is folly and leads to misery. The yogi knows that to love a person whilst fighting the evil in him is the right course to follow. The battle is won because he fights it with love. A loving mother will sometimes beat her child to cure it of a bad habit; in the same way a true follower of ahimsā loves his opponent.

Along with ahimsā go abhaya (freedom from fear) and akrodha (freedom from anger). Freedom from fear comes only to those who lead a pure life. The yogi fears none and none need fear him, because he is purified by the study of the Self. Fear grips a man and paralyses him. He is afraid of the future, the unknown and the unseen. He is afraid that he may lose his means of livelihood, wealth or reputation. But the greatest fear is that of death. The yogi knows that he is different from his body, which is a temporary house for his spirit. He sees all beings in the Self and the Self in all beings and therefore he loses all fear. Though the body is subject to sickness, age, decay and death, the spirit remains unaffected. To the yogi death is the sauce that adds zest to life. He has dedicated his mind, his reason and his whole life to the Lord. When he has linked his entire being to the Lord, what shall he then fear?

There are two types of anger (krodha), one of which debases the mind while the other leads to spiritual growth. The root of the first is pride, which makes one angry when slighted. This prevents the mind from seeing things in perspective and makes one's judgement defective. The yogi, on the other hand, is angry with himself when his mind stoops low or when all his learning and experience fail to stop him from folly. He is stern with himself when he deals with his own faults, but gentle with the faults of others. Gentleness of mind is an attribute of a yogi, whose heart melts at all suffering. In him gentleness for others and firmness for himself go hand in hand, and in his presence all hostilities are given up.

Satya. Satya or truth is the highest rule of conduct or morality. Mahātma Gandhi said: 'Truth is God and God is Truth.' As fire burns impurities and refines gold, so the fire of truth cleanses the yogi and burns up the dross in him.

If the mind thinks thoughts of truth, if the tongue speaks words of truth and if the whole life is based upon truth, then one becomes fit for union with the Infinite. Reality in its fundamental nature is love and truth and expresses itself through these two aspects. The yogi's life must conform strictly to these two facets of Reality. That is why ahimsā, which is essentially based on love, is enjoined. Satya presupposes perfect truthfulness in thought, word and deed. Untruthfulness in any form puts the sādhaka out of harmony with the fundamental law of truth.

Truth is not limited to speech alone. There are four sins of speech: abuse and obscenity, dealing in falsehoods, calumny or telling tales and lastly ridiculing what others hold to be sacred. The tale bearer is more poisonous than a snake. The control of speech leads to the rooting out of malice. When the mind bears malice towards none, it is filled with charity towards all. He who has learnt to control his tongue has attained self-control in a great measure. When such a person speaks he will be heard with respect and attention. His words will be remembered, for they will be good and true.

When one who is established in truth prays with a pure heart, then things he really needs come to him when they are really needed: he does not have to run after them. The man firmly established in truth gets the fruit of his actions without apparently doing anything. God, the source of all truth, supplies his needs and looks after his welfare.

Asteya. The desire to possess and enjoy what another has, drives a person to do evil deeds. From this desire spring the urge to steal and the urge to covet. Asteya (a = not, steya = stealing), or non-stealing includes not only taking what belongs to another without permission, but also using something for a different purpose to that intended, or beyond the time permitted by its owner. It thus includes misappropriation, breach of trust, mismanagement and misuse. The yogi reduces his physical needs to the minimum, believing that if he gathers things he does not really need, he is a thief. While other men crave for wealth, power, fame or enjoyment, the yogi has one craving and that is to adore the Lord. Freedom from craving enables one to ward off great temptations. Craving muddies the stream of tranquillity. It makes men base and vile and cripples them. He who obeys the commandment *Thou shalt not steal*, becomes a trusted repository of all treasures.

Brahmacharya. According to the dictionary brahmacharya means the life of celibacy, religious study and self-restraint. It is thought that the loss of semen leads to death and its retention to life. By the preservation of semen the yogi's body develops a sweet smell. So long as it is retained, there is no fear of death. Hence the injunction that it should be preserved by concentrated effort of the mind. The concept of brahmacharya is not one of negation, forced austerity and prohibition. According to Śankarāchārya, a brahmachārī (one who observes brahmacharya) is a man who is engrossed in the study of the sacred Vedic lore, constantly moves in Brahman and knows that all exists in Brahman. In other words, one who sees divinity in all is a brahmachārī. Patañjali, however, lays stress on continence of the body, speech and mind. This does not mean that the philosophy of Yoga is meant only for celibates. Brahmacharya has little to do with whether one is a bachelor or married and living the life of a householder. One has to translate the higher aspects of Brahmacharya in one's daily living. It is not necessary for one's salvation to stay unmarried and without a house. On the contrary, all the smṛtīs (codes of law) recommend marriage. Without experiencing human love and happiness, it is not possible to know divine love. Almost all the yogis and sages of old in India were married men with families of their own. They did not shirk their social or moral responsibilities. Marriage and parenthood are no bar to the knowledge of divine love, happiness and union with the Supreme Soul.

Dealing with the position of an aspirant who is a householder, the *Śiva Saṁhitā* says: Let him practise free from the company of men in a retired place. For the sake of appearances, he should remain in society, but not have his heart in it. He should not renounce the duties of his profession, caste or rank; but let him perform these as an instrument of the Lord, without any thought of the results. He succeeds by following wisely the method of Yoga; there is no doubt of it. Remaining in the midst of the family, always doing the duties of the householder, he who is free from merits and demerits and has restrained his senses, attains salvation. The householder practising Yoga is not touched by virtue or vice; if to protect mankind he commits any sin, he is not polluted by it. (Chapter V, verses 234–8.)

When one is established in brahmacharya, one develops a fund of vitality and energy, a courageous mind and a powerful intellect so that one can fight any type of injustice. The brahmachārī will use the forces he generates wisely: he will utilise the physical ones for doing the work of the Lord, the mental for the spread of culture and the intellectual for the growth of spiritual life. Brahmacharya is the battery that sparks the torch of wisdom.

Aparigraha. Parigraha means hoarding or collecting. To be free from hoarding is aparigraha. It is thus but another facet of asteya (non-stealing). Just as one should not take things one does not really need, so one should not hoard or collect things one does not require immediately. Neither should one take anything without working for it or as a favour from another, for this indicates poverty of spirit. The yogi feels that the collection or hoarding of things implies a lack of faith in God and in himself to provide for his future. He keeps faith by keeping before him the image of the moon. During the dark half of the month, the moon rises late when most men are asleep and so do not appreciate its beauty. Its splendour wanes but it does not stray from its path and is indifferent to man's lack of appreciation. It has faith that it will be full again when it faces the Sun and then men will eagerly await its glorious rising.

By the observance of aparigraha, the yogi makes his life as simple as possible and trains his mind not to feel the loss or the lack of anything. Then everything he really needs will come to him by itself at the proper time. The life of an ordinary man is filled with an unending series of disturbances and frustrations and with his reactions to them. Thus there is hardly any possibility of keeping the mind in a state of equilibrium. The sādhaka has developed the capacity to remain satisfied with whatever happens to him. Thus he obtains the peace which takes him beyond the realms of illusion and misery with which our world is saturated. He recalls the promise given by Śri Krishna to Arjuna in the ninth chapter of the *Bhagavad Gītā*: 'To those who worship Me alone with single-minded devotion, who are in harmony with Me every moment, I bring full security. I shall supply all their wants and shall protect them for ever.'

Niyama

Niyama are the rules of conduct that apply to individual discipline, while yama are universal in their application. The five niyama listed by Patañjali are: śaucha (purity), santoṣa (contentment), tapas (ardour or austerity), svādhyāya (study of the Self) and Iśvara praṇidhāna (dedication to the Lord).

Śaucha. Purity of body is essential for well-being. While good habits like bathing purify the body externally, āsana and prāṇāyāma cleanse it internally. The practice of āsanas tones the entire body and removes the toxins and impurities caused by over-indulgence. Prāṇāyāma cleanses and aerates the lungs, oxygenates the blood and purifies the nerves. But more important than the physical cleansing of the body is the cleansing of the mind of its disturbing emotions like hatred, passion, anger, lust, greed, delusion and pride. Still more important is the cleansing of the intellect (buddhi) of impure thoughts. The impurities of the mind are washed off in the waters of bhakti (adoration). The impurities of the intellect or reason are burned off in the fire of svādhyāya (study of the Self). This internal cleansing gives radiance and joy. It brings benevolence (saumanasya) and banishes mental pain, dejection, sorrow and despair (daurmanasya). When one is benevolent, one sees the virtues in others and not merely their faults. The respect which one shows for another's virtues, makes him self-respecting as well and helps him to fight his own sorrows and difficulties. When the mind is lucid, it is easy to make it one-pointed (ekāgra). With concentration, one obtains mastery over the senses (indriya-jaya). Then one is ready to enter the temple of his own body and see his real self in the mirror of his mind.

Besides purity of body, thought and word, pure food is also necessary. Apart from cleanliness in the preparation of food it is also necessary to observe purity in the means by which one procures it.

Food, the supporting yet consuming substance of all life, is regarded as a phase of Brahman. It should be eaten with the feeling that with each morsel one can gain strength to serve the Lord. Then food becomes pure. Whether or not to be a vegetarian is a purely personal matter as each person is influenced by the tradition and habits of the country in which he was born and bred. But, in course of time, the practitioner of yoga has to adopt a vegetarian diet, in order to attain one-pointed attention and spiritual evolution.

Food should be taken to promote health, strength, energy and life. It should be simple, nourishing, juicy and soothing. Avoid foods which are sour, bitter, salty, pungent, burning, stale, tasteless, heavy and unclean.

Character is moulded by the type of food we take and by how we eat it. Men are the only creatures that eat when not hungry and generally live to eat rather than eat to live. If we eat for flavours of the tongue, we over-eat and so suffer from digestive disorders which throw our systems out of gear. The yogi believes in harmony, so he eats for the sake of sustenance only. He does not eat too much or too little. He looks upon his body as the rest-house of his spirit and guards himself against over-indulgence.

Besides food, the place is also important for spiritual practices. It is difficult to practise in a distant country (away from home), in a forest, in a crowded city, or where it is noisy. One should choose a place where food is easily procurable, a place which is free from insects, protected from the elements and with pleasing surroundings. The banks of a lake or river or the sea-shore are ideal. Such quiet ideal places are hard to find in modern times; but one can at least make a corner in one's room available for practice and keep it clean, airy, dry and pest-free.

Santoṣa. Santoṣa or contentment has to be cultivated. A mind that is not content cannot concentrate. The yogi feels the lack of nothing and so he is naturally content. Contentment gives bliss unsurpassed to the yogi. A contented man is complete for he has known the love of the Lord and has done his duty. He is blessed for he has known truth and joy.

Contentment and tranquillity are states of mind. Differences arise among men because of race, creed, wealth and learning. Differences create discord and there arise conscious or unconscious conflicts which distract and perplex one. Then the mind cannot become one-pointed (ekāgra) and is robbed of its peace. There is contentment and tranquillity when the flame of the spirit does not waver in the wind of desire. The sādhaka does not seek the empty peace of the dead, but the peace of one whose reason is firmly established in God.

Tapas. Tapas is derived from the root 'tap' meaning to blaze, burn, shine, suffer pain or consume by heat. It therefore means a burning effort under all circumstances to achieve a definite goal in life. It involves purification, self-discipline and austerity. The whole science of character building may be regarded as a practice of tapas.

Tapas is the conscious effort to achieve ultimate union with the Divine and to burn up all desires which stand in the way of this goal. A worthy aim makes life illumined, pure and divine. Without such an aim, action and prayer have no value. Life without tapas, is like a heart without love. Without tapas, the mind cannot reach up to the Lord.

Tapas is of three types. It may relate to the body (kāyika), to speech (vāchika) or to mind (mānasika). Continence (brahmacharya) and non-violence (ahimsā) are tapas of the body. Using words which do not offend, reciting the glory of God, speaking the truth without regard for the consequences to oneself and not speaking ill of others are tapas of speech. Developing a mental attitude whereby one remains tranquil and balanced in joy and sorrow and retains self-control are tapas of the mind.

It is tapas when one works without any selfish motive or hope of reward and with an unshakable faith that not even a blade of grass can move without His will.

By tapas the yogi develops strength in body, mind and character. He gains courage and wisdom, integrity, straightforwardness and simplicity.

Svādhyāya. Sva means self and adhyāya means study or education. Education is the drawing out of the best that is within a person. Svādhyāya, therefore, is the education of the self.

Svādhyāya is different from mere instruction like attending a lecture where the lecturer parades his own learning before the ignorance of his audience. When people meet for svādhyāya, the speaker and listener are of one mind and have mutual love and respect. There is no sermonising and one heart speaks to another. The ennobling thoughts that arise from svādhyāya are, so to speak, taken into one's bloodstream so that they become a part of one's life and being.

The person practising svādhyāya reads his own book of life, at the same time that he writes and revises it. There is a change in his outlook on life. He starts to realise that all creation is meant for bhakti (adoration) rather than for bhoga (enjoyment), that all creation is divine, that there is divinity within himself and that the energy which moves him is the same that moves the entire universe.

According to Śri Vinobā Bhāve (the leader of the Bhoodan movement), svādhyāya is the study of one subject which is the basis or root of all other subjects or actions, upon which the others rest, but which itself does not rest upon anything.

To make life healthy, happy and peaceful, it is essential to study regularly divine literature in a pure place. This study of the sacred books of the world will enable the sādhaka to concentrate upon and solve the difficult problems of life when they arise. It will put an end to ignorance and bring knowledge. Ignorance has no beginning, but it has an end. There is a beginning but no end to knowledge. By svādhyāya the sādhaka understands the nature of his soul and gains communion with the divine. The sacred books of the world are for all to read. They are not meant for the members of one particular faith alone. As bees savour the nectar in various flowers, so the sādhaka absorbs things in other faiths which will enable him to appreciate his own faith better.

Philology is not a language but the science of languages, the study of which will enable the student to learn his own language better. Similarly, Yoga is not a religion by itself. It is the science of religions, the study of which will enable a sādhaka the better to appreciate his own faith.

Īśvara praṇidhāna. Dedication to the Lord of one's actions and will is Īśvara praṇidhāna. He who has faith in God does not despair. He has illumination (tejas). He who knows that all creation belongs to the Lord will not be puffed up with pride or drunk with power. He will not stoop for selfish purposes; his head will bow only in worship. When the waters of bhakti (adoration) are made to flow through the turbines of the mind, the result is mental power and spiritual illumination. While mere physical strength without bhakti is lethal, mere adoration without strength of character is like an opiate. Addiction to pleasures destroys both power and glory. From the gratification of the senses as they run after pleasures arise moha (attachment) and lobha (greed) for their repetition. If the senses are not gratified, then, there is śoka (sorrow). They have to be curbed with knowledge and forbearance; but to control the mind is more difficult. After one has exhausted one's own resources and still not succeeded, one turns to the Lord for help for He is the source of all power. It is at this stage that bhakti begins. In bhakti, the mind, the intellect and the will are surrendered to the Lord and the sādhaka prays: 'I do not know what is good for me. Thy will be done.' Others pray to have their own desires gratified or accomplished. In bhakti or true love there is no place for 'I' and 'mine'. When the feeling of 'I' and 'mine' disappears, the individual soul has reached full growth.

When the mind has been emptied of desires of personal gratification, it should be filled with thoughts of the Lord. In a mind filled with thoughts of personal gratification, there is danger of the senses dragging the mind after the objects of desire. Attempts to practise bhakti without emptying the mind of desires is like building a fire with wet fuel. It makes a lot of smoke and brings tears to the eyes of the person who builds it and of those around him. A mind with desires does not ignite and glow, nor does it generate light and warmth when touched with the fire of knowledge.

The name of the Lord is like the Sun, dispelling all darkness. The moon is full when it faces the sun. The individual soul experiences fullness (pūrṇatā) when it faces the Lord. If the shadow of the earth comes between the full moon and the sun there is an eclipse. If the feeling of 'I' and 'mine' casts its shadow upon the experience of fullness, all efforts of the sādhaka to gain peace are futile.

Actions mirror a man's personality better than his words. The yogi has learnt the art of dedicating all his actions to the Lord and so they reflect the divinity within him.

Āsana

The third limb of yoga is āsana or posture. Āsana brings steadiness, health and lightness of limb. A steady and pleasant posture produces mental equilibrium and prevents fickleness of mind. Āsanas are not merely gymnastic exercises; they are postures. To perform them one needs a clean airy place, a blanket and determination, while for other systems of physical training one needs large playing fields and costly equipment. Āsanas can be done alone, as the limbs of the body provide the necessary weights and counter-weights. By practising them one develops agility, balance, endurance and great vitality.

Āsanas have been evolved over the centuries so as to exercise every muscle, nerve and gland in the body. They secure a fine physique, which is strong and elastic without being muscle-bound and they keep the body free from disease. They reduce fatigue and soothe the nerves. But their real importance lies in the way they train and discipline the mind.

Many actors, acrobats, athletes, dancers, musicians and sportsmen also possess superb physiques and have great control over the body, but they lack control over the mind, the intellect and the Self. Hence they are in disharmony with themselves and one rarely comes across a balanced personality among them. They often put the body above all else. Though the yogi does not underrate his body, he does not think merely of its perfection but of his senses, mind, intellect and soul.

The yogi conquers the body by the practice of āsanas and makes it a fit vehicle for the spirit. He knows that it is a necessary vehicle for the spirit. A soul without a body is like a bird deprived of its power to fly.

The yogi does not fear death, for time must take its toll of all flesh. He knows that the body is constantly changing and is affected by childhood, youth and old age. Birth and death are natural phenomena but the soul is not subject to birth and death. As a man casting off worn-out garments takes on new ones, so the dweller within the body casting aside worn-out bodies enters into others that are new.

The yogi believes that his body has been given to him by the Lord not for enjoyment alone, but also for the service of his fellow men during every wakeful moment of his life. He does not consider it his property. He knows that the Lord who has given him his body will one day take it away.

By performing āsanas, the sādhaka first gains health, which is not mere existence. It is not a commodity which can be purchased with money. It is an asset to be gained by sheer hard work. It is a state of complete equilibrium of body, mind and spirit. Forgetfulness of physical and mental consciousness is health. The yogi frees himself from physical disabilities and mental distractions by practising āsanas. He surrenders his actions and their fruits to the Lord in the service of the world.

The yogi realises that his life and all its activities are part of the divine action in nature, manifesting and operating in the form of man. In the beating of his pulse and the rhythm of his respiration, he recognises the flow of the seasons and the throbbing of universal life. His body is a temple which houses the Divine Spark. He feels that to neglect or to deny the needs of the body and to think of it as something not divine, is to neglect and deny the universal life of which it is a part. The needs of the body are the needs of the divine spirit which lives through the body. The yogi does not look heaven-ward to find God for he knows that He is within, being known as the Antarātmā (the Inner Self). He feels the kingdom of God within and without and finds that heaven lies in himself.

Where does the body end and the mind begin? Where does the mind end and the spirit begin? They cannot be divided as they are inter-related and but different aspects of the same all-pervading divine consciousness.

The yogi never neglects or mortifies the body or the mind, but cherishes both. To him the body is not an impediment to his spiritual liberation nor is it the cause of its fall, but is an instrument of attainment. He seeks a body strong as a thunderbolt, healthy and free from suffering so as to dedicate it in the service of the Lord for which it is intended. As pointed out in the *Muṇḍakopaniṣad* the Self cannot be attained by one without strength, nor through heedlessness, nor without an aim. Just as an unbaked earthen pot dissolves in water the body soon decays. So bake it hard in the fire of yogic discipline in order to strengthen and purify it.

The names of the āsanas are significant and illustrate the principle of evolution. Some are named after vegetation like the tree (vṛkṣa) and the lotus (padma); some after insects like the locust (śalabha) and the scorpion (vṛśchika); some after aquatic animals and amphibians like the fish (matsya), the tortoise (kūrma), the frog (bheka or maṇḍūka) or the crocodile (nakra). There are āsanas called after birds like the cock (kukkuṭa), the heron (baka), the peacock (mayūra) and the swan (haṁsa). They are also named after quadrupeds like the dog (śvāna), the horse (vātāyana), the camel (uṣṭra) and the lion (siṁha). Creatures that crawl like the serpent (bhujaṅga) are not forgotten, nor is the human embryonic state (garbha-pinda) overlooked. Āsanas are named after legendary heroes like Vīrabhadra and Hanumān, son of the Wind. Sages like Bharadvāja, Kapila, Vasiṣṭha and Viśvāmitra are remembered by having āsanas named after them. Some āsanas are also called after gods of the Hindu pantheon and some recall the Avatārās, or incarnations of Divine Power. Whilst performing āsanas the yogi's body assumes many forms resembling a variety of creatures. His mind is trained not to despise any creature, for he knows that throughout the whole gamut of creation, from the lowliest insect to the most perfect sage, there breathes the same Universal Spirit, which assumes innumerable forms. He knows that the highest form is that of the Formless. He finds unity in universality. True āsana is that in which the thought of Brahman flows effortlessly and incessantly through the mind of the sādhaka.

Dualities like gain and loss, victory and defeat, fame and shame, body and mind, mind and soul vanish through mastery of the āsanas, and the sādhaka then passes on to prāṇāyāma, the fourth stage in the path of yoga. In prāṇāyāma practices the nostrils, nasal passages and membranes, the windpipe, the lungs and the diaphragm are the only parts of the body which are actively involved. These alone feel the full impact of the force of prāṇa, the breath of life. Therefore, do not seek to master prāṇāyāma in a hurry, as you are playing with life itself. By its improper practice respiratory diseases will arise and the nervous system will be shattered. By its proper practice one is freed from most diseases. Never attempt to practise prāṇāyāma alone by yourself. For it is essential to have the personal supervision of a Guru who knows the physical limitations of his pupil.

Prāṇāyāma

Just as the word yoga is one of wide import, so also is prāṇa. Prāṇa means breath, respiration, life, vitality, wind, energy or strength. It also connotes the soul as opposed to the body. The word is generally used in the plural to indicate vital breaths. Āyāma means length, expansion, stretching or restraint. Prāṇāyāma thus connotes extension of breath and its control. This control is over all the functions of breathing, namely, (1) inhalation or inspiration, which is termed pūraka (filling up); (2) exhalation or expiration, which is called rechaka (emptying the lungs), and (3) retention or holding the breath, a state where there is no inhalation or exhalation, which is termed kumbhaka. In Haṭha Yoga texts kumbhaka is also used in a loose generic sense to include all the three respiratory processes of inhalation, exhalation and retention.

A kumbha is a pitcher, water pot, jar or chalice. A water pot may be emptied of all air and filled completely with water, or it may be emptied of all water and filled completely with air. Similarly, there are two states of kumbhaka namely (1) when breathing is suspended after full inhalation (the lungs being completely filled with life-giving air), and (2) when breathing is suspended after full exhalation (the lungs being emptied of all noxious air). The first of these states, where breath is held after a full inhalation, but before exhalation begins, is known as antara kumbhaka. The second, where breath is held after a full exhalation, but before inhalation begins is known as bāhya kumbhaka. Antara means inner or interior, while bāhya means outer or exterior. Thus, kumbhaka is the interval or intermediate time between full inhalation and exhalation (antara kumbhaka) or between full exhalation and inhalation (bāhya kumbhaka). In both these types breathing is suspended and restrained.

Prāṇāyāma is thus the science of breath. It is the hub round which the wheel of life revolves. 'As lions, elephants and tigers are tamed very slowly and cautiously, so should prāṇa be brought under control very slowly in gradation measured according to one's capacity and physical limitations. Otherwise it will kill the practitioner,' warns the *Haṭha Yoga Pradīpikā* (chapter II, verse 16).

The yogi's life is not measured by the number of his days but by the number of his breaths. Therefore, he follows the proper rhythmic patterns of slow deep breathing. These rhythmic patterns strengthen the respiratory system, soothe the nervous system and reduce craving. As desires and cravings diminish, the mind is set free and becomes a fit vehicle for concentration. By improper practice of prāṇāyāma the pupil introduces several disorders into his system like hiccough, wind, asthma, cough, catarrh, pains in the head, eyes and ears and nervous irritation. It takes a long time to learn slow, deep, steady and proper inhalations and exhalations. Master this before attempting kumbhaka.

As a fire blazes brightly when the covering of ash over it is scattered by the wind, the divine fire within the body shines in all its majesty when the ashes of desire are scattered by the practice of prāṇāyāma.

'The emptying the mind of the whole of its illusion is the true rechaka (exhalation). The realisation that "I am Ātmā (spirit)" is the true pūraka (inhalation). And the steady sustenance of the mind on this conviction is the true kumbhaka (retention). This is true prāṇāyāma,' says Śankarāchārya.

Every living creature unconsciously breathes the prayer 'So'ham' (Saḥ = He : Aham = I – He, the Immortal Spirit, am I) with each inward breath. So also with each outgoing breath each creature prays 'Haṁsaḥ' (I am He). This ajapa-mantra (unconscious repetitive prayer) goes on for ever within each living creature throughout life. The yogi fully realises the significance of this ajapa-mantra and so is released from all the fetters that bind his soul. He offers up the very breath of his being to the Lord as a sacrifice and receives the breath of life from the Lord as his blessing.

Prāṇa in the body of the individual (jīvātmā) is part of the cosmic breath of the Universal Spirit (Paramātmā). An attempt is made to harmonise the individual breath (piṇḍa-prāṇa) with the cosmic breath (Brahmāṇḍa-prāṇa) through the practice of prāṇāyāma.

It has been said by Kariba Ekken, a seventeenth-century mystic; 'If you would foster a calm spirit, first regulate your breathing; for when that is under control, the heart will be at peace; but when breathing is spasmodic, then it will be troubled. Therefore, before attempting anything, first regulate your breathing on which your temper will be softened, your spirit calmed.'

The chitta (mind, reason and ego) is like a chariot yoked to a team of powerful horses. One of them is prāṇa (breath), the other is vāsanā (desire). The chariot moves in the direction of the more powerful animal. If breath prevails, the desires are controlled, the senses are held in check and the mind is stilled. If desire prevails, breath is in disarray and the mind is agitated and troubled. Therefore, the yogi masters the science of breath and by the regulation and control of breath, he controls the mind and stills its constant movement. In the practice of prāṇāyāma the eyes are kept shut to prevent the mind from wandering. 'When the prāṇa and the manas (mind) have been absorbed, an undefinable joy ensues.' (*Haṭha Yoga Pradīpikā*, chapter IV, verse 30.)

Emotional excitement affects the rate of breathing; equally, deliberate regulation of breathing checks emotional excitement. As the very object of Yoga is to control and still the mind, the yogi first learns prāṇāyāma to master the breath. This will enable him to control the senses and so reach the stage of pratyāhāra. Only then will the mind be ready for concentration (dhyāna).

The mind is said to be twofold – pure and impure. It is pure when it is completely free from desires and impure when it is in union with desires. By making the mind motionless and freeing it from sloth and distractions, one reaches the state of mindlessness (amanaska), which is the supreme state of samādhi. This state of mindlessness is not lunacy or idiocy but the conscious state of the mind when it is free from thoughts and desires. There is a vital difference between an idiot or a lunatic on the one hand, and a yogi striving to achieve a state of mindlessness on the other. The former is careless; the latter attempts to be carefree. It is the oneness of the breath and mind and so also of the senses and the abandonment of all conditions of existence and thought that is designated Yoga.

Prāṇa Vāyu. One of the most subtle forms of energy is air. This vital energy which also pervades the human body is classified in five main categories in the Haṭha Yoga texts according to the various functions performed by the energy. These are termed vāyu (wind) and the five main divisions are: prāṇa (here the generic term is used to designate the particular), which moves in the region of the heart and controls respiration; apāna, which moves in the sphere of the lower abdomen and controls the function of eliminating urine and faeces; samāna, which stokes the gastric fires to aid digestion; udāna, which dwells in the thoracic cavity and controls the intake of air and food; and vyāna, which pervades the entire body and distributes the energy derived from food and breath. There are also five subsidiary vāyūs. These are: nāga, which relieves abdominal pressure by belching; kūrma, which controls the movements of the eyelids to prevent foreign matter or too bright a light entering the eyes; kṛkara, which prevents substances passing up the nasal passages and down the throat by making one sneeze or cough; devadatta, which provides for the intake of extra oxygen in a tired body by causing a yawn, and lastly dhanaṁjaya, which remains in the body even after death and sometimes bloats up a corpse.

Pratyāhāra

If a man's reason succumbs to the pull of his senses he is lost. On the other hand, if there is rhythmic control of breath, the senses instead of running after external objects of desire turn inwards, and man is set free from their tyranny. This is the fifth stage of Yoga, namely, pratyāhāra, where the senses are brought under control.

When this stage is reached, the sādhaka goes through a searching self-examination. To overcome the deadly but attractive spell of sensual objects, he needs the insulation of adoration (bhakti) by recalling to his mind the Creator who made the objects of his desire. He also needs the lamp of knowledge of his divine heritage. The mind, in truth, is for mankind the cause of bondage and liberation; it brings bondage if it is bound to the objects of desire and liberation when it is free from objects. There is bondage when the mind craves, grieves or is unhappy over something. The mind becomes pure when all desires and fears are annihilated. Both the good and the pleasant present themselves to men and prompt them to action. The yogi prefers the good to the pleasant. Others driven by their desires, prefer the pleasant to the good and miss the very purpose of life. The yogi feels joy in what he is. He knows how to stop and, therefore, lives in peace. At first he prefers that which is bitter as poison, but he perseveres in his practice knowing well that in the end it will become as sweet as nectar. Others hankering for the union of their senses with the objects of their desires, prefer that which at first seems sweet as nectar, but do not know that in the end it will be as bitter as poison.

The yogi knows that the path towards satisfaction of the senses by sensual desires is broad, but that it leads to destruction and that there are many who follow it. The path of Yoga is like the sharp edge of a razor, narrow and difficult to tread, and there are few who find it. The yogi knows that the paths of ruin or of salvation lie within himself.

According to Hindu philosophy, consciousness manifests in three different qualities. For man, his life and his consciousness, together with the entire cosmos are the emanations of one and the same prakṛti (cosmic matter or substance) – emanations that differ in designation through the predominance of one of the guṇās. These guṇās (qualities or attributes) are:

1. Sattva (the illuminating, pure or good quality), which leads to clarity and mental serenity.
2. Rajas (the quality of mobility or activity), which makes a person active and energetic, tense and wilful, and
3. Tamas (the dark and restraining quality), which obstructs and counteracts the tendency of rajas to work and of sattva to reveal.

Tamas is a quality of delusion, obscurity, inertia and ignorance. A person in whom it predominates is inert and plunged in a state of torpor.

The quality of sattva leads towards the divine and tamas towards the demonic, while in between these two stands rajas.

The faith held, the food consumed, the sacrifices performed, the austerities undergone and the gifts given by each individual vary in accordance with his predominating guṇa.

He that is born with tendencies towards the divine is fearless and pure. He is generous and self-controlled. He pursues the study of the Self. He is non-violent, truthful and free from anger. He renounces the fruits of his labour, working only for the sake of work. He has a tranquil mind, with malice towards none and charity towards all, for he is free from craving. He is gentle, modest and steady. He is illumined, clement and resolute, being free from perfidy and pride.

A man in whom rajō-guṇa predominates has inner thirst and is affectionate. As he is passionate and covetous, he hurts others. Being full of lust and hatred, envy and deceit, his desires are insatiable. He is unsteady, fickle and easily distracted as well as ambitious and acquisitive. He seeks the patronage of friends and has family pride. He shrinks from unpleasant things and clings to pleasant ones. His speech is sour and his stomach greedy.

He that is born with demonic tendencies is deceitful, insolent and conceited. He is full of wrath, cruelty and ignorance. In such people there is neither purity, nor right conduct, nor truth. They gratify their passions. Bewildered by numerous desires, caught in the web of delusion, these addicts of sensual pleasures fall into hell.

The working of the mind of persons with different predominating gunās may be illustrated by their different ways of approach towards a universal commandment like 'Thou shalt not covet.' A man in whom tamō-guṇa predominates might interpret it thus: 'others should not covet what is mine, no matter how I obtained it. If they do, I shall destroy them.' The rajō-guṇa type is a calculating self-interested person who would construe the commandment as meaning: 'I will not covet others' goods lest they covet mine.' He will follow the letter of the law as a matter of policy, but not the true spirit of the law as a matter of principle. A person of sattvika temperament will follow both the letter and the spirit of the precept as a matter of principle and not of policy, as a matter of eternal value. He will be righteous for the sake of righteousness alone, and not because there is a human law imposing punishment to keep him honest.

The yogi who is also human is affected by these three guṇās. By his constant and disciplined study (abhyāsa) of himself and of the objects which his senses tend to pursue, he learns which thoughts, words and actions are prompted by tamas and which by rajas. With unceasing effort he weeds out and eradicates such thoughts as are prompted by tamas and he works to achieve a sattvika frame of mind. When the sattva-guṇa alone remains, the human soul has advanced a long way towards the ultimate goal.

Like unto the pull of gravity is the pull of the guṇās. As intensive research and rigorous discipline are needed to experience the wonder of weightlessness in space, so also a searching self-examination and the discipline furnished by Yoga is needed by a sādhaka to experience union with the Creator of space when he is freed from the pull of the guṇās.

Once the sādhaka has experienced the fullness of creation or of the Creator, his thirst (tṛṣṇā) for objects of sense vanishes and he looks at them ever after with dispassion (vairāgya). He experiences no disquiet in heat or cold, in pain or pleasure, in honour or dishonour and in virtue or vice. He treats the two imposters – triumph and disaster – with equanimity. He has emancipated himself from these pairs of opposites. He has passed beyond the pull of the guṇās and has become a guṇātīta (one who has transcended the guṇās). He is then free from birth and death, from pain and sorrow and becomes immortal. He has no self-identity as he lives experiencing the fullness of the Universal Soul. Such a man, scorning nothing, leads all things to the path of perfection.

Dhāraṇā

When the body has been tempered by āsanas, when the mind has been refined by the fire of prāṇāyāma and when the senses have been brought under control by pratyāhāra, the sādhaka reaches the sixth stage called dhāraṇā. Here he is concentrated wholly on a single point or on a task in which he is completely engrossed. The mind has to be stilled in order to achieve this state of complete absorption.

The mind is an instrument which classifies, judges and co-ordinates the impressions from the outside world and those that arise within oneself.

Mind is the product of thoughts which are difficult to restrain for they are subtle and fickle. A thought which is well guarded by a controlled mind brings happiness. To get the best out of an instrument, one must know how it works. The mind is the instrument for thinking and it is therefore necessary to consider how it functions. Mental states are classified in five groups. The first of these is the kṣipta state, where the mental forces are scattered, being in disarray and in a state of neglect. Here the mind hankers after objects, the ragō-guṇa being dominant. The second is the vikṣipta state, where the mind is agitated and distracted. Here there is a capacity to enjoy the fruits of one's efforts, but the desires are not marshalled and controlled. Then in the mūḍha state the mind is foolish, dull and stupid. It is confounded and at a loss to know what it wants and here the tamō-guṇa predominates. The fourth state of the mind is the ekāgra (eka = one; agra = foremost) state, where the mind is closely attentive and the mental faculties are concentrated on a single object or focussed on one point only, with the sattva-guṇa prevailing. The ekāgra person has superior intellectual powers and knows exactly what he wants, so he uses all his powers to achieve his purpose. At times the ruthless pursuit of the desired object, irrespective of the cost to others, can create great misery, and it often happens that even if the desired object is achieved it leaves behind a bitter taste.

Arjuna, the mighty bowman of the epic Mahābhārata, provides us with an example of what is meant by dhāraṇā. Once Droṇa, the preceptor of the royal princes, organised an archery contest to test their proficiency. They were called upon one by one to describe the target, which was pointed out to them. It was a nesting bird. Some princes described the grove of trees, others the particular tree or the bough on which the nest stood. When Arjuna's turn came, he described first the bird. Then he saw only its head, and lastly he could see nothing but the shining eye of the bird, which was the centre of the target chosen by Droṇa.

There is danger, however, of an ekāgra person becoming supremely egotistical. Where the senses start roaming unchecked, the mind follows suit. They cloud a man's judgement and set him adrift like a battered ship on a storm-tossed sea. A ship needs ballast to keep her on an even keel and the helmsman needs a star to steer her by. The ekāgra person needs bhakti (adoration of the Lord) and concentration on divinity to keep his mental equilibrium so that he goes on always in the right direction. He will not know happiness until the sense of 'I' and 'mine' disappears.

The last mental state is that of niruddha, where the mind (manas), intellect (buddhi) and ego (ahaṁkāra) are all restrained and all these faculties are offered to the Lord for His use and in His service. Here there is no feeling of 'I' and 'mine'. As a lens becomes more luminous when great light is thrown upon it and seems to be all light and undistinguishable from it, so also the sādhaka who has given up his mind, intellect and ego to the Lord, becomes one with Him, for the sādhaka thinks of nothing but Him, who is the creator of thought.

Without ekāgratā or concentration one can master nothing. Without concentration on Divinity, which shapes and controls the universe, one cannot unlock the divinity within oneself or become a universal man. To achieve this concentration, what is recommended is eka-tattva-abhyāsa or study of the single element that pervades all, the inmost Self of all beings, who converts His one form into many. The sādhaka, therefore, concentrates upon AUM, which is His symbol, to achieve ekāgratā.

Aum: According to Śri Vinobā Bhāve, the Latin word Omne and the Sanskrit word Aum are both derived from the same root meaning all and both words convey the concepts of omniscience, omnipresence and omnipotence. Another word for Aum is praṇava, which is derived from the root nu meaning to praise, to which is added the prefix pra denoting superiority. The word, therefore, means the best praise or the best prayer.

The symbol AUM is composed of three syllables, namely the letters A, U, M, and when written has a crescent and dot on its top. A few instances of the various interpretations given to it may be mentioned here to convey its meaning.

The letter A symbolises the conscious or waking state (jāgrata-avasthā), the letter U the dream state (svapna-avasthā) and the letter M the dreamless sleep state (suṣupta-avasthā) of the mind and spirit. The entire symbol, together with the crescent and the dot, stands for the fourth state (turīya-avasthā), which combines all these states and transcends them. This is the state of samādhi.

The letters A, U and M symbolise respectively speech (vak), the mind (manas) and the breath of life (prāṇa), while the entire symbol stands for the living spirit, which is but a portion of the divine spirit.

The three letters also represent the dimensions of length, breadth and depth, while the entire symbol represents Divinity, which is beyond the limitations of shape and form.

The three letters A, U and M symbolise the absence of desire, fear and anger, while the whole symbol stands for the perfect man (a sthita-prajñā), one whose wisdom is firmly established in the divine.

They represent the three genders, masculine, feminine and neuter, while the entire symbol represents all creation together with the Creator.

They stand for the three guṇās or qualities of sattva, rajas and tamas, while the whole symbol represents a guṇātīta, one who has transcended and gone beyond the pull of the guṇās.

The letters correspond to the three tenses – past, present and future – while the entire symbol stands for the Creator, who transcends the limitations of time.

They also stand for the teaching imparted by the mother, the father and the Guru respectively. The entire symbol represents Brahma Vidyā, the knowledge of the Self, the teaching which is imperishable.

The A, U and M depict the three stages of yogic discipline, namely, āsana, prāṇāyāma and pratyāhāra. The entire symbol represents samādhi, the goal for which the three stages are the steps.

They represent the triad of Divinity, namely, Brahmā – the creator, Viṣṇu – the Maintainer, and Śiva – the Destroyer of the universe. The whole symbol is said to represent Brahman from which the universe emanates, has its growth and fruition and into which it merges in the end. It does not grow or change. Many change and pass, but Brahman is the One that ever remains unchanged.

The letters A, U and M also stand for the mantra 'Tat Twam Asi' ('That Thou Art'), the realisation of man's divinity within himself. The entire symbol stands for this realisation, which liberates the human spirit from the confines of his body, mind, intellect and ego.

After realising the importance of AUM, the yogi focusses his attention on his beloved Deity adding AUM to the name of the Lord. The word AUM being too vast and too abstract, he unifies his senses, will, intellect, mind and reason by focussing on the name of the Lord and adding the word AUM with one pointed devotion and so experiences the feeling and meaning of the mantra.

The yogi recalls the verses of the *Muṇḍakopaniṣad*: 'Taking as a bow the great weapon of the Upaniṣad, one should put upon it an arrow sharpened by meditation. Stretching it with a thought directed to the essence of That, penetrate the Imperishable as the mark, my friend. The mystic syllable AUM is the bow. The arrow is the Self (Ātmā). Brahman is the target. By the undistracted man is It penetrated. One should come to be in It, as the arrow in the mark.'

Dhyāna

As water takes the shape of its container, the mind when it contemplates an object is transformed into the shape of that object. The mind which thinks of the all-pervading divinity which it worships, is ultimately through long-continued devotion transformed into the likeness of that divinity.

When oil is poured from one vessel to another, one can observe the steady constant flow. When the flow of concentration is uninterrupted, the state that arises is dhyāna (meditation). As the filament in an electric bulb glows and illumines when there is a regular uninterrupted current of electricity, the yogi's mind will be illumined by dhyāna. His body, breath, senses, mind, reason and ego are all integrated in the object of his contemplation – the Universal Spirit. He remains in a state of consciousness which has no qualification whatsoever. There is no other feeling except a state of SUPREME BLISS. Like a streak of lightning the yogi sees LIGHT that shines beyond the earth and the heavens. He sees the light that shines in his own heart. He becomes a light unto himself and others.

The signs of progress on the path of Yoga are health, a sense of physical lightness, steadiness, clearness of countenance and a beautiful voice, sweetness of odour of the body and freedom from craving. He has a balanced, serene and a tranquil mind. He is the very symbol of humility. He dedicates all his actions to the Lord and taking refuge in

Him, frees himself from the bondage of karma (action) and becomes a Jīvana Mukta (a Liberated Soul).

'What becomes of him who strives and fails to reach the end of Yoga, who has faith, but whose mind wanders away from Yoga?' To this query of Arjuna, the Lord Śri Krishna replied:

'No evil can befall a righteous man. He dwells long years in the heaven of those who did good, and then he is reborn in the house of the pure and the great. He may even be born in a family of illumined yogis; but to be born in such a family is most difficult in this world. He will regain the wisdom attained in his former life and strives ever for perfection. Because of his former study, practice and struggle which drive him ever onwards, the yogi ever strives with a soul cleansed of sin, attains perfection through many lives and reaches the supreme goal. The yogi goes beyond those who only follow the path of austerity, knowledge or service. Therefore, Arjuna, be thou a yogi. The greatest of all yogis is he who adores Me with faith and whose heart abides in Me.' (*Bhagavad Gītā*, chapter VI, verses 38 to 47.)

Samādhi

Samādhi is the end of the sādhaka's quest. At the peak of his meditation, he passes into the state of samādhi, where his body and senses are at rest as if he is asleep, his faculties of mind and reason are alert as if he is awake, yet he has gone beyond consciousness. The person in a state of samādhi is fully conscious and alert.

All creation is Brahman. The sādhaka is tranquil and worships it as that from which he came forth, as that in which he breathes, as that into which he will be dissolved. The soul within the heart is smaller than the smallest seed, yet greater than the sky, containing all works, all desires. Into this the sādhaka enters. Then there remains no sense of 'I' or 'mine' as the working of the body, the mind and the intellect have stopped as if one is in deep sleep. The sādhaka has attained true Yoga; there is only the experience of consciousness, truth and unutterable joy. There is a peace that passeth all understanding. The mind cannot find words to describe the state and the tongue fails to utter them. Comparing the experience of samādhi with other experiences, the sages say: 'Neti! Neti!'–'It is not this! It is not this!' The state can only be expressed by profound silence. The yogi has departed from the material world and is merged in the Eternal. There is then no duality between the knower and the known for they are merged like camphor and the flame.

There wells up from within the heart of the yogi the Song of the Soul, sung by Śankarāchārya in his *Ātma Ṣaṭkam.*

Song of the Soul

I am neither ego nor reason, I am neither mind nor thought,
I cannot be heard nor cast into words, nor by smell nor sight ever caught:
In light and wind I am not found, nor yet in earth and sky –
Consciousness and joy incarnate, Bliss of the Blissful am I.

I have no name, I have no life, I breathe no vital air,
No elements have moulded me, no bodily sheath is my lair:
I have no speech, no hands and feet, nor means of evolution –
Consciousness and joy am I, and Bliss in dissolution.

I cast aside hatred and passion, I conquered delusion and greed;
No touch of pride caressed me, so envy never did breed:
Beyond all faiths, past reach of wealth, past freedom, past desire,
Consciousness and joy am I, and Bliss is my attire.

Virtue and vice, or pleasure and pain are not my heritage,
Nor sacred texts, nor offerings, nor prayer, nor pilgrimage:
I am neither food, nor eating, nor yet the eater am I –
Consciousness and joy incarnate, Bliss of the Blissful am I.

I have no misgiving of death, no chasms of race divide me,
No parent ever called me child, no bond of birth ever tied me:
I am neither disciple nor master, I have no kin, no friend –
Consciousness and joy am I, and merging in Bliss is my end.

Neither knowable, knowledge, nor knower am I, formless is my form,
I dwell within the senses but they are not my home:
Ever serenely balanced, I am neither free nor bound –
Consciousness and joy am I, and Bliss is where I am found.

Part II

Yogasānas, Bandha and Kriyā

Hints, Cautions, Technique and Effects

(After the name of each āsana, there is a number with an asterisk. These numbers before an asterisk indicate the intensity of the āsana; the lower the number, the easier the āsana, the higher the number, the more difficult the āsana. The easiest is numbered 'one*', the most difficult 'sixty*'.)

Yogāsanas

Hints and Cautions for the Practice of Āsanas

The requisites

1. Without firm foundations a house cannot stand. Without the practice of the principles of yama and niyama, which lay down firm foundations for building character, there cannot be an integrated personality. Practice of āsanas without the backing of yama and niyama is mere acrobatics.

2. The qualities demanded from an aspirant are discipline, faith, tenacity and perseverance to practise regularly without interruptions.

Cleanliness and food

3. Before starting to practise āsanas, the bladder should be emptied and the bowels evacuated. Topsy-turvy poses help bowel movements. If the student is constipated or it is not possible to evacuate the bowels before the practice of āsanas, start with Śīrṣāsana and Sarvāṅgāsana and their variations. Attempt other āsanas only after evacuation. Never practise advanced āsanas without having first evacuated the bowels.

Bath

4. Āsanas come easier after taking a bath. After doing them, the body feels sticky due to perspiration and it is desirable to bathe some fifteen minutes later. Taking a bath or a shower both before and after practising āsanas refreshes the body and mind.

Food

5. Āsanas should preferably be done on an empty stomach. If this is difficult, a cup of tea or coffee, cocoa or milk may be taken before doing them. They may be practised without discomfort one hour after a very light meal. Allow at least four hours to elapse after a heavy meal before starting the practice. Food may be taken half an hour after completing the āsanas.

Time

6. The best time to practise is either early in the morning or late in the evening. In the morning āsanas do not come easily as the body is stiff. The mind, however, is still fresh but its alertness and determination

diminish as time goes by. The stiffness of the body is conquered by regular practice and one is able to do the āsanas well. In the evening, the body moves more freely than in the mornings, and the āsanas come better and with greater ease. Practice in the morning makes one work better in one's vocation. In the evening it removes the fatigue of the day's strain and makes one fresh and calm. Difficult āsanas should, therefore, be done in the morning when one has more determination and stimulative āsanas (like Śīrṣāsana, Sarvāṅgāsana and their variations and Paśchimottānāsana) should be practised in the evening.

Sun

7. Do not practise āsanas after being out in the hot sun for several hours.

Place

8. They should be done in a clean airy place, free from insects and noise.

9. Do not do them on the bare floor or on an uneven place, but on a folded blanket laid on a level floor.

Cautions

10. No undue strain should be felt in the facial muscles, ears and eyes or in breathing during the practice.

Closing of the eyes

11. In the beginning, keep the eyes open. Then you will know what you are doing and where you go wrong. If you shut your eyes you will not be in a position to watch the requisite movements of the body or even the direction in which you are doing the pose. You can keep your eyes closed only when you are perfect in a particular āsana for only then will you be able to adjust the bodily movements and feel the correct stretches.

Mirror

12. If you are doing the āsanas in front of a mirror, keep it perpendicular to the floor and let it come down to ground level, for otherwise the poses will look slanting due to the angle of the mirror. You will not be able to observe the movements or placing of the head and shoulders in the topsy-turvy poses unless the mirror reaches down to the floor.

The Brain

13. During the practice of āsanas, it is the body alone which should be active while the brain should remain passive, watchful and alert. If they are done with the brain, then you will not be able to see your own mistakes.

Breathing

14. In all the āsanas, the breathing should be done through the nostrils only and not through the mouth.

15. Do not restrain the breath while in the process of the āsana or while staying in it. Follow the instructions regarding breathing given in the technique sections of the various āsanas as described hereafter.

Śavāsana

16. After completing the practice of āsanas always lie down in Śavāsana for at least 10 to 15 minutes, as this will remove fatigue.

Āsanas and Prāṇāyāma

17. Read carefully the hints and cautions for the practice of prāṇāyāma before attempting it (see Part III). Prāṇāyāma may be done either very early in the morning before the āsanas or in the evening after completing them. If early in the morning, prāṇāyāma may be done first for 15 to 30 minutes: then a few minutes of Śavāsana, and after allowing some time to elapse, during which one may be engaged in normal activities, practise āsanas. If, however, these are done in the evening, allow at least half an hour to elapse before sitting for prāṇāyāma.

Special provisions for persons suffering from dizziness or blood pressure

18. Do not start with Śīrṣāsana and Sarvāṅgāsana if you suffer from dizziness or high blood pressure. First practise Paśchimottānāsana Uttānāsana, and Adhomukha Śvānāsana before attempting topsy-turvy poses like Śīrṣāsana and Sarvāṅgāsana and after doing these poses repeat Paśchimottānāsana, Adhomukha Śvānāsana and Uttānāsana in that order.

19. All forward bending poses are beneficial for persons suffering from either high or low blood pressure.

Special warning for persons affected by pus in the ears or displaced retina

20. Those suffering from pus in the ears or displacement of the retina should not attempt topsy-turvy poses.

Special provisions for women

21. *Menstruation:* Avoid āsanas during the menstrual period. But if the flow is in excess of normal, Upaviṣṭha Koṇāsana, Baddha Koṇāsana, Vīrāsana, Jānu Śīrṣāsana, Paśchimottānāsana and Uttānāsana may be performed with beneficial effect. On no account stand on your head during the menstrual period.

Pregnancy

22. All the āsanas can be practised during the first three months of pregnancy. All the standing poses and the forward bending āsanas may be done with mild movements, for at this time the spine should be made strong and elastic and no pressure should be felt on the abdomen. Baddha Koṇāsana and Upaviṣṭha Koṇāsana may be practised throughout pregnancy at any time of the day (even after meals, but not forward bending immediately after meals) as these two āsanas will strengthen the pelvic muscles and the small of the back and also reduce labour pains considerably. Prāṇāyāma without retention (kumbhaka) may be practised throughout pregnancy, as regular deep breathing will help considerably during labour.

After delivery

23. No āsanas should be done during the first month after delivery. Thereafter they may be practised mildly. Gradually increase the course as mentioned in Appendix I. Three months after delivery all āsanas may be practised with comfort.

Effects of āsanas

24. Faulty practice causes discomfort and uneasiness within a few days. This is sufficient to show that one is going wrong. If you cannot find the fault for yourself, it is better to approach a person who has practised well and get his guidance.

25. The right method of doing āsanas brings lightness and an exhilarating feeling in the body as well as in the mind and a feeling of oneness of body, mind and soul.

26. Continuous practice will change the outlook of the practiser. He will discipline himself in food, sex, cleanliness and character and will become a new man.

27. When one has mastered an āsana, it comes with effortless ease and causes no discomfort. The bodily movements become graceful. While performing āsanas, the student's body assumes numerous forms of life found in creation – from the lowliest insect to the most perfect sage – and he learns that in all these there breathes the same Universal Spirit – the Spirit of God. He looks within himself while practising and feels the presence of God in different āsanas which he does with a sense of surrender unto the feet of the LORD.

ĀSANAS

1. *Tāḍāsana* (also called Samasthiti) One* (Plate 1)

Tāḍa means a mountain. Sama means upright, straight, unmoved. Sthiti is standing still, steadiness. Tāḍāsana therefore implies a pose where one stands firm and erect as a mountain. This is the basic standing pose.

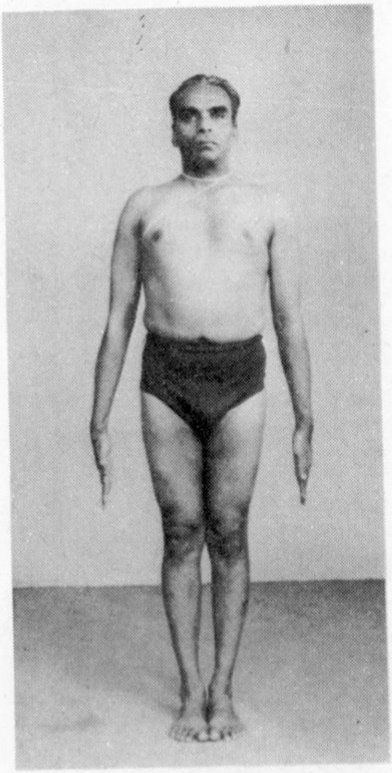

1

Technique

1. Stand erect with the feet together, the heels and big toes touching each other. Rest the heads of metatarsals on the floor and stretch all the toes flat on the floor.

2. Tighten the knees and pull the knee-caps up, contract the hips and pull up the muscles at the back of the thighs.

3. Keep the stomach in, chest forward, spine stretched up and the neck straight.

4. Do not bear the weight of the body either on the heels or the toes, but distribute it evenly on them both.

5. Ideally in Tāḍāsana the arms are stretched out over the head, but for the sake of convenience, one can place them by the side of the thighs.

Each of the standing poses described below can then be followed easily, starting with the pupil standing in Tāḍāsana with palms by the side of the thighs.

Effects

People do not pay attention to the correct method of standing. Some stand with the body weight thrown only on one leg, or with one leg turned completely sideways. Others bear all the weight on the heels, or on the inner or outer edges of the feet. This can be noticed by watching where the soles and heels of the shoes wear out. Owing to our faulty method of standing and not distributing the body weight evenly on the feet, we acquire specific deformities which hamper spinal elasticity. Even if the feet are kept apart, it is better to keep the heel and toe in a line parallel to the median plane and not at an angle. By this method, the hips are contracted, the abdomen is pulled in and the chest is brought forward. One feels light in body and the mind acquires agility. If we stand with the body weight thrown only on the heels, we feel the gravity changing; the hips become loose, the abdomen protrudes, the body hangs back and the spine feels the strain and consequently we soon feel fatigued and the mind becomes dull. It is therefore essential to master the art of standing correctly.

2. *Vṛkṣāsana* One* (Plate 2)

Vṛkṣa means a tree.

Technique

1. Stand in Tāḍāsana. (Plate 1)

2. Bend the right leg at the knee and place the right heel at the root of the left thigh. Rest the foot on the left thigh, toes pointing downwards.

3. Balance on the left leg, join the palms and raise the arms straight over the head. (Plate 2)

4. Stay for a few seconds in the pose breathing deeply. Then lower the arms and separate the palms, straighten the right leg and stand again in Tāḍāsana.

5. Repeat the pose, standing on the right leg, placing the left heel at the root of the right thigh. Stay for the same length of time on both sides, come back to Tāḍāsana (Plate 1) and relax.

Effects

The pose tones the leg muscles and gives one a sense of balance and poise.

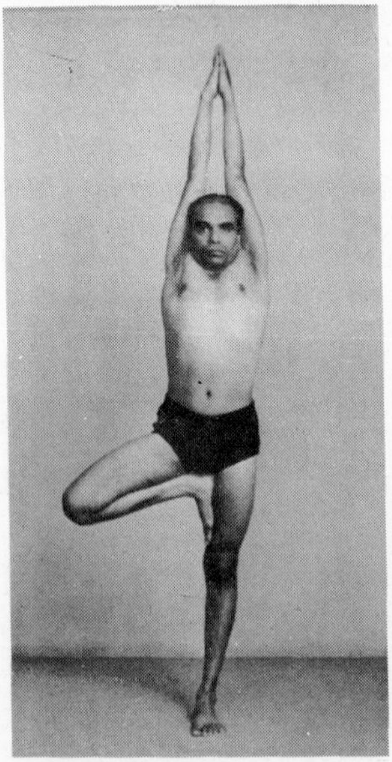

2

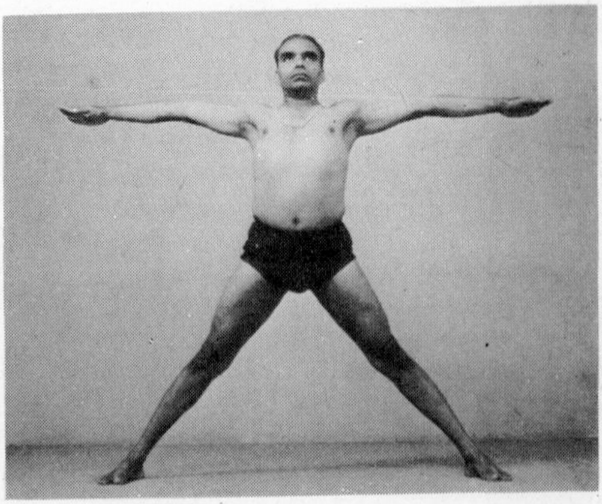

3

3. *Utthita Trikoṇāsana* Three* (Plates 4 and 5)

Utthita means extended, stretched. Trikoṇa (tri = three; koṇa = angle) is a triangle. This standing āsana is the extended triangle pose.

Technique

1. Stand in Tāḍāsana. (Plate 1)

2. Inhale deeply and with a jump spread apart the legs sideways 3 to 3½ feet. Raise the arms sideways, in line with the shoulders, palms facing down. Keep the arms parallel to the floor. (Plate 3)

3. Turn the right foot sideways 90 degrees to the right. Turn the left foot slightly to the right, keeping the left leg stretched from the inside and tightened at the knee.

4. Exhale, bend the trunk sideways to the right, bringing the right palm near the right ankle. If possible, the right palm should rest completely on the floor. (Plates 4 and 5)

5. Stretch the left arm up (as in the illustration), bringing it in line with the right shoulder and extend the trunk. The back of the legs, the back of the chest and the hips should be in a line. Gaze at the thumb of the

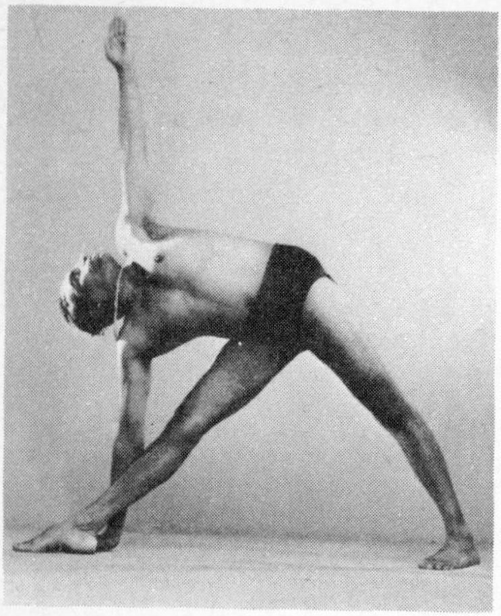

4

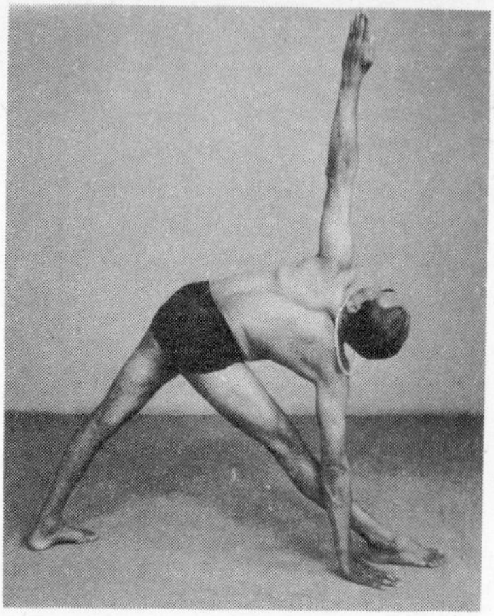

5

outstretched left hand. Keep the right knee locked tight by pulling up the knee-cap and keep the right knee facing the toes.

6. Remain in this position from half a minute to a minute, breathing deeply and evenly. Then lift the right palm from the floor. Inhale and return to position 2 above.

7. Now, turn the left foot sideways 90 degrees to the left, turn the right foot slightly to the left, keep both knees tight and continue from position 2 to 6, reversing all processes. Inhale and come to position 2. Hold the posture for the same length of time on the left side.

8. Exhale, and jump, coming back to Tāḍāsana. (Plate 1)

Effects

This āsana tones up the leg muscles, removes stiffness in the legs and hips, corrects any minor deformity in the legs and allows them to develop evenly. It relieves backaches and neck sprains, strengthens the ankles and develops the chest.

4. *Parivṛtta Trikoṇāsana* Five* (Plates 6 and 7)

Parivṛtta means revolved, turned round or back. Trikoṇa is a triangle. This is the revolving triangle posture. It is a counter pose to Uttihita Trikoṇāsana. (Plate 4)

Technique

1. Stand in Tāḍāsana. (Plate 1.) Take a deep inhalation and with a jump spread the legs apart sideways 3 to $3\frac{1}{2}$ feet. Raise the arms sideways, in line with the shoulders, palms facing down. (Plate 3)

2. Turn the right foot sideways 90 degrees to the right. Turn the left foot 60 degrees to the right, keeping the left leg stretched out and tightened at the knee.

3. Exhale, rotate the trunk along with the left leg in the opposite direction (to the right) so as to bring the left palm on the floor near the outer side of the right foot.

4. Stretch the right arm up, bringing it in line with the left arm. Gaze at the right thumb. (Plates 6 and 7)

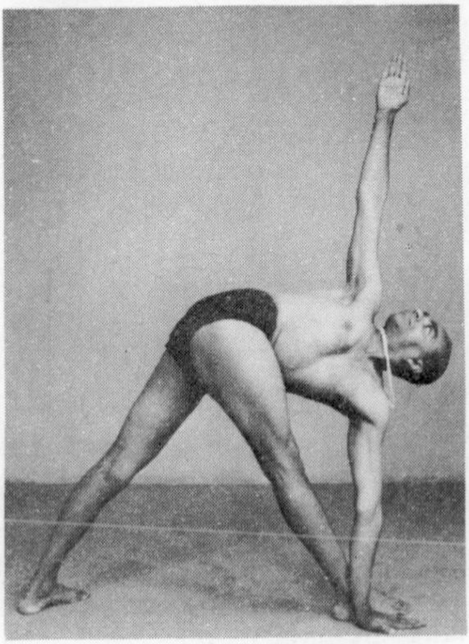

6

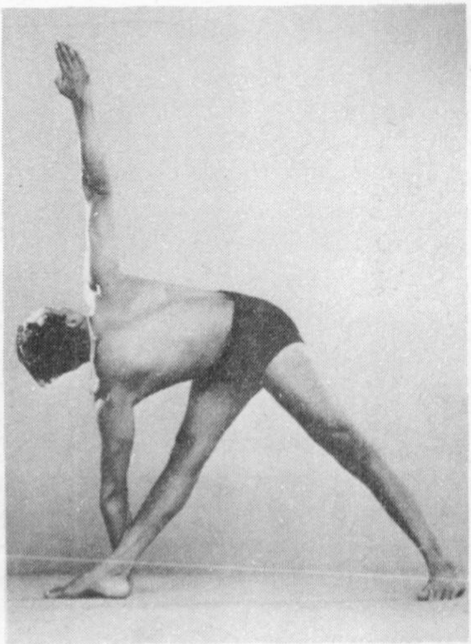

7

5. Keep the knees tight. Do not lift the toes of the right foot from the floor. Remember to rest the outer side of the left foot well on the floor.

6. Stretch both the shoulders and shoulder-blades.

7. Stay in this pose for half a minute with normal breathing.

8. Inhale, lift the left hand from the floor, rotate the trunk back to its original position and come back to position 1.

9. Exhale, repeat the pose on the left side by turning the left foot sideways 90 degrees to the left and the right foot 60 degrees to the left and place the right palm on the floor near the outer side of the left foot.

10. Stay in the pose on both sides for the same length of time, which can be adjusted by doing, say, three to four deep respirations on each side.

11. After completing the time, inhale, raise the trunk back to its original position, bring the toes to the front and keep the arms as in position 1.

12. Exhale and jump back to Tāḍāsana. (Plate 1.) This completes the āsana.

Effects

This āsana tones the thigh, calf and hamstring muscles. The spine and muscles of the back are also made to function properly, as the pose increases the blood supply round the lower part of the spinal region. The chest is expanded fully. The pose relieves pains in the back, invigorates the abdominal organs and strengthens the hip muscles.

5. *Utthita Pārśvakoṇāsana* Four* (Plates 8 and 9)

Pārśva means side or flank. Koṇa is an angle. This is the extended lateral angle pose.

Technique

1. Stand in Tāḍāsana. (Plate 1.) Take a deep inhalation and with a jump spread the legs apart sideways 4 to $4\frac{1}{2}$ feet. Raise the arms sideways, in line with the shoulders, palms facing down. (Plate 3)

2. While exhaling slowly, turn the right foot sideways 90 degrees to the right, and the left foot slightly to the right, keeping the left leg stretched out and tightened at the knee. Bend the right leg at the knee until the thigh and the calf form a right angle and the right thigh is parallel to the floor.

3. Place the right palm on the floor by the side of the right foot, the right armpit covering and touching the outer side of the right knee. Stretch the left arm out over the left ear. Keep the head up. (Plates 8 and 9)

4. Tighten the loins and stretch the hamstrings. The chest, the hips and the legs should be in a line and in order to achieve this, move the chest up and back. Stretch every part of the body, concentrating on the back portion of the whole body, specially the spine. Stretch the spine until all the vertebrae and ribs move and there is a feeling that even the skin is being stretched and pulled.

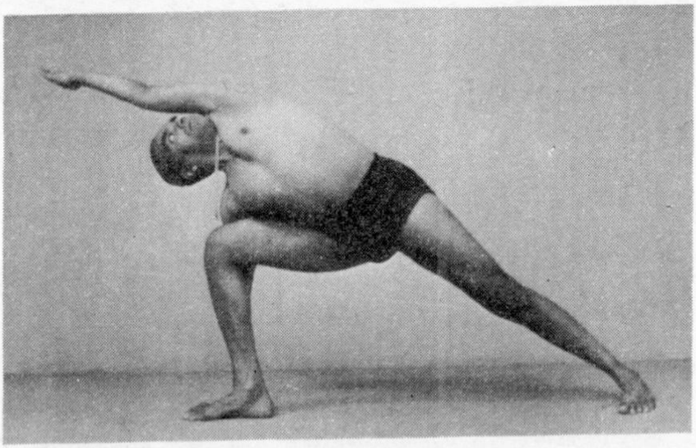

8

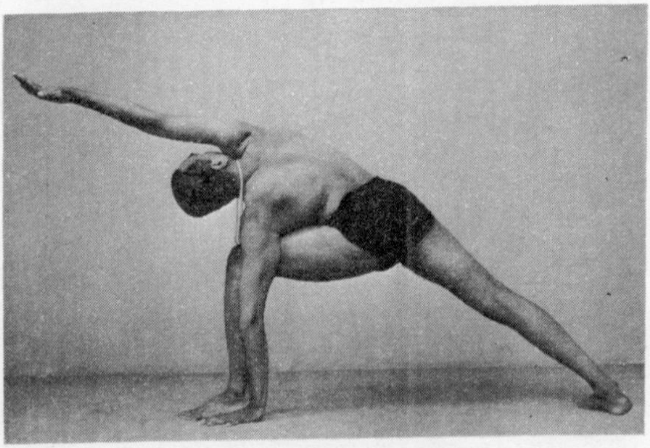

9

5. Remain in this pose from half a minute to a minute, breathing deeply and evenly. Inhale and lift the right palm from the floor.

6. Inhale, straighten the right leg and raise the arms as in position 1.

7. Continue with exhalation as in positions 2 to 5, reversing all processes, on the left side.

8. Exhale and jump back to Tāḍāsana. (Plate 1)

Effects

This āsana tones up the ankles, knees and thighs. It corrects defects in the calves and thighs, develops the chest and reduces fat round the waist and hips and relieves sciatic and arthritic pains. It also increases peristaltic activity and aids elimination.

6. *Parivṛtta Pārśvakoṇāsana* Eight* (Plates 10 and 11)

Parivṛtta means revolved, turned round or back. Pārśva means side or flank. Koṇa is an angle. This is the revolving lateral angle posture.

Technique

1. Stand in Tāḍāsana. (Plate 1)

2. Take a deep inhalation, and with a jump spread the legs apart sideways 4 to 4½ feet. Raise the arms sideways in line with the shoulders, palms down. (Plate 3)

3. Turn the right foot sideways 90 degrees to the right and the left foot 60 degrees to the right, keeping the left leg stretched out and tightened at the knee. Bend the right leg at the knee until the thigh and the calf form a right angle and the right thigh is parallel to the floor.

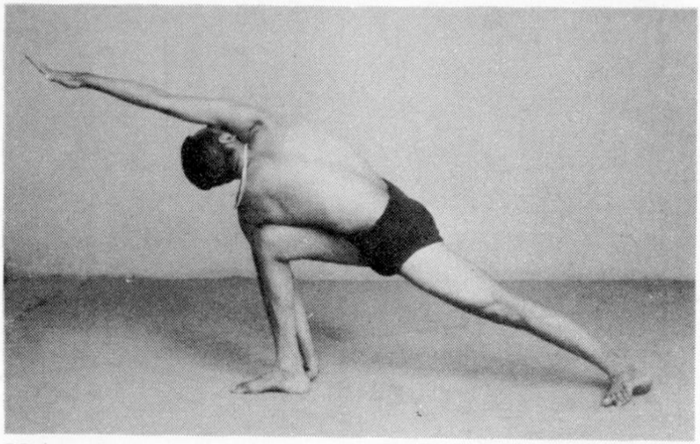

10

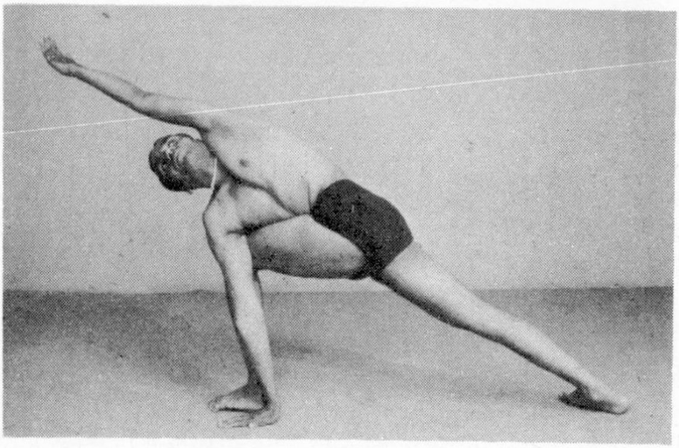

11

4. Exhale, and rotate the trunk and the left leg so as to bring the left arm over the right knee. Rest the left armpit on the outer side of the right knee, and place the left palm on the floor by the outer side of the right foot. (Plates 10 and 11)

5. Give a good twist to the spine (to the right), turn the trunk and bring the right arm over the right ear (as in the illustrations) and gaze up at the outstretched right arm. Keep the left knee tight throughout.

6. Hold this pose from half a minute to a minute, breathing deeply and evenly. Inhale, and lift the left palm from the floor. Raise the trunk and come back to position 2, by straightening the right leg and raising the arms.

7. Continue with exhalation on the left side, as in positions 3 to 5, reversing all processes.

8. In all cases where the movements are done first on one side and then on the other the time taken should be the same in each case. This general rule applies here.

Effects

This pose being a more intensified one than Parivṛtta Trikoṇāsana (Plate 6), has a greater effect. The hamstrings, however, are not stretched as much as in Parivṛtta Trikoṇāsana. The abdominal organs are more contracted and that aids digestion. The blood circulates well round the abdominal organs and the spinal column, and they are thus rejuvenated. The āsana helps to remove waste matter from the colon without strain.

7. *Vīrabhadrāsana I* Three* (Plate 14)

Dakṣa once celebrated a great sacrifice, but he did not invite his daughter Satī nor her husband Śiva, the chief of the gods. Satī, however, went to the sacrifice, but being greatly humiliated and insulted threw herself into the fire and perished. When Śiva heard this he was gravely provoked, tore a hair from his matted locks and threw it to the ground. A powerful hero named Vīrabhadra rose up and awaited his orders. He was told to lead Śiva's army against Dakṣa and destroy his sacrifice. Vīrabhadra and his army appeared in the midst of Dakṣa's assembly like a hurricane and destroyed the sacrifice, routed the other gods and priests and beheaded Dakṣa. Śiva in grief for Satī withdrew to Kailās and plunged into meditation. Satī was born again as Umā in the house of Himālaya. She strove once more for the love of Śiva and ultimately won his heart. The story is told by Kālidāsa in his great poem *Kumāra saṁbhava* (The Birth of the War-Lord).

This āsana is dedicated to the powerful hero created by Śiva from his matted hair.

Technique

1. Stand in Tāḍāsana. (Plate 1)

2. Raise both arms above the head; stretch up and join the palms. (Plate 12)

3. Take a deep inhalation and with a jump spread the legs apart sideways 4 to 4½ feet.

4. Exhale, turn to the right. Simultaneously turn the right foot 90 degrees to the right and the left foot slightly to the right. (Plate 13.) Flex the right knee till the right thigh is parallel to the floor and the right shin perpendicular to the floor, forming a right angle between the right thigh and the right calf. The bent knee should not extend beyond the ankle, but should be in line with the heel.

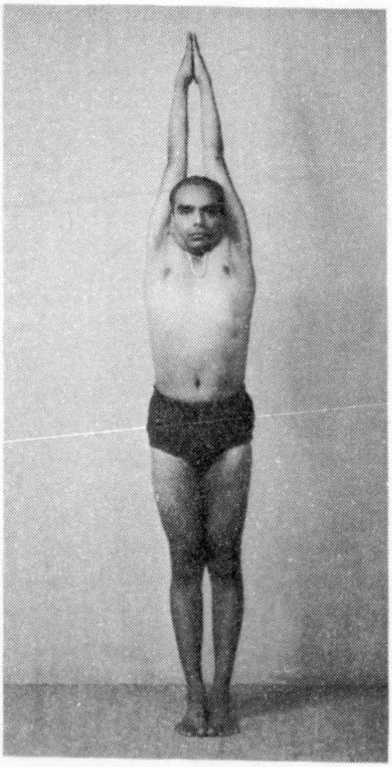

12

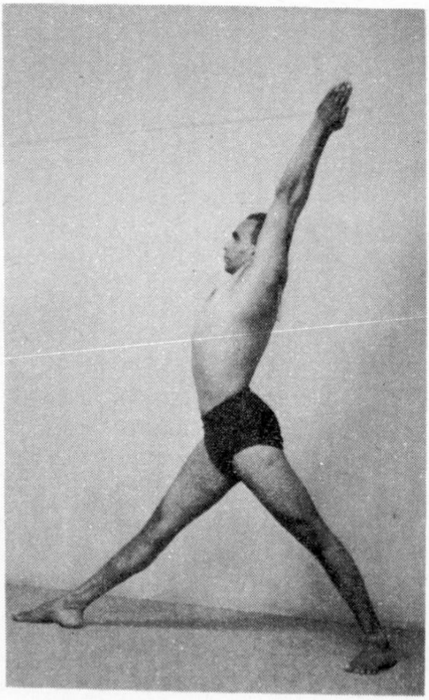

13

5. Stretch out the left leg and tighten at the knee.

6. The face, chest and right knee should face the same way as the right foot, as illustrated. Throw the head up, stretch the spine from the coccyx and gaze at the joined palms. (Plate 14)

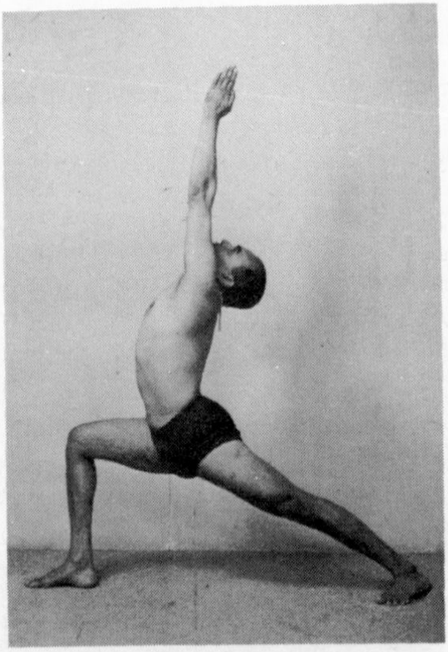

14

7. Hold the pose from 20 seconds to half a minute with normal breathing.

8. Repeat on the left side as in positions 4 to 6, reversing all processes.

9. Exhale and jump back to Tāḍāsana. (Plate 1)

*** All standing poses are strenuous, this pose in particular. It should not be tried by persons with a weak heart. Even people who are fairly strong should not stay long in this āsana.

Effects

In this pose the chest is fully expanded and this helps deep breathing. It relieves stiffness in shoulders and back, tones up the ankles and knees and cures stiffness of the neck. It also reduces fat round the hips.

8. *Vīrabhadrāsana II* One* (Plate 15)

Technique

1. Stand in Tāḍāsana. (Plate 1)

2. Take a deep inhalation, and with a jump spread the legs apart sideways 4 to 4½ feet. Raise the arms sideways in line with the shoulders, palms facing down. (Plate 3)

3. Turn the right foot sideways 90 degrees to the right and the left foot slightly to the right, keeping the left leg stretched out and tightened at the knee. Stretch the hamstring muscles of the left leg.

4. Exhale and bend the right knee till the right thigh is parallel to the floor, keeping the right shin perpendicular to the floor, thus forming a right angle between the right thigh and the right calf. The bent knee should not extend beyond the ankle, but should be in line with the heel. (Plate 15)

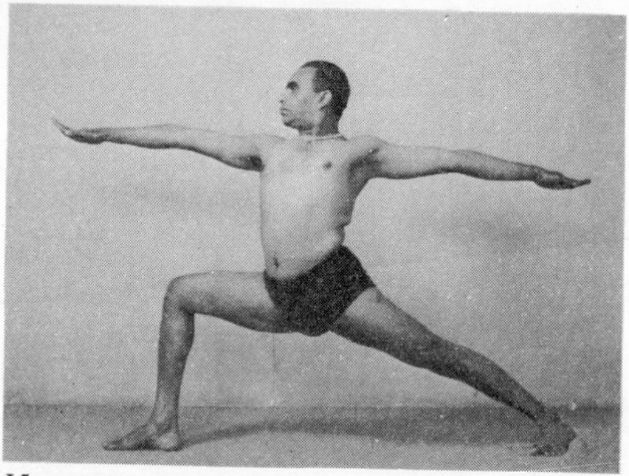

15

5. Stretch out the hands sideways, as though two persons are pulling you from opposite ends.

6. Turn the face to the right and gaze at the right palm. Stretch the back muscles of the left leg fully. The back of the legs, the dorsal region and the hips should be in one line.

7. Stay in the pose from 20 seconds to half a minute with deep breathing. Inhale and return to position 2.

8. Turn the left foot sideways 90 degrees to the left and the right foot slightly to the left, flex the left knee and continue from positions 3 to 6 on the left side, reversing all processes.

9. Inhale, again come back to position 2. Exhale and jump back to Tāḍāsana. (Plate 1)

Effects

Through this pose the leg muscles become shapely and stronger. It relieves cramp in the calf and thigh muscles, brings elasticity to the leg and back muscles and also tones the abdominal organs.

Mastery of the standing poses prepares the pupil for the advanced poses in forward bending, which can then be acquired with ease.

9. *Vīrabhadrāsana III* Five* (Plate 17)

This posture is an intensified continuation of Vīrabhadrāsana I. (Plate 14)

Technique

1. Stand in Tāḍāsana. (Plate 1)

2. Take a deep inhalation and with a jump spread the legs apart sideways 4 to $4\frac{1}{2}$ feet. (Plate 3)

3. Come to the final pose of Vīrabhadrāsana I on the right side. (Plate 14)

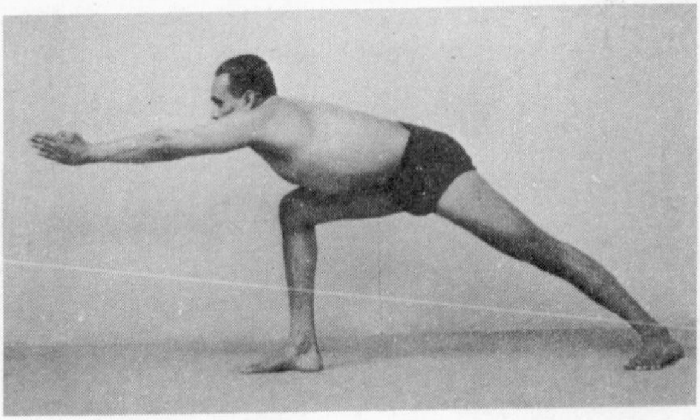

16

4. Exhale, bend the trunk forward and rest the chest on the right thigh. Keep the arms straight and the palms together. (Plate 16.) Rest in this position, taking two breaths.

5. Now exhale and simultaneously lift the left leg from the floor by swinging the body slightly forward and also straighten the right leg, making it stiff as a poker. Turn the left leg inwards so that the front is parallel to the floor. (Plate 17)

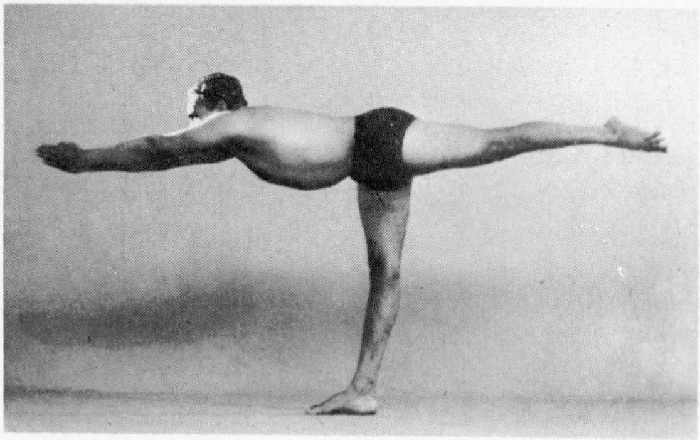

17

6. Hold in this pose from 20 to 30 seconds, with deep and even breathing.

7. While balancing, the whole body (except the right leg) is to be kept parallel to the floor. The right leg, which should be fully stretched and stiff, should be kept perpendicular to the floor. Pull the back of the right thigh and stretch the arms and the left leg as if two persons are pulling you from either end.

8. Exhale and come back to Vīrabhadrāsana I. (Plate 14)

9. Repeat the pose on the left side.

Effects

The illustration (Plate 17) conveys the harmony, balance, poise and power attained by practising this āsana. It helps to contract and tone the abdominal organs and makes the leg muscles more shapely and sturdy. It is recommended for runners, as it gives vigour and agility.

All the movements of this āsana improve one's bearing and carriage. When we stand badly, by throwing the weight on the heels, we retard symmetrical growth and hamper spinal elasticity. Standing with the weight on the heels causes the stomach to protrude and lessens bodily and mental agility. This āsana helps one to stand firmly on the soles of the feet, keeps the stomach muscles in and gives agility to the body and the mind.

10. *Ardha Chandrāsana* Five* (Plate 19)

Ardha means half. Chandra is the moon. The pose resembles the half moon, hence the name.

Technique

1. Stand in Tāḍāsana (Plate 1) and then do Utthita Trikoṇāsana, (Plate 4), following the technique described earlier.

2. After attaining Trikoṇāsana on the right side, exhale and place the right palm about a foot away from the right foot by bending the right knee and at the same time bringing the left foot near the right one. (Plate 18)

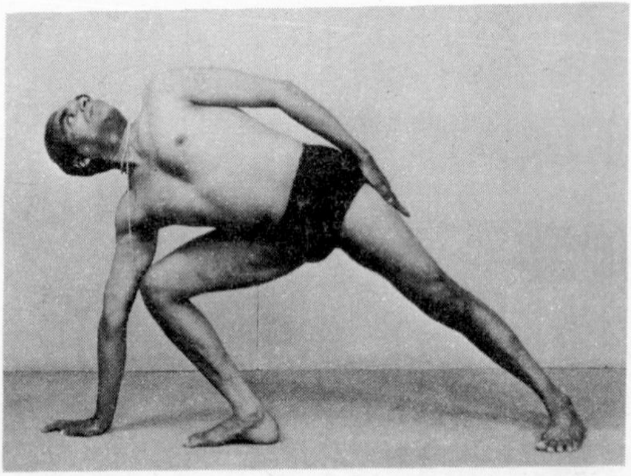

18

3. Wait in this position and take two breaths. Then exhale and raise the left leg from the floor, toes pointing up. Stretch the right hand and the right leg.

4. Place the left palm over the left hip and stretch up, keeping the shoulders well up. Turn the chest to the left and balance. (Plate 19)

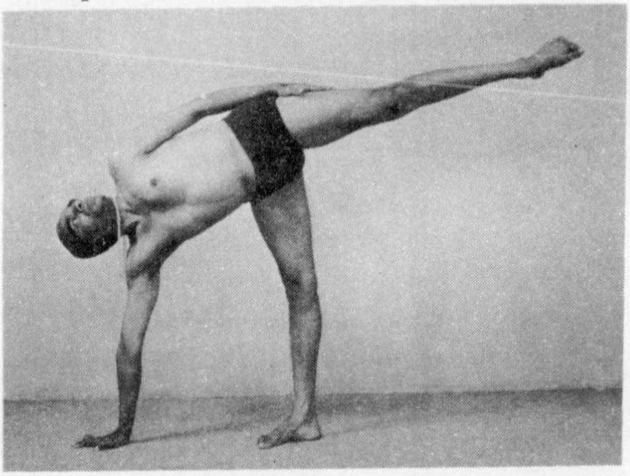

19

5. The weight of the body is borne on the right foot and hip. The right hand is only a support to control the balance.

6. Hold the pose from 20 to 30 seconds, breathing deeply and evenly. Then slide the left leg to the floor and go back to Trikoṇāsana. (Plate 4)

7. Repeat the pose on the left side.

Effects

The posture is beneficial for those whose legs are damaged or infected. It tones the lower region of the spine and the nerves connected with the leg muscles and it strengthens the knees. Along with other standing postures, this āsana cures gastric troubles.

Note. Those who feel weak and are exhausted by the standing poses should only practise Utthita Trikoṇāsana (Plate 4) and Utthita Pārśvakoṇāsana (Plate 8), as these two āsanas strengthen the body. The other standing āsanas should be done only by people who have built up their strength and whose bodies have become elastic.

11. *Utthita Hasta Pādānguṣṭhāsana* Sixteen* (Plate 23)

Utthita means extended. Hasta means the hand. Pādānguṣṭha is the big toe. This pose is done by standing on one leg, extending the other in front, holding the toe of the extended leg and resting the head on the leg.

Technique

1. Stand in Tāḍāsana. (Plate 1)

2. Exhale, raise the right leg by bending the knee and hold the big toe of the right foot between the thumb and the fore and middle fingers of the right hand.

3. Rest the left hand on the left hip and balance. (Plate 20.) Take two breaths.

4. Exhale, stretch the right leg forward and pull it. (Plate 21.) Take two breaths.

5. When you are firm in this position, hold the right foot with both hands and raise it still higher. (Plate 22.) Take two breaths.

6. Now, with an exhalation rest the head, then the nose and lastly the chin beyond the right knee. (Plate 23.) Stay in this position and take a few deep breaths.

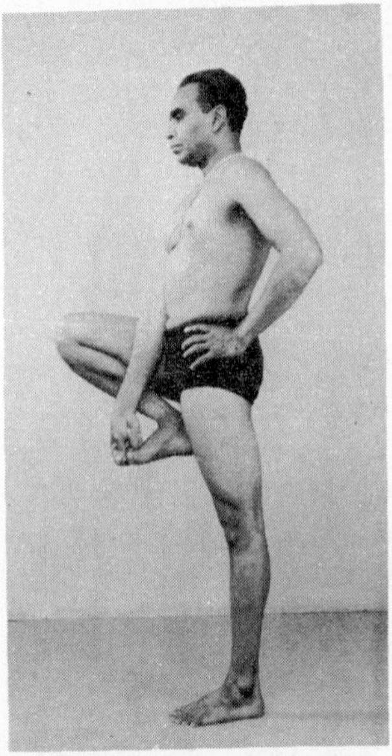
20

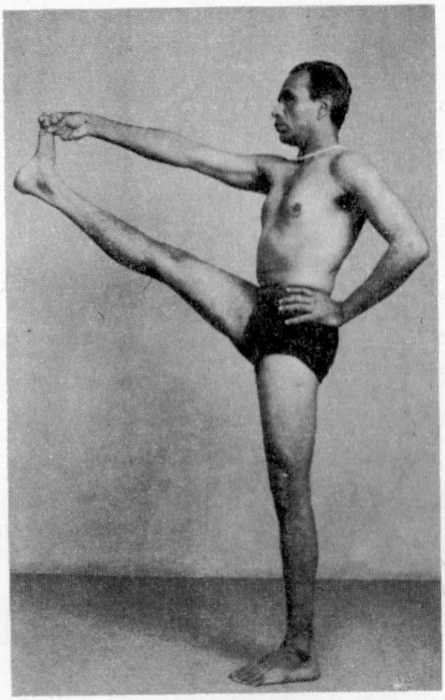
21

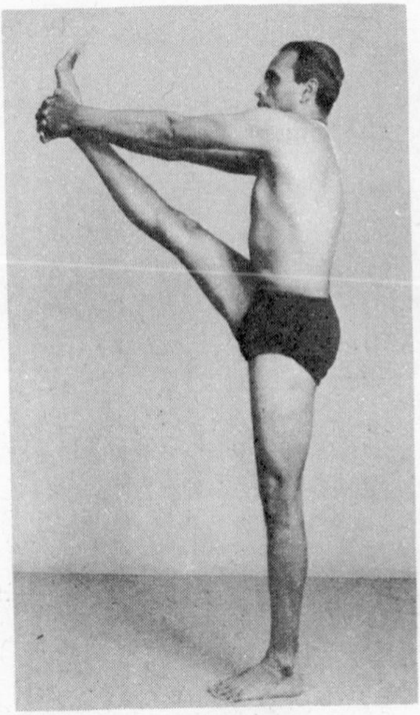
22

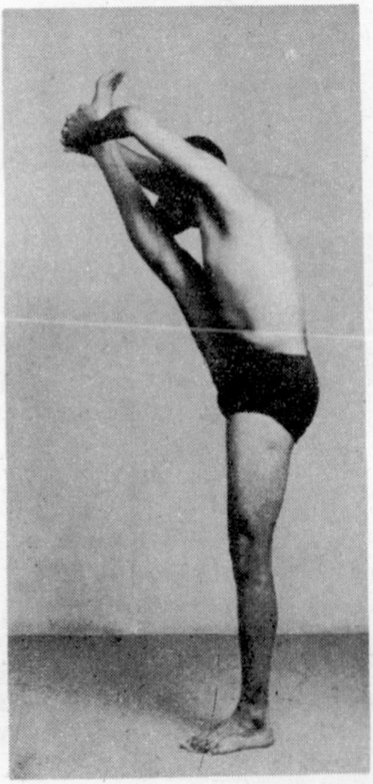
23

7. Exhale, release the hands and lower the right leg to the floor to return to Tāḍāsana. (Plate 1)

8. Repeat the pose on the other side, keeping the right leg on the floor and raising the left leg.

9. Balancing in positions 5 and 6 is difficult and cannot be attained without mastering position 4.

Effects

This āsana makes the leg muscles powerful and the balance gives one steadiness and poise.

12. *Pārśvōttānāsana* Six* (Plate 26)

Pārśva means side or flank. Uttāna (ut = intense, and tān = to extend, stretch, lengthen) means an intense stretch. The name implies a pose in which the side of the chest is stretched intensely.

Technique

1. Stand in Tāḍāsana. (Plate 1.) Inhale deeply and stretch the body forward.

2. Join the palms behind the back and draw the shoulders and elbows back.

3. Exhale, turn the wrists and bring both palms up above the middle of the back of the chest, the fingers at the level of the shoulder-blades. You are doing 'namaste' (the Indian gesture of respect by folding the hands) with your hands behind your back. (Plate 24)

4. Inhale and with a jump spread the legs apart sideways 3 to 3½ feet. Stay in this position and exhale.

5. Inhale and turn the trunk to the right. Turn the right foot 90 degrees sideways to the right keeping the toes and heel in a line with the trunk; turn the left foot with the leg 75 to 80 degrees to the right and keep the left foot stretched out and the leg tightened at the knee. Throw the head back. (Plate 25)

6. Exhale, bend the trunk forward and rest the head on the right knee. Stretch the back and gradually extend the neck until the nose, then the lips and lastly the chin touch and then rest beyond the right knee. (Plate 26.) Tighten both the legs by pulling the knee-caps up.

7. Stay in the pose from 20 seconds to half a minute with normal breathing. Then slowly move the head and trunk towards the left knee by swinging the trunk round the hips. At the same time turn the

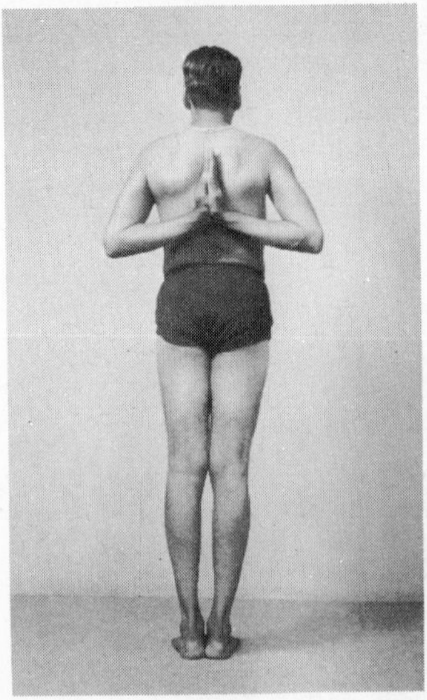

24

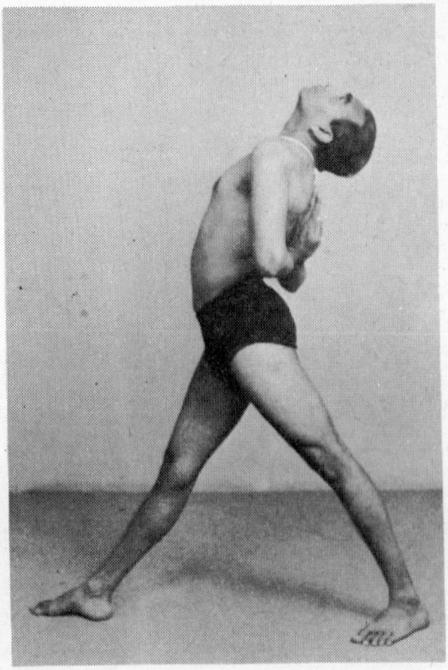

25

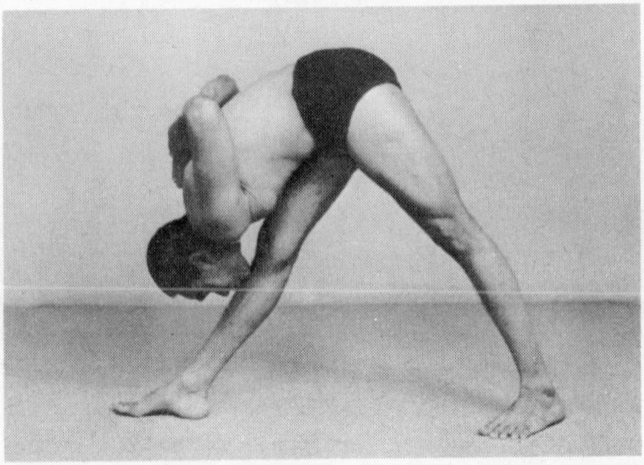

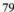

26

left foot 90 degrees towards the left and the right foot 75 to 80 degrees to the left. Now raise the trunk and head as far back as you can, without bending the right leg. This movement should be done with one inhalation.

8. Exhale, bend the trunk forward, rest the head on the left knee and gradually extend the chin beyond the left knee by stretching the neck as in position 6.

9. After holding the pose from 20 seconds to half a minute with normal breathing, inhale, move the head to the centre and the feet to their original position so that the toes point forward. Then raise the trunk up.

10. Exhale and jump back to Tāḍāsana (Plate 1), releasing the hands from the back.

11. If you cannot fold the hands together behind the back, just grip the wrist and follow the above technique. (Plates 27 and 28)

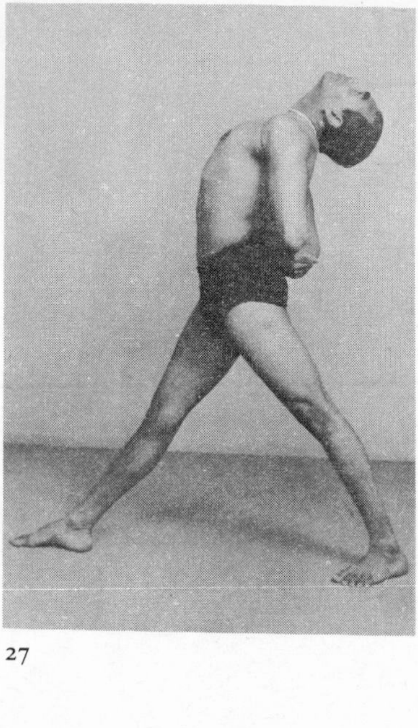

27

Effects

This āsana relieves stiffness in the legs and hip muscles and makes the hip joints and spine elastic. While the head is resting on the knees, the abdominal organs are contracted and toned. The wrists move freely and any stiffness there disappears. The posture also corrects round and drooping shoulders. In the correct pose, the shoulders are drawn well back and this makes deep breathing easier.

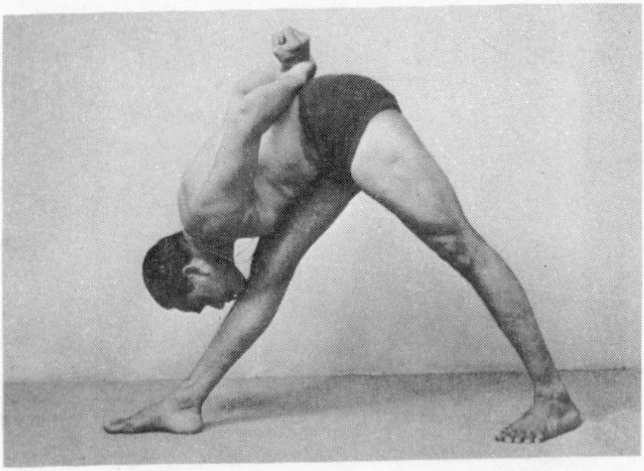

28

13. *Prasārita Pādōttānāsana I* Four* (Plates 33 and 34)

Prasārita means expanded, spread, extended. Pāda means a foot. The pose is one where the expanded legs are stretched intensely.

Technique

1. Stand in Tāḍāsana. (Plate 1)

2. Inhale, place the hands on the waist and spread the legs apart $4\frac{1}{2}$ to 5 feet. (Plate 29)

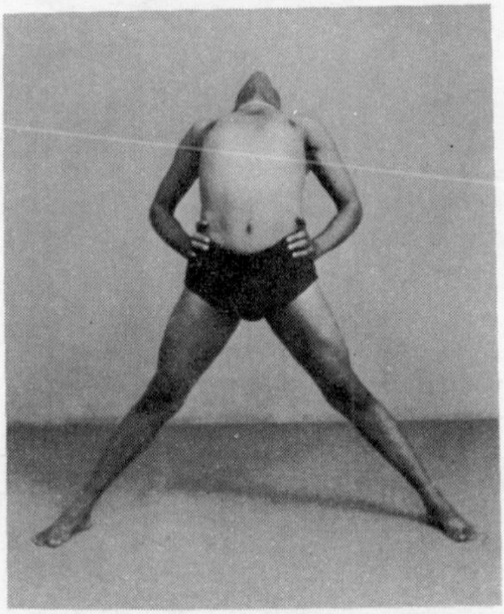

29

3. Tighten the legs by drawing up the knee-caps. Exhale, and place the palms on the floor in line with the shoulders between the feet. (Front view Plate 30)

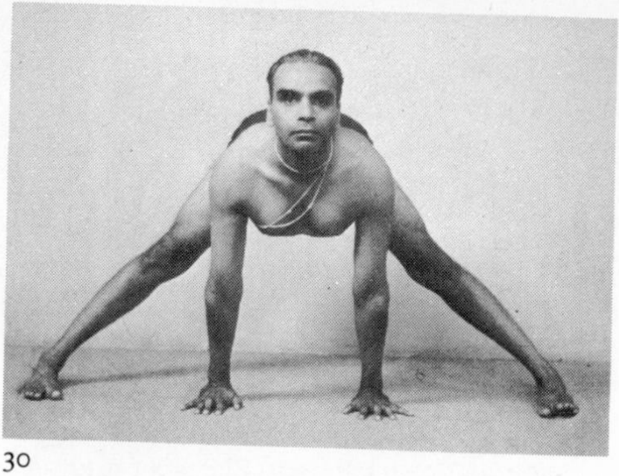

30

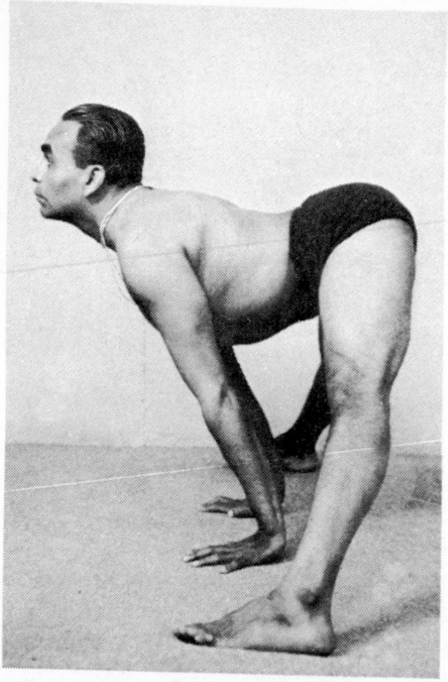

31

4. Inhale and raise the head up, keeping the back concave. (Side view Plates 31 and 32)

5. Exhale, bend the elbows and rest the crown of the head on the floor, keeping the weight of the body on the legs. (Plates 33 and 34.)

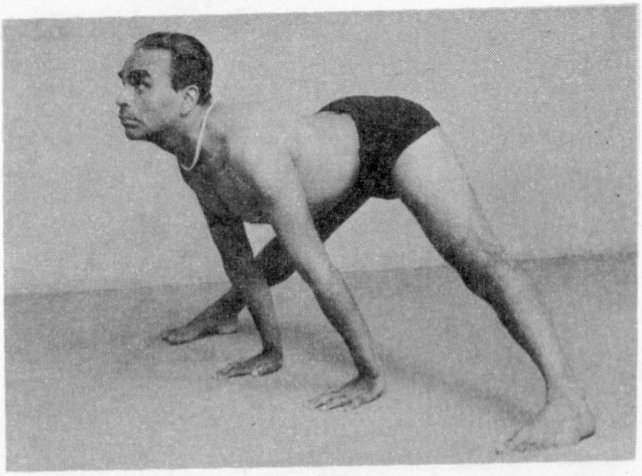

32

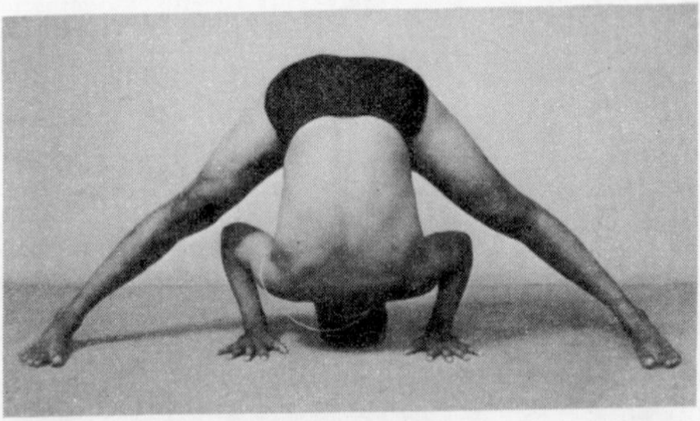

33

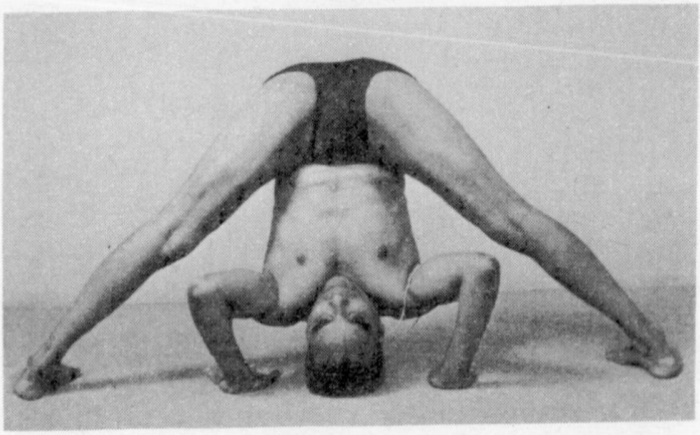

34

Do not throw the body weight on the head. Both feet, both palms and the head should be in a straight line.

6. Stay in the pose for half a minute, breathing deeply and evenly.

7. Inhale, raise the head from the floor and straighten the arms at the elbows. Keep the head well up by making the back concave as in position 4. (Plate 30)

8. Exhale and stand as in position 2. (Plate 29)

9. Jump back to Tāḍāsana. (Plate 1)

14. *Prasārita Pādōttānāsana II* Four* (Plates 35 and 36)

This is an advanced movement of the earlier pose. Here the hands are placed on the waist instead of on the floor (Plate 35), or are folded at the back as if one is doing 'namaste' behind the back (Plate 36) as described in Pārśvōttānāsana. (Plate 26.) In this movement the leg stretch is intensified.

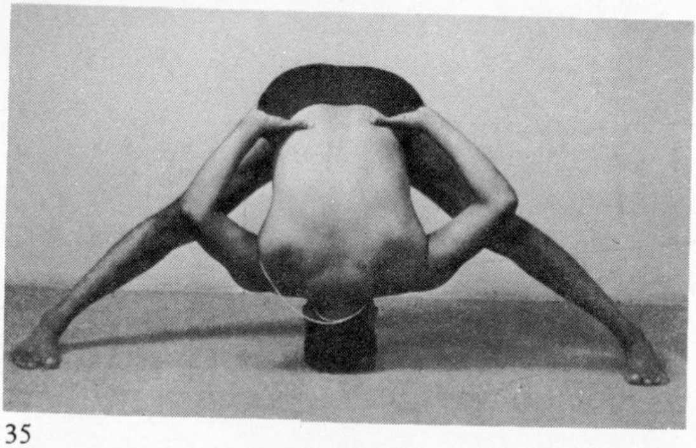

35

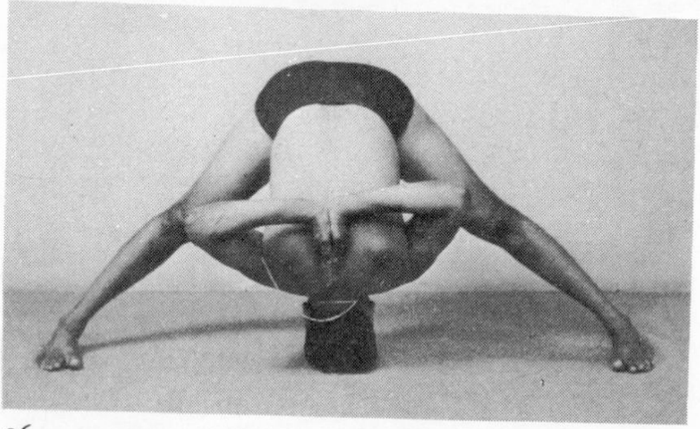

36

Effects

In this pose the hamstring and abductor muscles are fully developed, while blood is made to flow to the trunk and the head. People who cannot do Śīrṣāsana (Plate 184) can benefit from this pose, which increases digestive powers.

All the standing poses described above are necessary for beginners. As the pupil advances he attains better flexibility and then the standing poses can be dispensed with, though it is advisable to do them once a week. All these standing poses help to reduce the body weight.

15. *Parighāsana* Four* (Plate 39)

Parighā means a beam or bar used for shutting a gate. In this posture, the body resembles a cross beam used for locking a gate, hence the name of the pose.

Technique

1. Kneel on the floor with the ankles together.

2. Stretch the right leg sideways to the right and keep it in line with the trunk and the left knee. Turn the right foot sideways to the right, keeping the right leg stiff at the knee.

3. Extend the arms sideways with an inhalation. (Plate 37.) Take two breaths.

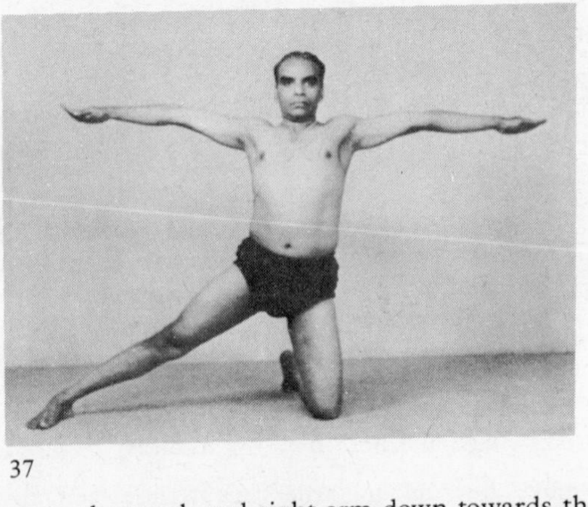

37

4. Exhale, move the trunk and right arm down towards the extended right leg. (Plate 38.) Rest the right forearm and wrist on the right shin and ankle respectively, the right palm facing up. The right ear will then rest on the right upper arm. Move the left arm over the head

and touch the right palm with the left. The left ear will then touch the left upper arm. (Plate 39)

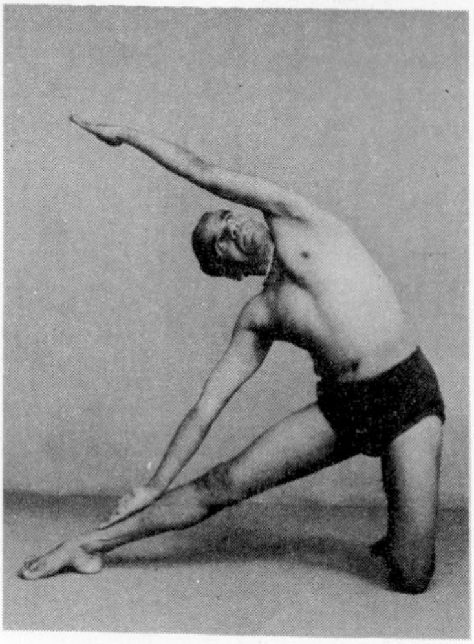

38

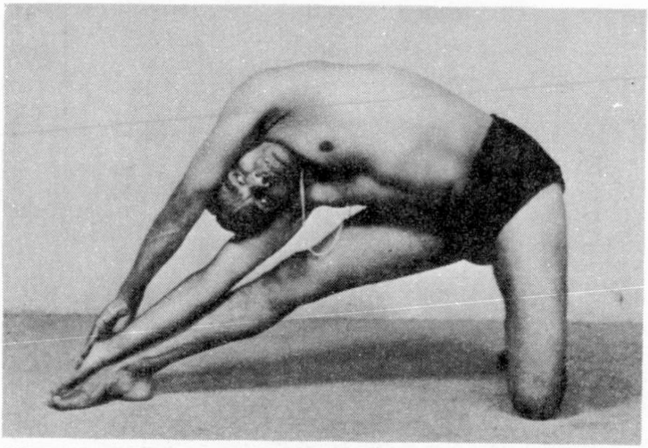

39

5. Stay in this position from 30 to 60 seconds, breathing normally.

6. Inhale, move the trunk and arms back to position 3. Bend the right leg and kneel on the floor, keeping the ankles together again.

7. Repeat the pose on the other side, substituting right for left and vice versa. Stay in the pose on both the sides for the same time.

Effects

In this posture the pelvic region is stretched. One side of the abdomen is extended while the other side is laterally flexed. This keeps the abdominal muscles and organs in condition and the skin round the abdomen will not sag but remain healthy. The sideways spinal movement will help persons suffering from stiff backs.

16. *Uṣṭrāsana* Three* (Plate 41)

Uṣṭra means a camel.

Technique

1. Kneel on the floor, keeping the thighs and feet together, toes pointing back and resting on the floor.

2. Rest the palms on the hips. Stretch the thighs, curve the spine back and extend the ribs. (Plate 40)

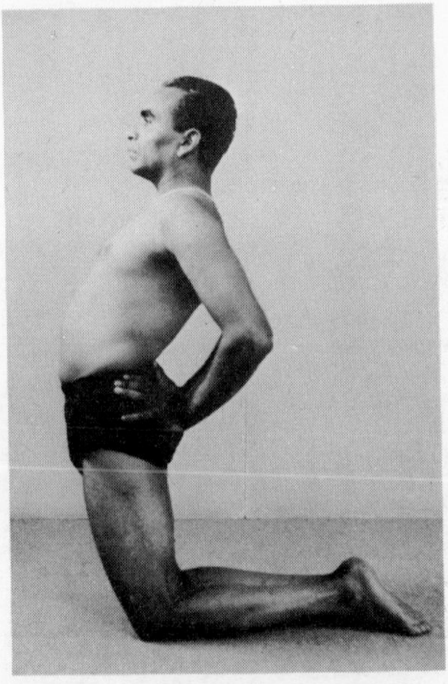

40

3. Exhale, place the right palm over the right heel and the left palm over the left heel. If possible, place the palms on the soles of the feet.

4. Press the feet with the palms, throw the head back and push the spine towards the thighs, which should be kept perpendicular to the floor.

5. Contract the buttocks and stretch the dorsal and the coccyx regions of the spine still further, keeping the neck stretched back. (Plate 41)

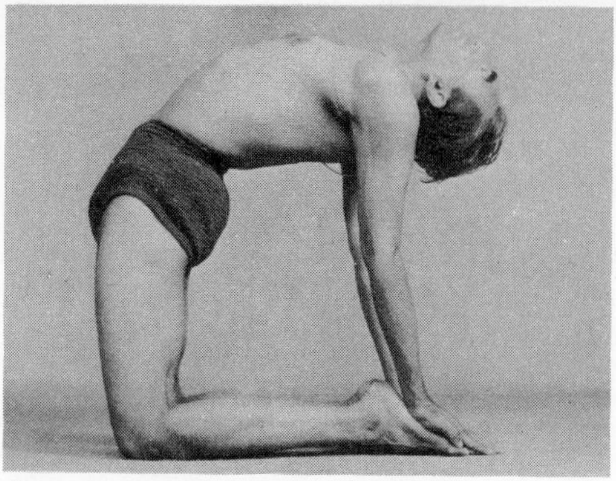

41

6. Remain in this position for about half a minute with normal breathing.

7. Release the hands one by one and rest them on the hips. (Plate 40.) Then sit on the floor and relax.

Effects

People with drooping shoulders and hunched backs will benefit by this āsana.

The whole spine is stretched back and is toned. This pose can be tried conveniently by the elderly and even by persons with spinal injury.

17. *Utkaṭāsana* Two* (Plate 42)

Utkaṭa means powerful, fierce, uneven. This āsana is like sitting on an imaginary chair.

Technique

1. Stand in Tāḍāsana (Plate 1), stretch the arms straight over the head and join the palms. (Plate 12)

2. Exhale, bend the knees and lower the trunk till the thighs are parallel to the floor. (Plate 42)

3. Do not stoop forward, but keep the chest as far back as possible and breathe normally.

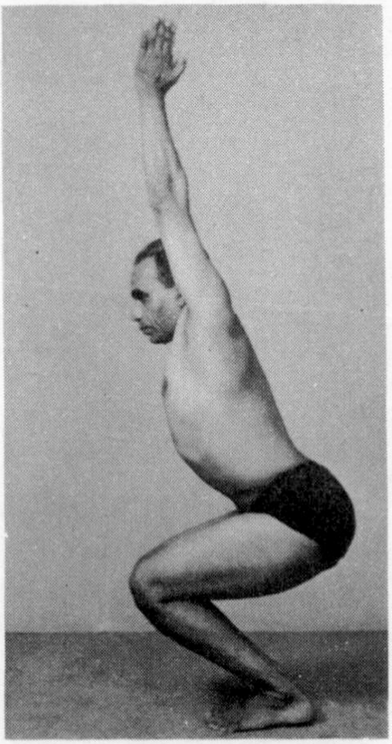

42

4. Stay in the pose for a few seconds, 30 being sufficient. It is difficult to balance in this pose.

5. Inhale, straighten the legs (Plate 12), lower the arms, come back to Tāḍāsana (Plate 1) and relax.

Effects

The pose removes stiffness in the shoulders and corrects any minor deformities in the legs. The ankles become strong and the leg muscles develop evenly. The diaphragm is lifted up and this gives a gentle massage to the heart. The abdominal organs and the back are toned, and the chest is developed by being fully expanded. It is a beneficial pose for horsemen.

18. *Pādānguṣṭhāsana* Three* (Plate 44)

Pāda means the foot. Anguṣṭha is the big toe. This posture is done by standing and catching the big toes.

Technique

1. Stand in Tāḍāsana. (Plate 1.) Spread the legs a foot apart.

2. Exhale, bend forward and hold the big toes between the thumbs and the first two fingers, so that the palms face each other. Hold them tight. (Plate 43)

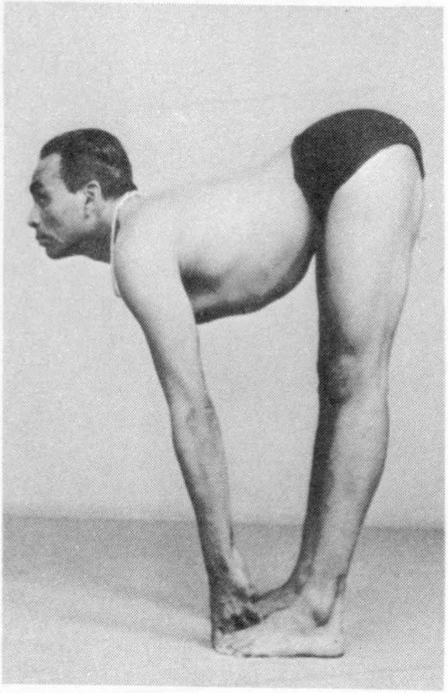

43

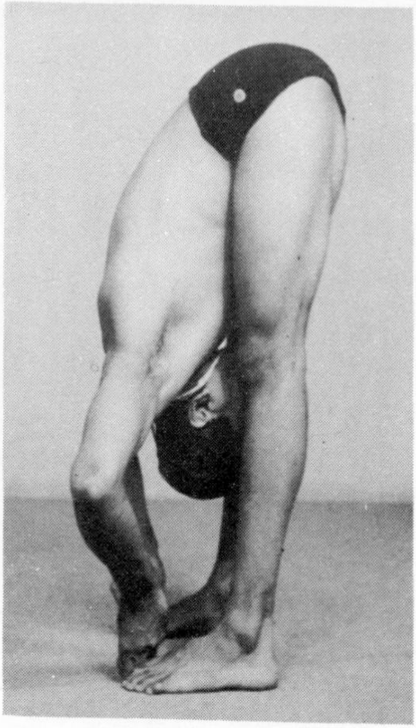

44

3. Keep the head up, stretch the diaphragm towards the chest and make the back as concave as possible. Instead of stretching down from the shoulders, bend forward from the pelvic region to get the concave shape of the back from the coccyx.

4. Keep the legs stiff and do not slacken the grip at the knees and toes. Stretch the shoulder-blades also. Take one or two breaths in this position.

5. Now exhale, and bring the head in between the knees by tightening the knees and pulling the toes without lifting them off the floor. (Plate 44.) Remain in this pose for about 20 seconds, maintaining normal breathing.

6. Inhale, come to position 2 (Plate 43), release the toes and stand up. Return to Tāḍāsana. (Plate 1)

19. *Pādahastāsana* Six* (Plate 46)

Pāda means the foot. Hasta means the hand. This posture is done by bending forward and standing on one's hands.

Technique

1. Stand in Tāḍāsana. (Plate 1.) Spread the legs a foot apart.

2. Exhale, bend forward and without bending the legs at the knees insert the hands under the feet so that the palms touch the soles. (Plate 45)

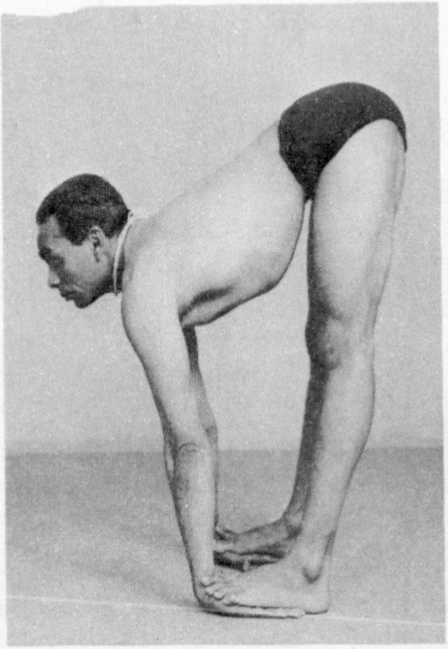

45

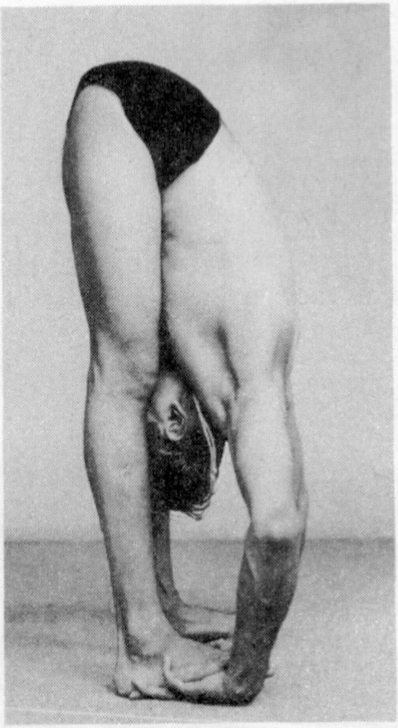

46

3. Keep the head up and make the back as concave as possible. Do not slacken the grip at the knees and take a few breaths in this position.

4. Now exhale, and move the head in between the knees by bending the elbows and pulling the feet up from the palms. (Plate 46.) Stay in the pose for about 20 seconds with normal breathing.

5. Inhale, raise the head and come back to position 2 (Plate 45), with the head well up. Take two breaths.

6. Inhale, stand up and return to Tāḍāsana. (Plate 1)

Effects of Pādānguṣṭhāsana and Pādahastāsana

The second āsana is more strenuous than the first, but the effects of both are the same. The abdominal organs are toned and digestive juices increase, while the liver and spleen are activated. Persons suffering from a bloating sensation in the abdomen or from gastric troubles will benefit by practising these two āsanas.

Slipped spinal discs can only be adjusted in the concave back position as in Plates 43 and 45. Do not bring the head in between the knees if you have a displaced disc. I have experimented with persons suffering from slipped discs and the concave back position proved a boon to them. It is imperative to get guidance from a guru (master) before trying this pose, because it may not be possible to achieve the concave back position immediately. One has to master other minor poses before attempting this one.

20. *Uttānāsana* Eight* (Plate 48)

Ut is a particle indicating deliberation, intensity. The verb tān means to stretch, extend, lengthen out. In this āsana, the spine is given a deliberate and an intense stretch.

Technique

1. Stand in Tāḍāsana (Plate 1), keeping the knees tight.

2. Exhale, bend forward and place the fingers on the floor. Then place the palms on the floor by the side of the feet, behind the heels. Do not bend the legs at the knees. (Plate 47)

3. Try to hold the head up and stretch the spine. Move the hips a little forward towards the head so as to bring the legs perpendicular to the floor.

4. Remain in this position and take two deep breaths.

5. Exhale, move the trunk closer to the legs and rest the head on the knees. (Plate 48)

6. Do not slacken the grip at the knees, but pull the knee-caps well up. Hold this position for a minute with deep and even breathing.

7. Inhale and raise the head from the knees, but without lifting the palms from the floor. (Plate 47)

8. After two breaths, take a deep inhalation, lift the hands from the floor and come back to Tāḍāsana. (Plate 1)

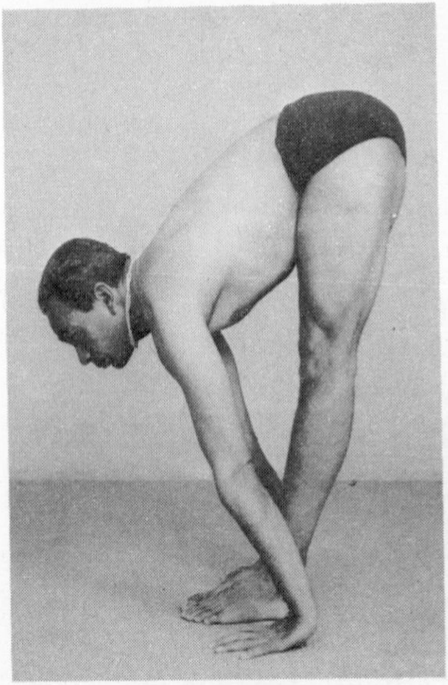

47

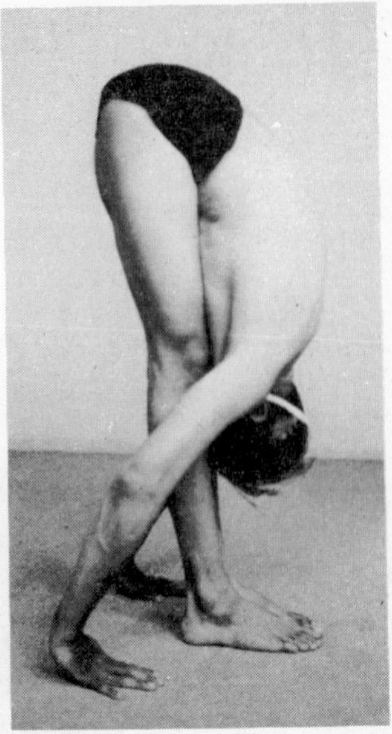

48

Effects

This āsana cures stomach pains and tones the liver, the spleen and the kidneys. It also relieves stomach pain during menstrual periods. The heart beats are slowed down and the spinal nerves rejuvenated. Any depression felt in the mind is removed if one holds the pose for two minutes or more. The posture is a boon to people who get excited quickly, as it soothes the brain cells. After finishing the āsana, one feels calm and cool, the eyes start to glow and the mind feels at peace.

Persons who feel heaviness in the head, flushing or any discomfort while attempting Śīrṣāsana (Plate 184), should do Uttānāsana first; then they will be able to do Śīrṣāsana (the head stand) with comfort and ease.

21. *Ūrdhva Prasārita Ekapādasana* Six* (Plate 49)

Ūrdhva means upright, above, high. Prasārita means extended, stretched out. Eka means one, pāda means the foot. This posture is done by standing on one leg, bending forward and lifting the other leg high up.

Technique

1. Stand in Tāḍāsana. (Plate 1)

2. Exhale and bend the trunk forward. With the left hand catch the back of the right ankle. Rest the right hand on the floor by the side of the right foot and the head or the chin on the right knee.

3. Lift the left leg as high up in the air as possible. Tighten both knees. Keep the toes of the lifted leg pointed upwards. The legs should remain straight so that the toes point straight ahead and do not tilt sideways. (Plate 49)

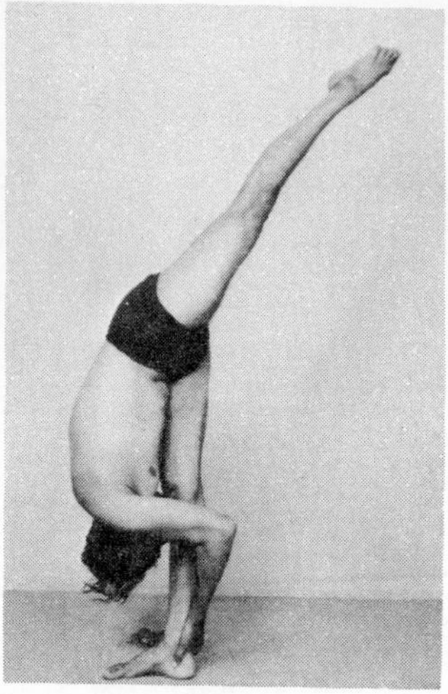

49

4. Stay in the pose for about 20 seconds, with even breathing. Inhale, bring the left leg down to the ground and come back to Tāḍāsana. (Plate 1)

5. Repeat the pose on the other side, keeping the left leg on the ground and the right leg up in the air. Stay in the pose for the same length of time on both sides.

Effects

This āsana tones the leg muscles and reduces fat around the hips.

22. *Ardha Baddha Padmōttānāsana* Nine* (Plate 52)

Ardha means half. Baddha means bound, restrained, caught, withheld. Padma is a lotus. Uttāna is an intense stretch.

Technique

1. Stand in Tāḍāsana. (Plate 1)

2. Inhale, raise the right leg from the floor, bend the right knee and rest the sole of the right foot on the left thigh.

3. Hold the right foot with the left hand, bring the right arm round the back and catch hold of the big toe of the right foot with the thumb and the fore and middle fingers of the right hand. (Plate 50)

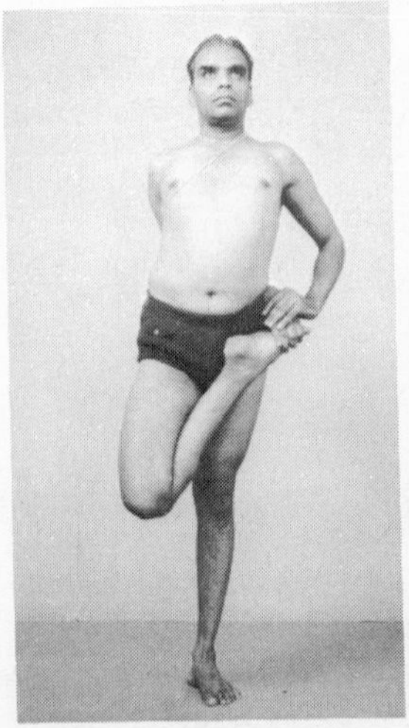

50

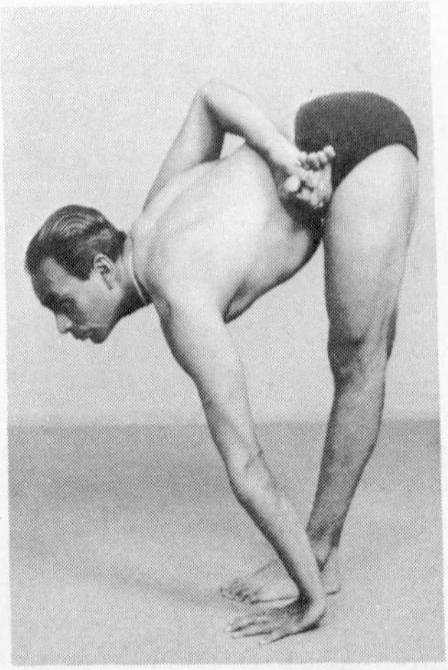

51

4. Release the left hand. Exhale, bend the trunk forward, place the left hand on the floor by the left foot (Plate 51), and keep the head up. Make the back as concave as possible. Take a few breaths.

5. Exhale, rest the head or the chin on the left knee. (Plate 52)

6. If the whole left palm cannot be placed on the floor, start with the tips of the fingers, then gradually place the fingers and lastly the whole palm on the floor. Similarly with the position of the head, first place the forehead on the left knee, then extend the neck to place the tip of the nose, then the lips and lastly the chin on the left knee. The progress from the head to the chin shows that the body is becoming more and more elastic.

7. After taking a few deep breaths in this pose, inhale and raise the trunk to position 4. (Plate 51.) Take two breaths.

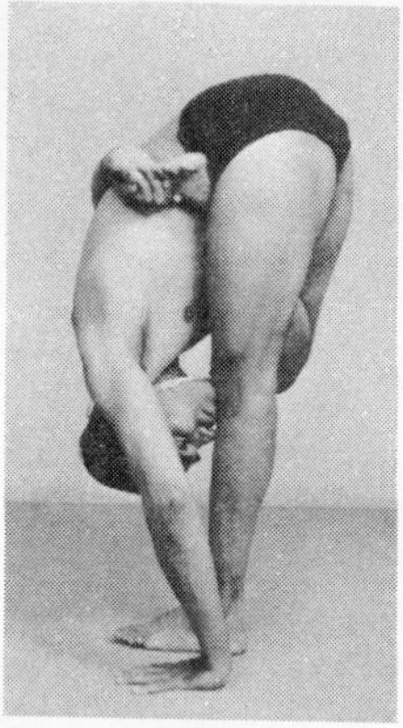

52

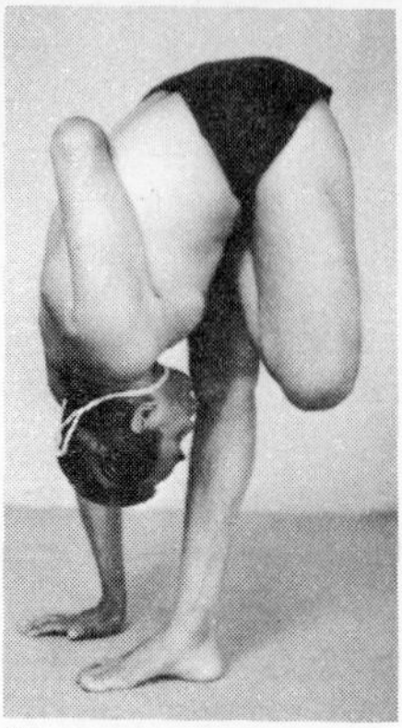

53

8. Inhale, lift the left palm from the floor and come to position 3. (Plate 50)

9. Release the left foot from the grip of the right hand and return to Tāḍāsana. (Plate 1)

10. Repeat on the other side, keeping the right leg on the floor, bending the left leg, placing the left foot on the right thigh, catching the left toe with the left hand from behind, bending forward and placing the right palm on the floor. (Plate 53)

11. If you cannot hold the toe with the hand from behind, place both the palms on the floor and follow the above technique. (Plates 54 and 55)

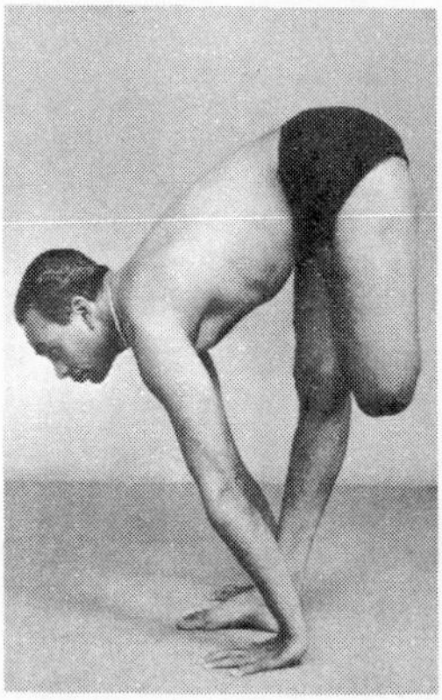

54

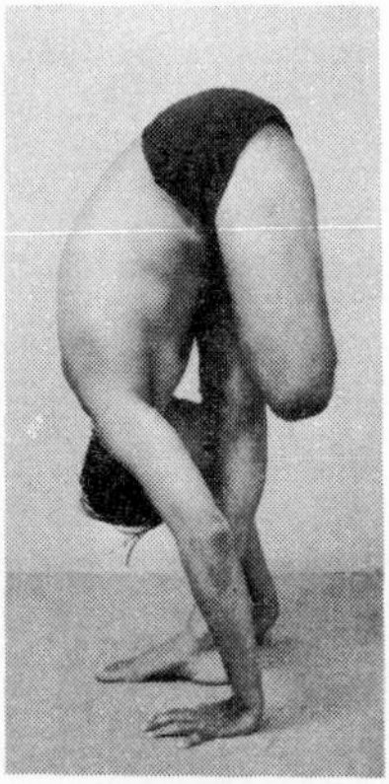

55

Effects

Stiffness of the knees is cured by this āsana. As the abdominal organs are contracted, digestive powers increase and the peristaltic activity helps to eliminate toxin creating waste matter. The pose helps one to move the shoulders further back. This expands the chest and helps in breathing freely and deeply.

23. *Garuḍāsana* One* (Plate 56)

Garuḍa means an eagle. It is also the name of the king of birds. Garuḍa is represented as the vehicle of Viṣṇu and as having a white face, an acquiline beak, red wings and a golden body.

Technique

1. Stand in Tāḍāsana. (Plate 1.) Bend the right knee.

2. Bring the left leg over the right thigh above the right knee and rest the back of the left thigh on the front of the right thigh.

3. Then move the left foot behind the right calf so that the left shin touches the right calf and the left big toe hooks just above the inner side of the right ankle. The left leg is now entwined around the right leg.

4. You are balancing on the right leg only; this will take some time to learn.

5. Bend the elbow and raise the arms to the level of the chest. Rest the right elbow on the front of the left upper arm near the elbow joint. Then move the right hand back to the right and the left hand back to the left and join the palms. The left arm will now be entwined around the right arm. (Plate 56)

6. Remain in this position for a few seconds, say about 15 to 20 with deep breathing. Then release the arms and legs and come back to Tāḍāsana. (Plate 1)

7. Repeat the pose, standing on the left leg and entwining the right leg around the left leg and the right arm around the left arm. Stay for an equal length of time on both the sides.

Effects

This āsana develops the ankles and removes stiffness in the shoulders. It is recommended for preventing cramps in the calf muscles. For removing cramps in the legs and for relieving pain the poses recommended are Garuḍāsana, Vīrāsana (Plate 89) and Bhekāsana, also called Maṇḍukāsana (Plate 100), described later.

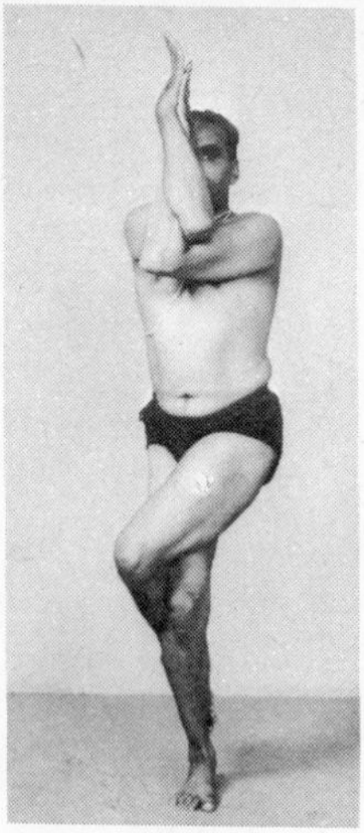

56

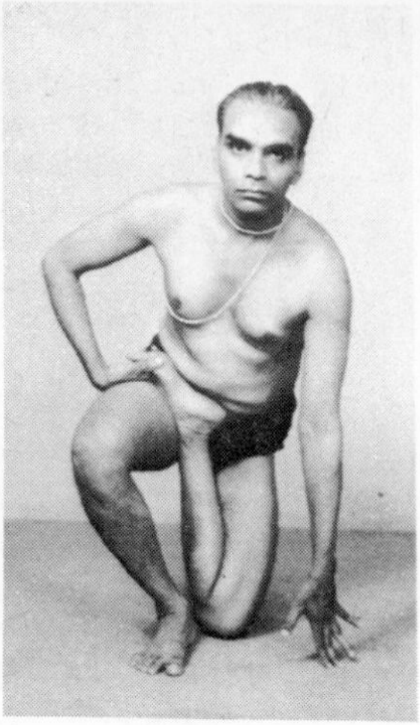

57

24. *Vātāyanāsana* Eleven* (Plate 58)

Vātāyana means a horse. The pose resembles a horse's face hence the name.

Technique

1. Sit on the floor, and place the left foot at the root of the right thigh in half Padmāsana.

2. Place the hands on the floor by the side of the hips. Exhale, raise the trunk off the floor and place the top of the left knee on the floor. Place the right foot near the bent left knee and keep the right thigh parallel to the floor. (Plate 57)

3. Stretch the pelvis forward, keep the left thigh perpendicular to the floor, raise the hands, straighten the back and balance the body. Do not stoop forward while maintaining the balance, but keep the back erect.

4. Bend the elbows and raise the arms to the level of the chest. Place the back of the upper right arm near the elbow on the front of the upper left arm above the elbow joint. Entwine the forearms round one another and join the palms. Hold this position for about 30 seconds with normal breathing. (Front view: Plate 58. Side view: Plate 59)

5. Release the arms, sit on the floor and straighten the legs.

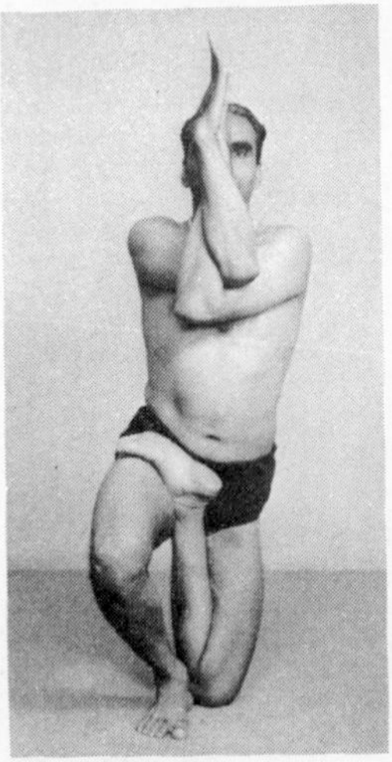

58

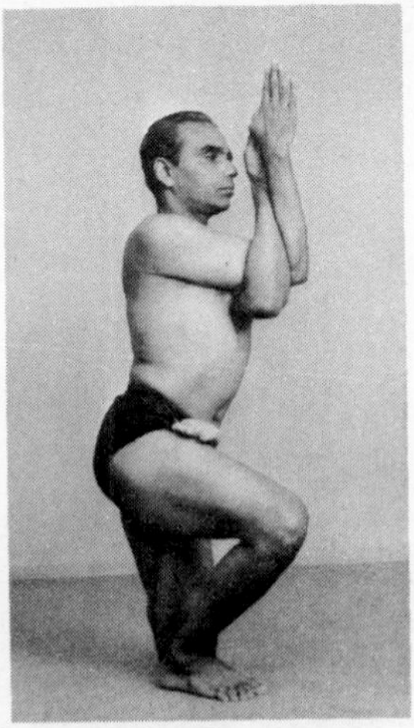

59

6. Repeat the pose on the other side. Here, place the right foot at the root of the left thigh, place the left foot near the bent right knee on the floor and entwine the arms in front of the chest so that the left arm is over the right near the elbow joint, and balance, keeping the left thigh parallel to the floor. Maintain the pose for an equal length of time on both sides. Then release the pose and relax on the floor.

7. In the beginning, it will be difficult to balance and the knees will be painful. With practice the pain disappears and the balance is achieved.

Effects

In this pose the hip joints receive proper circulation of the blood and minor deformity in the hips and thighs is corrected. The pose is also good for stiffness in the sacroiliac region.

25. *Śalabhāsana* One* (Plate 60)

Śalabhā means a locust. The pose resembles that of a locust resting on the ground, hence the name.

Technique

1. Lie full length on the floor on the stomach, face downwards. Stretch the arms back.

2. Exhale, lift the head, chest and legs off the floor simultaneously as high as possible. The hands should not be placed and the ribs should

not rest on the floor. Only the abdominal front portion of the body rests on the floor and bears the weight of the body. (Plate 60)

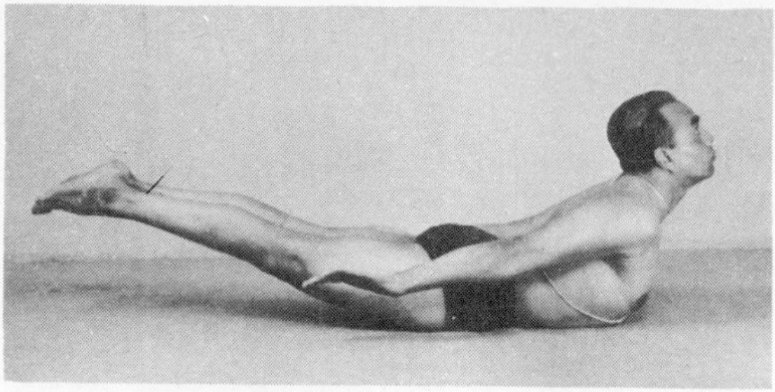

60

3. Contract the buttocks and stretch the thigh muscles. Keep both legs fully extended and straight, touching at the thighs, knees and ankles.

4. Do not bear the weight of the body on the hands but stretch them back to exercise the upper portion of the back muscles.

5. Stay in the position as long as you can with normal breathing.

6. In the beginning it is difficult to lift the chest and the legs off the floor, but this becomes easier as the abdominal muscles grow stronger.

Effects

The pose aids digestion and relieves gastric troubles and flatulence. Since the spine is stretched back it becomes elastic and the pose relieves pain in the sacral and lumbar regions. In my experience, persons suffering from slipped discs have benefited by regular practice of this āsana without recourse to enforced rest or surgical treatment. The bladder and the prostate gland also benefit from the exercise and remain healthy.

A variation of the pose may also be tried to relieve aches in the lower part of the back. Here, the legs are bent at the knees and the thighs are kept apart while the shins are kept perpendicular to the floor. Then with an exhalation, the thighs are lifted off the floor and brought closer together until the knees touch, the shins still being kept perpendicular. (Plate 61)

Verse 40 of the second chapter of the Gheraṇḍa Saṁhitā describes 26. *Makarāsana* (Plate 62) thus:
'Lie on the ground face down, the chest touching the earth and both legs stretched out: catch the head with the arms. This is the Crocodile Posture which increases bodily heat.' It is a variation of Śalabhāsana.

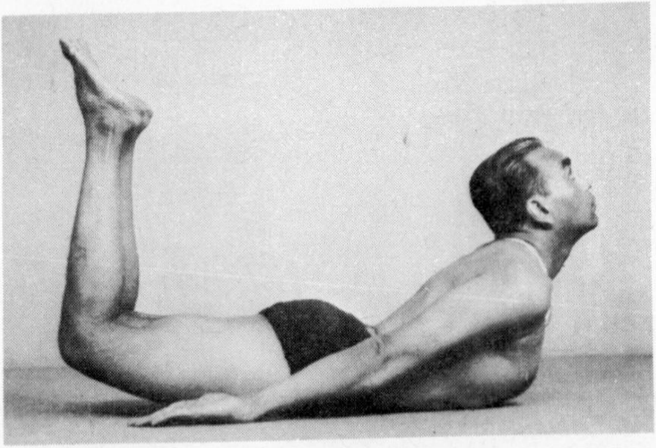

61

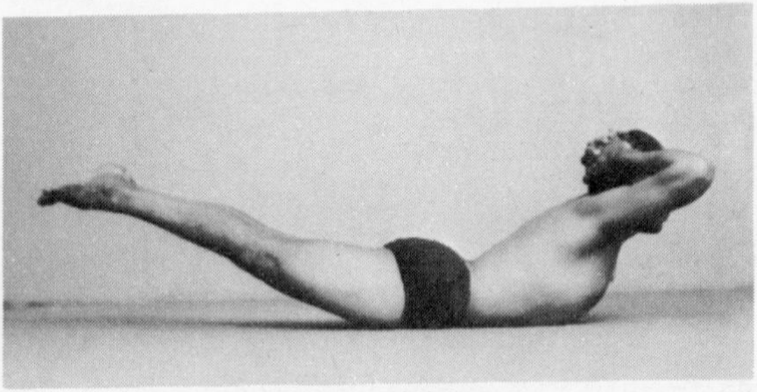

62

27. *Dhanurāsana* Four* (Plate 63)

Dhanu means a bow. The hands here are used like a bow-string to pull the head, trunk and legs up and the posture resembles a bent bow.

Technique

1. Lie full length on the floor on the stomach, face downwards.

2. Exhale and bend the knees. Stretch the arms back and hold the left ankle with the left hand and the right ankle with the right hand. Take two breaths.

3. Now exhale completely and pull the legs up by raising the knees above the floor, and simultaneously lift the chest off the floor. The arms and hands act like a bow-string to tauten the body like a bent bow. (Plate 63)

4. Lift up the head and pull it as far back as possible. Do not rest either

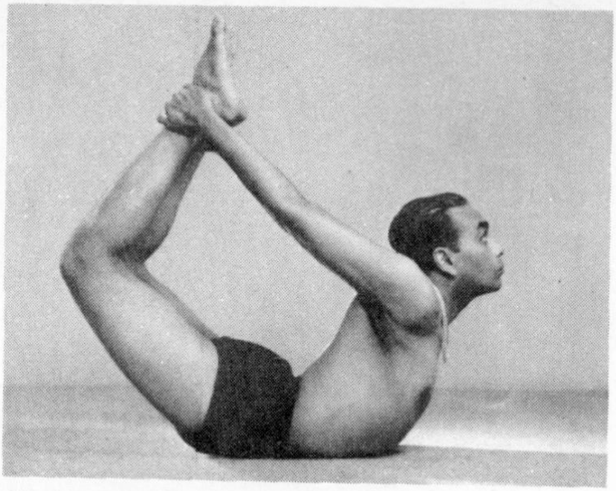

63

the ribs or the pelvic bones on the floor. Only the abdomen bears the weight of the body on the floor.

5. While raising the legs do not join them at the knees, for then the legs will not be lifted high enough. After the full stretch upwards has been achieved, join together the thighs, the knees and the ankles.

6. Since the abdomen is extended, the breathing will be fast, but do not worry about it. Stay in the pose to your capacity from 20 seconds to one minute.

7. Then, with an exhalation, release the ankles, stretch the legs straight, bring the head and the legs back to the floor and relax.

Effects

In this posture the spine is stretched back. Elderly people do not normally do this, so their spines get rigid. This āsana brings back elasticity to the spine and tones the abdominal organs. In my experience, persons suffering from slipped discs have obtained relief by the regular practice of Dhanurāsana and Śalabhāsana (Plate 60) without being forced to rest or to undergo surgical treatment.

28. *Pārśva Dhanurāsana* Four* (Plates 64 and 65)

Pārśva means sideways. In this variation of Dhanurāsana, one performs the posture lying on one's side.

Technique

1. Perform Dhanurāsana. (Plate 63)

2. Exhale, roll over to the right side and stretch the legs and chest. (Plate 64)

3. Inhale and come to position 1. Then exhale, and roll over to the left side. (Plate 65)

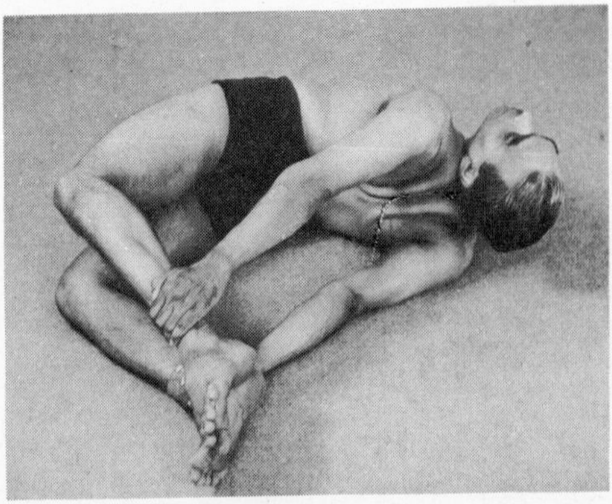

64

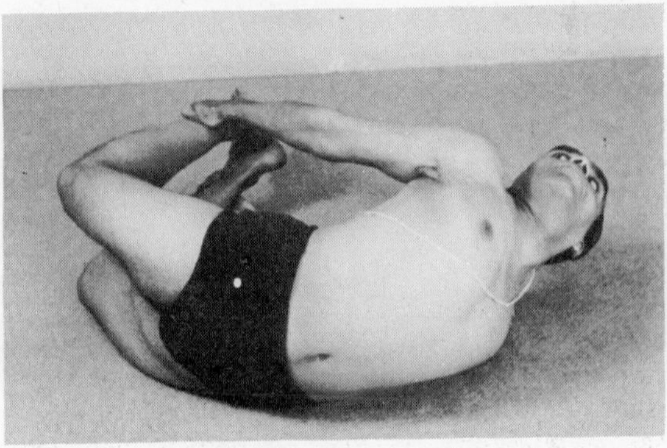

65

4. Stay on either side for the same length of time according to your capacity with normal breathing. Inhale, come back to Dhanurāsana, release the legs and relax.

5. In this pose, which is a more strenuous version of the earlier one, the ankles are inclined to slip from the hand grip. Therefore, grip the ankles more firmly.

Effects

The sideways roll in this posture massages the abdominal organs by pressing them against the floor.

29. *Chaturaṅga Daṇḍāsana* One* (Plate 67)

Chatur means four. Aṅga means a limb or a part thereof. Daṇḍa means a staff. Lie flat on the floor, face down and take the weight of the body on the palms and toes, exhale and keep the body parallel to the floor, stiff as a staff. The four limbs supporting the body are the hands and feet. The pose is similar to dips in western gymnastics.

Technique

1. Lie flat on the floor, face downwards.

2. Bend the elbows and place the palms by the side of the chest. Keep the feet about a foot apart.

3. With an exhalation, raise the whole body a few inches above the floor, balancing it on the hands and the toes. (Plate 66.) Keep the body stiff as a staff, parallel to the floor from head to heel and the knees taut. Stay for some time with normal breathing.

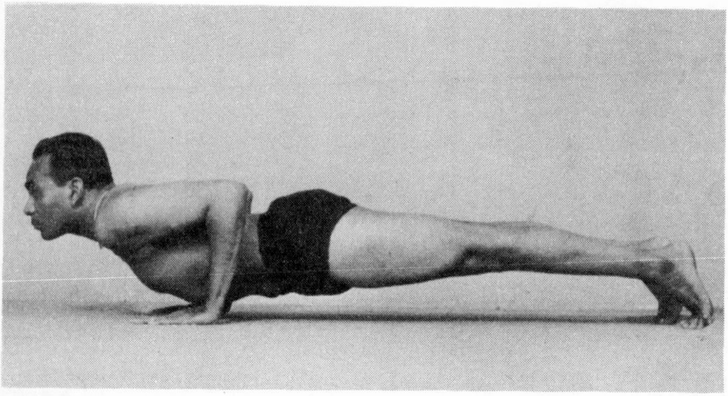

66

4. Then gradually extend the whole body forward so that the feet rest on the upper portion of the toes on the floor. (Plate 67)

5. Stay in the pose for about 30 seconds with normal or deep breathing. The movement may be repeated several times. Then relax on the floor.

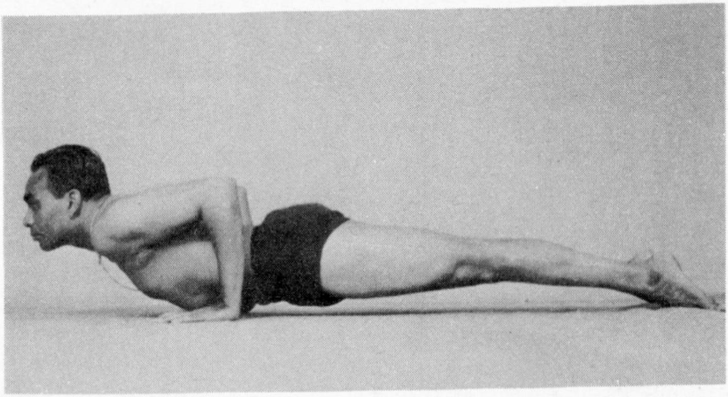

67

Effects

The pose strengthens the arms and the wrists develop mobility and power. It also contracts and tones the abdominal organs.

30. *Nakrāsana* Six* (Plates 68 to 71)

Nakra means a crocodile. This posture consists of several dynamic movements resembling those of a crocodile stalking its prey, hence the name.

Technique

1. Lie flat on the floor, face downwards.

2. Bend the elbows and place the palms by the side of the waist.

3. Keep the feet about one foot apart. Exhale, raise the whole body a few inches above the floor, balancing it on the palms and the toes. Keep the body stiff as a poker and the knees taut. The body should remain parallel to the floor. (Plate 68)

4. Take a few breaths and with an exhalation lunge the whole body a foot forward, lifting the hands and feet simultaneously off the floor. (Plates 69, 70 and 71.) After going a foot forward, take a few breaths. Then exhale and lunge forward again.

5. Repeat the forward lunges four or five times. At the end of each lunge, the position of the body should be as described in position 3 above. These movements resemble the lunges made by a crocodile stalking its prey. After each lunge, rest a few seconds taking deep breaths.

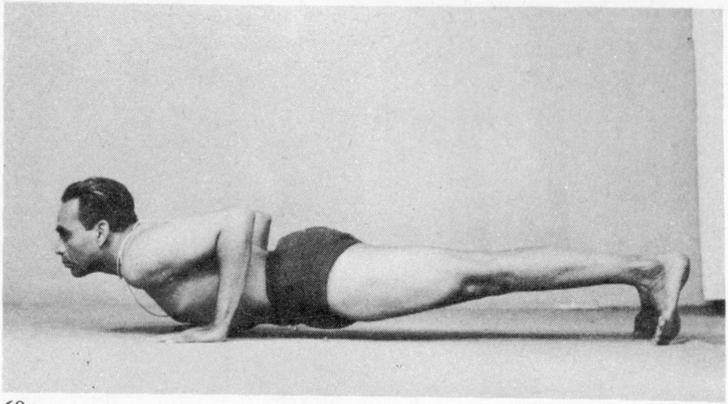

68

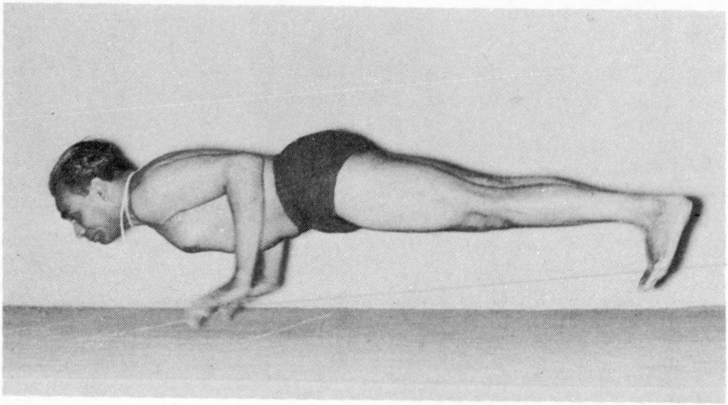

69

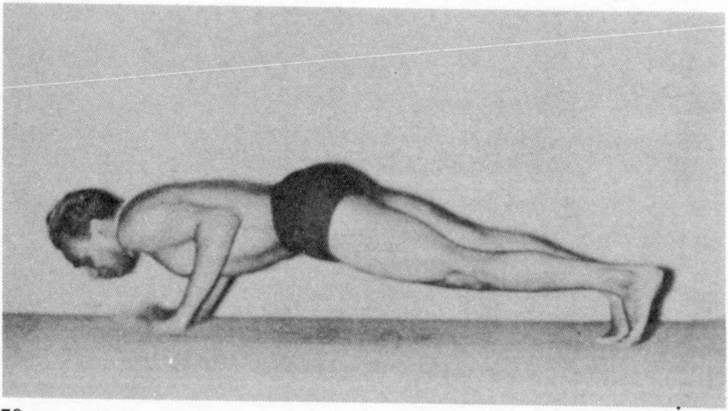

70

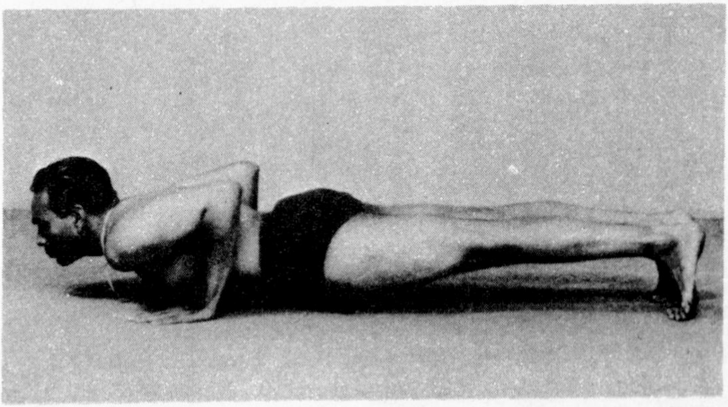

71

6. Now reverse the movements and with exhalations jump back about a foot at a time until you return to the position from where you started.

7. Rest the trunk on the floor and relax.

Effects

This āsana develops powerful wrists, throws off lethargy of the body and fatigue of the brain, rejuvenates the entire body and makes one feel lively and vigorous. Since the movements bring great pressure on the wrists, it is recommended that they be tried gradually, otherwise one is apt to sprain the wrists.

31. *Bhujaṅgāsana I* One* (Plate 73)

Bhujaṅga means a serpent. In this posture, lie flat on the floor, face downwards, lift the body up from the trunk and throw the head back like a serpent about to strike.

Technique

1. Lie on the floor face downwards. Extend the legs, keeping the feet together. Keep the knees tight and the toes pointing.

2. Rest the palms by the side of the pelvic region.

3. Inhale, press the palms firmly on the floor and pull the trunk up. (Plate 72.) Take two breaths.

4. Inhale, lift the body up from the trunk until the pubis is in contact with the floor and stay in this position with the weight on the legs and palms. (Plate 73)

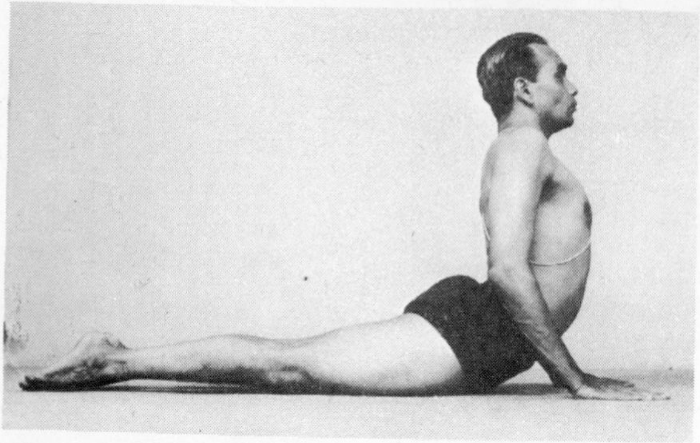

72

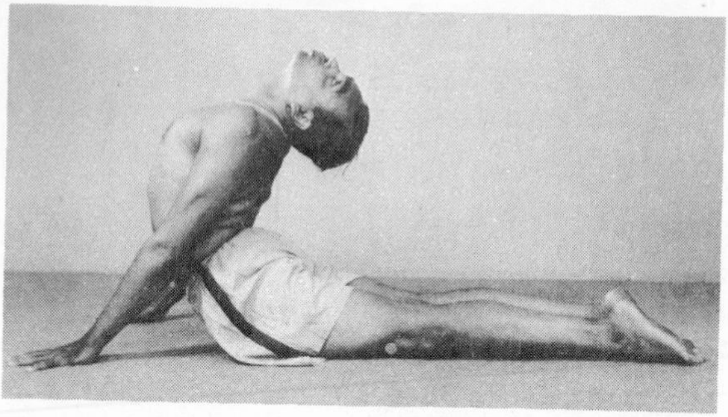

73

5. Contract the anus and the buttocks, tighten the thighs.

6. Maintain the pose for about 20 seconds, breathing normally.

7. Exhale, bend the elbows and rest the trunk on the floor. Repeat the pose two or three times and then relax.

Effects

The posture is a panacea for an injured spine and in cases of slight displacement of spinal discs the practice of this pose replaces the discs in their original position. The spinal region is toned and the chest fully expanded.

32. *Ūrdhva Mukha Śvānāsana* One* (Plate 74)

Ūrdhva Mukha means having the mouth upwards. Śvāna means a dog. The pose resembles a dog stretching itself with the head up in the air, hence the name.

Technique

1. Lie on the floor on the stomach, face downwards.

2. Keep the feet about one foot apart. The toes should point straight back. Place the palms on the floor by the side of the waist, the fingers pointing to the head.

3. Inhale, raise the head and trunk, stretch the arms completely and push the head and trunk as far back as possible, without resting the knees on the floor.

4. Keep the legs straight and tightened at the knees, but do not rest the knees on the floor. The weight of the body rests on the palms and toes only. (Plate 74)

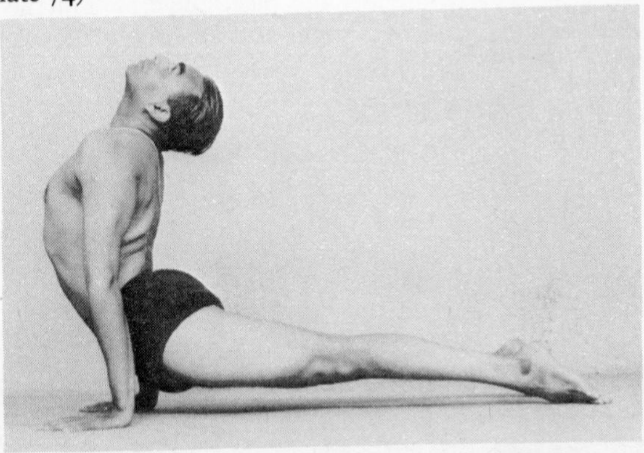

74

5. The spine, thighs and calves should be fully stretched, and the buttocks contracted tight. Push the chest forward, stretch the neck fully and throw the head as far back as possible. Stretch also the back portions of the arms.

6. Stay in the pose from half a minute to a minute with deep breathing.

7. Bend the elbows, release the stretch and rest on the floor.

Effects

The pose rejuvenates the spine and is specially recommended for people suffering from a stiff back. The movement is good for persons with lumbago, sciatica and those suffering from slipped or prolapsed discs of the spine. The pose strengthens the spine and cures backaches. Due to chest expansion, the lungs gain elasticity. The blood circulates properly in the pelvic region and keeps it healthy.

33. *Adho Mukha Śvānāsana* Five* (Plate 75)

Adho Mukha means having the face downwards. Śvāna means a dog. The pose resembles a dog stretching itself with head and forelegs down and the hind legs up, hence the name.

Technique

1. Lie full length on the floor on the stomach, face downwards. The feet should be kept one foot apart.

2. Rest the palms by the side of the chest, the fingers straight and pointing in the direction of the head.

3. Exhale and raise the trunk from the floor. Straighten the arms, move the head inwards towards the feet and place the crown of the head on the floor, keeping the elbows straight and extending the back. (Side view: Plate 75. Back view: Plate 76)

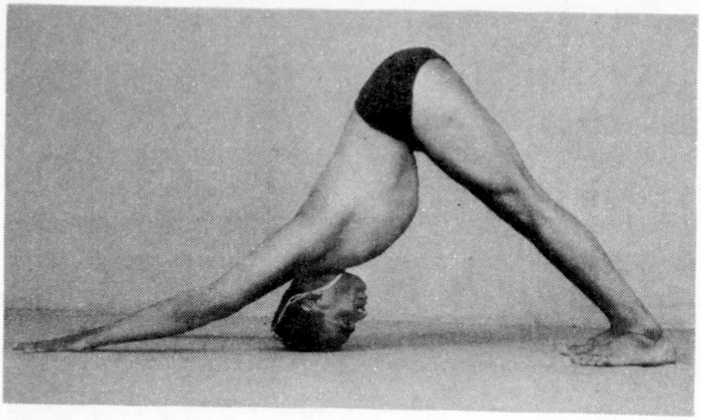

75

4. Keep the legs stiff and do not bend the knees but press the heels down. The heels and soles of the feet should rest completely on the floor, while the feet should be parallel to each other, the toes pointing straight ahead.

5. Stay in the pose for about a minute with deep breathing. Then with an exhalation lift the head off the floor, stretch the trunk forward and lower the body gently to the floor and relax.

Effects

When one is exhausted, a longer stay in this pose removes fatigue and brings back the lost energy. The pose is especially good for runners who get tired after a hard race. Sprinters will develop speed and lightness in the legs. The pose relieves pain and stiffness in the heels and helps to

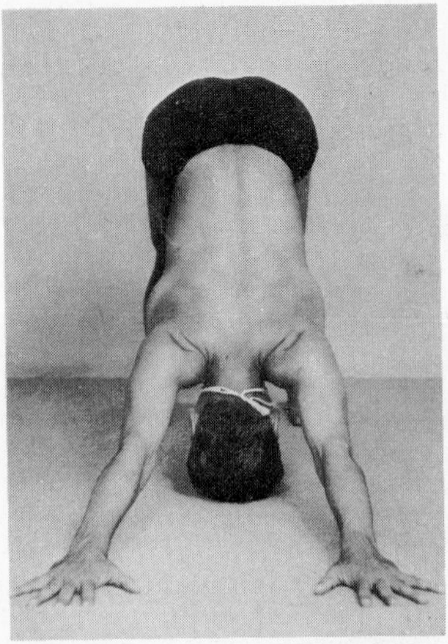

76

soften calcaneal spurs. It strengthens the ankles and makes the legs shapely. The practice of this āsana helps to eradicate stiffness in the region of the shoulder-blades, and arthritis of the shoulder joints is relieved. The abdominal muscles are drawn towards the spine and strengthened. As the diaphragm is lifted to the chest cavity the rate of the heart beat is slowed down. This is an exhilarating pose.

Those who are afraid to do Śīrṣāsana (Plate 184) can conveniently practise this position. As the trunk is lowered in this āsana it is fully stretched and healthy blood is brought to this region without any strain on the heart. It rejuvenates the brain cells and invigorates the brain by relieving fatigue.

Persons suffering from high blood pressure can do this pose.

34. *Paripūrṇa Nāvāsana* Two* (Plate 78)

Paripūrṇa means entire or complete. The posture here resembles that of a boat with oars, hence the name.

Technique

1. Sit on the floor with the legs stretched straight in front. Place the palms on the floor by the hips, the fingers pointing to the feet. Stretch the hands straight and keep the back erect. This position is called:

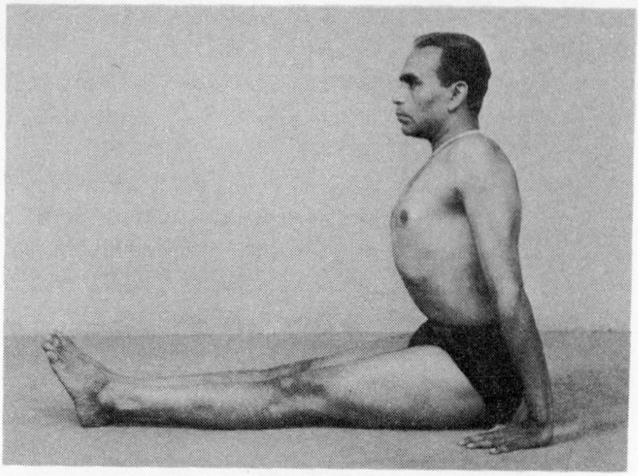

77

35. *Daṇḍāsana* Two★ (Plate 77) (Daṇḍa = a staff or rod)

2. Exhale, recline the trunk slightly back and simultaneously raise the legs from the floor and keep them stiff as a poker with the knees tight and the toes pointing forwards. Balance is maintained only on the buttocks and no part of the spine should be allowed to touch the floor, from which the legs should be kept at an angle of 60 to 65 degrees. The feet are higher than the head and not level with it as in Ardha Nāvāsana. (Plate 79)

3. Remove the hands from the floor and stretch the arms forward, keeping them parallel to the floor and near the thighs. The shoulders and the palms should be on one level, and the palms should face each other. (Plate 78)

4. Stay in the pose for half a minute, with normal breathing. Gradually increase the time to one minute. One feels the effect of the exercise after only 20 seconds.

5. Then exhale, lower the hands, rest the legs on the floor and relax by lying on the back.

Effects

This āsana gives relief to persons who feel a bloating sensation in the abdomen due to gas and also to those suffering from gastric complaints. It reduces fat around the waistline and tones the kidneys.

36. *Ardha Nāvāsana* Two★ (Plate 79)

Ardha means half. Nāva is a ship, boat or vessel. This posture resembles the shape of a boat, hence the name.

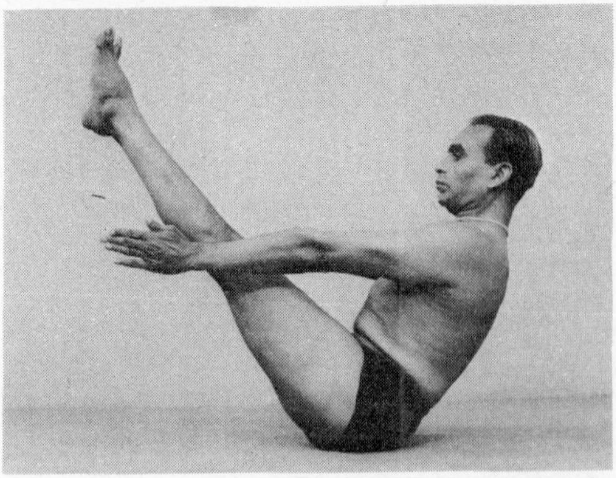

78

Technique

1. Sit on the floor. Stretch the legs out in front and keep them straight. (Plate 77)

2. Interlock the fingers and place them on the back of the head just above the neck.

3. Exhale, recline the trunk back and simultaneously raise the legs from the floor, keeping the knees tight and the toes pointed. The balance of the body rests on the buttocks and no part of the spine should be allowed to touch the floor. (Plate 79.) One feels the grip on the muscles of the abdomen and the lower back.

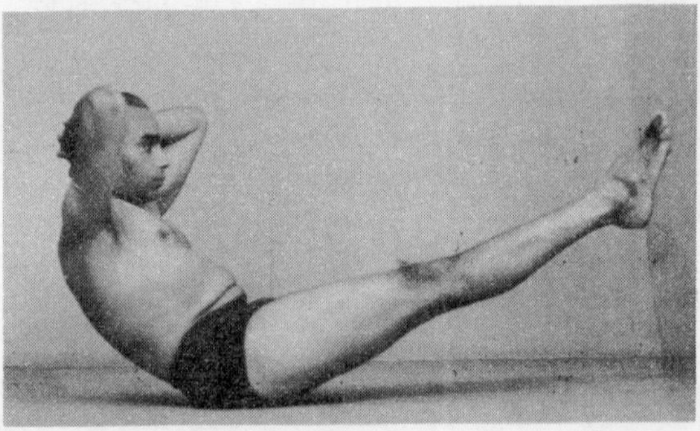

79

4. Keep the legs at an angle of about 30 to 35 degrees from the floor and the crown of the head in line with the toes.

5. Hold this pose for 20 to 30 seconds with normal breathing. A stay for one minute in this posture indicates strong abdominal muscles.

6. Do not hold the breath during this āsana, though the tendency is always to do it with suspension of breath after inhalation. If the breath is held, the effect will be felt on the stomach muscles and not on the abdominal organs. Deep inhalation in this āsana would loosen the grip on the abdominal muscles. In order to maintain this grip, inhale, exhale and hold the breath and go on repeating this process but without breathing deeply. This will exercise not only the abdominal muscles but the organs also.

7. The difference between Ardha Nāvāsana and Paripūrṇa Nāvāsana should be noted; in the latter, the legs are moved higher and the distance between them and the stomach is less than in the former.

Effects

The effects of Ardha Nāvāsana and that of Paripūrṇa Nāvāsana (Plate 78) differ due to the position of the legs. In Paripūrṇa Nāvāsana the exercise is effective on the intestines; whereas, Ardha Nāvāsana works on the liver, gall bladder and spleen.

In the beginning, the back is too weak to bear the strain of the pose. When power to retain the pose comes, it indicates that the back is gaining strength. A weak back is a handicap in many ways, especially to women as they need strong backs for child-bearing. These two āsanas coupled with lateral twistings of the spine will help to strengthen the back.

The importance of having a healthy lower back can be realised if we watch old people when they sit down, get up and walk, for consciously or unconsciously they support their backs with their hands. This indicates that the back is weak and cannot withstand the strain. As long as it is strong and needs no support, one feels young though advanced in age. The two āsanas bring life and vigour to the back and enable us to grow old gracefully and comfortably.

37. *Gomukhāsana* Two* (Plate 80)

Go means a cow. Mukha means face. Gomukha means one whose face resembles a cow. It also means a kind of a musical instrument, narrow at one end and broad at the other like the face of a cow.

Technique

1. Sit on the floor with the legs stretched straight in front. (Plate 77)

2. Place the palms on the floor and raise the seat.

3. Bend the left knee back and sit on the left foot. Remove the hands

from the floor, raise the right leg and place the right thigh over the left one. Raise the buttocks and with the help of the hands bring the ankles and the back of the heels together till they touch each other.

4. Rest the ankles, keeping the toes pointing back.

5. Raise the left arm over the head, bend it at the elbow and place the left palm below the nape of the neck between the shoulders. Lower the right arm, bend it at the elbow and raise the right forearm up behind the back until the right hand is level with and between the shoulder-blades. Clasp the hands behind the back between the shoulders. (Front view: Plate 80. Back view: Plate 81)

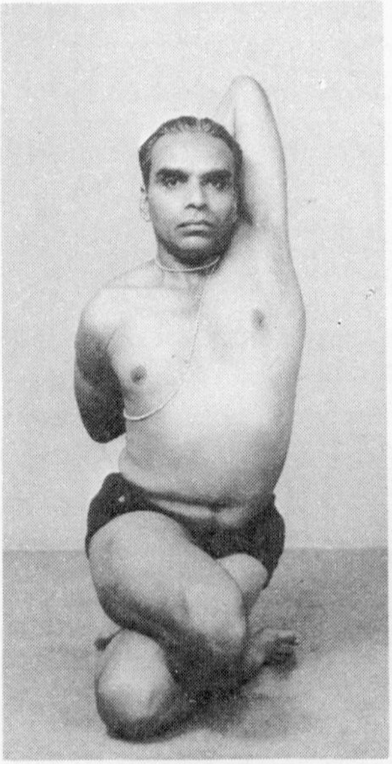

80

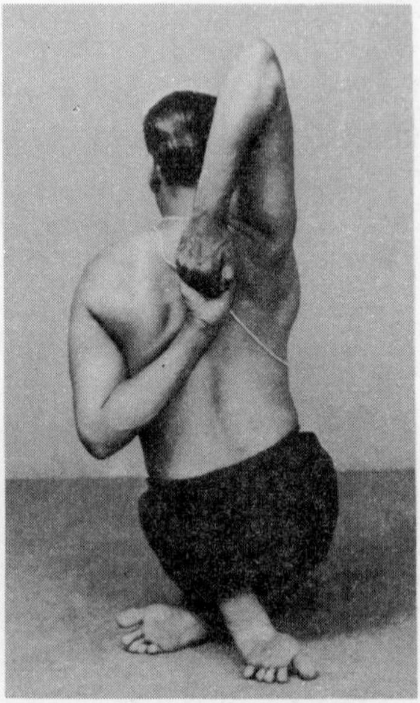

81

6. Hold this position from 30 to 60 seconds breathing normally. Keep the neck and head erect and look straight ahead.

7. Unclasp the hands, straighten the legs and repeat the pose on the other side for the same length of time by inserting 'left' for 'right' and vice versa. Then unclasp the hands at the back, straighten the legs and relax.

Effects

The pose cures cramp in the legs and makes the leg muscles elastic.

The chest is well expanded and the back becomes erect. The shoulder joints move freely and the latissimus dorsi are fully extended.

38. *Lolāsana* Six* (Plate 83)

Lola means tremulous, moving to and fro or dangling like an ear-ring. In this posture the legs and feet are kept as in Gomukhāsana. (Plate 80.) The hands are placed on the floor by the side of the hips and the body is raised up and supported only by the hands and wrists. Then one balances swaying slightly forward and backward, the movement resembling that of a dangling pendant.

Technique

1. Sit on the floor with the legs stretched straight in front. (Plate 77)

2. Place the palms on the floor by the side of the hips.

3. Raise the seat, bend the right knee back, place the right sole beneath the left buttock and sit on it.

4. Bend the left knee back and again raising the seat, place the left sole beneath the right buttock and sit on it.

5. The feet will be crossed so that the right shin is above the left calf. Keep the toes pointing backwards. (Plate 82)

6. Take a few breaths. Exhale, raise the trunk and legs off the floor and balance on the hands, stretching out the arms. (Plate 83.) Gently rock the trunk and legs forwards and backwards. Breathe normally.

7. Rest on the floor and uncross the legs.

8. Recross the legs the other way and again balance on the hands.

9. Balance as long as possible.

Effects

This āsana strengthens the wrists and hands, the muscles of the back and the abdominal organs. It makes the leg muscles elastic and the minor muscles of the arms will be developed and toned.

39. *Siddhāsana* One* (Plate 84)

Siddha means a semi-divine being supposed to be of great purity and holiness, and to possess supernatural faculties called siddhis. Siddha means also an inspired sage, seer or prophet.

'The Siddhas say that as among niyamas, the most important is not to harm anyone, and among the yamas a moderate diet, so is Siddhāsana among the āsanas.'

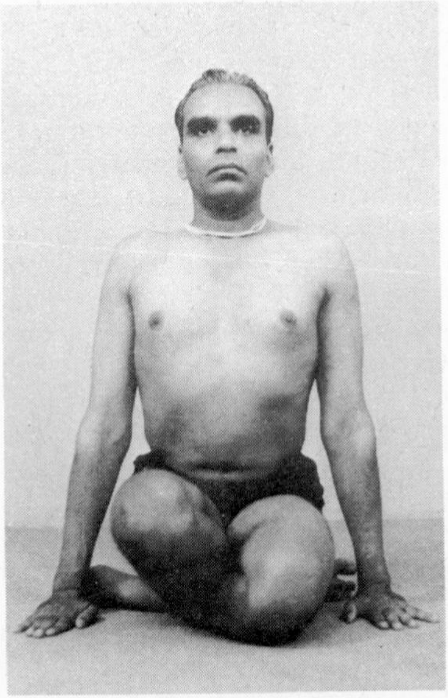
82

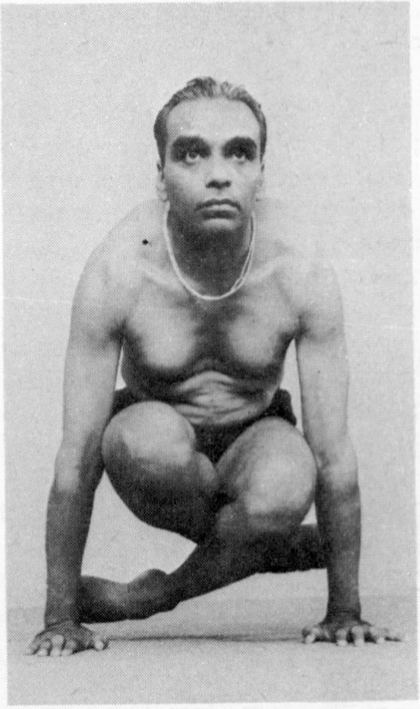
83

'Of the 84 lacs of āsanas, one should always practise Siddhāsana. It purifies 72,000 nāḍīs.' (Nāḍīs are channels in the human body through which nervous energy passes.)

'The yogin practising contemplation upon Ātman and observing a moderate diet, if he practises Siddhāsana for twelve years, obtains the yoga siddhis.' (Ātman means the Self and the supreme Soul. Siddhīs are supernatural faculties.)

'When Siddhāsana is mastered, the Unmanī Avasthā (Samādhi) that gives delight follows without effort and naturally.'

The soul has three avasthās or conditions which are included in a fourth. They are waking, dreaming, sleeping and what is called Turīya. 'The first condition is that of wakefulness, where the self is conscious of the common world of gross objects. It enjoys gross things. Here the dependence of body is predominant. The second condition is that of dreaming, where the self enjoys subtle things, fashioning for itself a new world of forms from the material of its waking experience. The spirit is said to roam freely unfettered by the bonds of the body. The third condition is that of sound sleep, where we have neither dreams nor desires. It is called suṣupti. In it the soul is said to become temporarily one with Brahman and to enjoy bliss. In deep sleep we are lifted above all desires and freed from the vexations of spirit.... The soul is divine in origin, though clogged with the flesh. In sleep it is said to be released from the shackles of the body and to regain its own nature.... But this (that is, the eternal dreamless sleep) is likely to be confused with sheer unconsciousness.... The highest is not this dreamless sleep, but another, a fourth state of the soul, a pure intuitional consciousness where there is no knowledge of objects internal or external. In deep sleep the spirit dwells in a region far above the changeful life of sense in absolute union with Brahman. The turīya condition brings out the positive aspect of the negative emphasised in the condition of deep sleep.' – Radhakrishnan in *Philosophy of the Upanishads*. This fourth condition has been thus described in the Māṇḍūkya Upanishad as follows: 'The fourth, say the wise, is not subjective experience, nor objective experience, nor experience intermediate between the two, nor is it a negative condition which is neither consciousness nor unconsciousness. It is not the knowledge of the senses, nor is it relative knowledge, nor yet inferential knowledge. Beyond the senses, beyond understanding, beyond all expression, is the fourth. It is pure unitary consciousness, wherein all awareness of the world and of multiplicity is completely obliterated. It is the supreme good. It is One without a second. It is the Self. Know it alone!'

'Rāja-Yoga, Samādhi, Unmanī, Manomanī, Immortality, Concentration, Śūnyāśūnya (void and yet non-void), Parama Pāda (the Supreme State), Amanaska (suspended operation of the mind), Advaita (non-duality), Nirālamba (without support), Nirañjana (pure), Jīvanmukti (emancipated state), Sahajāvasthā (natural state) and Turīyā (literally the Fourth), all mean the same thing. As a grain of salt thrown into water unites and becomes one with it, a like union between the Mind and the Ātman is Samādhi. When Prāṇa and Manas (mind) are annihilated (absorbed), the state of harmony then arising is called Samādhi.' – *Haṭha Yoga Pradīpikā*, chapter IV, verses 3 to 6.

There is no āsana like Siddha, no kumbhaka like Kevala, no mudrā like Khecharī, and no laya (absorption of the mind) like Nāda.

(Khecharī Mudrā, literally roaming through space, is described in the *Gheraṇḍa Saṁhitā* as follows in verses 25 to 28 of the third chapter: 'Cut the lower tendon of the tongue and move the tongue constantly; rub it with fresh butter, and draw it out (to lengthen it) with an iron instrument. By practising this always, the tongue becomes long and when it reaches the space between the eyebrows, then Khecharī is accomplished. Then (the tongue being lengthened) practise turning it up and back so as to touch the palate, till at length it reaches the holes of the nostrils opening into the mouth. Close those holes with the tongue (thus stopping inspiration), and gaze on the space between the eyebrows.

This is called Khecharī. By this practice there is neither fainting, nor hunger, nor thirst, nor laziness. There comes neither disease, nor decay, nor death. The body becomes divine.')

(Nāda is the inner mystical sound. Verses 79 to 101 of the fourth chapter describes it in great detail with a variety of similes. Yoga is defined as control over the aberrations of the mind. In order to control the mind it is necessary that it should first be absorbed in concentration of some object, then it is gradually withdrawn from that object and made to look within one's own self. This is where the yogi is asked to concentrate upon the inner mystical sounds. 'The mind is like a serpent, forgetting all its unsteadiness by hearing Nāda, it does not run away anywhere.' Gradually as Nāda becomes latent so does the mind along with it. 'The fire, catching the wood, is extinguished along with it (after burning it up); and so the mind also, working with Nāda, becomes latent along with it.')

Technique

1. Sit on the floor, with legs stretched straight in front. (Plate 77)

2. Bend the left leg at the knee. Hold the left foot with the hands, place the heel near the perineum and rest the sole of the left foot against the right thigh.

3. Now bend the right leg at the knee and place the right foot over the left ankle, keeping the right heel against the pubic bone.

4. Place the sole of the right foot between the thigh and the calf of the left leg.

5. Do not rest the body on the heels.

6. Stretch the arms in front and rest the back of the hands on the knees so that the palms face upwards. Join the thumbs and the forefingers and keep the other fingers extended. (Plate 84)

7. Hold this position as long as you can, keeping the back, neck and head erect and the vision indrawn as if gazing at the tip of the nose.

8. Release the feet and relax for some time. Then repeat the pose for the same length of time, now placing the right heel near the perineum first and then the left foot over the right ankle as described above.

Effects

This posture keeps the pubic region healthy. Like Padmāsana (Plate 104), it is one of the most relaxing of āsanas. The body being in a sitting posture is at rest, while the position of the crossed legs and erect back

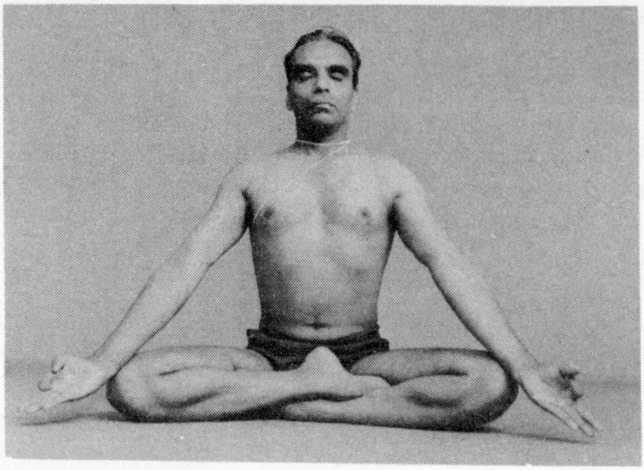

84

keeps the mind attentive and alert. This āsana is also recommended for the practice of prāṇāyāma and for meditation.

From the purely physical point of view, the āsana is good for curing stiffness in the knees and ankles. In it the blood circulates in the lumbar region and the abdomen, and this tones the lower region of the spine and the abdominal organs.

40. *Vīrāsana* One* (Plate 89)

Vīra means a hero, warrior, champion. This sitting posture is done by keeping the knees together, spreading the feet and resting them by the side of the hips.

The pose is good for meditation and prāṇāyāma.

Technique

1. Kneel on the floor. Keep the knees together and spread the feet about 18 inches apart.

2. Rest the buttocks on the floor, but not the body on the feet. The feet are kept by the side of the thighs, the inner side of each calf touching the outer side of its respective thigh. Keep the toes pointing back and touching the floor. Keep the wrists on the knees, palms facing up, and join the tips of the thumbs and forefingers. Keep the other fingers extended. Stretch the back erect. (Back view: Plate 88. Front view: Plate 89)

3. Stay in this position as long as you can, with deep breathing.

4. Then rest the palms on the knees for a while. (Side view: Plate 90)

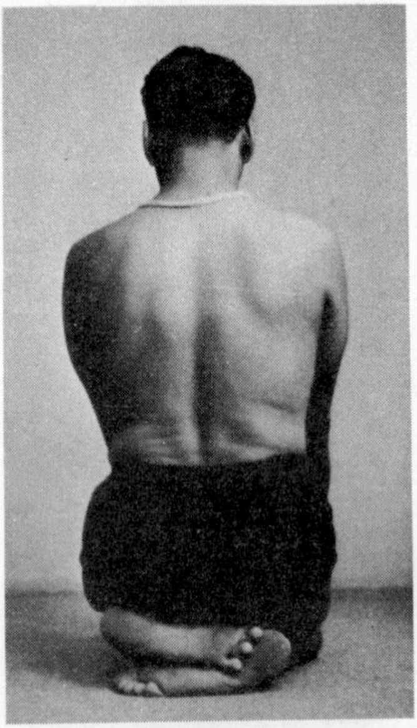

85

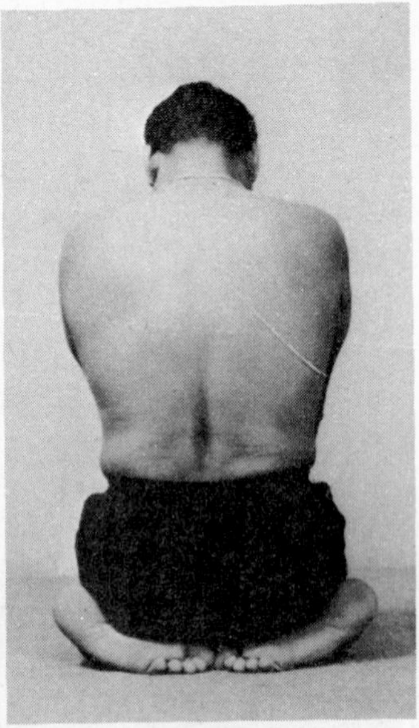

86

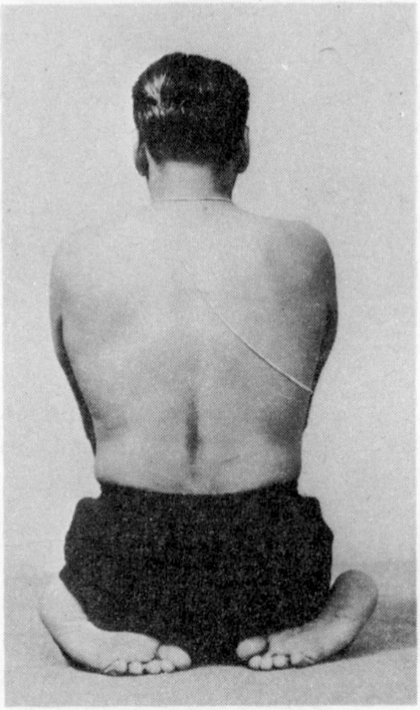

87

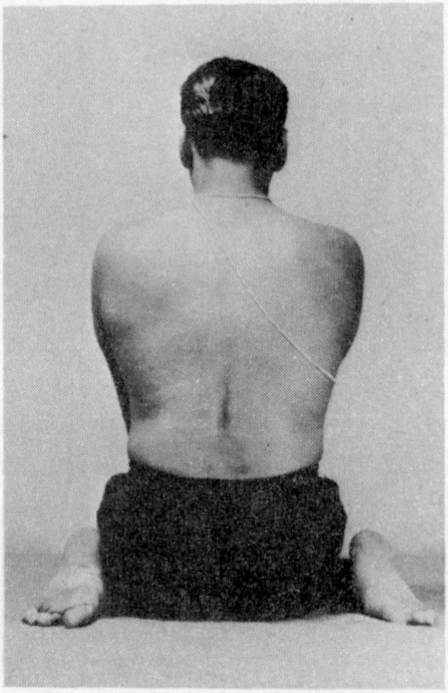

88

5. Now interlock the fingers and stretch the arm straight over the head, palms up. (Plate 91)

6. Stay in this position for a minute with deep breathing.

7. Exhale, release the fingerlock, place the palms on the soles, bend forward and rest the chin on the knees. (Plate 92)

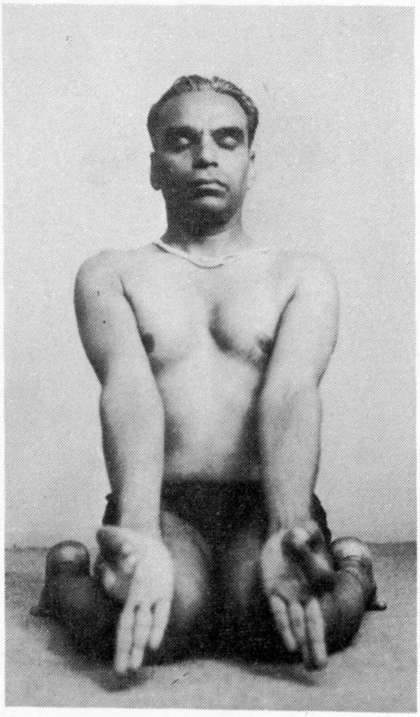

89

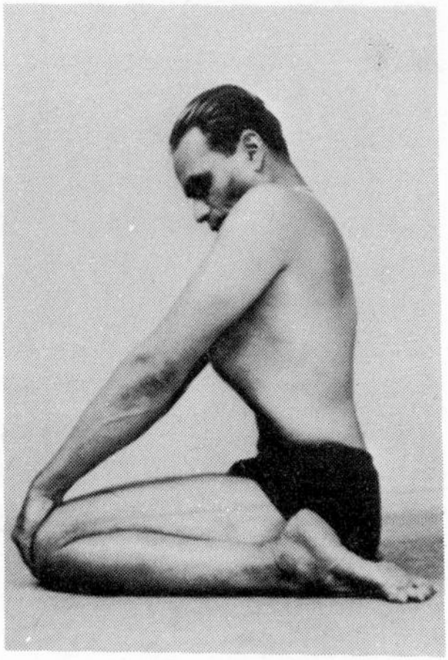

90

8. Stay in this position for a minute with normal breathing.

9. Inhale, raise the trunk up, bring the feet forward and relax.

10. If you find it difficult to perform the pose as described above, try placing the feet one above the other and rest the buttocks on them. (Plate 85.) Gradually move the toes further apart, separate the feet (Plates 86 and 87) and bring them to rest outside the thighs. Then, in time the buttocks will rest properly on the floor and the body will not rest on the feet.

Effects

The pose cures rheumatic pains in the knees and gout, and is also good for flat feet. Due to the stretching of the ankles and the feet, proper arches will be formed. This, however, takes a long time and requires

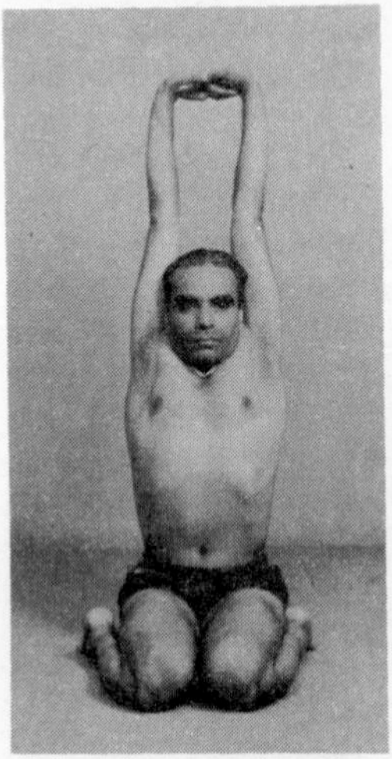

91

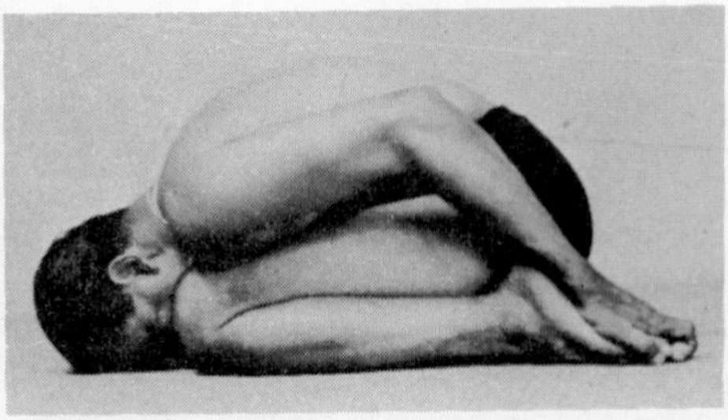

92

daily practice of the pose for a few minutes for several months. Those suffering from pain in the heels or growth of calcaneal spurs there will get relief and the spurs will gradually disappear.

The pose can even be done immediately after food and will relieve heaviness in the stomach.

41. *Supta Vīrāsana* Two* (Plate 96)

Supta means lying down. In this āsana one reclines back on the floor and stretches the arms behind the head.

Technique

1. Sit in Vīrāsana. (Plate 89)

2. Exhale, recline the trunk back and rest the elbows one by one on the floor. (Plate 93)

3. Relieve the pressure on the elbows one after the other by extending the arms.

4. At first rest the crown of the head on the floor. (Plate 94.) Gradually rest the back of the head and then the back on the floor. (Plate 95.) Take the arms over the head and stretch them out straight. (Plate 96.) Hold this pose as long as you can while breathing deeply. Then place the arms beside the trunk, press the elbows to the floor and sit up again with an exhalation.

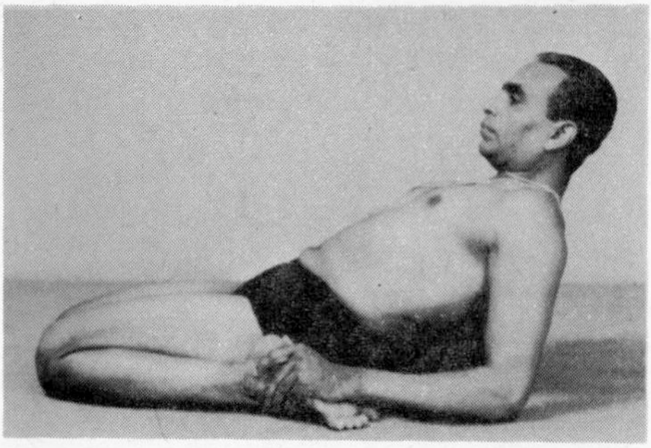
93

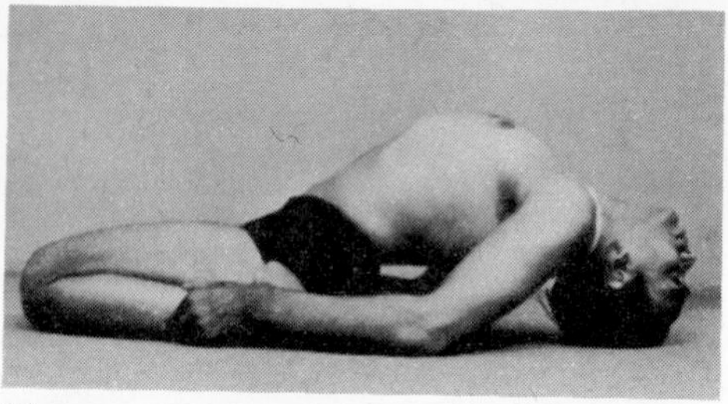
94

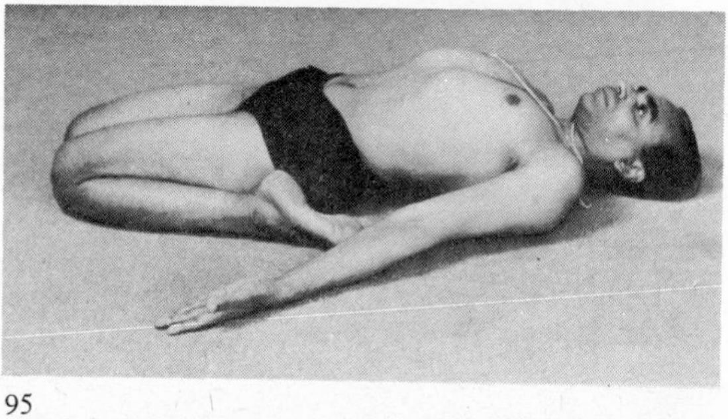
95

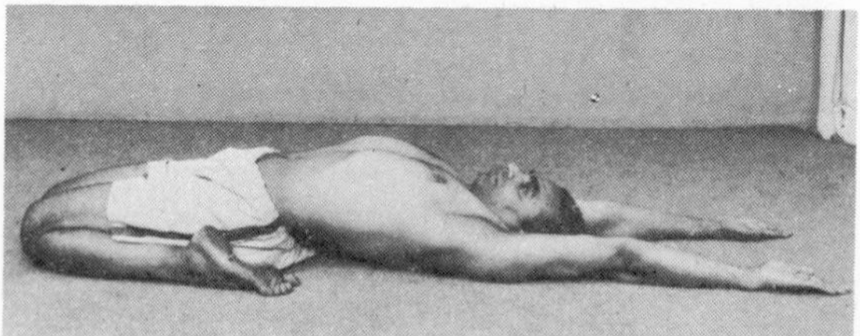
96

5. The hands may be stretched over the head or placed beside the thighs. When they are stretched over the head, do not raise the shoulder-blades from the floor.

6. Beginners may keep the knees apart.

Effects

This āsana stretches the abdominal organs and the pelvic region. People whose legs ache will get relief from holding this pose for 10 to 15 minutes and it is recommended to athletes and all who have to walk or stand about for long hours. It can be done after meals and if before retiring at night the legs feel rested next morning. Several of my pupils who were cadets at the National Defence Academy after long route marches found great relief by combining this āsana with Sarvāngāsana I. (Plate 223)

42. *Paryankāsana* Two* (Plate 97)

Paryanka means a bed, couch or sofa. This āsana is a continuation of Supta Vīrāsana. (Plate 96.) In it the body resembles a couch, hence the name.

Technique

1. Sit in Vīrāsana. (Plate 89)

2. Exhale and recline on the back. (Plate 93.) Lift the neck and the chest and arching the back up rest only the crown of the head on the floor. (Plate 94.) No part of the trunk should be on the floor.

3. Bend the arms at the elbows. Hold with the right hand the left upper arm near the elbow and with the left hand the right upper arm near the elbow. Rest the folded arms on the floor behind the head. (Plate 97)

4. Stay in the pose for a minute with even breathing.

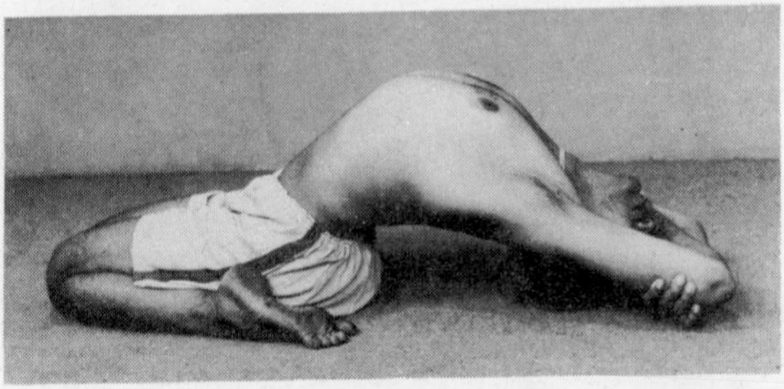

97

5. Inhale, rest the trunk and neck on the floor, release the hands and sit up in Vīrāsana. (Plate 89)

6. Then straighten the legs one by one, lie flat on the back and relax.

Effects

As in Matsyāsana (Plate 113) and Paryankāsana the dorsal region is fully extended so that the lungs are well expanded. The neck muscles are stretched and the thyroids and parathyroids are stimulated so that they function properly. Those who cannot perform Matsyāsana will derive the same benefit from this exercise.

Whereas Vīrāsana (Plate 89) and Supta Vīrāsana (Plate 96) can be done at any time, even immediately after taking food, Paryankāsana cannot be done immediately after a meal.

43. *Bhekāsana* (also called Maṇḍūkāsana) Four* (Plate 100)

Bheka means a frog. The action in this āsana resembles that of a frog, hence the name.

Technique

1. Lie full length on the floor on the stomach, face downwards. Stretch the arms back.

2. Exhale, bend the knees and move the heels towards the hips. Hold the sole of the right foot with the right hand and the sole of the left foot with the left hand. (Plate 98.) Take two breaths. Exhale, lift the head and trunk from the floor and look up.

3. Now turn the hands so that the palms touch the upper part of the feet and the toes and fingers point to the head. (Plate 99.) Push the

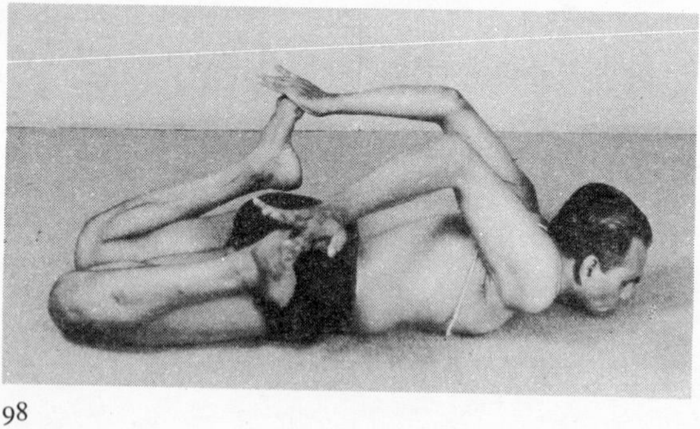

98

hands further down and bring the toes and heels closer to the ground. Keep the arms from the wrists to the elbows perpendicular. (Plate 100.) When the knees and ankles become flexible, the heels can be made to touch the floor.

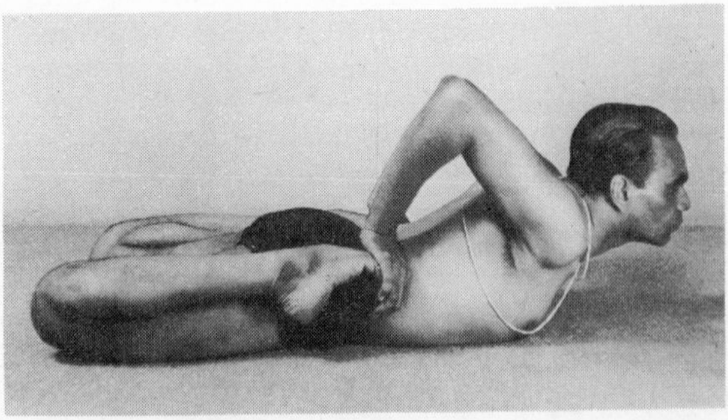

99

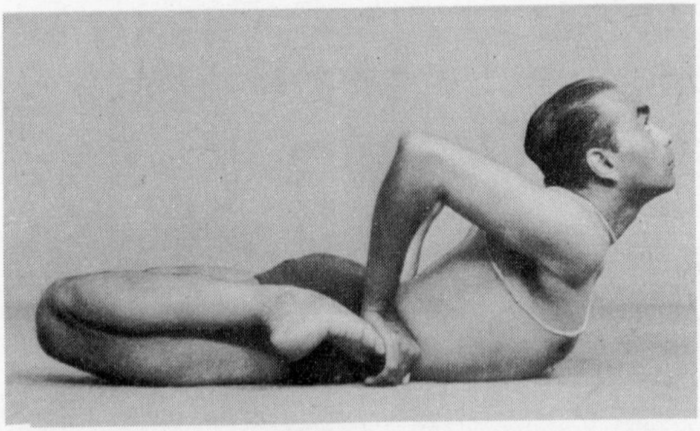

100

4. Remain in the pose from 15 to 30 seconds, but do not hold the breath. Exhale, release the palms from the feet, stretch the legs and relax.

Effects

The abdominal organs benefit from the exercise as they are pressed against the floor. The knees become firmer and the pose relieves pain in the knee joints due to rheumatism and gout. It also gives relief when there is any internal derangement of the knee joints. The pressure of the hands on the feet creates a proper arch and so cures flat feet. It helps sprained ankles and strengthens them. The pose also relieves pain in the heels. By continued practice of this āsana, the heels become softer. Persons suffering from calcaneal spurs in the heels benefit from it as well as from Vīrāsana. (Plate 89)

44. *Baddha Koṇāsana* Three* (Plate 102)

Baddha means caught, restrained. Koṇa means an angle. In this posture, sit on the floor, bring the heels near the perineum, catch the feet and widen the thighs until the knees touch the floor on either side. This is how Indian cobblers sit.

Technique

1. Sit on the floor with the legs stretched straight in front. (Plate 77)

2. Bend the knees and bring the feet closer to the trunk.

3. Bring the soles and heels of the feet together and catching the feet near the toes, bring the heels near the perineum. The outer sides of both feet should rest on the floor, and the back of the heels should touch the perineum.

4. Widen the thighs and lower the knees until they touch the floor.

5. Interlock the fingers of the hands, grip the feet firmly, stretch the spine erect and gaze straight ahead or at the tip of the nose. (Plate 101.) Hold the pose as long as you can.

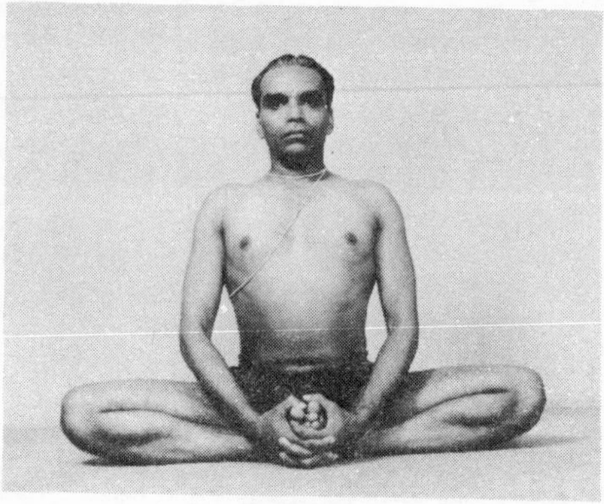

101

6. Place the elbows on the thighs and press them down. Exhale, bend forward, rest the head, then the nose and lastly the chin on the floor. (Plate 102.) Hold this position from half a minute to a minute with normal breathing.

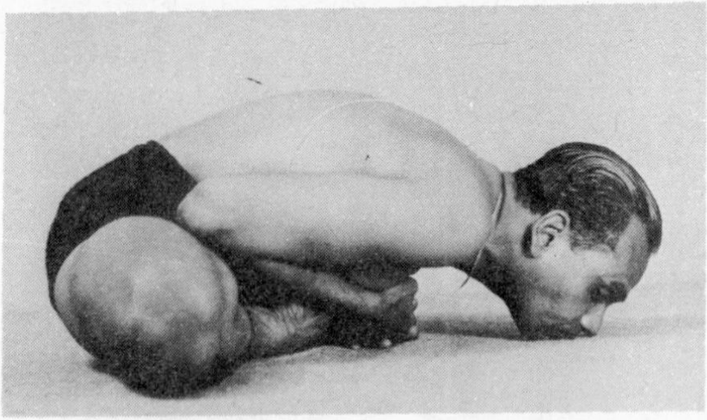

102

7. Inhale, raise the trunk from the floor and come back to position 5. (Plate 101)

8. Then release the feet, straighten the legs and relax.

Effects

The pose is specially recommended for those suffering from urinary disorders. The pelvis, the abdomen and the back get a plentiful supply of blood and are stimulated. It keeps the kidneys, the prostate and the urinary bladder healthy. It is well known that diseases of the urinary tract are rarely found among the Indian cobblers and the reason for that is that they sit all day in this pose.

It relieves sciatic pain and prevents hernia. If practised regularly, it relieves pain and heaviness in the testicles.

The pose is a blessing to women. Coupled with Sarvāngāsana I (Plate 223) and its cycle (Plates 235 to 271) it checks irregular menstrual periods and helps the ovaries to function properly. It is found that pregnant women who sit daily in this pose for a few minutes will have much less pain during delivery and will be free from varicose veins. (It is recommended for pregnant women in Dr Grantly Dick Reed's book *Childbirth Without Fear.*)

Along with Padmāsana (Plate 104) and Vīrāsana (Plate 89) this āsana is recommended for Prāṇāyāma practice and for meditation. When sitting in meditation in this pose the palms should be folded in front of the chest (Plate 103), but to do this with the back erect requires practice. This āsana can be done without fear even after meals as long as the head is not rested on the floor.

45. *Padmāsana* Four* (Plate 104)

Padma means a lotus. This is the lotus posture, one of the most

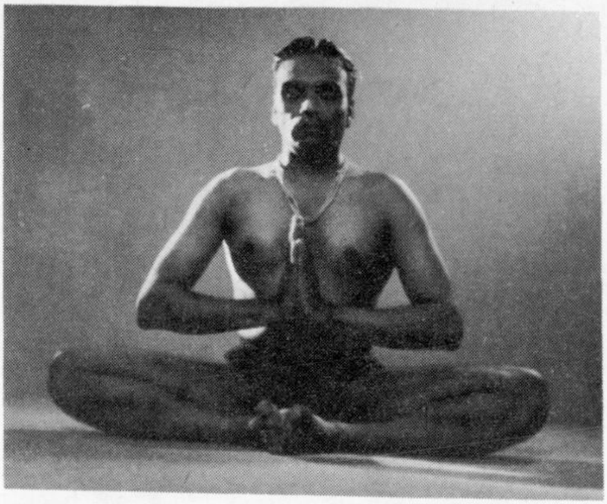

103

important and useful āsanas. It is the posture for meditation and the Buddha is often depicted in it.

Verse 48 of the first chapter of the *Haṭha Yoga Pradīpikā* describes the posture and the practice of breath control while seated in it thus:

'Assuming Padmāsana and having placed the palms one upon another, fix the chin firmly upon the breast and contemplating upon Brahman, frequently contract the anus and raise the apāna up; by similar contraction of the throat force the prāna down. By this he obtains unequalled knowledge through the favour of Kuṇḍalinī (which is roused by this process).'

Kuṇḍalinī is the Divine Cosmic Energy in bodies. It is symbolised by a coiled and sleeping serpent in the lowest bodily centre at the base of the spinal column. This latent energy has to be awakened and made to go up the spine to the brain through Suṣumnā Nāḍi, a channel through which nervous energy passes, and through the six chakrās, the subtle centres in the body, the fly-wheels in the nervous system of the human machine. The awakening of Kuṇḍalinī is discussed in detail in Arthur Avalon's (Sir John Woodroffe's) book entitled *The Serpent Power*.

This is one of the basic postures and is often used in the variations of Śīrṣāsana and Sarvāngāsana.

Technique

1. Sit on the floor with the legs straight. (Plate 77)

2. Bend the right leg at the knee, hold the right foot with the hands and place it at the root of the left thigh so that the right heel is near the navel.

3. Now bend the left leg, and holding the left foot with the hands place it over the right at the root, the heel being near the navel. The soles of the feet should be turned up. This is the basic Padmāsana pose. (Plate 104)

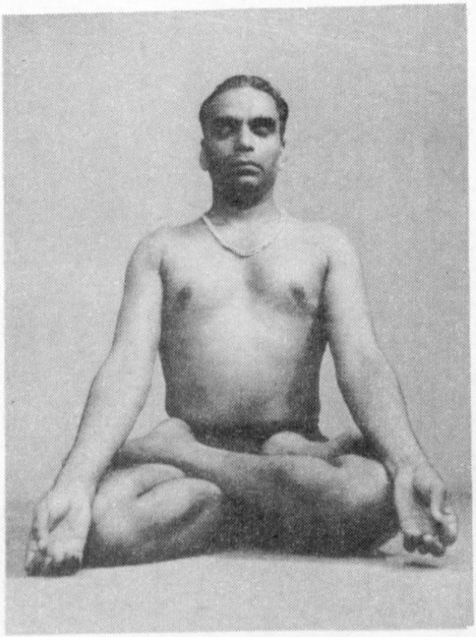

104

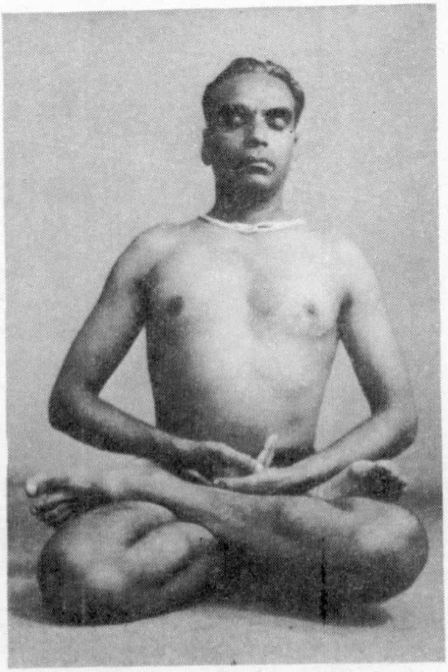

105

4. People not used to sitting on the floor seldom have flexible knees. At the start they will feel excruciating pain around the knees. By perseverance and continued practice the pain will gradually subside and they can then stay in the pose comfortably for a long time.

5. From the base to the neck the spine should remain erect. The arms may be stretched out, the right hand being placed on the right knee and the left hand on the left knee. The forefingers and the thumbs are bent and touch each other. Another way of placing the hands is in the middle where the feet cross each other with one palm upon the other. (Plate 105)

6. Change the leg position by placing the left foot over the right thigh and the right foot over the left thigh. This will develop the legs evenly.

Effects

After the initial knee pains have been overcome, Padmāsana is one of the most relaxing poses. The body being in a sitting posture, it is at rest without being sloppy. The position of the crossed legs and the erect back keeps the mind attentive and alert. Hence it is one of the āsanas recommended for practising prāṇāyāma (breath control).

On the purely physical level, the pose is good for curing stiffness in the knees and ankles. Since the blood is made to circulate in the lumbar region and the abdomen, the spine and the abdominal organs are toned.

46. *Ṣaṇmukhī Mudrā* Four* (Plate 106)

Ṣaṇ means six and mukha means the mouth. Ṣaṇmukha is the name of the six-headed god of war, also known as Kārtikeya. Mudrā means a seal or closing up.

The posture is also called Parāngmukhī Mudrā (facing inwards), Sāmbhavī Mudrā (Sambhu is the name of Siva, father of Kārtikeya. Hence, Śāmbhava is the progeny of Śiva), also as Yoni Mudrā. Yoni means the womb, the source. The mudrā is so called because the aspirant looks within himself to find the very source of his being.

Technique

1. Sit in Padmāsana. (Plate 104.) Keep the spine erect and the head level.

2. Raise the hands to the face. Lift the elbows to the level of the shoulders, place the thumbs on the ear-holes so as to cut off external sounds. If the thumbs in the ear-hole cause pain, push the tragus (the small prominence at the entrance of the external ear) over the ear-holes and press it with the thumbs.

3. Close the eyelids, but turn the eyes up. Place the index and middle fingers on the closed lids so that the first two phalanges only press the entire eyeball. Do not, however, press the cornea. Pull the eyelids down with the middle finger. Push the upper part of the eyelids below the eyebrow upwards with the index fingers. Gently press the eyes at both the corners.

4. Equal pressure should be maintained on the ears and the eyes.

5. With the tips of the ring fingers press both nostrils equally. The nasal passages are thus narrowed for slow, deep, steady, rhythmic and subtle breathing.

6. The little fingers are placed on the upper lip where they can check the rhythmic flow of the breath.

7. Stay in this position as long as you can, drawing the vision inwards. (Plate 106)

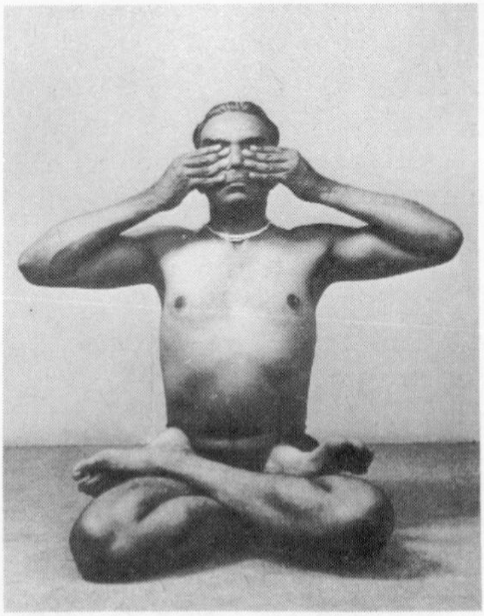

106

Effects

The senses are turned inwards and the rhythmic breathing calms the mind's wandering. This brings a feeling of inner peace and one hears the divine voice of his self within, 'Look here! look within! not outside, for the source of all peace is within yourself.' The posture thus prepares the practitioner for the fifth stage of yoga, Pratyāhāra, where he attempts to free himself from the thraldom of the senses and to prevent them from running after their desires.

47. *Parvatāsana* Four* (Plate 107)

Parvata means a mountain. In this variation of Padmāsana the arms are stretched over the head with the fingers interlocked.

Technique

1. Sit in Padmāsana. (Plate 104)

2. Interlock the fingers, and stretch the hands vertically up over the head. Keep the head bent forward with the chin on the breast bone.

3. Stretch the arms up from the latissimus dorsi (near the floating ribs at the back) and the shoulder-blades. The palms should face upwards. (Plate 107)

4. Hold the pose for a minute or two with deep and even breathing. Change the crossing of the legs and the interlock of the fingers and repeat the pose, keeping the back erect.

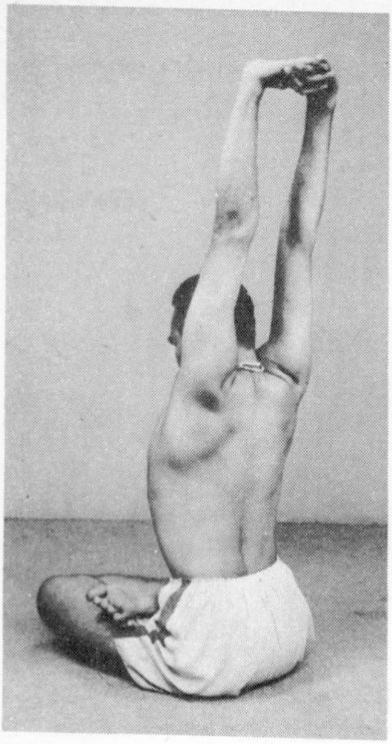

107

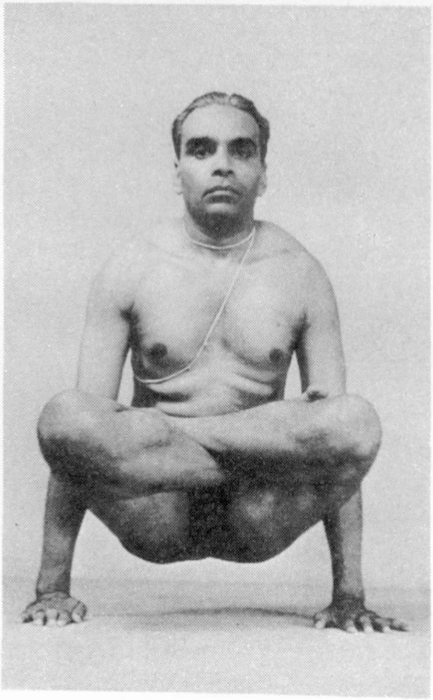

108

Effects

The āsana relieves rheumatic pains and stiffness in the shoulders. It helps free movement and to develop the chest. The abdominal organs are drawn in and the chest expands fully.

48. *Tolāsana* Four* (Plate 108)

Tola means a pair of scales. This pose resembles one pan of the scales, hence the name.

Technique

1. Sit in Padmāsana. (Plate 104)

2. Rest the palms on the floor beside the hips. Exhale, raise the trunk and balance only on the hands, stretching out the arms (Plate 108)

3. Rest on the floor, uncross the legs, recross them the other way and again balance on the hands.

4. Balance as long as possible.

Effects

This āsana strengthens the wrists, hands and abdominal walls.

49. *Siṃhāsana I* One* (Plate 109)

Siṃha means a lion. This āsana is dedicated to Narasiṃha (Nara = man: Siṃha = lion), the Man-Lion Incarnation of Viṣṇu. It is related that the demon king Hiraṇya Kaśipu had obtained a boon from Brahmā ensuring that he would not be killed by day or night, in or out of his house, on land or water, by God, man or beast. The demon king then persecuted both gods and men, including his pious son Prahlāda, who was an ardent devotee of Viṣṇu. Prahlāda was subjected to a variety of cruelties and ordeals, but by the favour of Viṣṇu he remained unscathed and preached with greater faith and vigour the omnipresence, omniscience and omnipotence of Lord Viṣṇu. In a fit of exasperation Hiraṇya Kaśipu asked his son why, if Viṣṇu was omnipresent, he could not see Him in the pillar of his palace hall. The demon king contemptuously kicked the pillar to convince his son of the absurdity of his faith. When Prahlāda called upon Viṣṇu for help, the Lord burst from the pillar in a fearful form, the top half being a lion and the lower half a man. It was then dusk, when it was neither day nor night. The Lord lifted Hiraṇya Kaśipu in the air, seated Himself on the threshold, placed the demon king on His thigh and tore him to pieces. Narasiṃha Avatār is often depicted in Indian sculpture and one such powerful group can be seen in the Ellora caves.

There are two variations of this āsana. The first, described in the technique given below, follows the texts, whereas the second variation, which is more strenuous to perform but which has greater beneficial effects, is described later as Siṃhāsana II. (Plate 110)

Technique

1. Sit on the floor, with the legs stretched straight in front. (Plate 77)

2. Raise the seat, bend the right knee and place the right foot under the left buttock. Then bend the left knee and place the left foot under the right buttock. The left ankle should be kept under the right one.

3. Sit on the heels with the toes pointing back.

4. Then bring the weight of the body on the thighs and knees.

5. Stretch the trunk forward and keep the back erect.

6. Place the right palm on the right knee and the left palm on the

left knee. Stretch the arms straight and keep them stiff. Spread the fingers and press them against the knees.

7. Open the jaws wide and stretch the tongue out towards the chin as far as you can. (Plate 109)

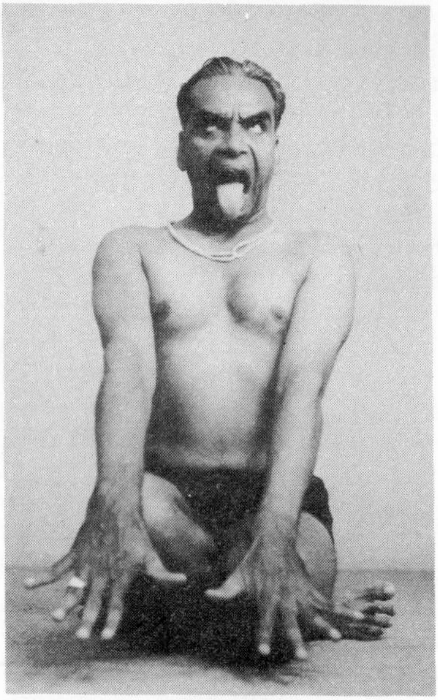

109

8. Gaze at the centre of the eyebrows or at the tip of the nose. Stay in the pose for about 30 seconds, breathing through the mouth.

9. Withdraw the tongue into the mouth, lift the hands from the knees and straighten the legs. Then repeat the pose, first placing the left foot under the right buttock and then the right foot under the left buttock.

10. Stay for an equal length of time on both sides.

Effects

The pose cures foul breath and cleans the tongue. After continued practice speech becomes clearer so this āsana is recommended to stammerers. It also helps one to master the three Bandhas (see Part III).

50. *Siṃhāsana II* Six* (Plate 110)

Technique

1. Sit in Padmāsana. (Plate 104)

2. Extend the arms in front and place the palms on the floor, fingers pointing forward.

3. Stand on the knees and then push the pelvic region to the floor.

4. Stretch the back by contracting the buttocks, keeping the arms fully stretched. The weight of the body rests on the palms and knees only. Open the mouth and stretch the tongue out towards the chin as far as you can. (Front view: Plate 110. Side view: Plate 111)

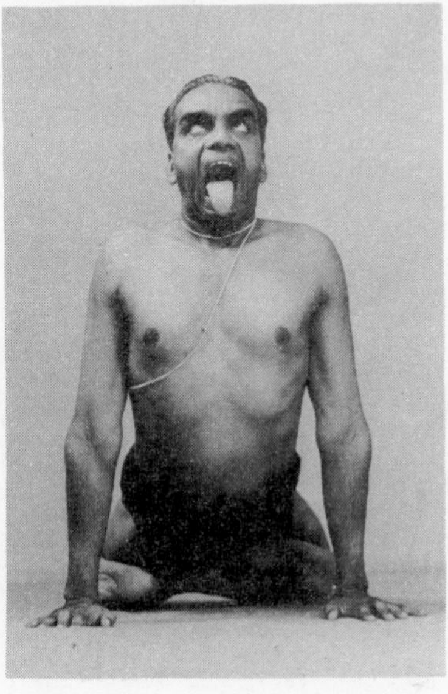

110

5. Gaze at the centre of the eyebrows or at the tip of the nose and keep the pose for about 30 seconds. Breathe through the mouth.

6. Sit in Padmāsana (Plate 104) and lift the hands off the floor. Then interchange the position of the legs, perform Padmāsana again and repeat the pose for the same length of time.

Effects

The pose exercises the liver and controls the flow of bile. It cures

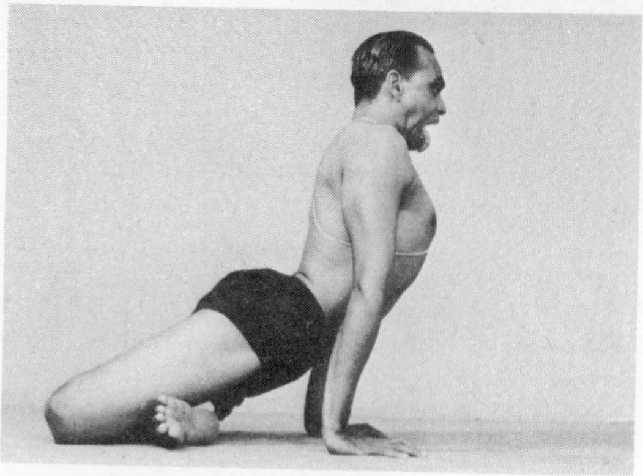

111

foul breath, the tongue becomes cleaner and words are enunciated more clearly. It is, therefore, recommended to persons who stammer.

The āsana relieves a painful coccyx and helps to set it when displaced.

51. *Matsyāsana* Five* (Plate 113)

Matsya means a fish. This posture is dedicated to Matsya the Fish Incarnation of Viṣṇu, the source and maintainer of the universe and of all things. It is related that once upon a time the whole earth had become corrupt and was about to be overwhelmed by a universal flood. Viṣṇu took the form of a fish and warned Manu (the Hindu Adam) of the impending disaster. The fish then carried Manu, his family and the seven great sages in a ship, fastened to a horn on his head. It also saved the Vedas from the flood.

Technique

1. Sit in Padmāsana. (Plate 104)

2. Lie flat on the back with the legs on the floor.

3. Exhale, arch the back by lifting the neck and the chest, take the head back and rest the crown on the floor. Drag the head further back by holding the crossed legs with the hands and increase the back arch. (Plate 112)

4. Now take the hands from the legs, bend the arms, hold the elbows with the hands and rest the forearms on the floor behind the head. (Plate 113)

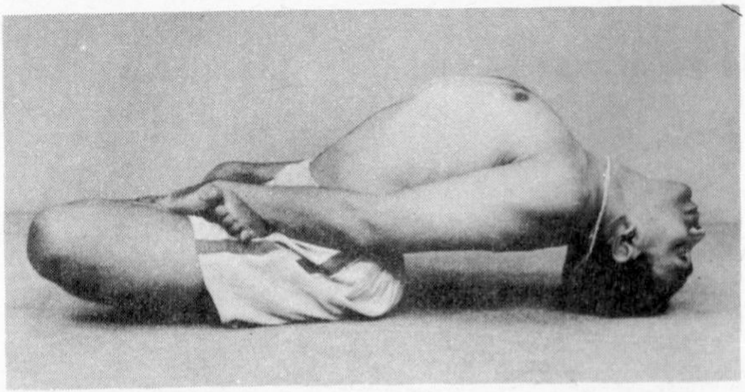

112

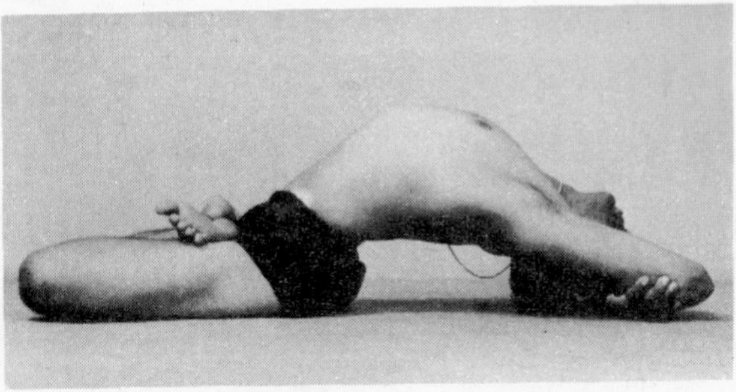

113

5. Stay in this position from 30 to 60 seconds while breathing deeply.

6. Rest the back of the head on the floor, lie flat on the back, inhale and then come up to Padmāsana, release the legs and relax.

7. Recross the legs the other way and repeat the pose for the same length of time.

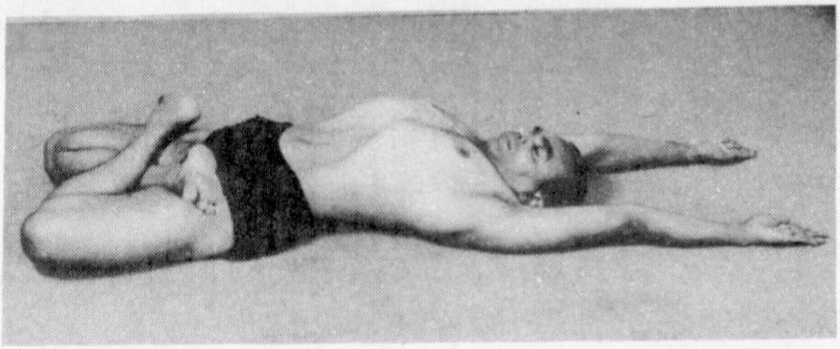

114

8. If positions 3 and 4 are difficult to achieve, lie flat on the back with the arms stretched straight over the head. (Plate 114)

Effects

The dorsal region is fully extended in this posture and the chest is well expanded. Breathing becomes fuller. The thyroids benefit from the exercise due to the stretching of the neck. The pelvic joints become elastic. The āsana relieves inflamed and bleeding piles.

52. *Kukkuṭāsana* Six* (Plate 115)

Kukkuṭa means a cock, which this posture resembles.

Technique

1. Sit in Padmāsana. (Plate 104)

2. Insert the hands in the space between the thigh and calf near the knees. Start with the fingers and gradually push the hands down up to the elbows.

3. Exhale, raise the body off the floor and balance on the palms keeping the thumbs together. Maintain the balance as long as you can with normal breathing. (Plate 115)

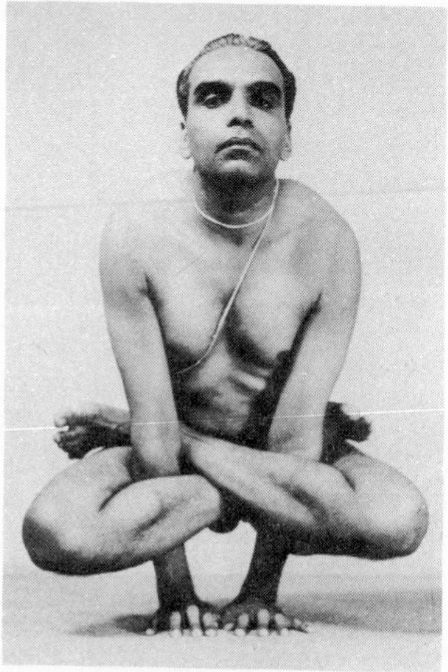

115

4. Rest on the floor, release the hands, change the crossing of the legs and repeat the pose.

Effects

This posture strengthens the wrists and abdominal walls.

53. *Garbha Piṇḍāsana* Seven* (Plate 116)

Garbha Piṇḍa means an embryo in the womb (garbha = womb; piṇḍa = embryo). In this variation of Padmāsana, insert the hands and arms in the space between the calves and thighs until the elbows are bent. The arms are then bent up and the hands brought close to the ears. The pose then resembles that of a human foetus in the womb, the differences being that the embryo's head is down, while the legs are up and not folded in Padmāsana. The name of the posture indicates that the ancient sages knew about the growth of the human foetus in the mother's womb though the medical instruments at their disposal were limited.

Technique

1. Sit in Padmāsana. (Plate 104)

2. Insert the hands in the space between the thighs and calves, each on its own side.

3. Push the arms forwards till the elbows can be easily bent.

4. Then, with an exhalation, lift the thighs off the floor, balance the body on the coccyx (the tail bone) and catch the ears with the fingers. (Plate 116)

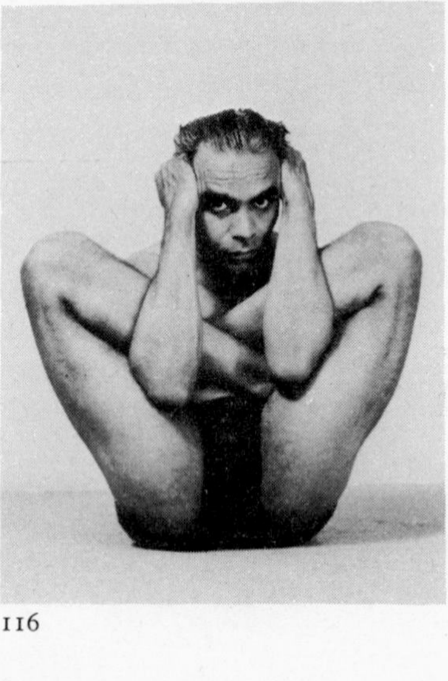

116

5. Remain in the pose for about 15 to 30 seconds with normal breathing. Lower the legs, release the arms from between the legs one by one, straighten the legs and relax.

6. Change the crossing of the legs and repeat the pose.

Effects

In this posture the abdominal organs are contracted completely and the blood is made to circulate well round the organs. This keeps them in trim.

54. *Gorakṣāsana* Ten* (Plate 117)

Gorakṣa means a cowherd. It is a difficult balancing pose and one feels elated even if one can only balance for a few seconds.

Technique

1. Perform Padmāsana (Plate 104), stretch the arms forward and place them on the floor.

2. Rest on the hands and raise the hips from the floor.

3. Stretch the trunk up vertically and stand with the top part of the knees on the floor.

4. Stretch the thighs and balance gradually by lifting the hands one by one from the floor.

5. When balance is secured, fold the hands in front of the chest and hold the position as long as you can. (Plate 117)

6. Place the hands on the floor, sit down and release the legs.

7. Change the leg position and repeat the pose for the same length of time.

Effects

In addition to the benefits of Padmāsana (Plate 104), one achieves a sense of balance. The coccyx (the tail bone) gets elasticity by the practice of this pose.

55. *Baddha Padmāsana* Six* (Plate 118)

Baddha means caught, restrained. In this position the hands are crossed at the back and the big toes are caught from behind. The body is caught between the crossed legs in front and the crossed hands behind, hence the name.

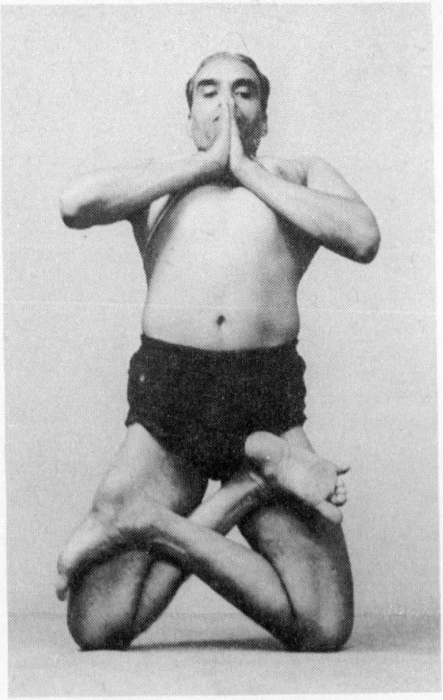

117

Technique

1. Sit in Padmāsana. (Plate 104)

2. Exhale, swing the left arm back from the shoulders and bring the hand near the right hip. Catch the left big toe, hold the position and inhale.

3. Similarly, with an exhalation, swing the right arm back from the shoulder, bring it near the left hip and catch the right big toe. (Front view: Plate 118. Back view: Plate 119)

4. If the toes are difficult to catch stretch the shoulders back, so that the shoulder-blades are brought near each other. A little practice in swinging the arms back with an exhalation will enable one to catch the big toes.

5. If the right foot is placed first over the left thigh and then the left foot over the right thigh, catch the left big toe first and then the right big toe. If, on the other hand, the left foot is placed over the right thigh first and then the right foot over the left thigh, catch the right big toe first and then the left big toe. Catch first the big toe of the foot which is uppermost.

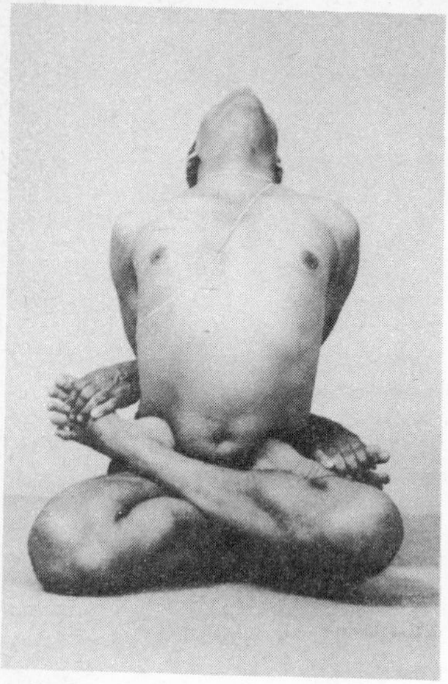

118

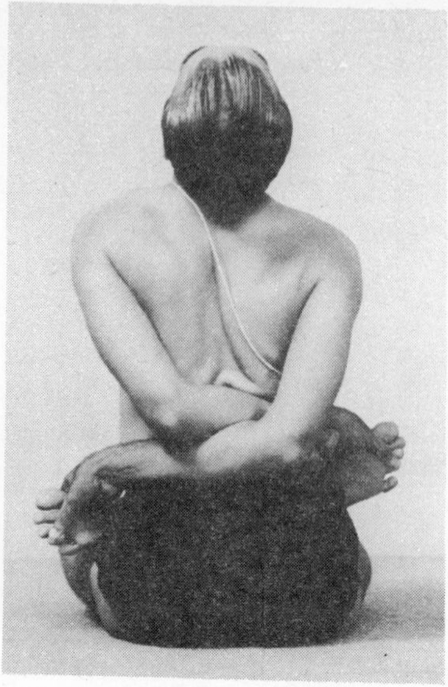

119

6. Throw the head as far back as possible and take a few deep breaths.

7. Inhale deeply, and then with an exhalation bend the trunk forward from the hips and rest the head on the floor, without releasing the toes from the hand grip. Bending the head forward in Baddha Padmāsana (Plate 118) and touching it on the floor is called:

56. *Yoga Mudrāsana* Six* (Plate 120)

This āsana is especially useful in awakening Kuṇḍalinī.

8. Also move the head on to the right and left knees alternately with an exhalation. (Plates 121 and 122)

Effects

Crossing the hands behind the back expands the chest and increases the range of shoulder movements. Yoga Mudrāsana (Plate 120) intensifies the peristaltic activity and pushes down the accumulated waste matter in the colon and thereby relieves constipation and increases digestive power.

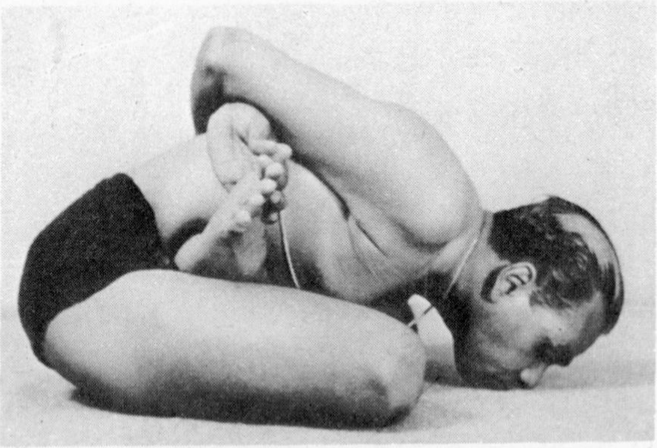

120

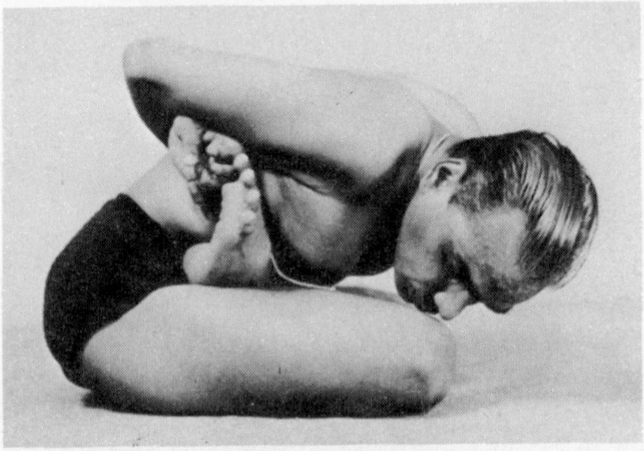

121

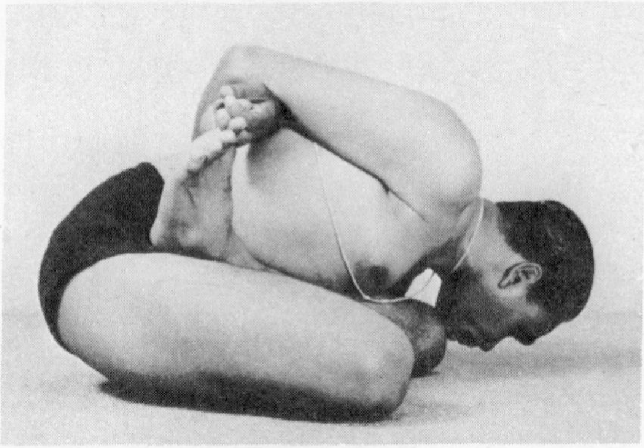

122

57. *Supta Vajrāsana* Twelve* (Plate 124)

Supta means lying down. Vajra means a thunderbolt, the weapon of Indra, king of the gods. This is a difficult āsana and requires great practice.

Technique

1. Sit in Padmāsana. (Plate 104.) Then perform Baddha Padmāsana. (Plate 118)

2. Exhale, raise the knees and thighs off the floor and recline back on the floor. (Plate 123.) Take two breaths.

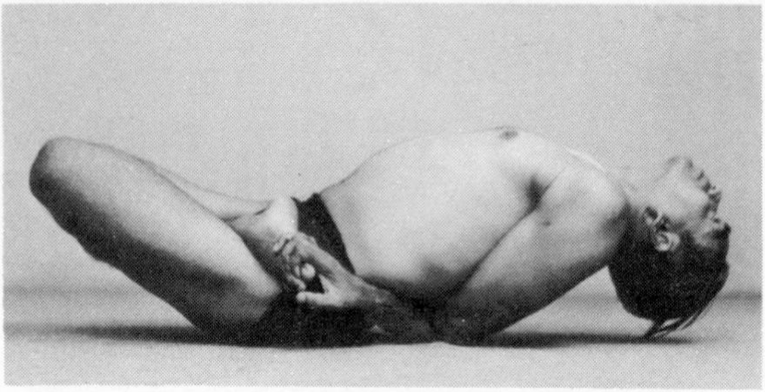

123

3. Stretch the neck back to rest the crown of the head on the floor, and arch the chest and trunk up.

4. Without releasing the grip on the toes throughout, exhale and lower the knees and thighs back to the floor. (Plate 124.) Then the crown of the head, the elbows and crossed arms behind the back and the buttocks will be the only parts of the body touching the floor.

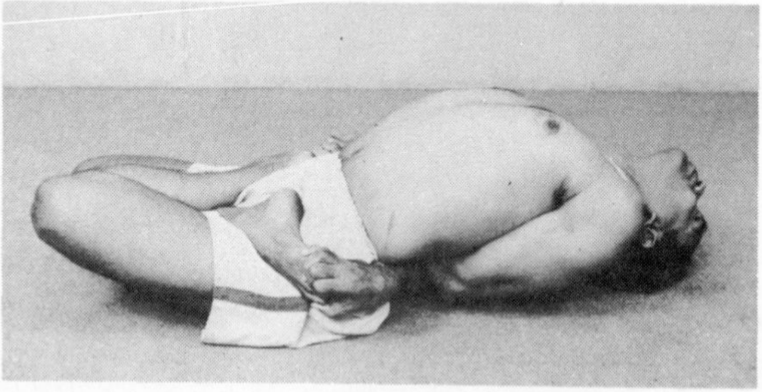

124

5. Stay in the pose for a few seconds. Exhale, release the grips on the toes, uncross the hands at the back and sit up again in Padmāsana. (Plate 104.) Then straighten the legs and relax.

6. Change the leg position and repeat the pose.

Effects

The dorsal region is fully extended in this posture and so the chest is expanded fully. Due to the stretch of the neck the thyroids benefit by the exercise. The pelvic joints become elastic. Once the pose is mastered, Matsyāsana (Plate 113) will appear to be child's play.

58. *Mahā Mudrā* Five* (Plate 125)

Mahā means great or noble. Mudrā means shutting, closing or sealing. In this sitting posture the apertures at the top and bottom of the trunk are held fast and sealed.

Technique

1. Sit on the floor with the legs stretched straight in front. (Plate 77)

2. Bend the left knee and move it to the left, keeping the outer side of the left thigh and the left calf on the floor.

3. Place the left heel against the inner side of the left thigh near the perineum. The big toe of the left foot should touch the inner side of the right thigh. The angle between the extended right leg and the bent left leg should be a right angle of 90 degrees.

4. Stretch the arms forward towards the right foot and hook the big toe with the thumbs and forefingers.

5. Lower the head to the trunk until the chin rests in the hollow between the collar bones just above the breast-bone.

6. Keep the spine fully stretched and do not allow the right leg to tilt to the right.

7. Inhale completely. Tighten the entire abdomen from the anus to the diaphragm. Pull the abdomen back towards the spine and also up towards the diaphragm.

8. Relax the abdominal tension, then exhale, again inhale and hold the breath, maintaining the abdominal grip. Hold this posture as stated above from one to three minutes. (Plate 125)

9. Relax the abdominal tension, exhale, raise the head, release the hands and straighten the bent leg.

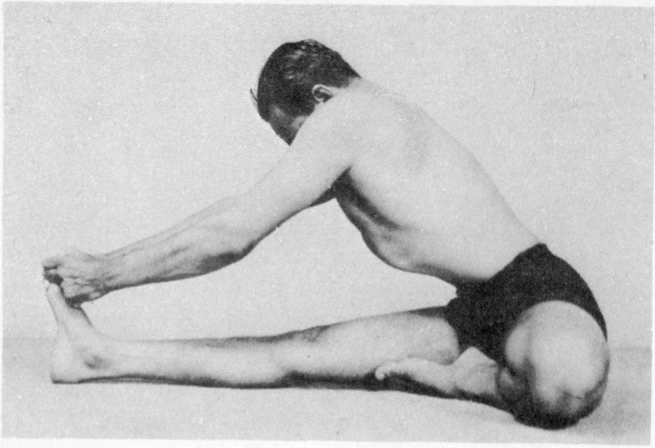

125

10. Repeat on the other side, keeping the left leg straight and the right one bent for an equal length of time.

Effects

This āsana tones the abdominal organs, the kidneys and adrenal glands. Women suffering from a prolapsed womb find relief as it pulls the womb up to its original position. Persons suffering from spleen ailments and from enlargement of the prostate gland will benefit by staying in this pose longer. It cures indigestion.

'This Mahāmudrā destroys death and many other pains.' 'There is nothing that one cannot eat or has to avoid (if one has practised it). All food regardless of taste and even when deadly poisonous is digested.' 'He who practises Mahāmudrā, overcomes consumption, leprosy, piles, enlargement of the spleen, indigestion and other complaints of long duration.' (*Haṭha Yoga Pradīpikā*, chapter 3, verses 14, 16 and 17.)

59. *Jānu Śīrṣāsana* Five* (Plate 127)

Jānu means the knee. Śīrṣa is the head. In this posture sit with one leg stretched out on the ground and the other bent at the knee. Then catch the extended foot with both the hands and place the head on that knee.

Technique

1. Sit on the floor, with legs stretched straight in front. (Plate 77)

2. Bend the left knee and move it to the left, keeping the outer side of left thigh and the left calf on the floor.

3. Place the left heel against the inner side of the left thigh near the perineum. The big toe of the left foot should touch the inner side of the right thigh. The angle between the two legs should be obtuse. Do not keep the left knee in line with the left thigh at a right angle to the extended right leg. Try and push the left knee as far back as possible, so that the body is stretched from the bent leg.

4. Extend the arms forward towards the right foot and hold it with the hands. First catch the toes of the right foot, then gradually catch the sole, then the heel and finally extend the arms and catch the wrist of one hand with the other, beyond the outstretched foot. (Plate 126)

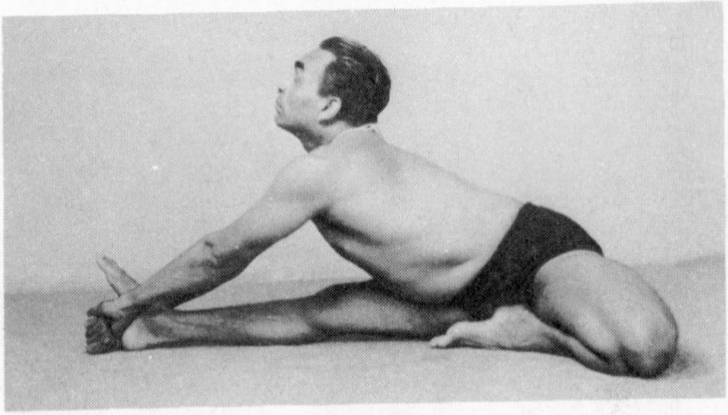

126

5. Keep the right leg stretched throughout by tightening the knee. See that the back of the right knee rests on the floor.

6. Exhale, move the trunk forward by bending and widening the elbows, and rest first the forehead, then the nose, then the lips and lastly the chin beyond the right knee. (Plate 127.) Then rest on either side of the right knee. (Plates 128 and 129.) The right foot will tilt to the right in the beginning. Do not allow the leg to tilt.

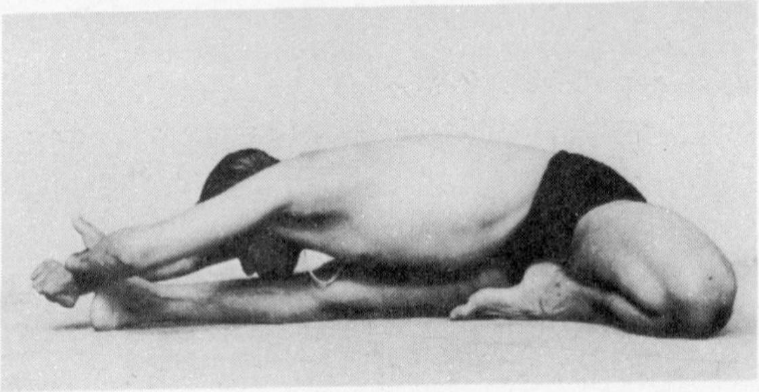

127

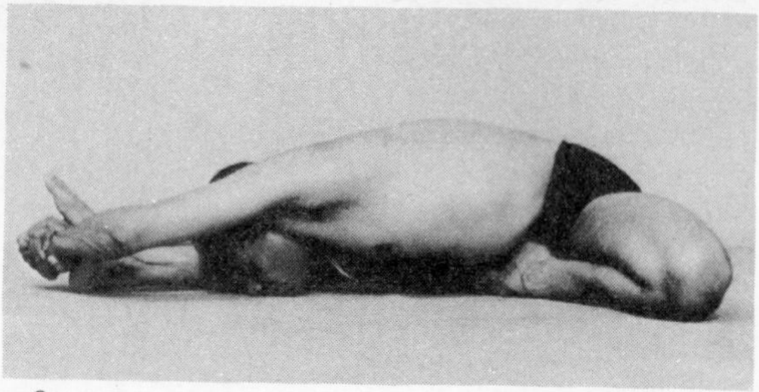

128

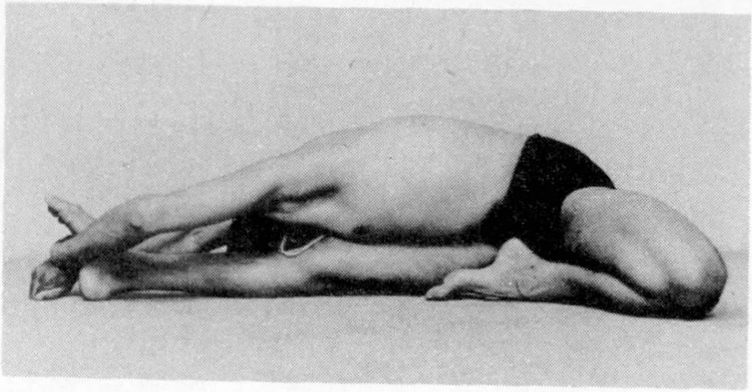

129

7. Stretch the back fully, pull the trunk forward and keep the chest against the right thigh.

8. Stay in this position with deep breathing from half a minute to a minute. One can also do the pose holding the breath after each exhalation.

9. Inhale, raise the head and trunk, straighten the arms and gaze up for a few seconds, extending the spine and trying to make it concave. (Plate 126)

10. Release the hand grip on the right foot, straighten the left leg and come back to position 1.

11. Repeat the pose keeping the left leg stretched out and bending the right leg at the knee. Stay in the pose for the same length of time on both the sides.

Effects

This āsana tones the liver and the spleen and thereby aids digestion. It also tones and activates the kidneys, the effect on which can be felt while one is performing the pose as explained above.

Persons suffering from enlargement of the prostate gland will benefit by staying longer in this pose. They should practise this āsana along with Sarvāngāsana. (Plate 223)

The pose is also recommended for people suffering from low fever for a long time.

60. *Parivṛtta Jānu Śīrṣāsana* Nine* (Plate 132)

Parivṛtta means turned round, revolved, jānu means the knee and śīrṣa the head. In this variation of Jānu Śīrṣāsana one leg is extended on the ground, the other is bent at the knee, the trunk is twisted round, the extended foot is caught with both hands and the back of the head is placed on the knee of the extended leg by bending the spine back.

Technique

1. Sit on the floor with the legs stretched straight in front. (Plate 77)

2. Bend the left knee and move it to the left, keeping the outer side of the left thigh and the left calf on the floor.

3. Place the left heel against the inner side of the left thigh near the perineum. The big toe of the left foot should touch the inner side of the right thigh. The angle between the two legs should be obtruse. Extend the left knee as far back as possible.

4. Twist the trunk to the left.

5. Stretch the right arm towards the extended right leg. Turn the right forearm and wrist so that the right thumb points to the floor and the right little finger points up. Then, with the right hand hold the inner side of the right foot. (Plate 130)

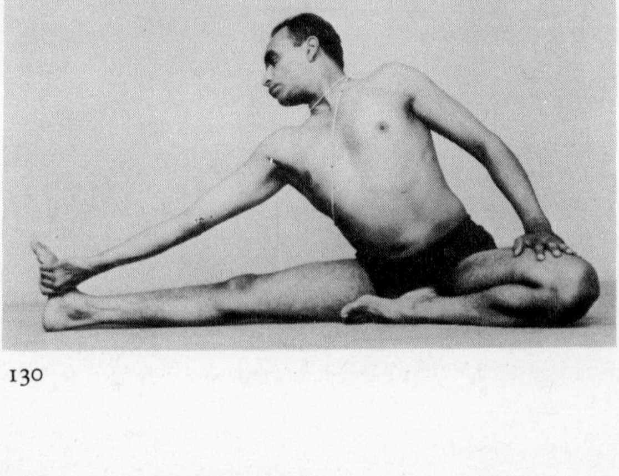

130

6. Throw the trunk back, stretch the left arm over the head keeping the wrist up, and with the left hand hold the outer side of the extended right foot. Here also the left thumb points to the floor and the little finger points up. (Plate 131)

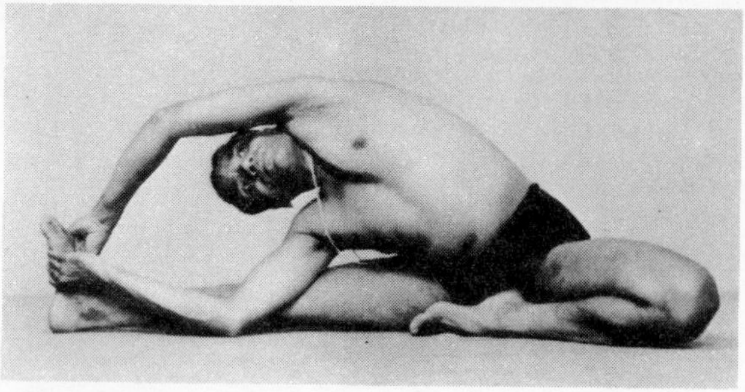

131

7. Bend and widen the elbows. Exhale, turn the trunk up, move the head in between the arms and rest the back of the head on the right knee. Try to touch the inner side of the right knee joint with the back of the right shoulder so that the back of the ribs on the right side rests on the right knee. Extend the bent left knee still further and stretch the left side of the ribs. (Plate 132)

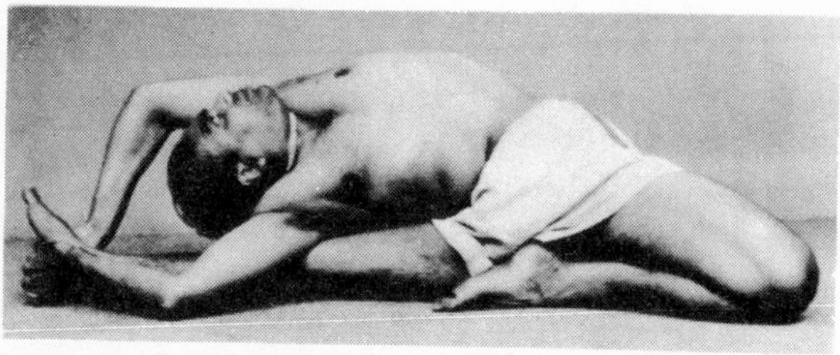

132

8. Maintain the pose for about 20 seconds. The breathing will be short and fast due to the contraction of the abdomen.

9. Inhale, release the hands, move the trunk back to its original position so that you face the extended right leg, raise the head and straighten the left leg to come to position 1.

10. Repeat the pose on the other side. Here bend the right knee and keep the left leg straight. Twist the trunk to the right until you face the bent right knee and extend the left arm towards the left foot. Then

turn the left forearm and the left wrist so that the left thumb points to the floor. With the left hand catch the inner side of the left foot, bring the right arm over the head and catch the outer side of the left foot near the heel. Then rest the back of the head on the left knee and try to touch the inner side of the left knee with the back of the left shoulder so that the back of the left side ribs rests on the left knee and stretch the right side of the ribs. Remain on this side for the same length of time.

Effects

In addition to the effects stated in the note on Jānu Śīrṣāsana (Plate 127), this pose stimulates the blood circulation to the spine and relieves backaches. In Jānu Śīrṣāsana the abdominal organs are contracted, here they are stretched on both sides. This is a very invigorating pose.

61. *Ardha Baddha Padma Paschimottānāsana* Eight* (Plate 135)

Ardha means half, baddha means caught, restrained and padma a lotus. Paschimottānāsana (Plate 160) is the posture where the back of the whole body is intensely stretched.

Technique

1. Sit on the floor, with the legs stretched straight in front. (Plate 77)

2. Bend the left leg at the knee, and place the left foot over the right thigh. The left heel should press the navel and the toes should be stretched and pointing. This is the half lotus posture.

3. Bring the left arm round the back from behind and with an exhalation catch the big toe of the left foot. If the toe cannot be grasped easily, swing back the left shoulder.

4. After holding the left big toe, move the bent left knee nearer to the extended right leg. Stretch the right arm forward and catch the right foot with the right hand, the palm touching the sole. (Plates 133 and 134)

5. Inhale, stretch the back and gaze up for a few seconds, without releasing the grip on the left big toe.

6. Exhale, move the trunk forward by bending the right elbow outwards. Rest the forehead, then the nose, then the lips and lastly the chin on the right knee. (Plate 135)

7. In the initial stages, the knee of the extended leg will be lifted off the floor. Tighten the thigh muscles and rest the entire back of the extended right leg on the floor.

8. Stay in this position from 30 to 60 seconds, breathing evenly.

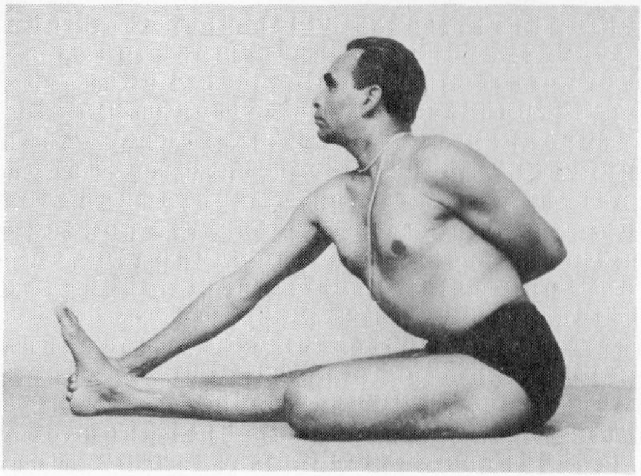
133

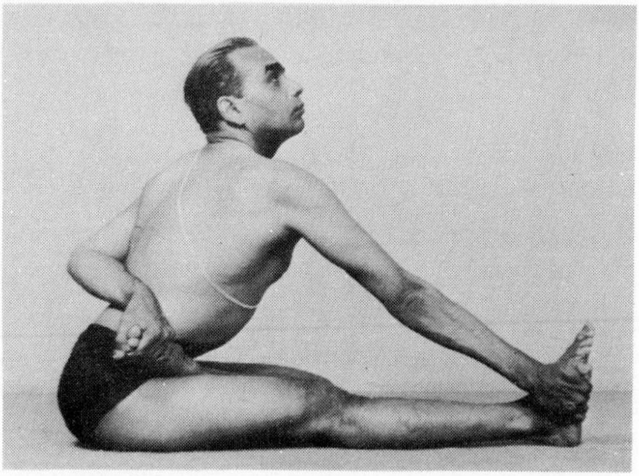
134

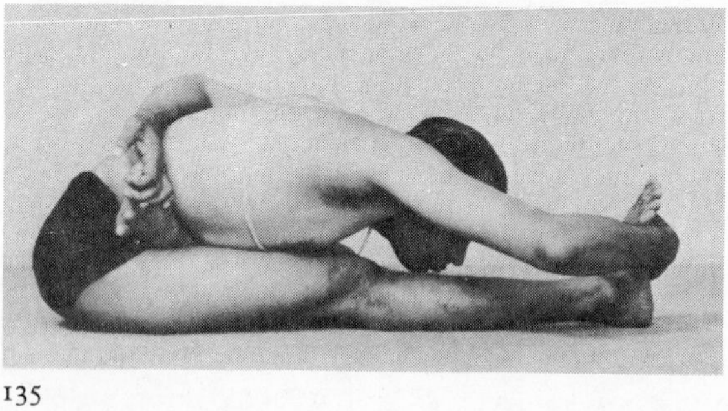
135

9. Inhale, raise the head and trunk, release the hands, straighten the left leg and come to position 1.

10. Repeat the pose on the other side, keeping the left leg stretched out on the ground, bending the right knee and placing the right foot on the left thigh. Stay for the same length of time on both sides.

11. If you cannot hold the toe with the hand from behind, hold the extended leg with both hands and follow the above technique. (Plates 136 and 137)

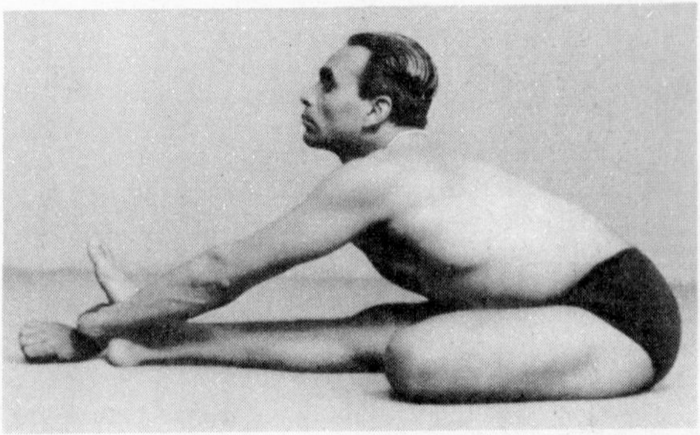

136

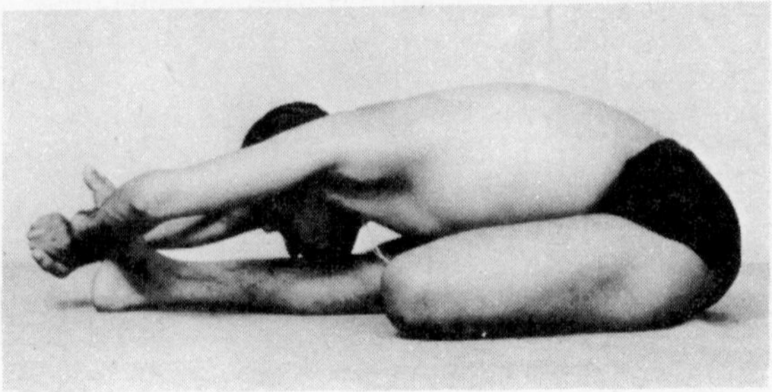

137

Effects

Due to the half lotus pose, the knees become flexible enough to execute the full lotus pose. While placing the chin on the knee of the extended leg, the bent knee is brought close to the stretched leg. This gives a good pull to the navel and abdominal organs. Blood is made to flow round the navel and the genital organs. The navel is considered to be a nerve centre, and the Svādhiṣṭhāna Chakra, one of the purificatory fly-wheels in the human nervous system, is situated there. This chakra corresponds to the hypo-gastric plexus. The pose is recommended for persons with rounded and drooping shoulders.

62. *Triaṅgā Mukhaikapda Paschimottānāsana* Five* (Plate 139)

Trianga means three limbs or parts thereof. In this posture the three parts are the feet, knees and buttocks. Mukhaikapāda (a compound of three words, mukha = face, eka = one, and pāda = leg or foot) corresponds to the face (or mouth) touching one (extended) leg. In Paschimottānāsana (Plate 160) the back of the whole body is intensely stretched.

Technique

1. Sit on the floor, with the legs stretched straight in front. (Plate 77)

2. Bend the right leg at the knee and move the right foot back. Place the right foot by the side of the right hip joint, keep the toes pointing back and rest them on the floor. The inner side of the right calf will touch the outer side of the right thigh.

3. Balance in this position, throwing the weight of the body on the bent knee. In the beginning, the body tilts to the side of the outstretched leg, and the foot of the outstretched leg also tilts outwards. Learn to balance in this position, keeping the foot and toes stretched and pointing forward.

4. Now hold the left foot with both the palms, gripping the sides of the sole. If you can, then extend the trunk forward and hook the wrists round the outstretched left foot. (Plate 138.) Take two deep breaths. It usually takes several months before one can hook the wrists in this way, so do not despair after the first few attempts.

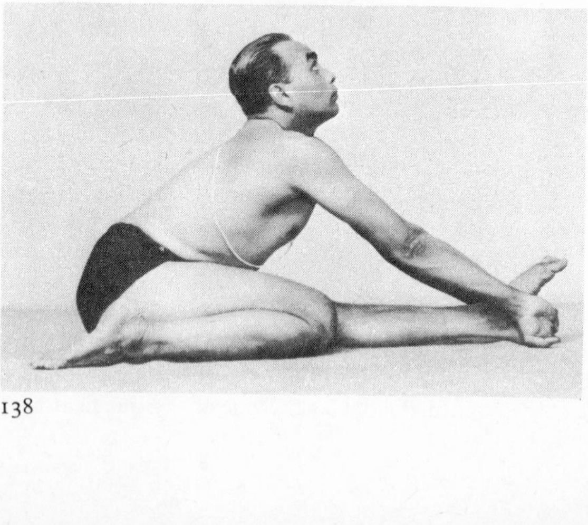

138

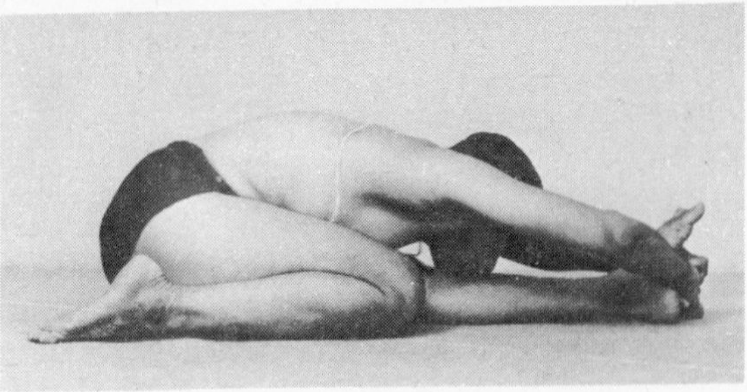

139

5. Join the knees, exhale and bend forward. Rest first the forehead, then the nose, next the lips and ultimately the chin on the left knee. (Plate 139.) To achieve this, widen the elbows and push the trunk forward with an exhalation.

6. Do not rest the left elbow on the floor. In the beginning, one loses balance and topples over to the side of the extended leg. The trunk should, therefore, be slightly bent towards the side of the bent leg and the weight of the body should be taken by the bent knee.

7. Stay in this position from half a minute to a minute, breathing evenly.

8. Inhale, raise the head and trunk, release the hands, straighten the right leg and come to position 1.

9. Repeat the pose on the other side, keeping the right leg stretched out on the ground, bending the left knee and placing the left foot by the left hip joint. Stay for the same length of time on both sides.

Effects

This āsana is recommended for persons suffering from dropped arches and flat feet. It cures sprains in the ankle and the knee, and any swelling in the leg is reduced.

Along with Jānu Śīrṣāsana (Plate 127) and Ardha Baddha Padma Paschimottānāsana (Plate 135), this āsana tones the abdominal organs and keeps them free from sluggishness. We abuse our abdominal organs by over-indulgence or by conforming to social etiquette. Abdominal organs cause a majority of diseases and ancient sages emphasised that their health was essential for longevity, happiness and peace of mind. These forward bending āsanas keep the abdominal organs healthy and in trim. Apart from keeping the muscles in shape, they work on the organs as well.

63. *Krounchāsana* Ten* (Plates 141 and 142)

Krouncha means a heron. It is also the name of a mountain, said to be the grandson of Himālaya and to have been pierced by Kārtikeya, the god of war, and by Paraśurāma, the sixth incarnation of Viṣṇu. In this sitting posture, one leg is bent back at the knee and the foot is placed against the side of the hip joint, while the other leg is raised up vertically, its foot being held by the hands. The chin is then placed on the knee of the vertical leg. The raised leg resembles the outstretched neck and head of a heron, also a precipice. Hence the name.

Technique

1. Sit on the floor, with the legs stretched straight in front. (Plate 77)

2. Bend the right leg at the knee and move the right foot back. Place the right foot by the side of the hip joint, keep the toes pointing back and rest all of them on the floor. The inner side of the right calf will touch the outer side of the right thigh. Join the knees together.

3. Exhale, bend the left knee, hold the left foot with both hands and raise the left leg up vertically. (Plate 140)

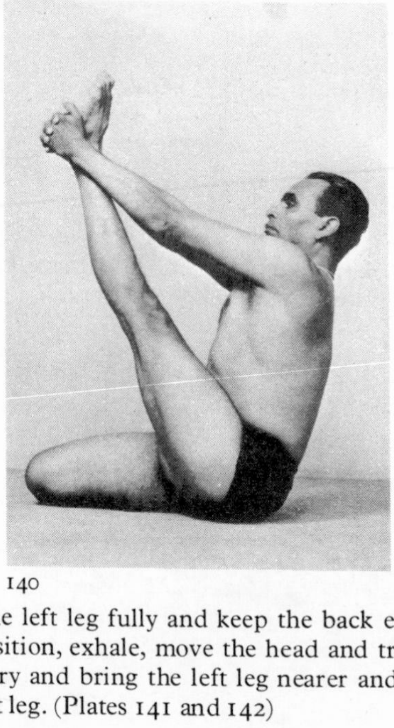

140

4. Stretch out the left leg fully and keep the back erect. After a few breaths in this position, exhale, move the head and trunk forward and at the same time try and bring the left leg nearer and rest the chin on the knee of the left leg. (Plates 141 and 142)

5. Hold this position for 20 to 30 seconds, with deep breaths. Do not lift the bent knee off the floor while the chin is touching the knee of the lifted leg.

6. Inhale, move the head and trunk back (Plate 140), lower the left leg, release the hands, bring the right leg straight forward and return to position 1.

7. Repeat the pose on the other side, bending the left knee and placing

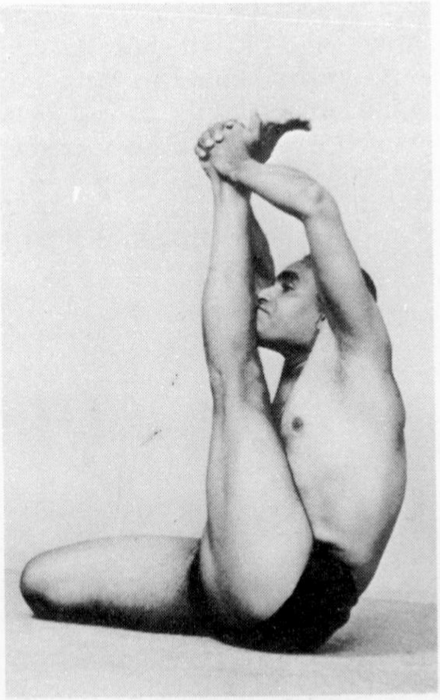

141

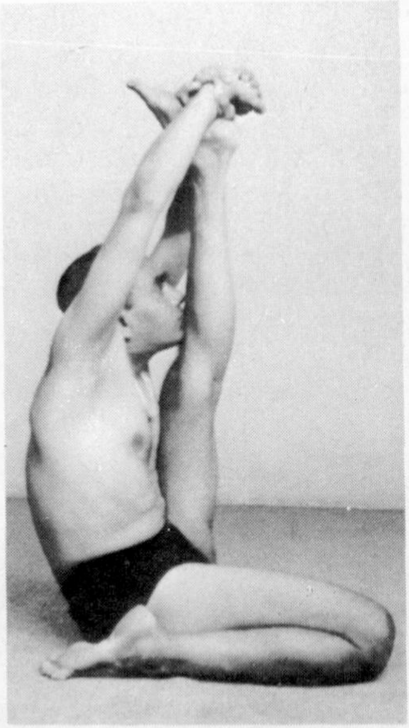

142

the left foot by the left hip joint and raising the right leg up. Stay for an equal length of time on this side also.

Effects

The pose can be done as a continuation of Triang Mukhaikapāda Paschimottānāsana (Plate 139). It is harder to do than Paschimottānāsana (Plate 160) and therefore its effects are greater. It gives a full extension to the leg and exercises the muscles of the legs. The abdominal organs are also rejuvenated.

64. *Marīchyāsana I* Five* (Plate 144)

This āsana is dedicated to the sage Marīchi, son of the Creator, Brahmā. Marīchi was the grandfather of Sūrya (the Sun God).

Technique

1. Sit on the floor with the legs stretched straight in front. (Plate 77)

2. Bend the left knee and place the sole and heel of the left foot flat on the floor. The shin of the left leg should be perpendicular to the floor and the calf should touch the thigh. Place the left heel near the perineum. The inner side of the left foot should touch the inner side of the outstretched right thigh.

3. Stretch the left shoulder forward till the left armpit touches the perpendicular left shin. Turn the left arm round the left shin and thigh, bend the left elbow and throw the left forearm behind the back at the level of the waist. Then move the right hand behind the back and clasp the left hand with the right at the wrist or vice versa. If that is not possible then clasp the palms or the fingers. (Plate 143)

4. Now, turn the spine to the left, keeping the outstretched right leg

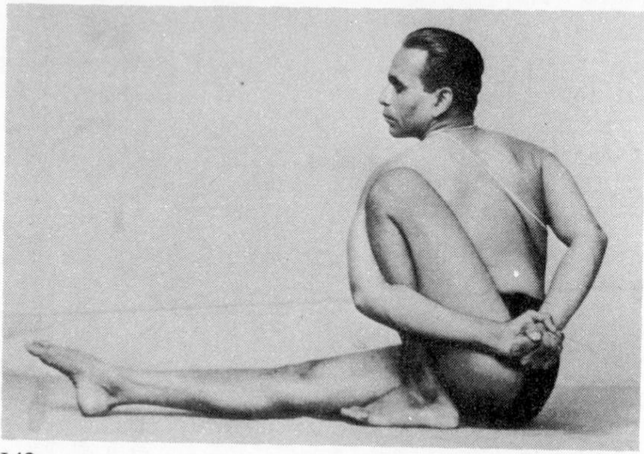

143

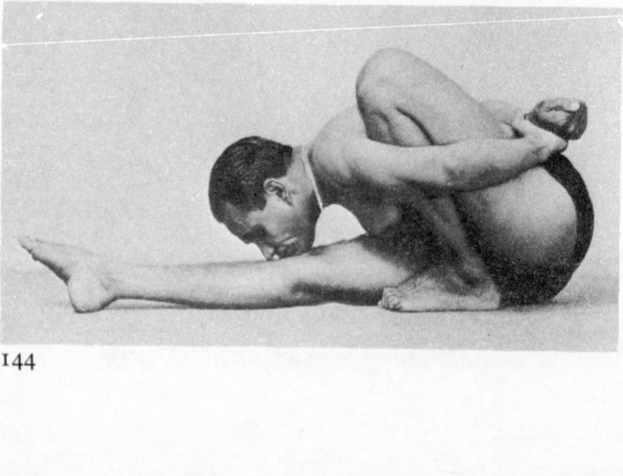

144

straight. Remain in this position gazing at the outstretched right big toe and take a few deep breaths.

5. Exhale, and bend forward. Rest the forehead, then the nose, next the lips and lastly the chin on the right knee. (Plate 144.) While in this position, keep both shoulders parallel to the floor and breathe normally. Stay in the pose for about 30 seconds and see that the back of the entire extended leg rests on the floor throughout.

6. Inhale, raise the head from the right knee (Plate 143), release the hands, straighten the left leg and come to position 1.

7. Repeat the pose on the other side for an equal length of time.

Effects

The fingers gain in strength by the practice of this āsana. In the preceding āsanas (namely, Jānu Śīrṣāsana (Plate 127), Ardha Baddha Padma Paschimottānāsana (Plate 135) and Triang Mukhaikapāda Paschimottānāsana (Plate 139) the abdominal organs are made to contract by gripping a leg with the hands. In this pose the hands do not hold the legs. To bend forward and to rest the chin on the knee of the extended leg the abdominal organs have to contract vigorously. This creates a better circulation of blood round the abdominal organs and keeps them healthy. In the beginning it is very difficult to bend forward at all after gripping both hands behind the back, but it comes with practice. The dorsal region of the spine is also exercised in this pose.

Note. The four poses, Jānu Śīrṣāsana, Ardha Baddha Padma Paschimottānāsana, Triang Mukhaikapāda Paschimottānāsana and Marīchyāsana I, are preparatory poses for the correct Paschimottānāsana. (Plate 161.) It is difficult for many to get a good grip on the feet in Paschimottānāsana (Plate 160) even after several attempts. These four āsanas give one sufficient elasticity in the back and legs so that one gradually achieves the correct Paschimottānāsana (Plate 161) as described later. Once this is done with ease, these four āsanas can be practised once or twice a week instead of daily.

65. *Marīchyāsana II* Six* (Plates 146 and 147)

Technique

1. Sit on the floor, with the legs stretched straight in front. (Plate 77)

2. Bend the left leg at the knee and place the left foot at the root of the right thigh. The left heel should press the navel and the toes be stretched and pointing. The left leg is now in half Padmāsana.

3. Bend the right leg at the knee. Place the sole and heel of the right foot flat on the floor. Keep the shin of the right leg perpendicular, so that

the right thigh and the right calf touch each other and the right heel touches the perineum.

4. Bend slightly forward, stretch the right shoulder forward until the right armpit touches the perpendicular right shin. With an exhalation, curl the right arm round the right shin and thigh, bend the right elbow and turn the right forearm behind the back at the level of the waist. Then move the left hand behind the back and clasp the right hand with the left at the wrist. (Plate 145)

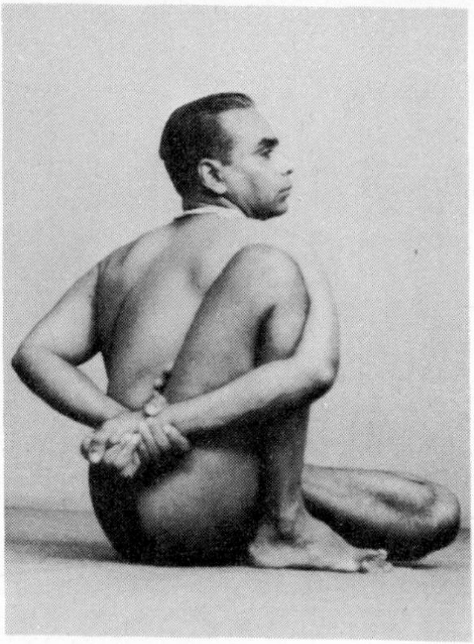

145

5. Stretch the spine up and hold this position for a few seconds, breathing deeply.

6. Exhale, move the trunk and head forward and rest the head on the bent left knee. Then extend the neck and rest the chin on the left knee. (Plates 146 and 147.) Repeat this movement three or four times, inhaling while coming up and exhaling while going down.

7. Inhale, move the head and trunk up, release the hands, straighten the legs, and then repeat the pose on the other side for the same length of time.

Effects

As this pose is an intensified form of Marīchyāsana I (Plate 144), its effects are greater. The heel at the navel puts extra pressure on the abdomen so that the abdominal organs are toned better and grow stronger and digestive power increases.

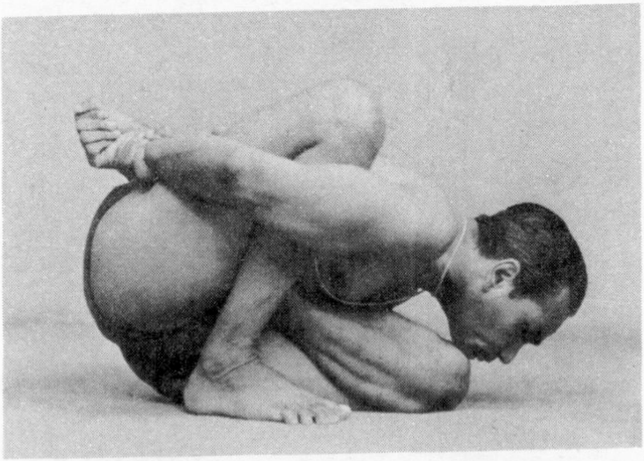

146

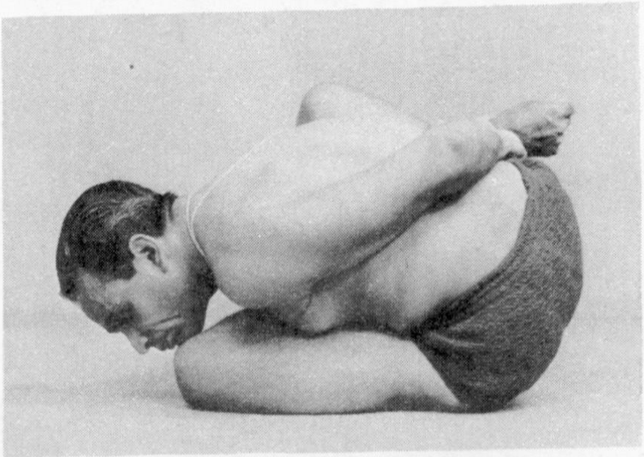

147

66. *Upaviṣṭha Koṇāsana* Nine* (Plate 151)

Upaviṣṭha means seated. Koṇa means an angle.

Technique

1. Sit on the floor with the legs stretched straight in front. (Plate 77)

2. Move the legs sideways one by one and widen the distance between them as far as you can. Keep the legs extended throughout and see that the back of the entire legs rests on the floor.

3. Catch the big toes between the respective thumbs and index and middle fingers.

4. Keep the spine erect and extend the ribs. Pull the diaphragm up and hold the pose for a few seconds with deep breaths. (Plate 148)

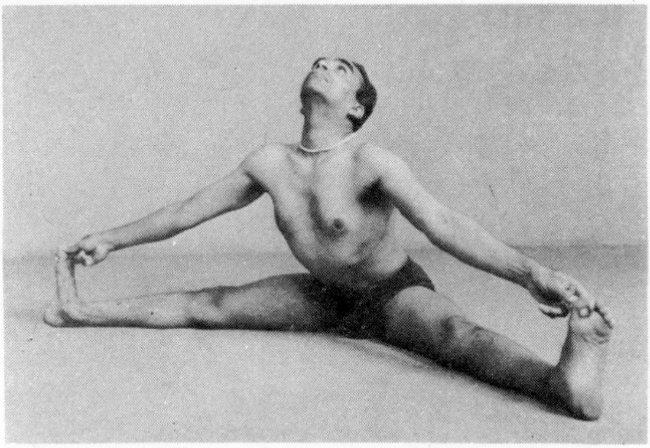

148

5. Exhale, bend forward and rest the head on the floor. (Plate 149.) Then extend the neck and place the chin on the floor. (Plate 150)

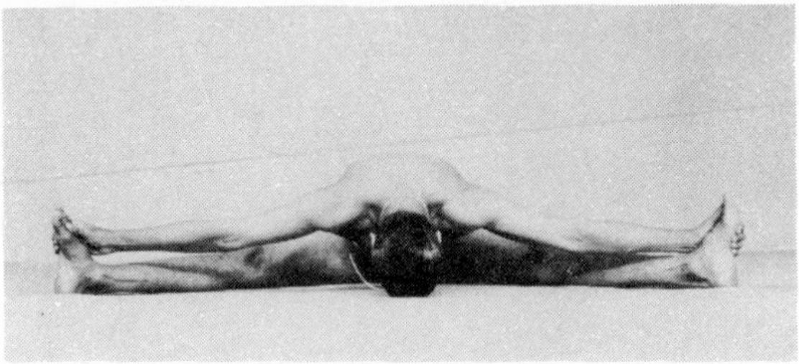

149

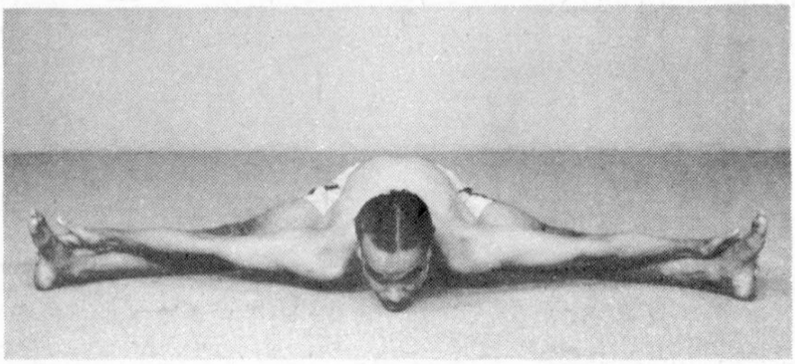

150

6. Then, clasp the feet with the hands and try to rest the chest on the floor. (Plate 151.) Stay in this position from 30 to 60 seconds with normal breathing.

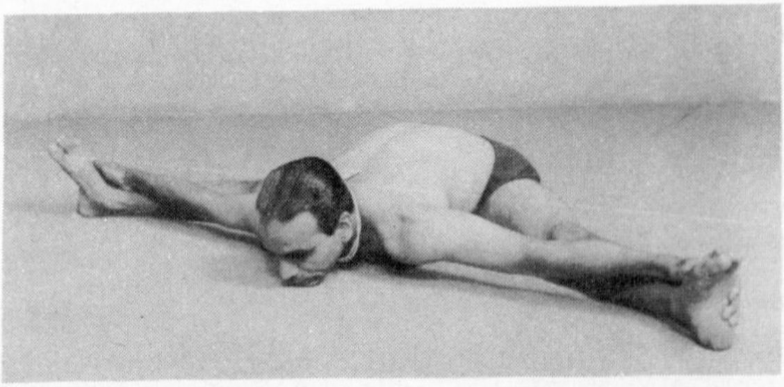

151

7. Inhale, raise the trunk off the floor (Plate 148) and release the hold on the feet, bring them together and relax.

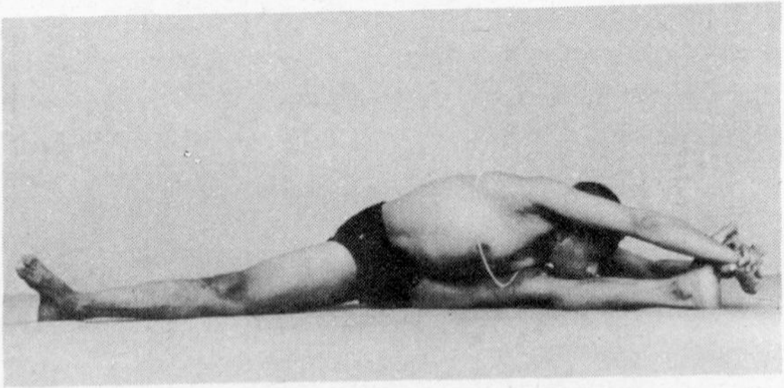

152

8. Hold the left foot with both hands, exhale and rest the chin on the left knee. (Plate 152.) Inhale and raise the head and trunk. Now catch the right foot and with an exhalation rest the chin on the right knee. Inhale, raise the head and trunk, release the hands, bring the feet together and relax.

Effects

The āsana stretches the hamstrings and helps the blood to circulate properly in the pelvic region and keeps it healthy. It prevents the development of hernia of which it can cure mild cases and relieves sciatic pains. Since the āsana controls and regularises the menstrual flow and also stimulates the ovaries, it is a boon to women.

67. *Paschimottānāsana* Six* (Plate 161)

(Also called Ugrāsana or Brahmacharyāsana)
Paschima literally means the west. It implies the back of the whole body from the head to the heels. The anterior or eastern aspect is the front of the body from the face down to the toes. The crown of the head is the upper or northern aspect while the soles and heels of the feet form the lower or southern aspect of the body. In this āsana the back of the whole body is intensely stretched, hence the name.

Ugra means formidable, powerful and noble. Brahmacharya means religious study, self-restraint and celibacy.

Technique

1. Sit on the floor with the legs stretched straight in front. Place the palms on the floor by the side of the hips. Take a few deep breaths. (Plate 77)

2. Exhale, extend the hands and catch the toes. Hold the right big toe between the right thumb and the index and middle fingers and likewise the left big toe. (Plate 153)

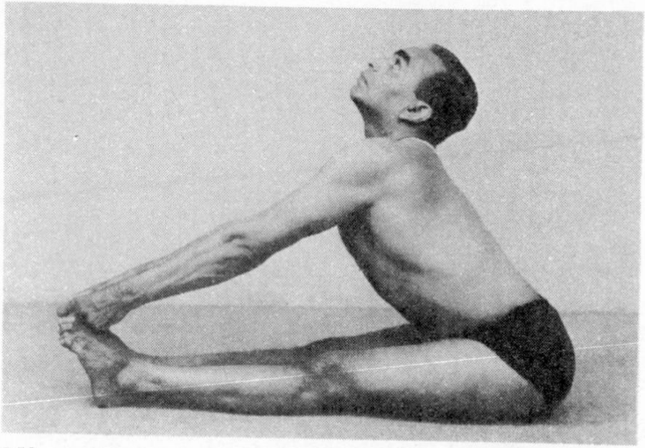

153

3. Extend the spine and try to keep the back concave. To start with the back will be like a hump. This is due to stretching the spine only from the area of the shoulders. Learn to bend right from the pelvic region of the back and also to extend the arms from the shoulders. Then the hump will disappear and the back will become flat as in Plate 153. Take a few deep breaths.

4. Now exhale, bend and widen the elbows, using them as levers, pull the trunk forward and touch the forehead to the knees. (Plate 154.)

Gradually rest the elbows on the floor, stretch the neck and trunk, touch the knees with the nose and then with the lips. (Plate 155)

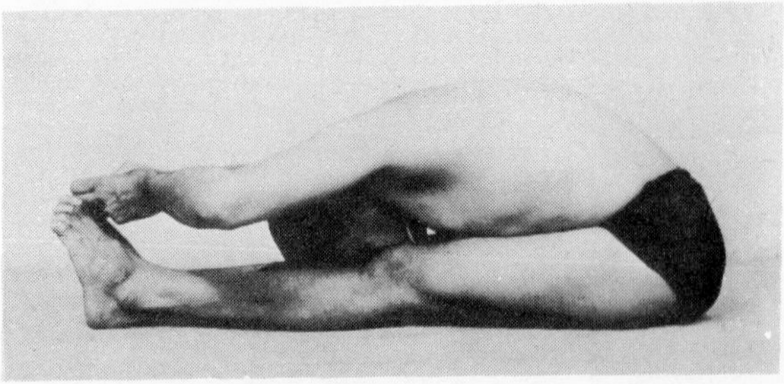

154

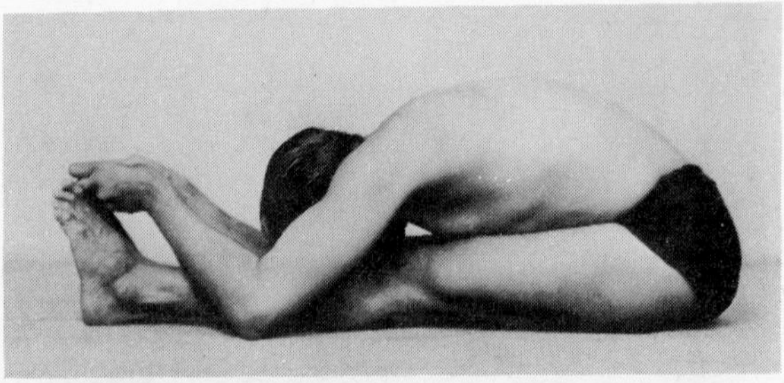

155

5. When this becomes easy, make a further effort to grip the soles and rest the chin on the knees. (Plate 156)

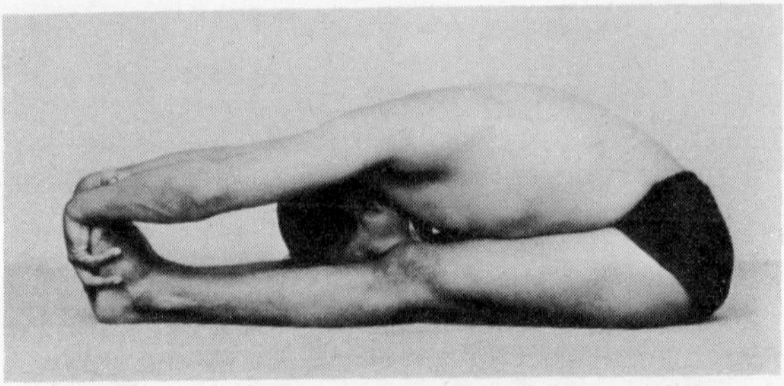

156

6. When this also becomes easy, clasp the hands by interlocking the fingers and rest the chin on the shins beyond the knees. (Plate 157)

7. When position 6 becomes easy, grip the right palm with the left hand

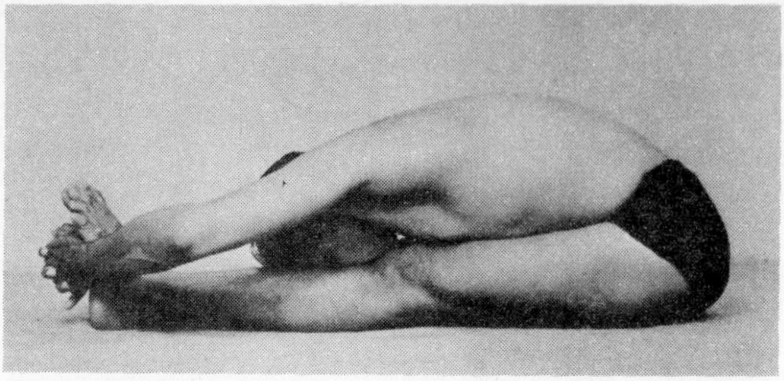

157

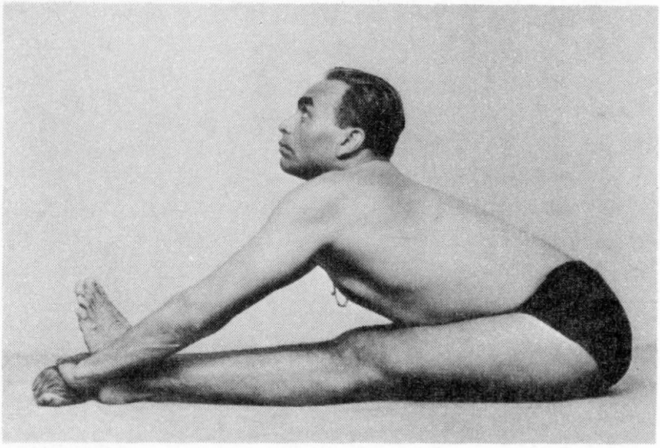

158

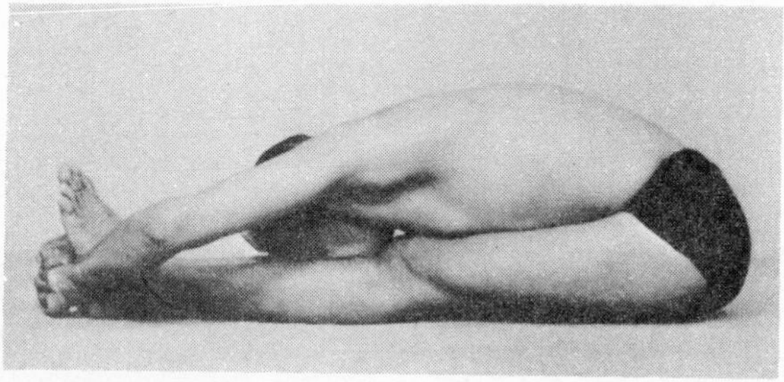

159

or the left palm with the right hand beyond the outstretched feet and keep the back concave. (Plate 158.) Take a few deep breaths.

8. Exhale and rest the chin on the shins beyond the knees. (Plate 159)

9. If position 8 also becomes easy, hold the right wrist with the left hand or the left wrist with the right hand and rest the chin on the shins beyond the knees. (Plate 160)

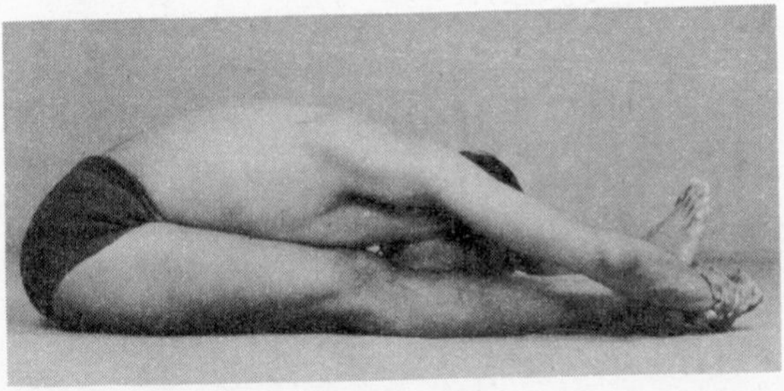

160

10. See that the back of the legs at the knee joints rests firmly on the ground. In the initial stages the knees will be lifted off the floor. Tighten the muscles at the back of the thighs and pull the trunk forward. Then the back of the knee joints will rest on the floor.

11. Try and stay in whichever of the above positions you can achieve from 1 to 5 minutes, breathing evenly.

12. Advanced pupils may extend the hand straight, rest the palms on the floor, join the thumbs beyond the outstretched feet and rest the chin on the shins beyond the knees. (Plate 161.) Stay for a minute or two with even breathing.

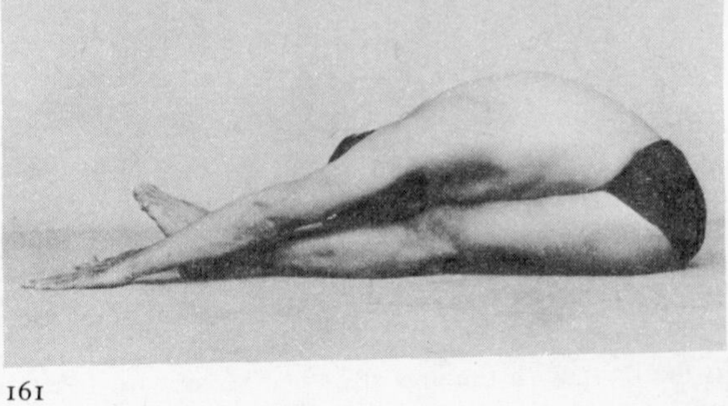

161

13. Inhale, raise the head from the knees and relax.

14. One does not feel any weight on the back in correct Paschimottanāsana. (Plate 162)

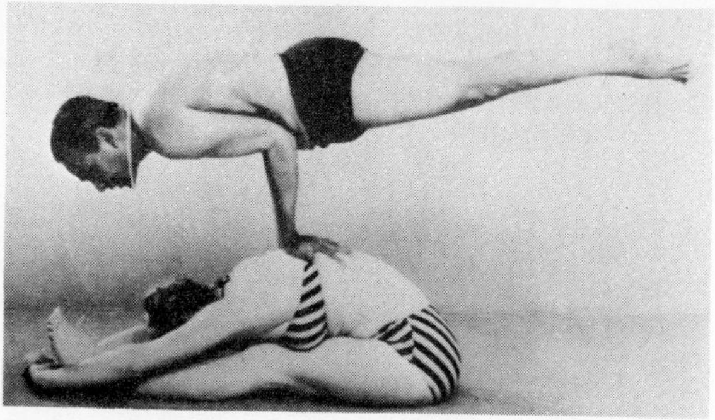

162

Effects

This āsana tones the abdominal organs and keeps them free from sluggishness. It also tones the kidneys, rejuvenates the whole spine and improves the digestion.

The spines of animals are horizontal and their hearts are below the spine. This keeps them healthy and gives them great power of endurance. In humans the spine is vertical and the heart is not lower than the spine, so that they soon feel the effects of exertion and are also susceptible to the heart diseases. In Paschimottānāsana the spine is kept straight and horizontal and the heart is at a lower level than the spine. A good stay in this pose massages the heart, the spinal column and the abdominal organs, which feel refreshed and the mind is rested. Due to the extra stretch given to the pelvic region more oxygenated blood is brought there and the gonad glands absorb the required nutrition from the blood. This increases vitality, helps to cure impotency and leads to sex control. Hence, this āsana was called Brahmacharyāsana. Brahmacharya means celibacy and a Brahmachāri is one who has controlled the sex appetite.

68. *Parivṛtta Paschimottānāsana* Nine* (Plate 165)

Parivṛtta means turned around, revolved. Paschima literally means the west and refers to the back of the entire body from the head to the heels. Uttāna means an intense stretch. In this variation of Paschimottānāsana the trunk is twisted on one side.

Technique

1. Sit on the floor with the legs stretched straight in front. Keep the

knees tight and the legs touching each other at the knees, ankles, heels and big toes. (Plate 77)

2. Exhale, extend the right arm towards the left foot. Twist the right forearm and the right wrist so that the right thumb points to the floor and the right little finger points up. Then with the right hand hold the outer side of the left foot. Take a breath.

3. Now, exhale, extend the left arm over the right forearm keeping the left wrist up. Twist the left forearm and the left wrist so that the left thumb points to the floor and the left little finger points up. Hold the outer side of the right foot (Plate 163) and take a breath.

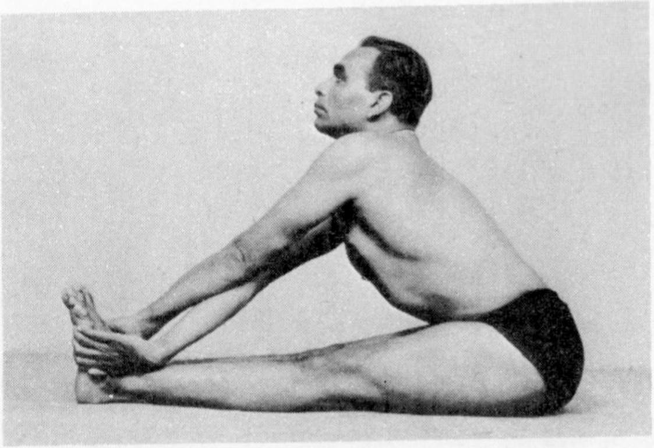

163

4. Exhale, twist the trunk about 90 degrees to the left by bending and widening the elbows. (Plate 164.) Take a breath. Exhale again, move the head between the arms and look up. The back portion of the upper right arm near the armpit will rest across the left knee. Try and rest the right side ribs on the left thigh. (Front view: Plate 165. Back view: Plate 166.) Due to the lateral twist of the trunk, breathing will be fast. Hold the pose for about 20 seconds.

5. Inhale, release the hands and move the trunk back to its original position. (Plate 163)

6. Now twist the trunk to the right and repeat the pose for the same length of time, following the technique given above, but substituting the word 'left' for the word 'right' and the word 'right' for the word 'left'.

Effects

This invigorating posture tones the abdominal organs and keeps them

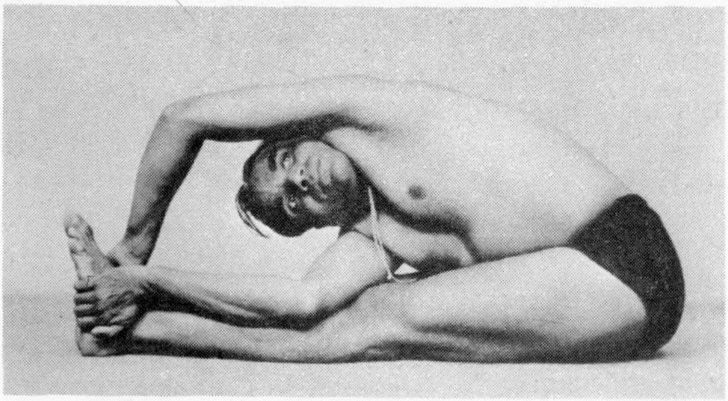

164

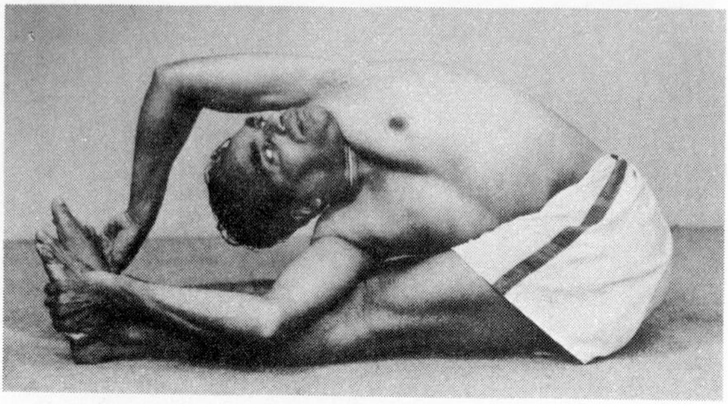

165

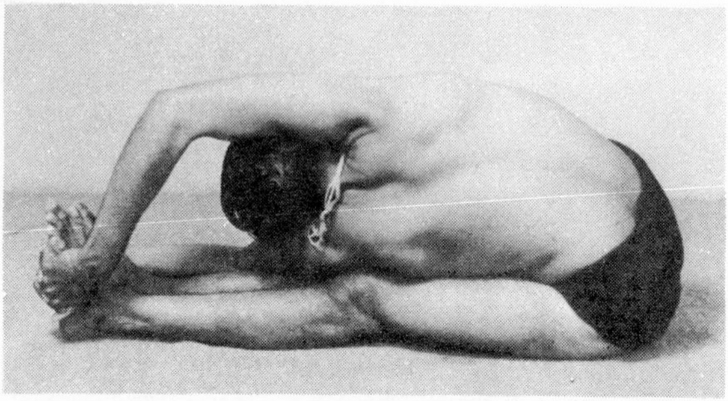

166

free from sluggishness. It also tones the kidneys and rejuvenates the entire spine, while the digestion is improved. The lateral twist stimulates blood circulation in the spine and relieves backaches. Due to the stretch of the pelvic region, more oxygenated blood is brought there and the gonad glands absorb the required nutrition from the blood. This increases vitality, helps to cure impotency and promotes sex control.

69. *Ūrdhva Mukha Paschimottānāsana I* Ten* (Plate 168)

Ūrdhva (upwards) and Mukha (face, mouth) when used together mean having the face upwards. Paschimottānāsana is the intense posterior stretch.

Technique

1. Sit on the floor with the legs stretched straight in front. (Plate 77)

2. Flex the knees and bring the feet closer to the buttocks.

3. Catch the toes with the hands, exhale and stretch the legs up in the air, straighten them at the knees, pull the knee-caps towards the thighs and balance on the buttocks, keeping the spine as concave as you can. This position is called:

70. *Ubhaya Pādānguṣṭhāsana* Three* (Plate 167)

(Ubhaya = both, pādānguṣṭha = big toe)
To start with one rolls over backwards to the floor, and it takes some time and practice to learn to balance on the buttocks alone. Stay in the pose from 30 to 60 seconds with normal breathing.

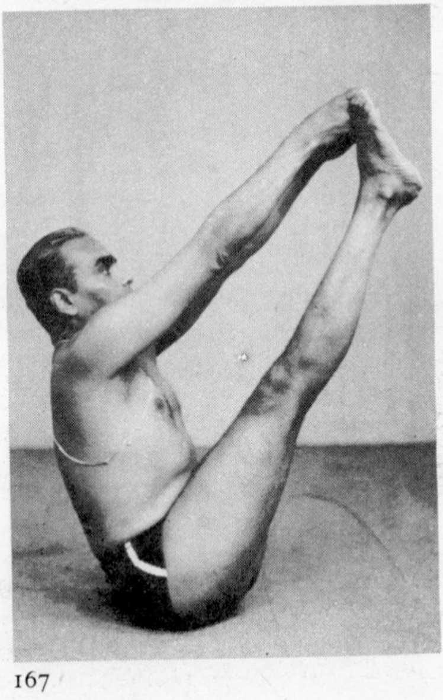

167

4. After securing the balance, release the toes and hold the heels.

5. When this becomes easy, interlock the fingers behind the extended feet and balance. Then without disturbing the position of the legs, move the head and trunk nearer to them, stretch the neck up and with an exhalation rest the forehead on the knees. (Plate 168.) Now stretch the legs up to the full extent and also the spine. Hold the pose for about 30 seconds with normal breathing.

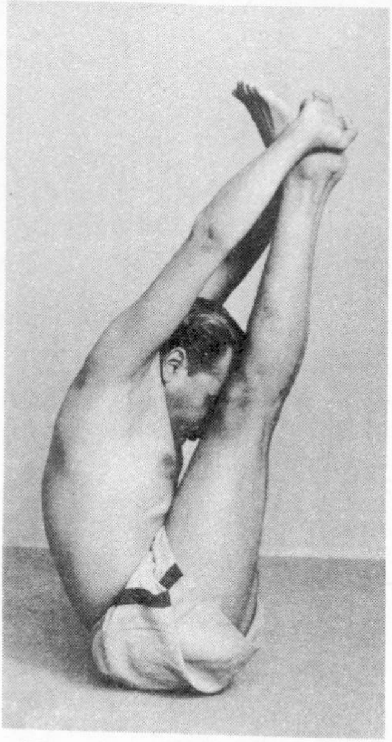

168

6. Inhale, release the hands, bend the legs, rest them on the floor and relax.

71. *Ūrdhva Mukha Paschimottānāsana II* Ten* (Plate 170)

Technique

1. Lie flat on the floor or carpet and place the hands straight over the head. (Plate 276)

2. Stretch the legs straight, tighten the knees and take a few deep breaths.

3. Exhale and slowly raise the legs together and bring them over the head.

4. Interlock the fingers, clasp the soles and stretch the legs straight up with the knees kept tight. Rest the entire back on the floor. (Plate 169.) Take three deep breaths.

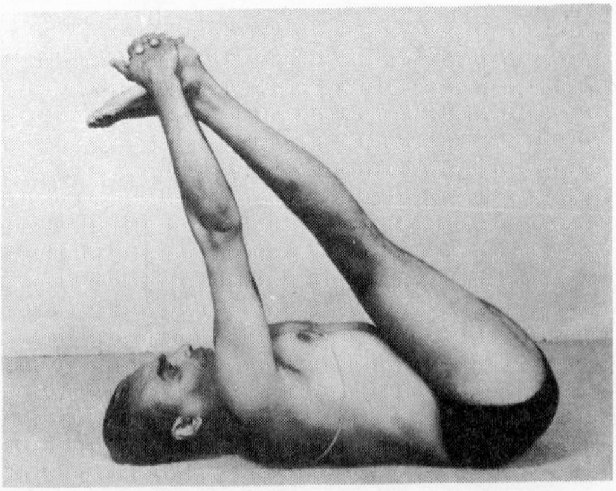

169

5. Exhale, lower the legs towards the floor beyond the head by widening the elbows. Try and keep the pelvis as near the floor as possible. Keep the legs tightened at the knees throughout. Rest the chin on the knees. (Plate 170)

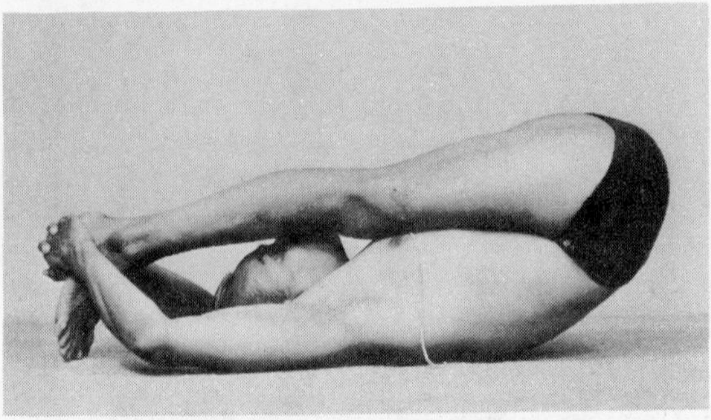

170

6. Stay in the position from 30 to 60 seconds, breathing evenly.

7. Exhale and move the legs to the original position. (Plate 169)

8. Inhale, release the hands, bring the legs straight to the floor (Plate 276) and relax.

Effects

The pose helps balance and poise. The legs stretch fully which makes the thighs and calves shapely. The benefits are the same as those of Paschimottānāsana (Plate 160), and in addition this pose prevents hernia and relieves severe backaches.

72. *Pūrvottānāsana* One* (Plate 171)

Pūrva literally means the East. It means the front of the whole body from the forehead to the toes. Uttāna means an intense stretch. In this posture, the whole front of the body is stretched intensely.

Technique

1. Sit on the floor with the legs stretched straight in front. Place the palms on the floor by the hips, with the fingers pointing in the direction of the feet. (Plate 77)

2. Bend the knees and place the soles and heels on the floor.

3. Take the pressure of the body on the hands and feet, exhale and lift the body off the floor. Straighten the arms and the legs and keep the knees and elbows tightened. (Plate 171)

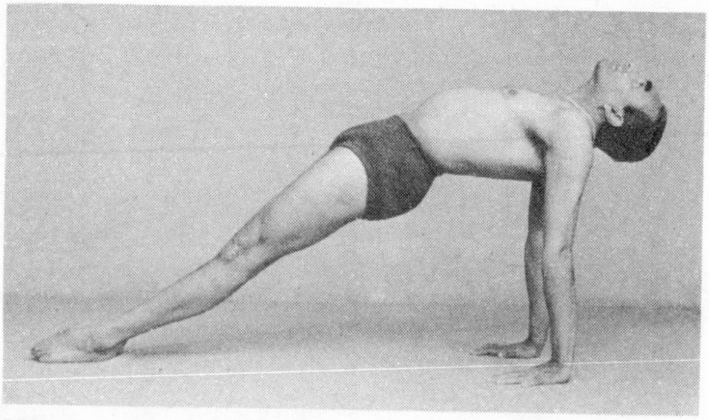

171

4. The arms will be perpendicular to the floor from the wrists to the shoulders. From the shoulders to the pelvis, the trunk will be parallel to the floor.

5. Stretch the neck and throw the head as far back as possible.

6. Stay in this posture for one minute, breathing normally.

7. Exhale, bend the elbows and knees, lower the body to sit on the floor and relax.

Effects

This posture strengthens the wrists and ankles, improves the movement of the shoulder joints and expands the chest fully. It gives relief from the fatigue caused by doing other strenuous forward bending āsanas.

73. *Ākarṇa Dhanurāsana* Eleven* (Plates 173 and 175)

Karṇa means the ear. The prefix ā expresses the sense of near to, towards. Dhanu means a bow. In this posture, the left foot is pulled up till the heel touches the ear as an archer pulls the bow-string, while the other hand holds the right big toe, this leg lying straight on the floor. In the second movement the raised leg is straightened up until it is almost perpendicular, the big toe being held throughout by the hand like an extended bow.

The āsana is given below in two movements.

Technique

1. Sit on the floor with the legs stretched straight in front. (Plate 77)

2. Hold the right big toe between the right thumb and the index and middle fingers. Similarly hold the left big toe. (Plate 153)

3. Exhale, bend the left elbow and lift the left foot up by bending the knee. (Plate 172.) Take a breath. Now exhale and pull the left foot up until the heel is close to the left ear. At the same time draw the left arm back from the shoulder. (Plate 173.) Do not let go of the right big toe. Keep the right leg extended throughout and see that the back of the entire leg rests on the floor. The extended right leg should not bend at the knee.

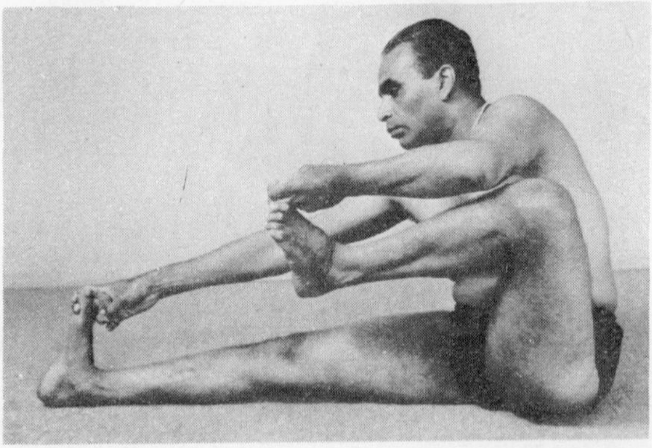

172

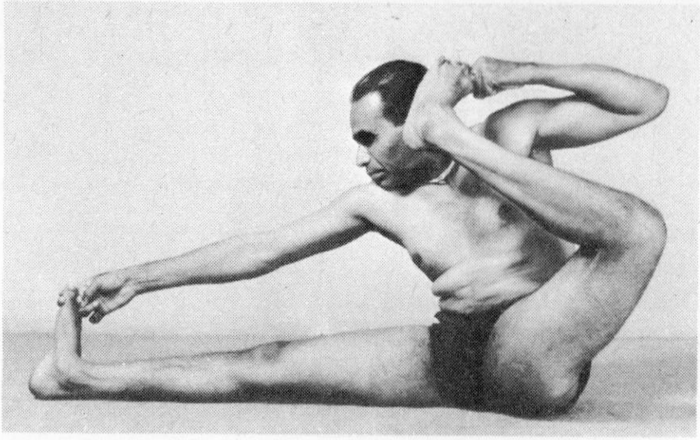

173

4. Hold this position from 15 to 20 seconds with normal breathing. This is the first movement.

5. Now exhale and stretch the left leg up vertically. (Plate 174.) Take a breath. Exhale, draw the leg further back until it touches the left ear. (Plate 175.) Continue to grip the toes of both feet and fully extend both legs. Do not bend them at the knees. It takes some time to learn to balance in this second movement. Remain in this position from 10 to 15 seconds, breathing normally.

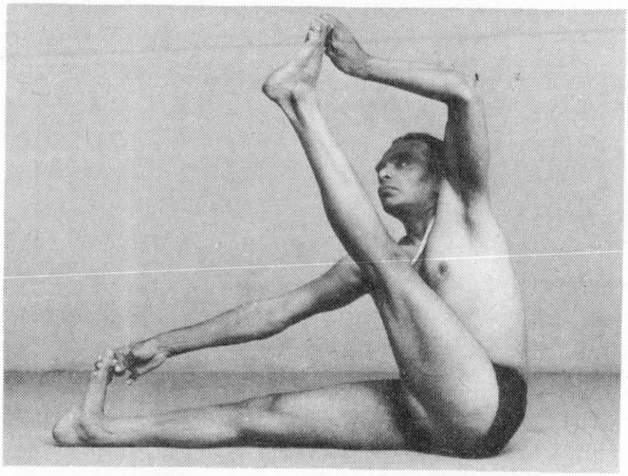

174

6. Exhale, bend the left leg at the knee and bring the left heel to the left ear as in position 3 above. (Plate 173.) Then lower the left leg to the floor and keep both legs stretched on the floor. (Plate 153)

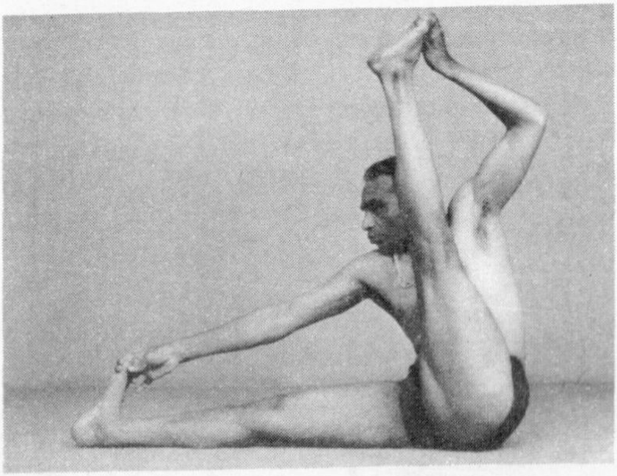

175

7. Repeat the pose on the right side, pulling the right foot towards the right ear and raising it up vertically near the right ear, while keeping the left leg straight on the floor. Do not relax the hand grip of the toes. Maintain the position on both sides for an equal length of time. Then release the hands and relax.

Effects

The practice of this posture makes the leg muscles very flexible. The abdominal muscles are contracted and this helps to move the bowels. Minor deformities in the hip joints are adjusted. The lower portion of the spine is exercised. The pose is full of grace. It should be practised until it comes effortlessly and gives the appearance of a trained archer discharging arrows from his bow.

74. *Sālamba Śīrṣāsana I* Four* (Plates 184, 185 and 190)

Sālamba means with support. Śīrṣa means the head. This is the head stand pose, one of the most important Yogic āsanas. It is the basic posture. It has several variations, which are described later as the Śīrṣāsana cycle. Its mastery gives one balance and poise, both physically and mentally. The technique of doing it is given at length in two parts; the first is for beginners, the second for those who can remain balanced in the pose. Attention is specially directed to the hints on Śīrṣāsana given after the two techniques.

Technique for beginners

1. Spread a blanket fourfold on the floor and kneel near it.

2. Rest the forearms on the centre of the blanket. While doing so take care that the distance between the elbows on the floor is not wider than the shoulders.

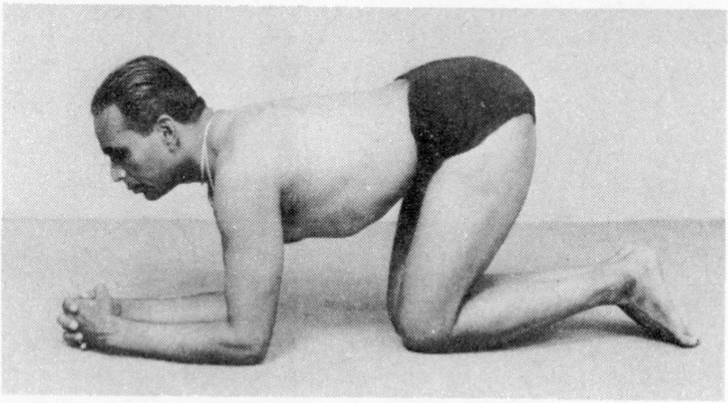

176

3. Interlock the fingers right up to the finger-tips (Plate 176), so that the palms form a cup. Place the sides of the palms near the little fingers on the blanket. While going up on to your head or balancing, the fingers should be kept tightly locked. If they are left loose, the weight of the body falls on them and the arms ache. So remember to lock them well.

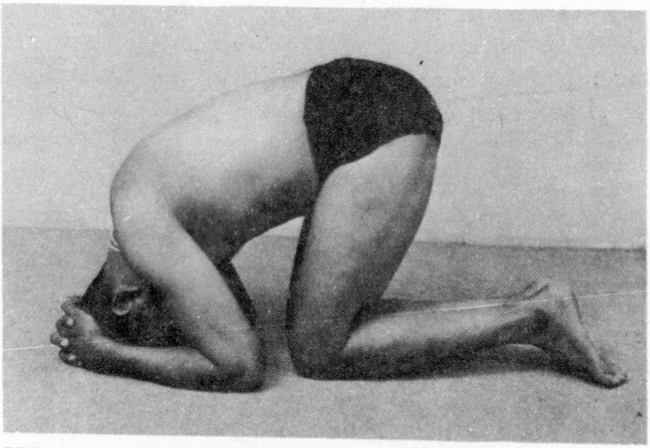

177

4. Rest the crown of the head only on the blanket, so that the back of the head touches the palms which are cupped. (Plate 177.) Do not rest the forehead nor the back but only the crown of the head on the blanket. To do this move the knees towards the head.

5. After securing the head position, raise the knees from the floor by moving the toes closer to the head. (Plate 178)

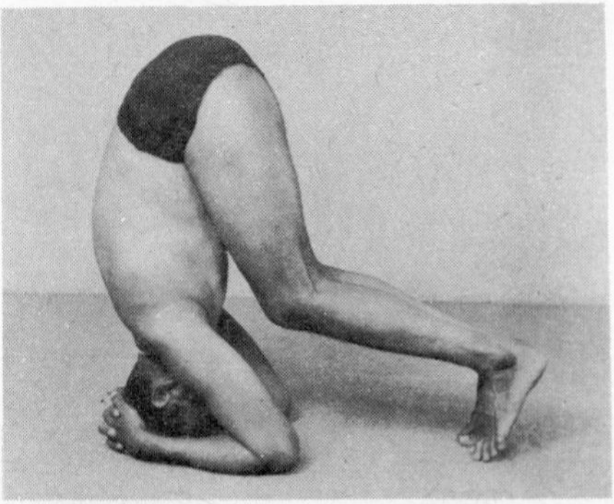
178

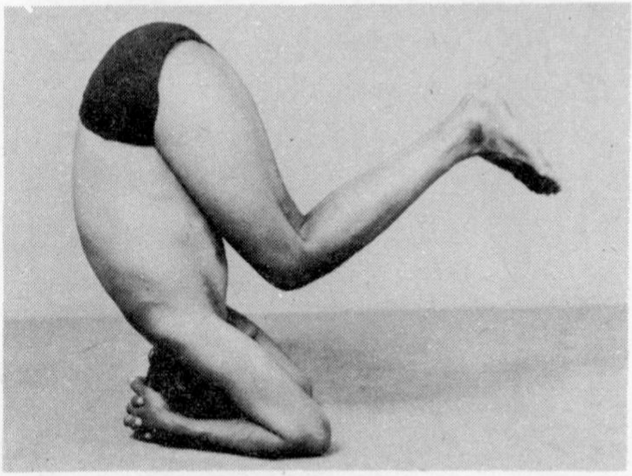
179

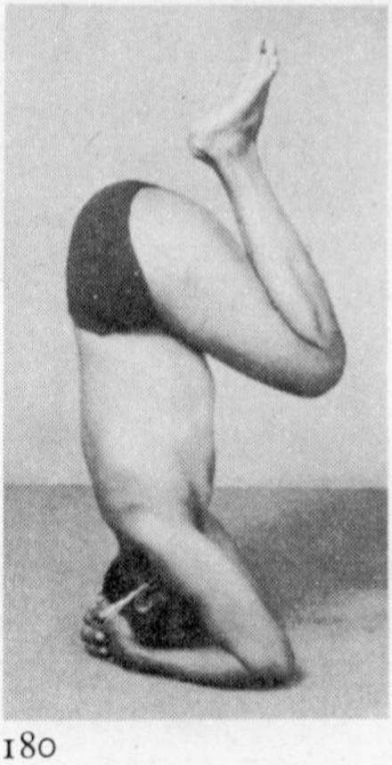
180

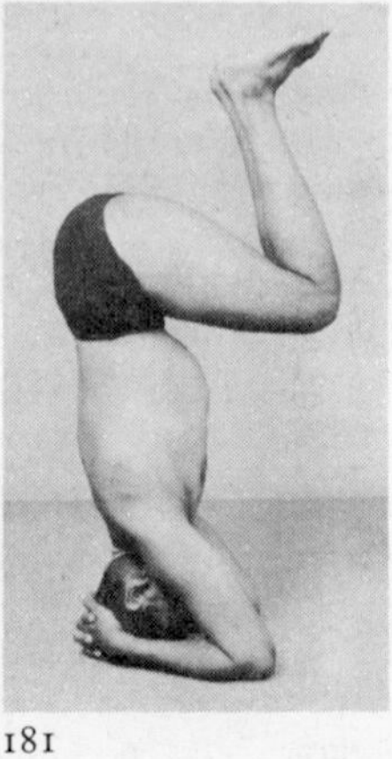
181

6. Exhale, take a gentle swing from the floor and lift the legs off the ground with bent knees. (Plate 179.) Take the swing in such a way that both feet leave the floor simultaneously. When once this position is secured, follow the various stages of the leg movements as in Plates 180, 181, 182 and 183, step by step.

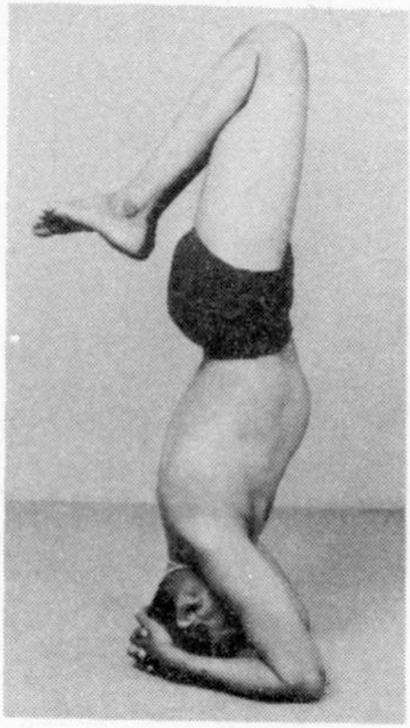

182

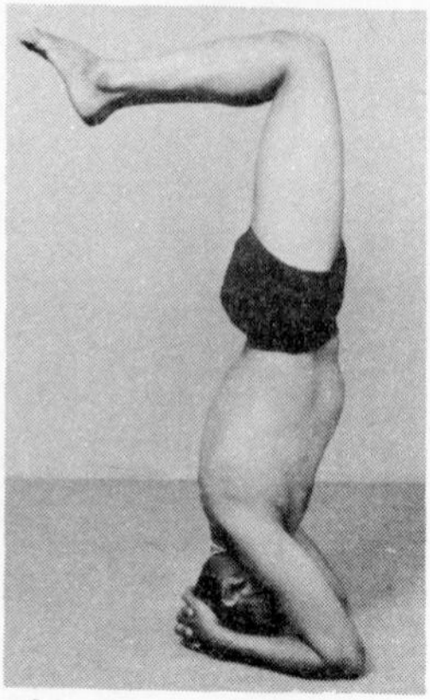

183

7. Stretch the legs and stand on the head, keeping the whole body perpendicular to the floor. (Front view: Plate 184. Back view: Plate 185. Side view: Plate 190)

8. After staying in the final position to capacity, from one to five minutes, flex the knees and slide down to the floor in the reverse order as in Plates 183, 182, 181, 180, 179, 178 and 177.

9. A beginner must have the assistance of a friend or do the āsana against a wall. While practising against a wall, the distance between it and the head should not be more than 2 or 3 inches. If the distance is greater, the spine will curve and the stomach will protrude. The weight of the body will be felt on the elbows and the position of the head may change. The face will appear to be flushed and the eyes either strained or puffed. It is, therefore, advisable for a beginner to do the head stand in a corner where two walls meet, placing the head some 2 to 3 inches from either wall.

10. While doing the head stand against a wall or in a corner, the beginner should exhale, swing the legs up, support the hips against the side of the wall and move the feet up. In a corner, he can touch the heels to either side of the walls. He should then stretch the back vertically up, gradually leave the support of the wall and learn to

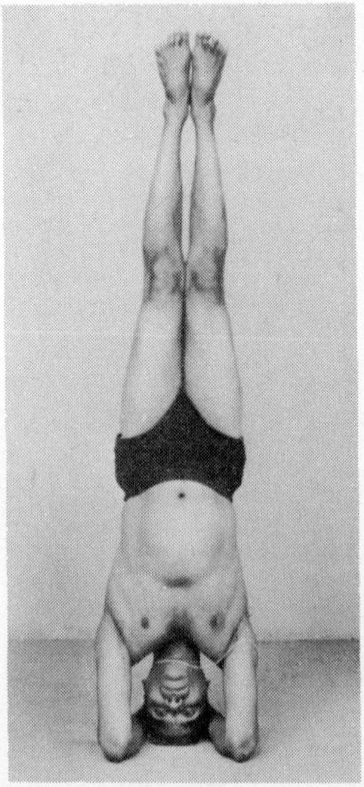
184

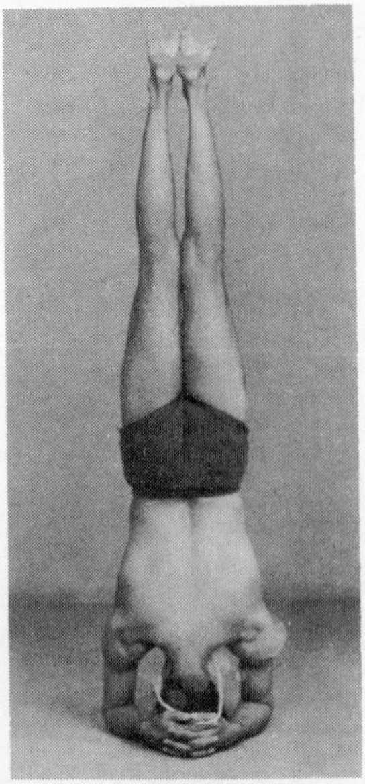
185

master the balance. While coming down, he can rest the feet and hips against the wall, slide down and kneel, resting his knees on the floor. The movements of coming down and going up should be done with an exhalation.

11. The advantage which the beginner has of balancing in a corner is that his head and legs will be in the right angle formed by the walls, and he will be sure of his right position. This will not be the case if he balances against a straight wall. For while his balance is insecure he may sway from the wall, or his body may tilt or swing to the stronger side, while his legs may rest against the wall with a bend either at the waist or the hips. The beginner will not be in a position to know that he has tilted to one side, much less to correct it. In time he may learn to balance on the head, but by habit his body may still tilt or his head may not be straight. It is as hard to correct a wrong pose in the head stand as it is to break a bad habit. Moreover this wrong posture may well lead to aches and pains in the head, neck, shoulders and back. But the two walls of a corner will help the beginner to keep the āsana symmetrical.

12. When once balance is secured, it is advisable to come down to the floor with the legs straight (that is, without bending the knees

at all) and with a backward action of the hips. At first, it is not possible to go up and come down without bending the legs, but the correct method should be learnt. Once the beginner has confidence in the head stand, he will find it more beneficial to go up and down with the legs together and straight, without any jerks.

13. It takes time for the beginner to become oriented to his surroundings while he is balancing on his head. Everything will seem at first to be completely unfamiliar. The directions and instructions will appear confusing and he will find it an effort to think clearly or to act logically. This is due to fear of a fall. The best way to overcome fear is to face with equanimity the situation of which one is afraid. Then one gets the correct perspective, and one is not frightened any more. To topple over while learning the head stand is not as terrible as we imagine. If one overbalances, one should remember to loosen the interlocked fingers, relax, go limp and flex the knees. Then one will just roll over and smile. If the fingers are not loosened they will take the jerk of the fall which will be painful. If we do not relax and go limp while falling we hit the floor with a hard bump. If we flex the knees, we are unlikely to graze them in the fall. After one has learnt to balance against a wall or in a corner, one should try the head stand in the middle of the room. There will be a few spills and one must learn the art of falling as indicated above. Learning to do Śīrṣāsana in the middle of a room gives the beginner great confidence.

Technique for those who can balance Eight*

1. Follow the technique described for beginners from positions 1 to 4.

2. After securing the head position, stretch the legs straight by raising the knees from the floor. Move the toes nearer to the head and try to press the heels to the floor, keeping the back erect. (Plate 186)

3. Stretch the dorsal or middle region of the spine and stay in this position for about 30 seconds while breathing evenly.

4. Exhale, raise the heels and take the toes off the floor with a backward movement of the hips. Raise both legs simultaneously, keeping them poker stiff. (Plate 187.) Take a breath.

5. Again with an exhalation move the legs up until they are parallel to the floor. This position is called:

75. *Ūrdhvā Daṇḍāsana* Eight* (Plate 188)

(Ūrdhvā = up, daṇḍa = a staff)
Stay in this position for 10 seconds with normal breathing.

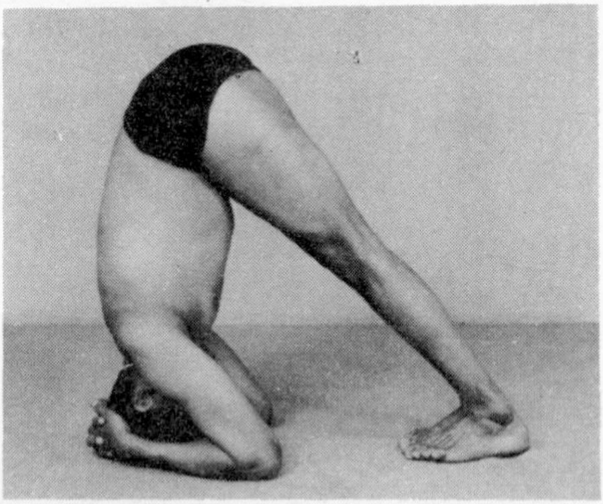

186

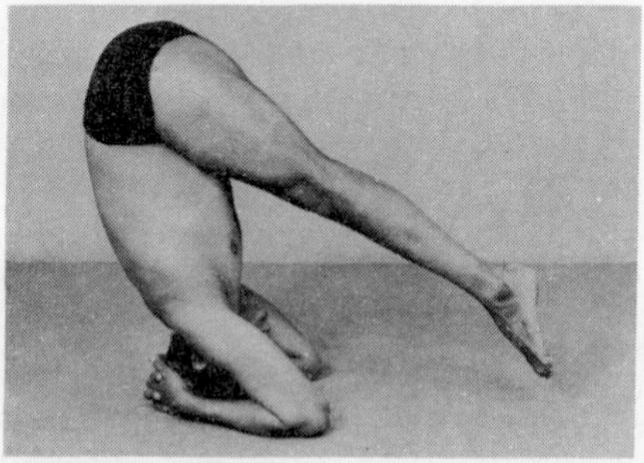

187

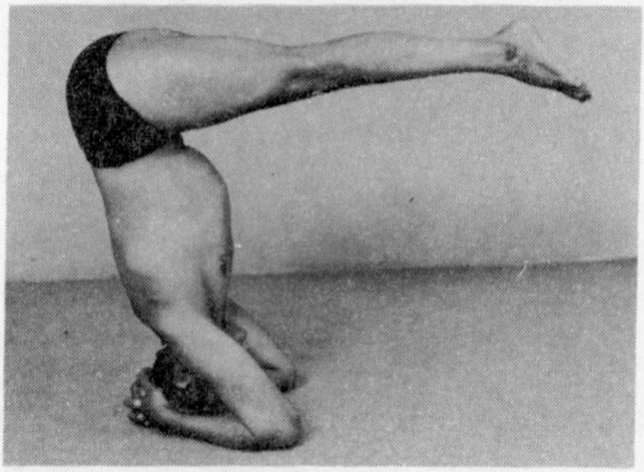

188

6. Exhale, move the legs up as in Plate 189, and then pull them up to the vertical position. (Side view: Plate 190.) Stay in this pose from 1 to 5 minutes while breathing evenly.

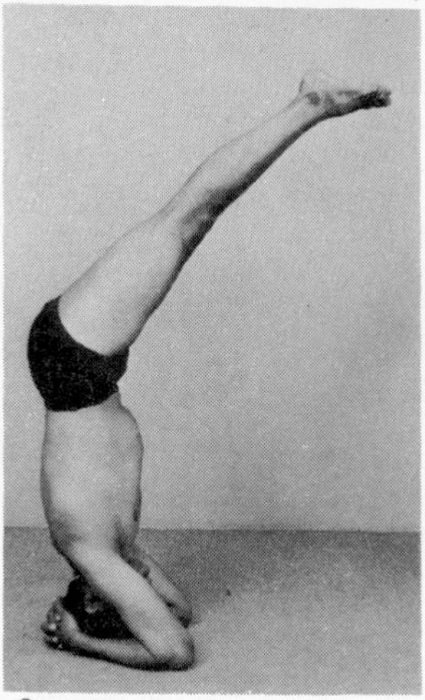

189

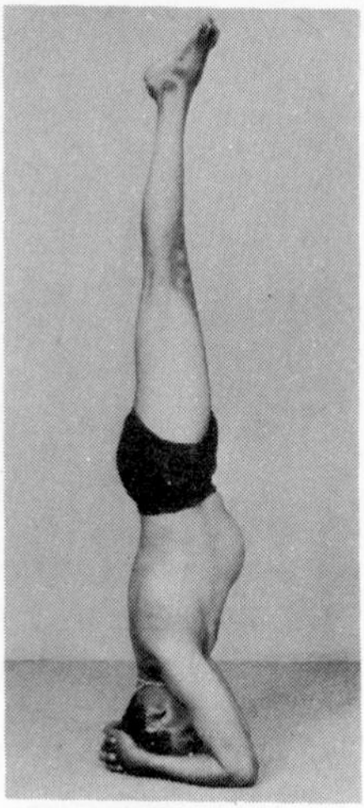

190

7. Come down gradually, observing the above technique in a reverse order. (Plates 189, 188, 187 and 186.) Rest the feet on the floor, bend the knees and raise the head from the floor or blanket.

8. While coming down, it is advisable to stay in Ūrdhvā Daṇḍāsana according to capacity up to one minute while breathing normally. In this position, the neck and trunk will not be perpendicular to the floor but will sway slightly backwards. The neck, shoulders and spine will be put to a very great strain and in the initial stages one cannot stay with the legs parallel to the floor for more than a few seconds. The stay will become longer as the neck, shoulders, abdomen and spine become stronger.

Hints on Śīrṣāsana

1. In Śīrṣāsana the balance alone is not important. One has to watch from moment to moment and find out the subtle adjustments. When we stand on our feet, we need no extra effort, strength or attention, for the position is natural. Yet the correct method of standing affects our bearing and carriage. It is, therefore, necessary to master the correct method as pointed out in the note on Tāḍāsana. In Śīrṣāsana also, the correct position should be mastered, as a faulty posture in this āsana will lead to pains in the head, neck and back.

2. The whole weight of the body should be borne on the head alone and not on the forearms and hands. The forearms and hands are to be used only for support to check any loss of balance. In a good pose you feel a circle, about the size of an Indian rupee, of the head in contact with the blanket on the floor.

3. The back of the head, the trunk, the back of the thighs and the heels should be in a line perpendicular to the floor and not inclined to one side. The throat, chin and breast-bone should be in one line, otherwise the head will tilt to one side or move forward. As regards the interlocked hands behind the head, the palms should not be stuck into the head. The upper and the lower sides of the palms should be in a line, otherwise the crown of the head will not rest on the floor correctly.

4. The elbows and the shoulders should be in a line and the elbows should not be widened. The shoulders should be kept as high above the floor as possible by moving them up and stretching them sideways. In order to learn the correct shoulder stretch, release the interlocked fingers and remove the hands from behind the head and widen the wrists from the forearms, keeping the elbows stationary. Place the wrists on the floor with the palms facing up, touch the shoulders with the fingers, keeping the wrists on the floor and maintain the balance. (Plate 191.) This will not only improve the balance but also prepare you for the other Śīrṣāsana poses described later.

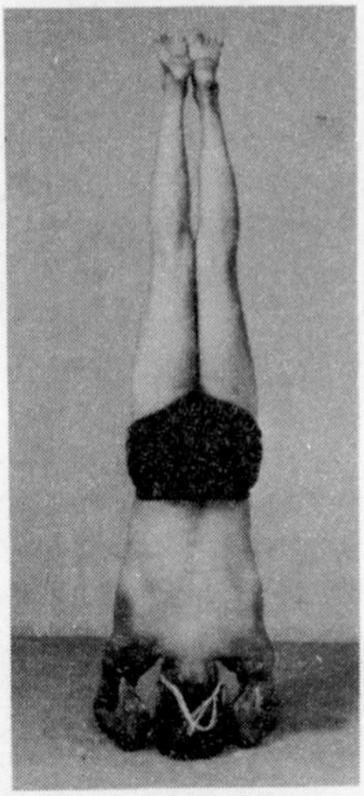

191

5. As to the position of the trunk, the dorsal region should be pushed forward as well as up. The lumbar (waist) and pelvic regions should not be pushed forward, while the trunk from the shoulders to the pelvis should be kept perpendicular. If the pelvic area juts forward, it means that you are bearing the weight of the body not on the head alone but also on the elbows for you have not stretched the dorsal region (the chest) correctly. When viewed from the side, the body from the neck to the heels should appear straight.

6. As far as possible try and join the thighs, knees, ankles and toes. Stretch the legs fully, especially the back of the knees and thighs. If the legs swing back tighten the knees and the lower median portion of the abdomen above the pubes. This will keep the legs perpendicular. Keep the toes pointing up. If the legs swing forward, stretch the dorsal region and push the pelvic area slightly back until it is in line with the shoulders. The body will then feel light and the pose will be exhilarating.

7. While going up or holding the head stand the eyes should never become bloodshot. If they do, the pose is faulty.[1]

8. The time limit for Śīrṣāsana depends upon individual capacity and the time at one's disposal. One can hold it comfortably from 10 to 15 minutes. A beginner can do it for 2 minutes and go up to 5 minutes. It is always difficult for a beginner to balance for one minute, but once he succeeds he can be sure that from then on he will be able to master Śīrṣāsana soon.

9. While going up or coming down, move both legs together, inch by inch. All the movements should be done with exhalation. Inhale while waiting in a position. The effect of going down and coming up straight without bending the legs at the knees is that harmonious slow movement is gained and the flow of blood to the head is controlled. The face does not flush from jerky and fast movements, as the flow of blood to the waist and the legs is also controlled. Then there is no danger of losing balance from giddiness or numbness of the feet when one stands up immediately after the head balance. In course of time the whole movement of going up, staying and coming down should become as effortless as possible. In a perfect Śīrṣāsana your body feels completely stretched and at the same time you experience a feeling of complete relaxation.

[1] I have taught this pose to a lady of 65 who was suffering from glaucoma. Now she finds the eyes are completely rested and the pain in them is much lessened. Medical examination revealed that the tension in the eyeballs had decreased. I am mentioning this to prove the value of the correct head stand.

10. It is always safe to perfect Sarvāngāsana (Plate 223) first before attempting Śīrṣāsana. If the standing poses described earlier (Plates 1 to 36) and the various movements of Sarvangāsana and Halāsana (Plates 234 to 271) are mastered first, Śīrṣāsana will come without much effort. If these elementary āsanas have not been mastered, the period taken to learn Śīrṣāsana will be longer.

11. After one has learnt to balance in Śīrṣāsana, however, it is preferable to perform Śīrṣāsana and its cycle (Plates 190 to 218) first before practising any other āsana. This is because one cannot balance or hold the head stand if the body is exhausted by doing other poses or if the breathing becomes fast and shaky. Once the body is tired or the breathing is not free and easy, the body will shake and it will be difficult to maintain the balance. It is always better to do Śīrṣāsana first when one is fresh.

12. Śīrṣāsana and its cycle should always be followed by Sarvāngāsana and its cycle. It has been observed that people who devote themselves to Śīrṣāsana alone without doing the Sarvāngāsana poses are apt to lose their temper over trifling things and become irritated quickly. The practice of Sarvāngāsana coupled with Śīrṣāsana checks this trait. If Sarvāngāsana is the Mother, then Śīrṣāsana may be regarded as the Father of all āsanas. And just as both parents are necessary for peace and harmony in a home, so the practice of both these āsanas is essential to keep the body healthy and the mind tranquil and peaceful.

Effects of Śīrṣāsana

The ancient books have called Śīrṣāsana the king of all āsanas and the reasons are not hard to find. When we are born, normally the head comes out first and then the limbs. The skull encases the brain, which controls the nervous system and the organs of sense. The brain is the seat of intelligence, knowledge, discrimination, wisdom and power. It is the seat of Brahman, the soul. A country cannot prosper without a proper king or constitutional head to guide it; so also the human body cannot prosper without a healthy brain.

The *Bhagavad-Gītā* says: 'Harmony (sattva), mobility (rajas), inertia (tamas), such are the qualities, matter-born; they bind fast, O great armed one (Arjuna), the indestructible dweller in the body.' (Fourteenth Discourse, verse 5.) All these qualities stem from the brain, and sometimes one quality prevails and sometimes the others. The head is the centre of sattvic qualities which control discrimination; the trunk of Rājasic qualities which control passion, emotion and actions; and the region below the diaphragm of tāmasic qualities which control sensual pleasures like the enjoyment of food and drink, and the thrills and pleasures of sex.

Regular practice of Śīrṣāsana makes healthy pure blood flow through the brain cells. This rejuvenates them so that thinking power increases and thoughts become clearer. The āsana is a tonic for people whose brains tire quickly. It ensures a proper blood supply to the pituitary and pineal glands in the brain. Our growth, health and vitality depend on the proper functioning of these two glands.

People suffering from loss of sleep, memory and vitality have recovered by the regular and correct practice of this āsana and have become fountains of energy. The lungs gain the power to resist any climate and stand up to any work, which relieves one from colds, coughs, tonsillitis, halitosis (foul breath) and palpitations. It keeps the body warm. Coupled with Sarvāngāsana movements (Plates 234 to 271), it is a boon to people suffering from constipation. Regular practice of Śīrṣāsana will show marked improvement in the haemoglobin content of the blood.

It is not advisable to start with Śīrṣāsana and Sarvāngāsana when one suffers from high or low blood pressure.

Regular and precise practice of Śīrṣāsana develops the body, disciplines the mind and widens the horizons of the spirit. One becomes balanced and self-reliant in pain and pleasure, loss and gain, shame and fame and defeat and victory.

The Śīrṣāsana Cycle

In Śīrṣāsana there is a variety of movements which can be practised at one stretch after staying in Sālamba Śīrṣāsana I (Plate 184) for not less than 5 minutes according to one's capacity. One may practise for 5 to 15 minutes and then perform these various movements for 20 to 30 seconds on each side at a time.

76. *Sālamba Śīrṣāsana II* Five* (Plate 192)

Technique

1. Spread a blanket fourfold on the floor and kneel near it.

2. Place the right palm on the floor just outside the right knee, and the left palm just outside the left knee. The palms should be parallel to each other and the fingers should point straight towards the head. The distance between the palms on the floor should not be wider than the width of the shoulders.

3. Move the knees towards the head and place the crown on the centre of the blanket.

4. After securing the head position, stretch the legs straight by raising the knees from the floor. Move the toes still closer to the head and press the heels to the floor, keeping the back erect.

5. Stretch the dorsal region of the spine by pushing the chest forward and hold this position for a few seconds. Take 3 to 4 breaths.

6. Exhale, take a gentle swing from the floor and lift the legs off it by flexing the knees. Both feet should leave the floor together. When this position is secured, stretch the legs up, exhale, keep the toes pointing up, tighten at the knees and balance. (Plate 192)

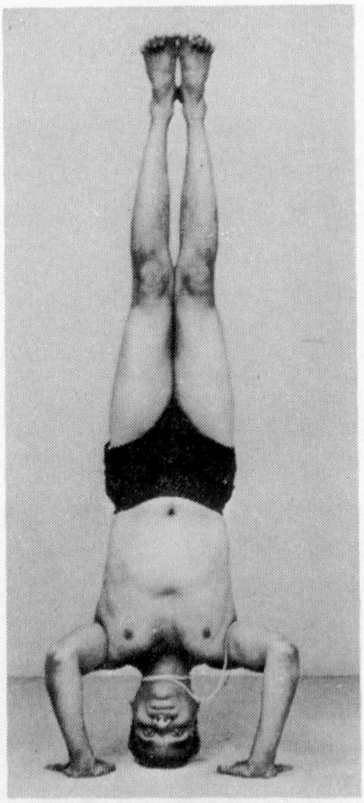

192

7. In the balancing position only the crown of the head and the two hands are on the floor. From the wrists to the elbows the forearms are to be kept perpendicular to the floor and parallel to each other. From the elbows to the shoulder the upper arms should be kept parallel to the floor and to each other.

8. Follow the rest of the technique and hints given under Sālamba Śīrṣāsana I for those who can balance.

9. Mastery of this variation of the head stand is essential for learning the other advanced āsanas like Bakāsana (Plate 410), Ūrdhva Kukku-

ṭāsana (Plate 419), Gālavāsana (Plates 427 and 428) and Kouṇḍinyāsana (Plate 438), etc.

The Śīrṣāsana Cycle (continued)

77. *Sālamba Śīrṣāsana III* Eight* (Plates 194 and 195)

Technique

1. Kneel on the floor near the blanket. Widen the knees about one foot.

2. Invert the palms and place them on the blanket between the knees so that the fingers point to the feet. The forearms from the wrist to the elbow should be kept perpendicular to the floor and parallel to each other. The distance between the palms should not be wider than that between the shoulders.

3. Rest the crown of the head on the blanket just behind the wrists. The forehead will face the inner side of the wrists. The head should be placed in the centre of the two hands, so that the crown is equidistant from the palms on the floor.

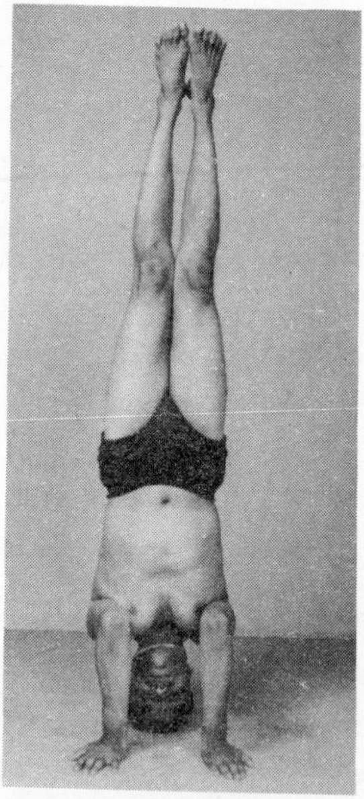

193

4. Press the wrists and palms down firmly, exhale, raise the feet from the floor, lift the legs up to a perpendicular position and balance. Do not widen the elbows, but try and bring them as close as possible. (Plate 193)

5. Balance in this position for a minute with normal breathing and then exhale and gently lower the legs to the floor.

6. After learning to balance in this variation of Śīrṣāsana, try to bring the hands as near to each other as possible until the sides of the palms and the little fingers touch each other. (Front view: Plate 194. Side view: Plate 195.) Also learn to go up and come down, keeping the legs straight without bending at the knees. (Plates 196 and 197.) This variation of Śīrṣāsana will give firmness and confidence in balance.

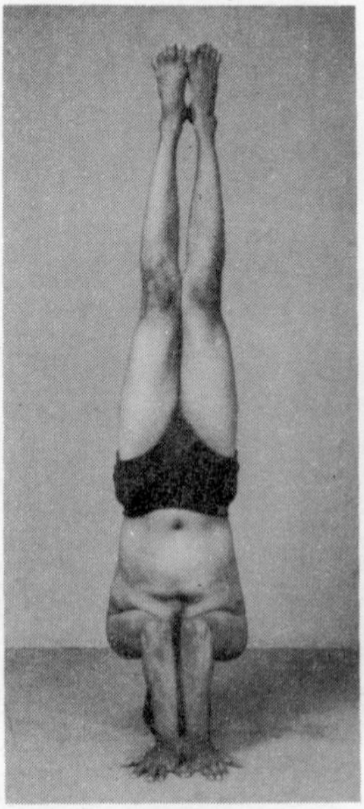

194

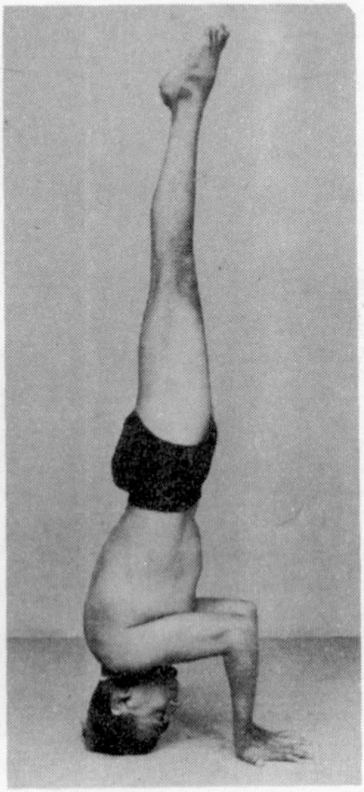

195

78. *Baddha Hasta Śīrṣāsana* Four* (Plate 198)

Baddha means bound, caught, restrained. Hasta means hand. This is a variation of the head stand.

Technique

1. Spread a blanket fourfold on the floor, and kneel near it.

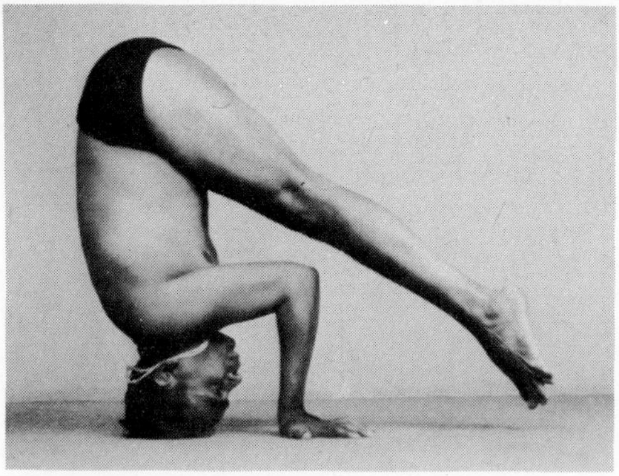

196

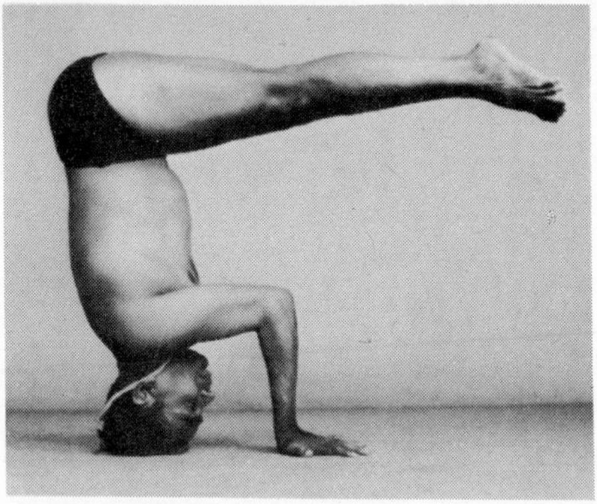

197

2. Fold the arms in front of the chest and catch the right upper arm near the elbow joint with the left hand. Similarly catch the left upper arm with the right hand.

3. Rest the elbows and the folded forearms on the blanket. Bend forward and place the crown of the head on the blanket just beyond the folded forearms. The forehead will be just behind the locked forearms.

4. Raise the knees from the floor and stretch the legs out straight.

5. After securing the weight on the head and elbows, press the forearms down, exhale, gently push the trunk slightly back without losing the hand grip and pull the legs up off the floor. (Plate 198)

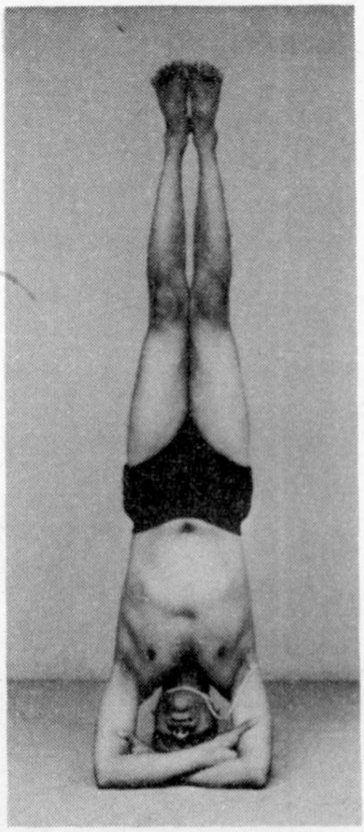

198

6. While the legs are going up to the perpendicular, the neck bears the weight of the body and feels the strain. Move the legs up until you feel lightness on the back of the neck and forearms and stretch the dorsal region of the trunk forward. When you feel the lightness, be sure that the body is straight. Follow the technique and hints given for Sālamba Śīrṣāsana I for those who can balance.

7. Remain erect in the head stand for a minute. Then exhale, draw the hips slightly back without lifting the elbows and gently lower the legs to the floor. Try to keep the legs straight and do not bend them at the knees while lowering them.

79. *Mukta Hasta Śīrṣāsana* Six* (Plates 200 and 201)

Mukta means free. Hasta means hand. This is the most difficult variation of Śīrṣāsana to master. When it comes comfortably, one is a perfect master of the head stand. It is comparatively easy to balance in this āsana, but it is extremely difficult to go up and come down keeping the the legs straight without bending them at the knees.

Technique

1. Spread a balanket fourfold on the floor and kneel near it.

2. Bend the trunk forward and rest the crown of the head on the blanket.

3. Stretch the arms straight out in front of the chest towards the feet and rest the back of the wrists on the floor. Keep the arms straight at the elbows with the palms up. The distance between the wrists should be the same as that between the shoulders.

4. Raise the trunk until it is perpendicular to the floor. Press the wrists gently against the floor, exhale and raise the feet. (Plate 199.) Tighten the legs and slowly raise them up until they are perpendicular. (Side view: Plate 200)

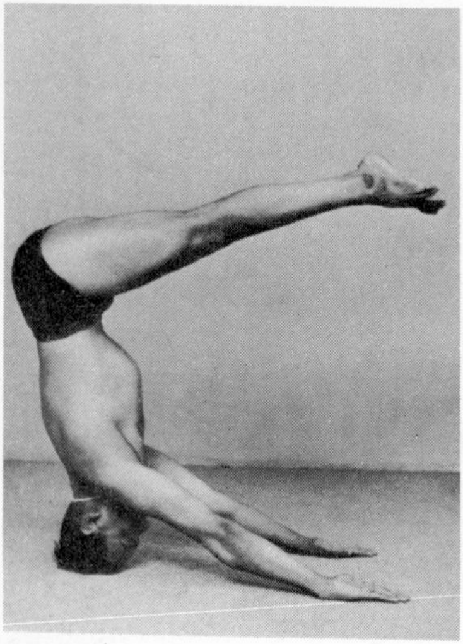

199

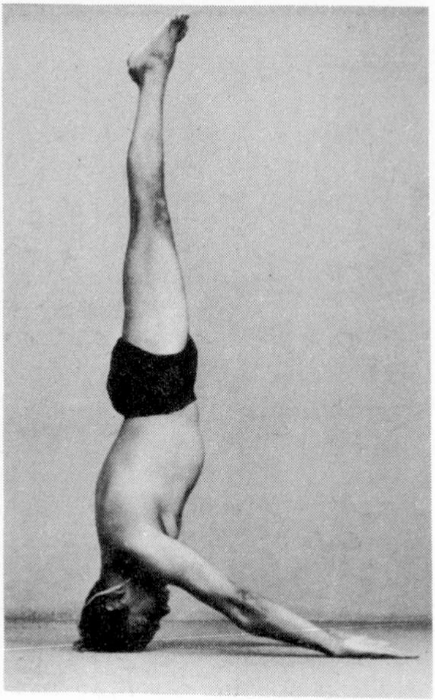

200

5. Stay in the pose for a minute with normal breathing. Keep the arms straight, stretch the elbows and extend the shoulders as high as possible from the floor, without disturbing the position of the wrists. (Front view: Plate 201)

6. Exhale, swing the hips slightly back and bring the legs down to the floor gradually, with the weight of the body thrown slightly on the wrists.

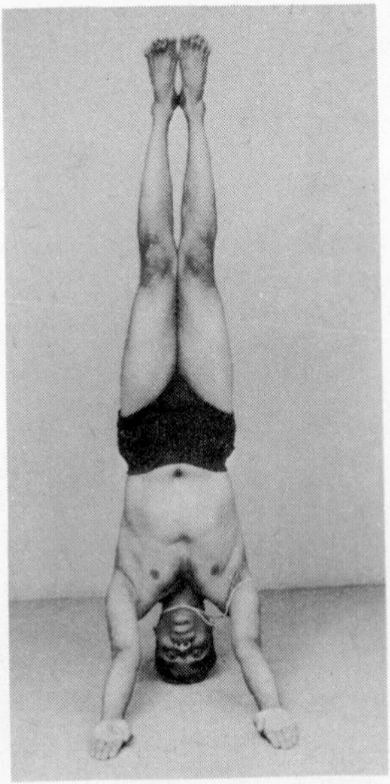

201

7. Then lift the head up from the floor, sit down and relax.

Note. Once mastery over the variations of Śīrṣāsana is secured, it is possible to change the position of the hands while balancing on the head only. One need not then come down again to change the position of the hands. One should learn this gradually, otherwise one is apt to strain the neck and shoulders.

80. *Pārśva Śīrṣāsana* Eight* (Plates 202 and 203)

Pārśva means side or flank. In this variation of Śīrṣāsana, the trunk and legs are turned sideways on either side while balancing without disturbing the position of the head or hands.

Technique

1. From the straight Sālamba Śīrṣāsana I (Plate 184), exhale and move the spine with a twist to the right; except the head and the hands turn the body sideways. (Front view: Plate 202. Back view: Plate 203)

2. The legs and navel should face sideways 90 degrees to their original positions as in the illustrations. One should feel the stretch near the region of the floating ribs.

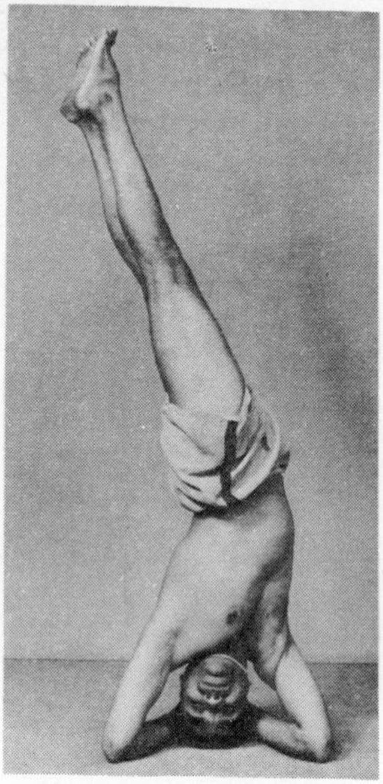

202

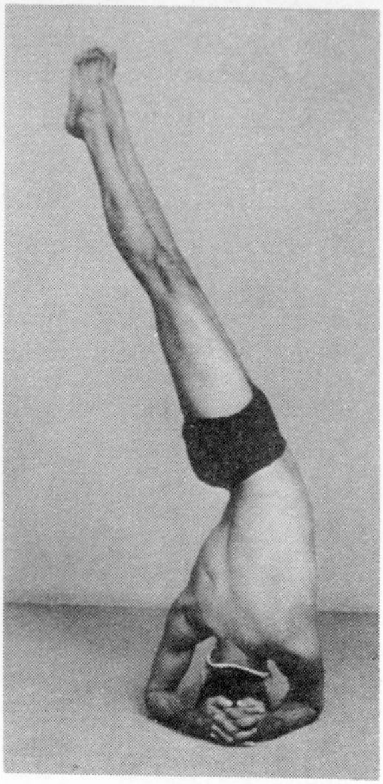

203

3. Hold the pose from 20 to 30 seconds with normal breathing.

4. Exhale, come back to the straight Sālamba Śīrṣāsana I. Take a breath, exhale and repeat the pose on the left side for the same length of time. Exhale and come to the straight position of Sālamba Śīrṣāsana I.

Effects

This āsana makes the spine strong and elastic.

81. *Parivṛttaikapāda Śīrṣāsana* Ten* (Plates 205, 206 and 207)

Parivṛtta means revolved, turned round. Eka means one and pāda the leg. In this variation of Śīrṣāsana, the legs are spread apart and the trunk and legs are then turned sideways on either side, while maintaining the balance without disturbing the position of the head or the hands.

Technique

1. After completing Pārśva Śīrṣāsana (Plate 202), spread the legs apart, move the right leg forward and the left leg back evenly. (Plate 204.) Then exhale, twist the spine to the left so that the legs move sideways clockwise through 90 degrees. (Side view: Plate 205)

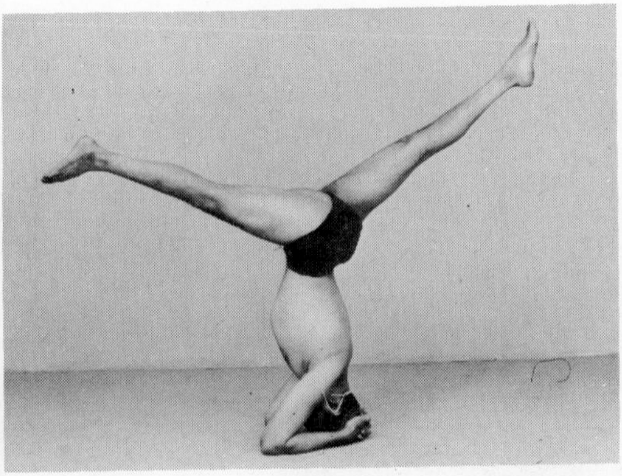

204

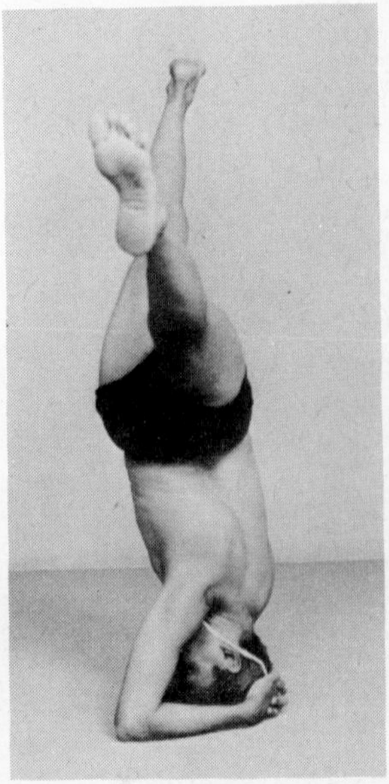

205

2. After turning sideways, keep the legs poker stiff by tightening the hamstring muscles, knees and calves.

3. Spread the legs still wider and stay in that position from 20 to 30 seconds trying to breathe normally.

4. Exhale, come to the straight Sālamba Śīrṣāsana I. Now, move the left leg forward and the right leg back, twist the spine to the right so that the legs move sideways anti-clockwise through 90 degrees. (Front view: Plate 206. Back view: Plate 207.) Stay in that position for the same length of time. Exhale and return to Sālamba Śīrṣāsana I.

Effects

This āsana develops the leg muscles and tones the kidneys, bladder, prostate and intestines.

82. *Eka Pāda Śīrṣāsana* Eleven* (Plates 208 and 209)

Eka means one. Pāda is the leg. This variation of Śīrṣāsana is done by lowering one leg to the floor in front of the head, holding the other leg up vertically.

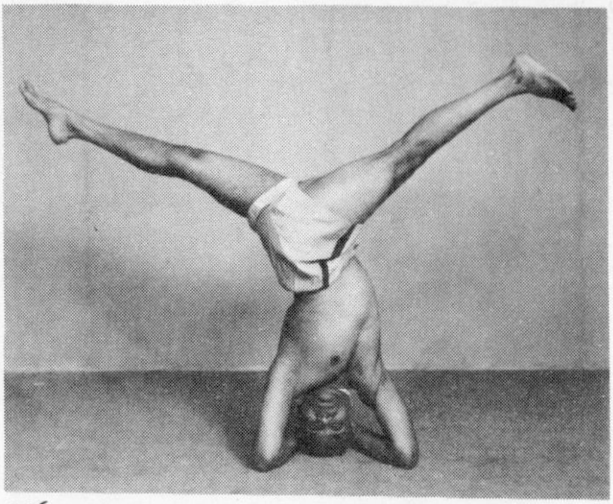

206

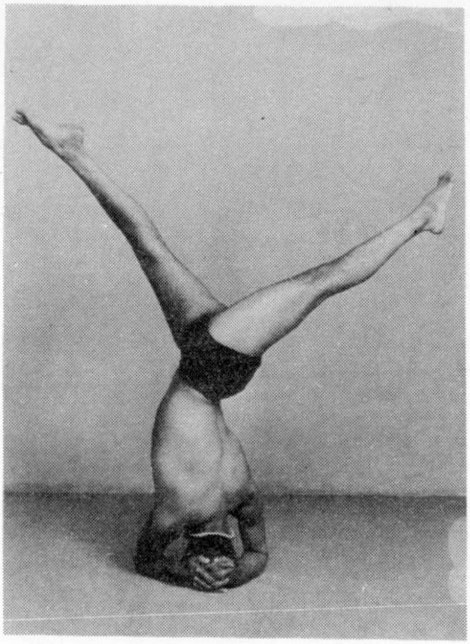

207

Technique

1. After staying according to your capacity in Sālamba Śīrṣāsana I, exhale, and move the right leg down to the floor in front of the head. (Side view: Plate 208)

2. While the right leg is being lowered and is resting on the floor, the left leg should be held up vertically as in Śīrṣāsana.

3. In the beginning, the neck feels tremendous strain. The left leg is also dragged down forwards. To overcome this, keep the legs rigid at the

knees and stretch the muscles at the back of the thighs of both the legs. Also tighten the muscles of the lower median portion of the abdomen.

4. The knees and toes of both legs should be in a line and should not tilt sideways.

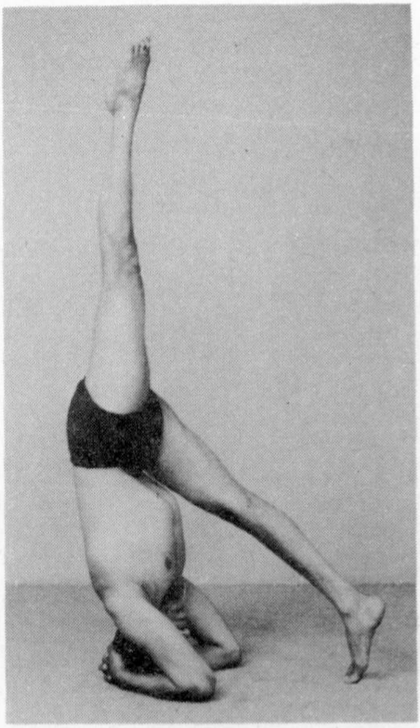
208

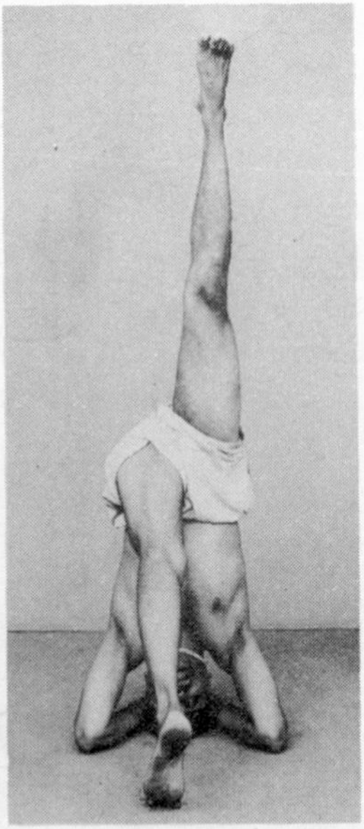
209

5. Stay in the pose from 10 to 20 seconds with deep breathing. Exhale, and lift the right leg up to Śīrṣāsana.

6. After staying in Śīrṣāsana for some time, lower the left leg to the floor (Front view: Plate 209) and after keeping it on the floor for the same length of time, exhale and go back to Śīrṣāsana.

7. While lowering and raising the legs, keep them straight and do not bend at the knees. If the knees are bent one loses the head balance.

Effects

This is a difficult pose, so it may not be possible to touch the floor in the beginning. Gradually as the legs become more elastic and the back gets stronger, the legs will touch and then rest on the floor without loss of the head balance. This āsana strengthens the neck and also the abdominal walls. The abdominal organs are contracted and made to function well.

83. *Pārśvaika Pāda Śīrṣāsana* Twelve* (Plate 210)

Pārśva means sideways. Eka is one and pāda is the leg. In this pose, one leg is lowered to the floor sideways in line with the head, while the other leg remains vertically up.

Technique

1. Do this position after completing Eka Pāda Śīrṣāsana (Plates 208 and 209) as described earlier.

2. Exhale and lower the right leg sideways to the right, placing it on the floor in line with the head. (Plate 210.) Keep the left leg erect as in Śīrṣāsana.

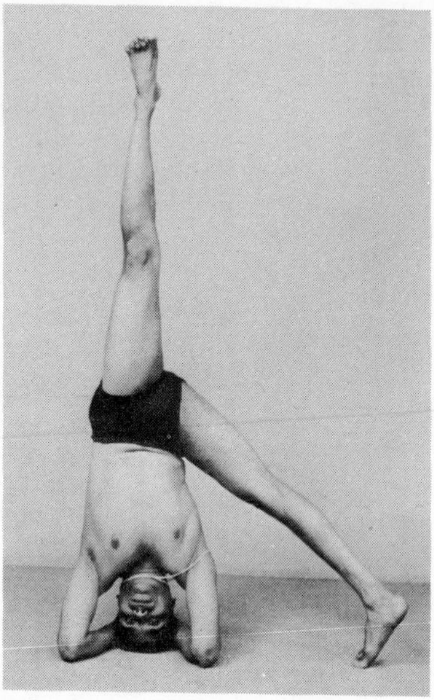

210

3. It is more difficult to hold the head stand in this position than in Eka Pāda Śīrṣāsana. To balance on the head in this pose, stretch the muscles at the back of the thighs of both the legs, tighten the knees and muscles of the groin in the iliac region of the abdomen on the side of the lowered leg.

4. Stay in this position for 10 to 20 seconds with deep breathing. Stretch the hamstrings and thighs and with an exhalation move the right leg to the Śīrṣāsana position.

5. Stay in Śīrṣāsana for some time and then exhale, lower the left leg sideways to the floor until it rests in line with the head. Maintain the pose for the same length of time here also. Then exhale, and return to Śīrṣāsana.

6. Do not bend the knees while lowering or raising the legs or you will lose balance.

Effects

This āsana makes the neck, abdominal walls and thighs powerful. It tones and strengthens the intestines and the spine.

84. *Ūrdhva Padmāsana in Śīrṣāsana* Six* (Plate 211)

Ūrdhva means above or high. Padmāsana (Plate 104) is the lotus pose described earlier. In this variation, Padmāsana is done in the head stand.

Technique

1. This pose is to be done after the Eka Pāda (Plates 208 and 209) and Pārśvaika Pāda Śīrṣāsanas. (Plate 210.) After completing these two positions cross the legs as in Padmāsana. First place the right foot over the left thigh and the left foot over the right thigh.

2. Press the knees closer to each other and stretch the thighs up vertically. (Plate 211)

3. Hold this position for half a minute with deep and even breaths. Then, exhale and extend the thighs as far back as possible. (Plate 212)

4. Uncross the legs and return to Śīrṣāsana. Now cross the legs the other way, first placing the left foot over the right thigh and then the right foot over the left thigh. Stay like this also for half a minute and then extend the thighs back.

5. While stretching the thighs up do not change the position of the head or the neck.

Effects

This posture gives an extra pull to the dorsal region, the ribs and the pelvic region. Consequently, the chest is fully expanded and blood circulates properly in the pelvic region. To give an added stretch, one can perform the pose by giving the trunk a lateral twist while doing the head stand. This is called:

85. *Pārśva Ūrdhva Padmāsana in Śīrṣāsana* Seven* (Plates 213 to 216)

(Pārśva means flank.)

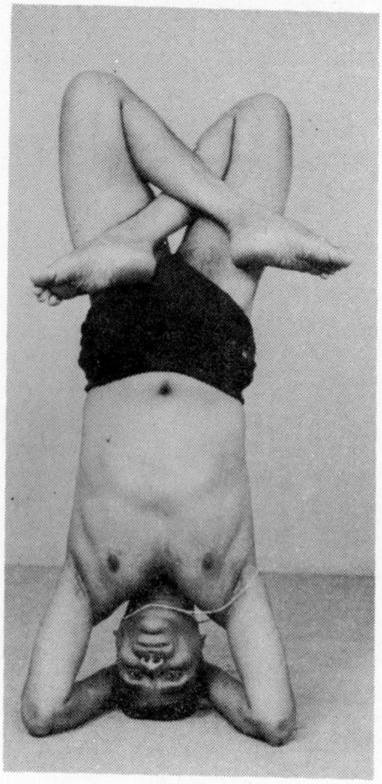

211

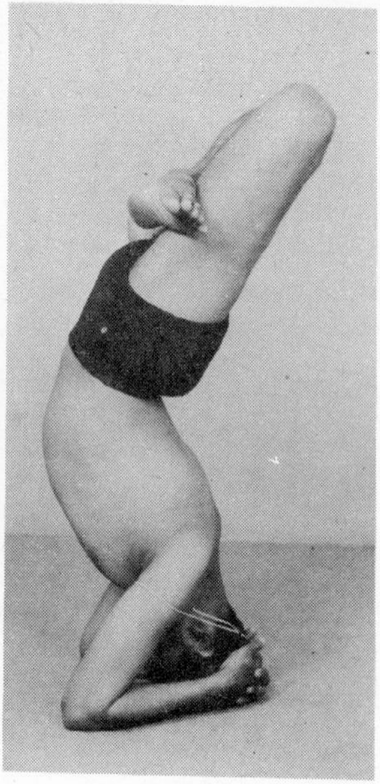

212

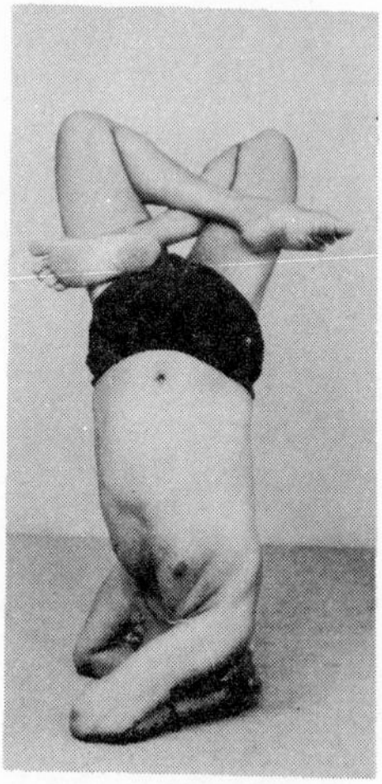

213

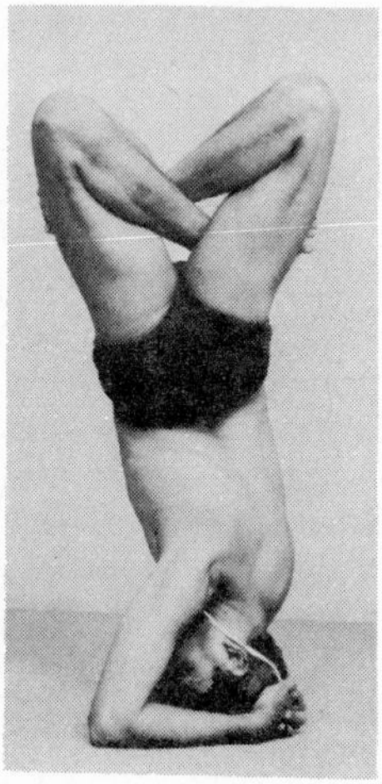

214

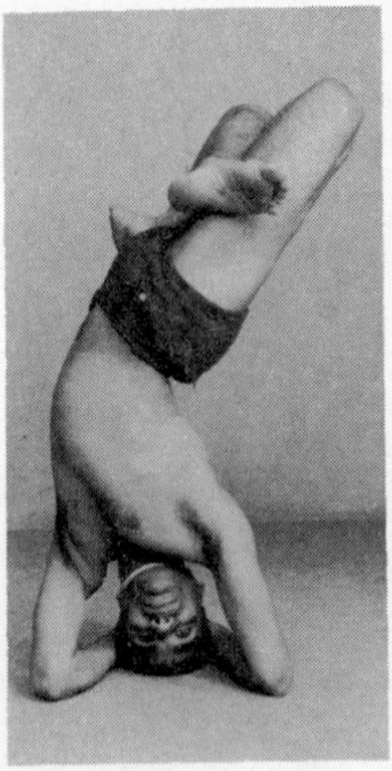

215

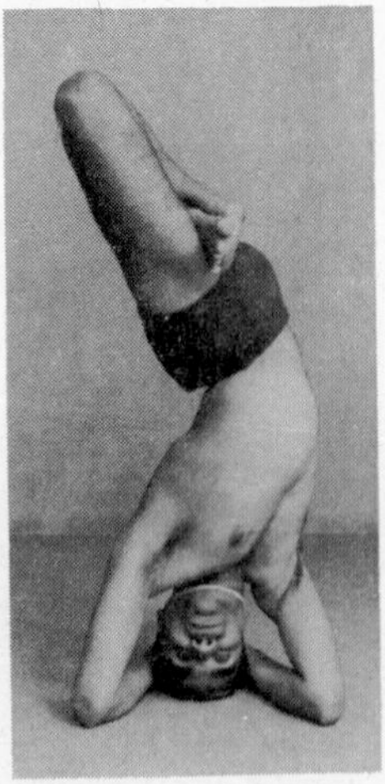

216

86. *Piṇḍāsana in Śīrṣāsana* Six* (Plate 218)

Piṇḍa means an embryo. From Padmāsana in the head stand (Plate 211), the hips are flexed and the legs are lowered to touch the armpits.

Technique

1. Do Padmāsana in Śīrṣāsana as described above. (Plate 211.) Exhale, flex the hips (Plate 217) and take two breaths. Again with an exhalation lower the legs till they touch the arms near the armpits. (Plate 218)

2. Stay in this position from 20 to 30 seconds with normal breathing.

3. Inhale, go back to Ūrdhva Padmāsana, uncross the legs and stay in Śīrṣāsana for some time. Then cross the legs the other way and repeat the pose.

4. Relax the crossed legs one by one, stretch them back to Śīrṣāsana and then lower them gradually and straight to the floor with an exhalation.

Effects

This pose has the same effects as the earlier one. Further the abdominal organs are toned by contraction and an additional supply of blood.

87. *Sālamba Sarvāṅgāsana I* Two* (Plates 223, 224 and 234)

Ālamba means a prop, a support and sa together with or accompanied by. Sālamba, therefore, means supported or propped up. Sarvānga (Sarva = all, whole, entire, complete; anga = limb or body) means the

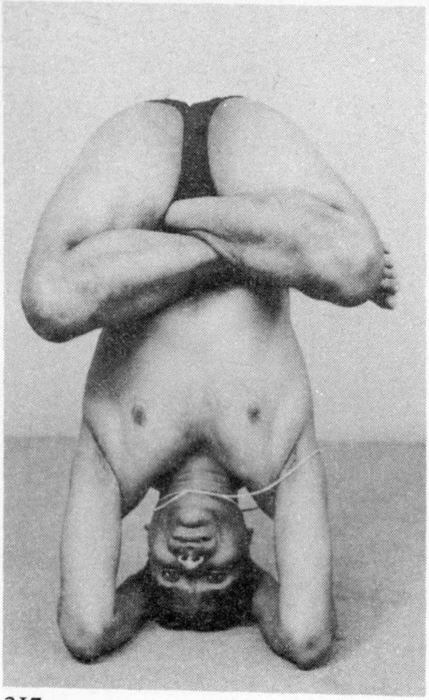

217

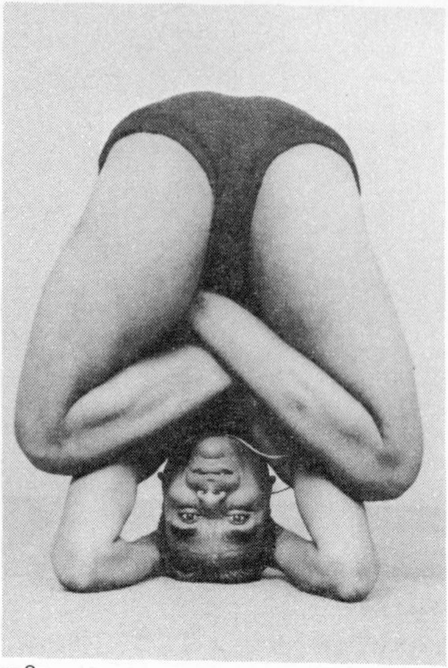

218

entire body or all the limbs. In this pose the whole body benefits from the exercise, hence the name.

Technique for beginners

1. Lie flat on the back on the carpet keeping the legs stretched out, tightened at the knees. Place the hands by the side of the legs, palms down. (Plate 219.) Take a few deep breaths.

2. Exhale, bend the knees and move the legs towards the stomach till the thighs press it. (Plate 220.) Take two breaths.

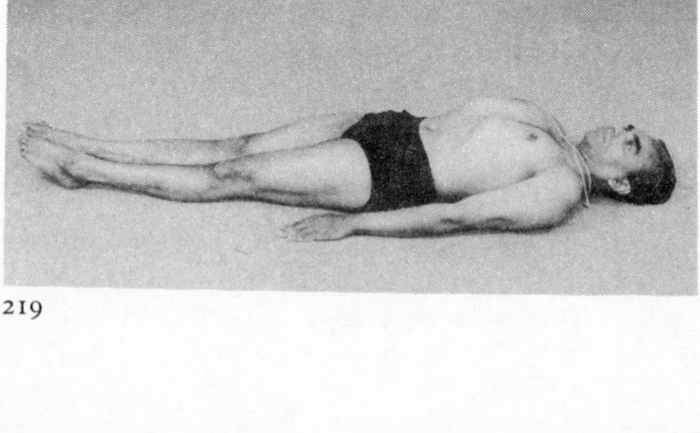

219

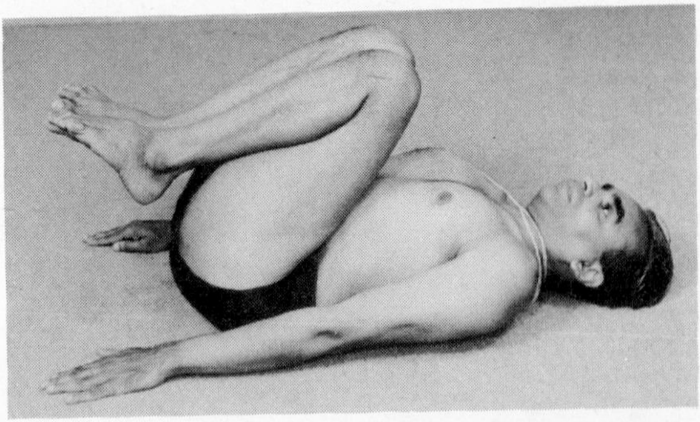

220

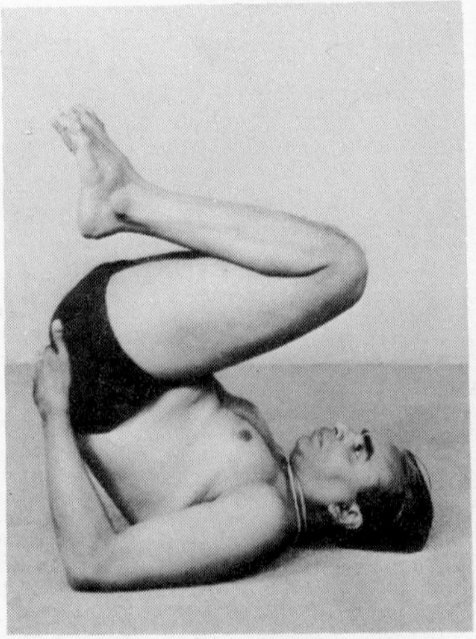

221

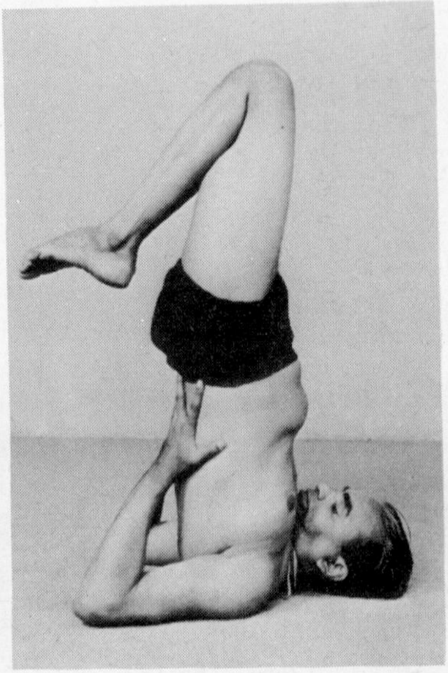

222

3. Raise the hips from the floor with an exhalation and rest the hands on them by bending the arms at the elbows. (Plate 221.) Take two breaths.

4. Exhale, raise the trunk up perpendicularly supported by the hands until the chest touches the chin. (Plate 222)

5. Only the back of the head and the neck, the shoulders and the backs of the arms up to the elbows should rest on the floor. Place the hands in the middle of the spine as in Plate 222. Take two breaths.

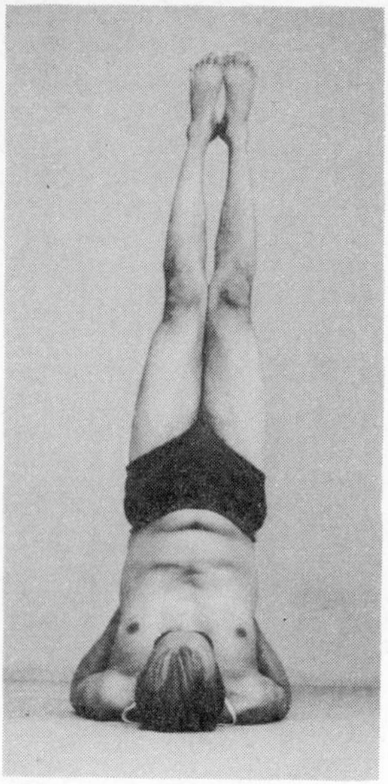

223

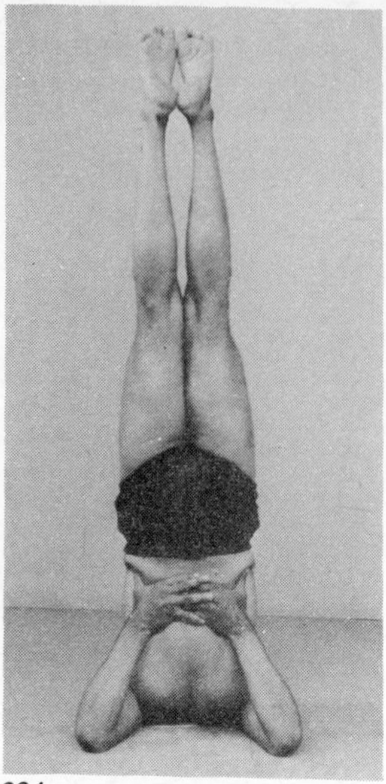

224

6. Exhale and stretch the legs straight with the toes pointing up. (Front view: Plate 223. Back view: Plate 224)

7. Stay in this position for 5 minutes with even breathing.

8. Exhale, gradually slide down, release the hands, lie flat and relax.

9. If you cannot do the āsana without support use a stool and follow the technique. See Plate 225.

Technique for advanced pupils

1. Lie flat on the back on the carpet.

2. Keep the legs stretched out, tightened at the knees. Place the hands by the side of the legs, palms down. (Plate 219)

3. Take a few deep breaths. Exhale slowly and at the same time raise both legs together and bring them at a right angle to the body as in Plates 226, 227 and 228. Remain in this position and inhale, keeping the legs steady.

4. Exhale, again raise the legs further up by lifting the hips and back from the floor, pressing the palms gently against the floor as in Plates 229, 230 and 231.

5. When the whole trunk is raised off the ground, bend the elbows

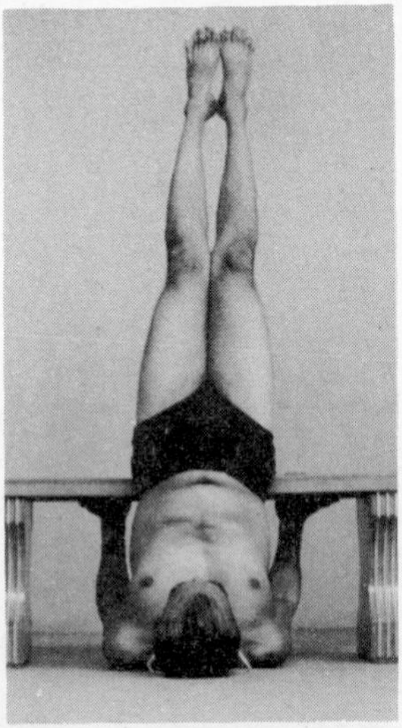

225

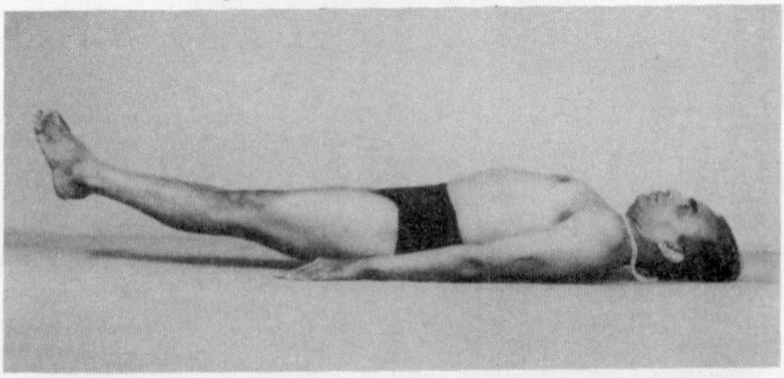

226

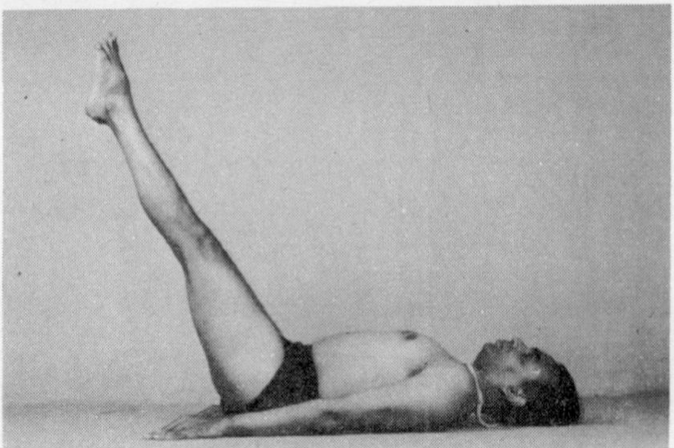

227

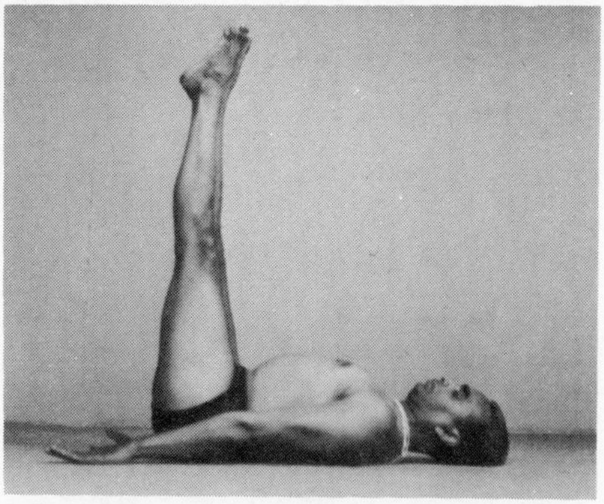

228

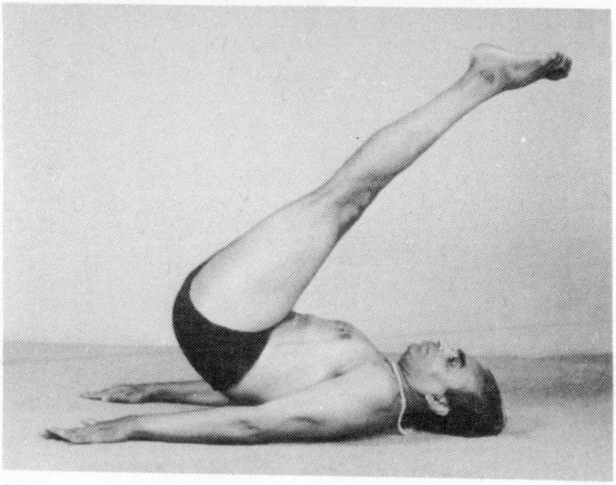

229

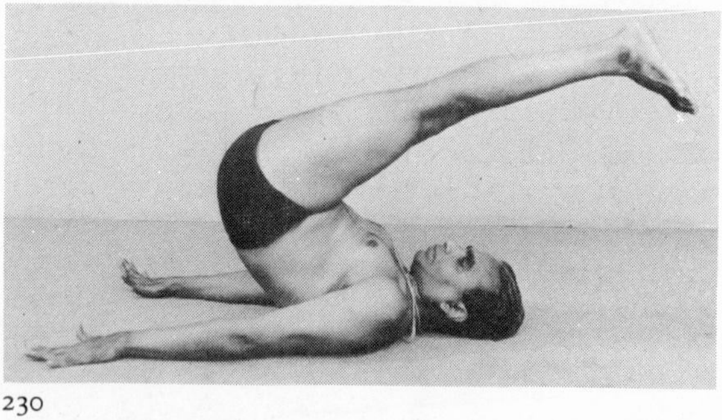

230

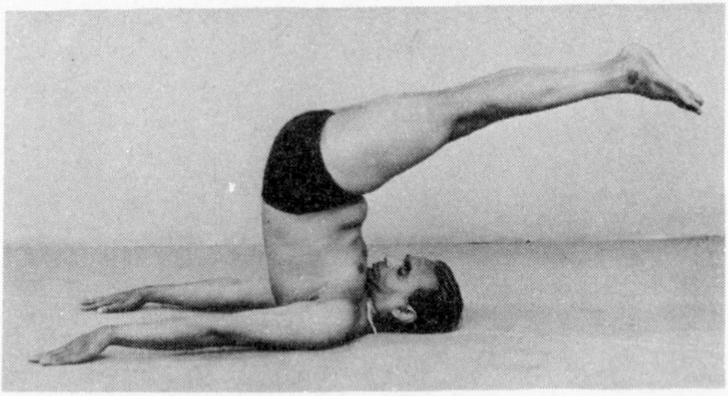

231

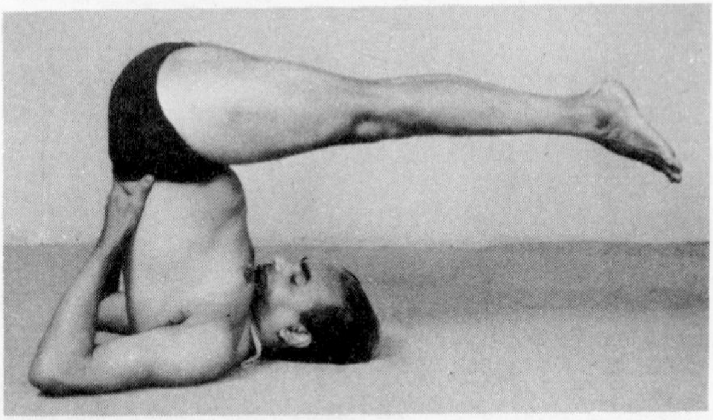

232

and place the palms on the back of the ribs, resting the shoulders well on the floor. (Plate 232)

6. Utilise the palm pressure and raise the trunk and legs up vertically as in Plate 233 so that the breast-bone presses the chin to form a firm chinlock. The contraction of the throat and pressing the chin against the breast-bone to form a firm chinlock is known as Jālandhara Bandha. Remember to bring the chest forward to touch the chin and not to bring the chin towards the chest. If the latter is done, the spine is not stretched completely and the full effect of this āsana will not be felt.

7. Only the back of the head and neck, the shoulders and the upper portion of the arms up to the elbows should rest well on the floor. The remainder of the body should be in one straight line, perpendicular to the floor. This is the final position. (Side view: Plate 234)

8. In the beginning, there is a tendency for the legs to swing out of the perpendicular. To correct this, tighten the back thigh muscles and stretch up vertically.

9. The elbows should not be placed wider than the shoulders. Try

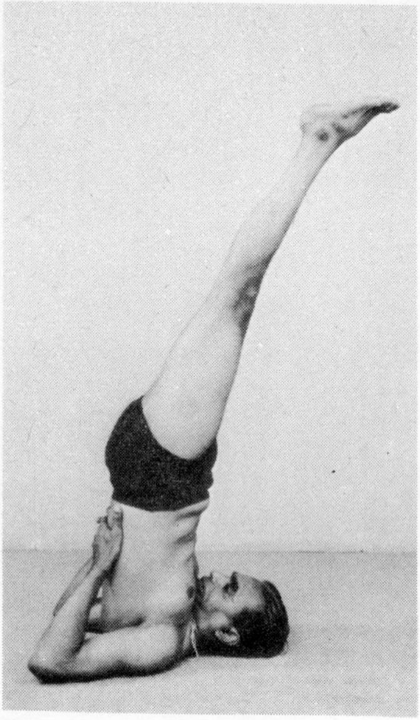

233

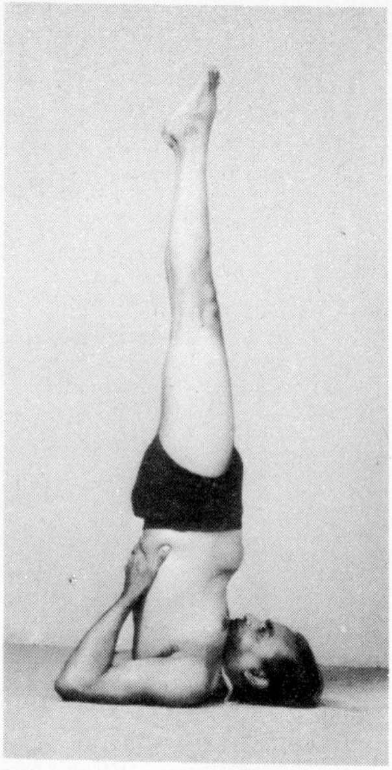

234

and stretch the shoulders away from the neck and also to bring the elbows close to each other. If the elbows are widened, the trunk cannot be pulled up properly and the pose will look imperfect. Also see that the neck is straight with the centre of the chin resting on the sternum. In the beginning, the neck moves sideways and if this is not corrected, it will cause pain and injure the neck.

10. Remain in this pose for not less than 5 minutes. Gradually increase the time to 15 minutes; this will have no ill effects.

11. Release the hands, slide down to the floor, lie flat and relax.

As the weight of the whole body is borne on the neck and shoulders and as the hands are used to support the weight this āsana is called Sālamba Sarvāngāsana. In Sarvāngāsana there are various movements which can be done in addition to the basic pose described above.

Effects

The importance of Sarvāngāsana cannot be over-emphasised. It is one of the greatest boons conferred on humanity by our ancient sages. Sarvāngāsana is the Mother of āsanas. As a mother strives for harmony and happiness in the home, so this āsana strives for the harmony and happiness of the human system. It is a panacea for most common ailments. There are several endocrine organs or ductless glands in the human system which bathe in blood, absorb the nutriments from the blood and secrete hormones for the proper functioning of a balanced and well developed body and brain. If the glands fail to function properly, the hormones are not produced as they should be and the body starts to deteriorate. Amazingly enough many of the āsanas have a direct effect on the glands and help them to function properly. Sarvāngāsana does this for the thyroid and parathyroid glands which are situated in the neck region, since due to the firm chinlock their blood supply is increased. Further, since the body is inverted the venous blood flows to the heart without any strain by force of gravity. Healthy blood is allowed to circulate around the neck and chest. As a result, persons suffering from breathlessness, palpitation, asthma, bronchitis and throat ailments get relief. As the head remains firm in this inverted position, and the supply of the blood to it is regulated by the firm chinlock, the nerves are soothed and headaches – even chronic ones – disappear. Continued practice of this āsana eradicates common colds and other nasal disturbances. Due to the soothing effect of the pose on the nerves, those suffering from hypertension, irritation, shortness of temper, nervous breakdown and insomnia are relieved. The change in bodily gravity also affects the abdominal organs so that the bowels move freely and constipation vanishes. As a result the system is freed from toxins and one feels full of energy. The āsana is recommended for urinary disorders and uterine displacement, menstrual trouble, piles and hernia. It also helps to relieve epilepsy, low vitality and anaemia. It is no over-statement to say that if a person regularly practises Sarvāngāsana he will feel new vigour and strength, and will be happy and confident. New life will flow into him, his mind will be at peace and he will feel the joy of life. After a long illness, the practice of this āsana regularly twice a day brings back lost vitality. The Sarvāngāsana cycle activates the abdominal organs and relieves people suffering from stomach and intestinal ulcers, severe pains in the abdomen and colitis.

People suffering from high blood pressure should not attempt Sālamba Sarvāngāsana I unless they do Halāsana (Plate 244) first and can stay in it for not less than 3 minutes.

Halāsana is described on p. 216 (Plate 244).

The Sarvāngāsana Cycle

These various movements can be practised at one stretch after staying in Sarvāngāsana I (Plate 223) from 5 to 10 minutes or more according to capacity; do them for 20 to 30 seconds at a time each side except Halāsana, which should last from 3 to 5 minutes at a stretch.

88. *Sālamba Sarvāngāsana II* Three* (Plate 235)

This position is slightly harder than the first one.

Technique

1. Do Sālamba Sarvāngāsana I. (Plate 223)

2. Release the hands from the back of the trunk, interlock the fingers, turn the wrists and extend the arms. The thumbs will then touch the floor and the palms will face outwards. (Plate 235.) The head will be on one side of the vertically extended body and the arms will be on the other side.

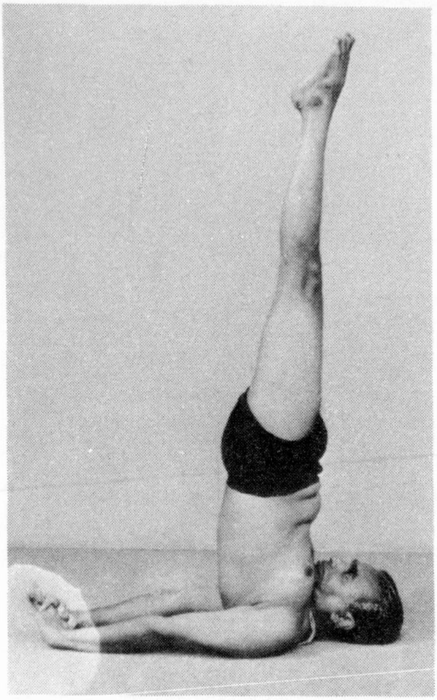

235

3. Keep the legs and back as steady as possible.

4. This pose can be done for a minute after doing Sarvāngāsana I.

Effects

As the balance is maintained by stretching the back muscles and as the weight of the body falls on the back of the neck, the back and the neck gain strength. The arm muscles are also toned.

89. *Nirālamba Sarvāngāsana I* Three* (Plate 236)

Ālamba means a prop, a support, while nir conveys the sense of away from, without, free from. Nirālamba, therefore, means without support. This variation of Sarvāngāsana is harder than the earlier two, as in it the body is not supported by the arms and the body weight and balance are maintained by the muscles of the neck, back and abdomen, which are thus strengthened.

Technique

1. Do Sālamba Sarvāngāsana I. (Plate 223)

2. Release the hands, bring them over the head, rest the extended arms on the floor on the same side of the vertical body as the head, and balance. (Plate 236)

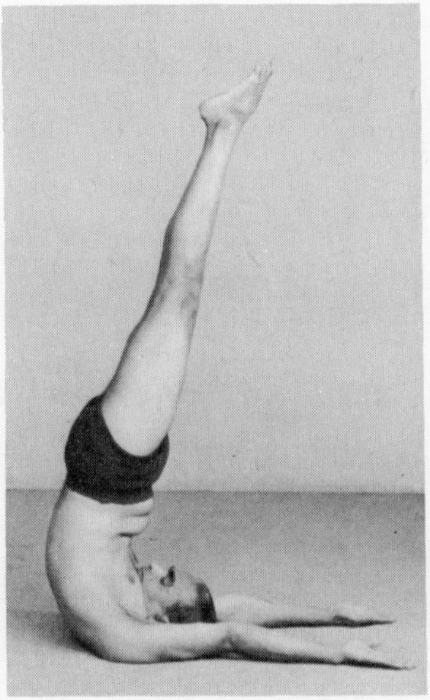

236

3. This pose can also be held for a minute.

90. *Nirālamba Sarvāngāsana II* Four* (Plate 237)

This is the hardest of the Sarvāngāsana poses. It enables one to extend the spinal vertebrae more than in the other Sarvāngāsanas and thus helps one to achieve a perfect Sālamba Sarvāngāsana. (Plate 223)

Technique

1. From the previous pose, raise the hands and place the palms on or by the side of the knees. (Plate 237.) Do not rest the legs on the palms.

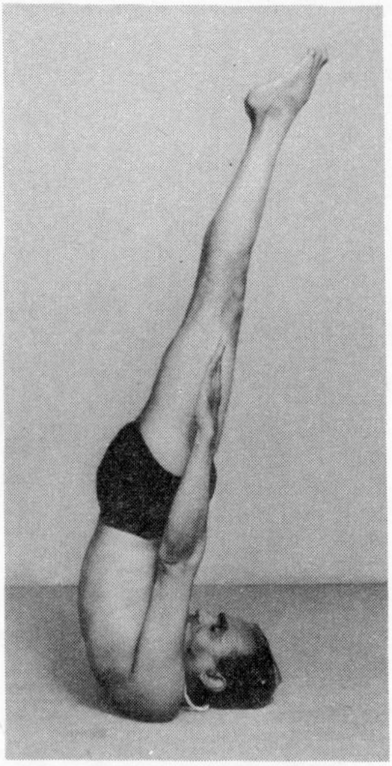

237

2. Stay in the pose for a minute. Then move into Sālamba Sarvāṅgāsana I for some time, slide into Halāsana (Plate 244) and continue the other Sarvāṅgāsana movements one after the other.

Effects

By practising these various Sarvāṅgāsana movements, the entire body is toned by an increase in the flow of blood and by the elimination of toxin-forming waste matter. These āsanas stimulate one like tonics. After convalescing one can practise them for speedier recovery from weakness.

91. *Halāsana* Four* (Plate 244)

Hala means a plough, the shape of which this posture resembles, hence the name. It is a part of Sarvāṅgāsana I and a continuation thereof.

Technique

1. Do Sālamba Sarvāngāsana I (Plate 223) with a firm chinlock.

2. Release the chinlock, lower the trunk slightly, moving the arms and legs over the head and resting the toes on the floor. (Plate 238)

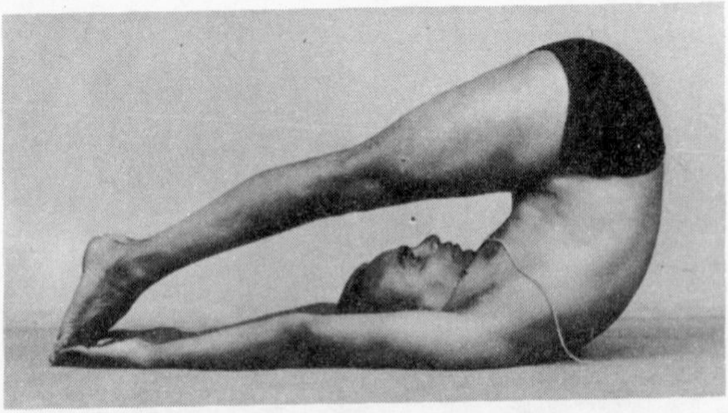

238

3. Tighten the knees by pulling up the hamstring muscles at the back of the thighs and raise the trunk. (Plate 239)

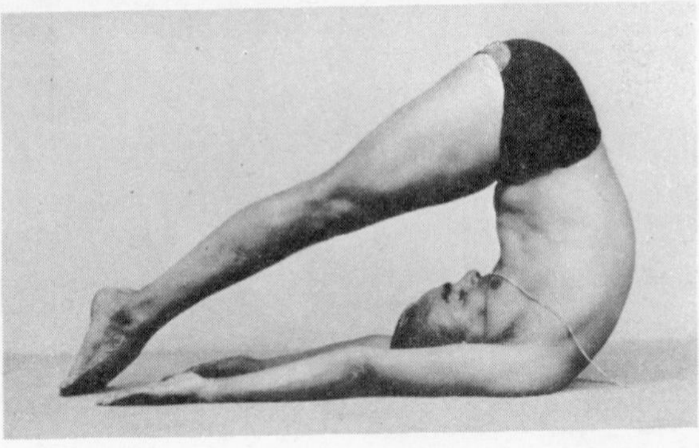

239

4. Place the hands in the middle of the back and press it to keep the trunk perpendicular to the floor. (Plate 240)

5. Stretch the arms on the floor in the direction opposite to that of the legs. (Plate 241)

6. Hook the thumbs and stretch the arms and legs. (Plate 242)

7. Interlock the fingers (Plate 243) and turn the wrists so that the thumbs rest on the floor. (Plate 244.) Stretch the palms along with the

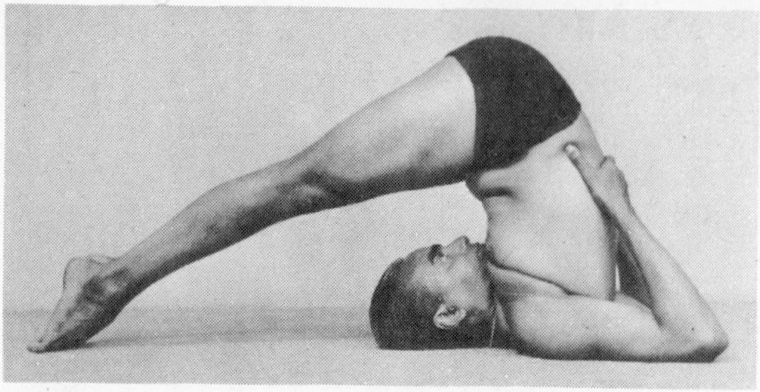

240

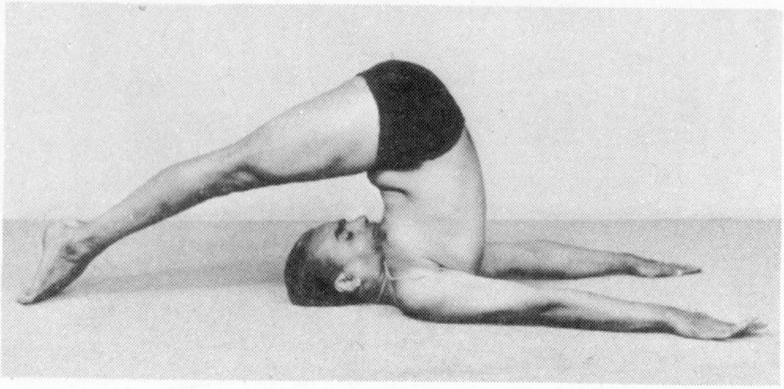

241

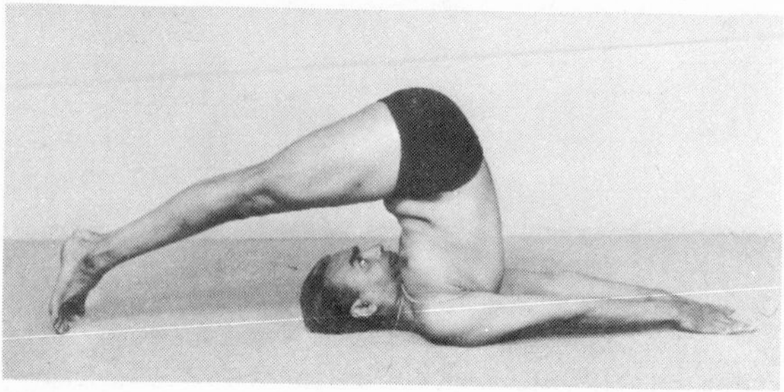

242

fingers, tighten the arms at the elbows and pull them from the shoulders.

8. The legs and the hands are stretched in opposite directions and this stretches the spine completely.

9. While interlocking the fingers, it is advisable to change the interlock. Suppose that the right thumb touches the floor first, maintain the position for a minute. Then release the grip and bring the left thumb

first on the floor, follow the interlock, finger by finger, and stretch out the arms for the same length of time. This will lead to harmonious development and elasticity of both the shoulders, elbows and wrists.

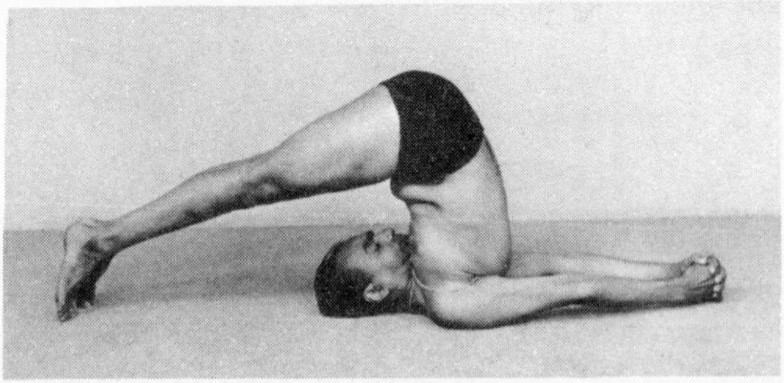

243

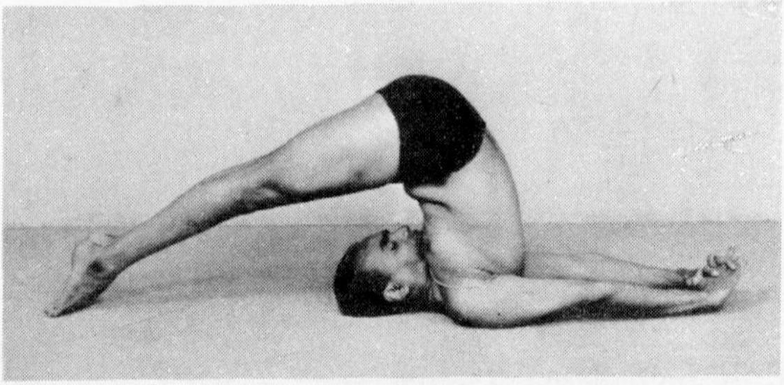

244

10. In the beginning interlocking will be difficult. By gradual practice of the above mentioned positions, you will interlock the fingers easily.

11. In the beginning it is also difficult to keep the toes firmly on the floor behind the head. If you lengthen the timing and stretch of Sarvāngāsana I (Plate 223) before going into Halāsana, the toes will remain longer on the floor.

12. Remain in the attainable pose from one to five minutes with normal breathing.

13. Release the hands. Raise the legs up to Sarvāngāsana I and gradually slide down to the floor. Lie flat on the back and relax.

Effects

The effect of Halāsana is the same as that of Sarvāngāsana I. (Plate 223.) In addition, the abdominal organs are rejuvenated due to contraction. The spine receives an extra supply of blood due to the forward bend and this helps to relieve backache. Cramps in the hands are cured by interlocking and stretching the palms and fingers. People suffering from stiff shoulders and elbows, lumbago and arthritis of the back find relief in this āsana. Griping pain in the stomach due to wind is also relieved and lightness is felt immediately.

The pose is good for people with a tendency for high blood pressure. If they perform Halāsana first and then Sarvāngāsana I, they will not feel the rush of blood or the sensation of fullness in the head.

Halāsana is a preparatory pose to Paschimottānāsana. (Plate 160.) If one improves in Halāsana, the resulting mobility of the back will enable one to perform Paschimottānāsana well.

Note. For persons suffering from high blood pressure the following technique is recommended for doing Halāsana before they attempt Sālamba Sarvāngāsana I.

1. Lie flat on the back on the floor.

2. Exhale, slowly raise the legs to a perpendicular position and stay there breathing normally for about 10 seconds.

3. Exhale, bring the legs over and beyond the head and touch the toes on the floor. Keep the toes on the floor and the legs stiff at the knees.

4. If you have difficulty in keeping the toes on the floor, then place a chair or a stool behind the head and rest the toes on it.

5. If the breathing becomes heavy or fast do not rest the toes on the floor, but on a stool or chair. Then fullness or pressure is not felt in the head.

6. Extend the arms over the head, keep them on the floor and stay in this position with normal breathing for 3 minutes.

7. Throughout the āsana, gaze at the tip of the nose with the eyes shut.

92. *Karṇapīdāsana* One* (Plate 246)

Karṇa means the ear. Pīda means pain, discomfort or pressure. This is a variant of Halāsana and can be done along with it.

Technique

1. Do Halāsana (Plate 244) and after completing the time limit for that pose, flex the knees and rest the right knee by the side of the right ear and the left knee by the side of the left.

2. Both knees should rest on the floor, pressing the ears.

3. Keep the toes stretched out and join the heels and toes. Rest the

hands either on the back of the ribs (Plate 245) or interlock the fingers and stretch out the arms (Plate 246) as in Halāsana.

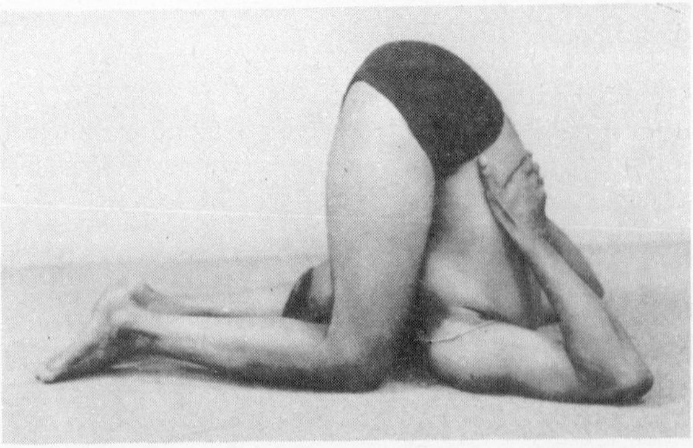

245

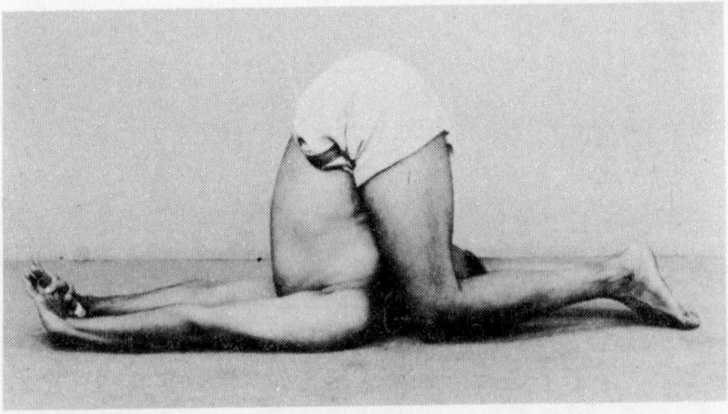

246

4. Remain in this position for half a minute or a minute with normal breathing.

Effects

This āsana rests the trunk, heart and legs. The spine is stretched more while bending the knees, and this helps the circulation of blood round the waistline.

93. *Supta Koṇāsana* Two* (Plate 247)

Supta means lying down and koṇa an angle. It is a variation of Halāsana in which the legs are spread apart.

Technique

1. From Karṇapīḍāsana (Plate 246), stretch the legs straight and spread the legs as far apart as you can.

2. Pull the trunk up and tighten the knees.

3. Hold the right toe with the right hand and the left toe with the left one. Keep the heels up. After gripping the toes, move the dorsal region of the spine still further up and extend the hamstring muscles. (Plates 247 and 248)

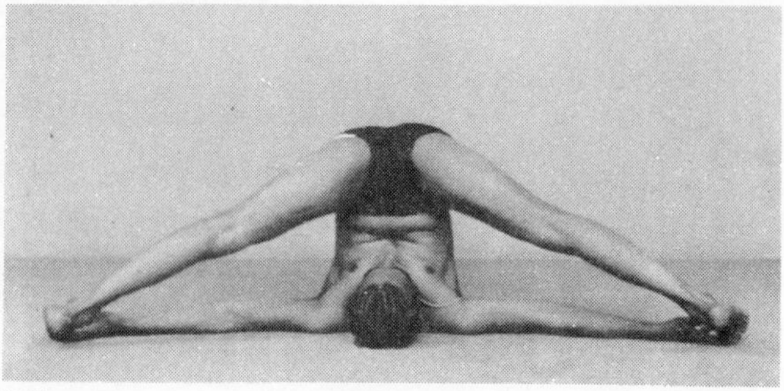

247

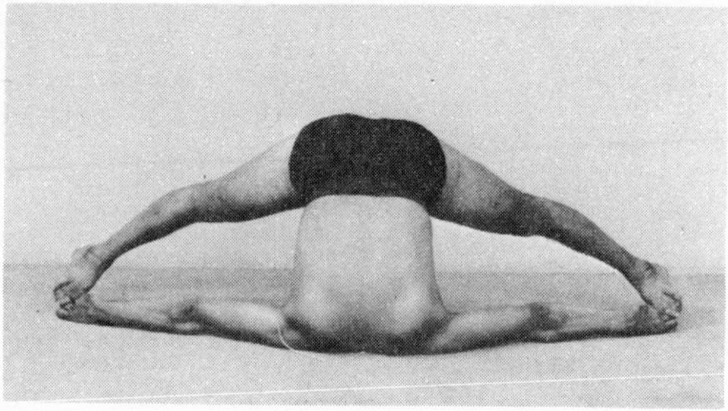

248

4. Stay in the pose from 20 to 30 seconds with normal breathing.

Effects

This pose tones the legs and helps to contract the abdominal organs.

94. *Pārśva Halāsana* Four* (Plate 249)

In Halāsana (Plate 244) both the legs rest behind the head. In this pose they rest sideways on one side of and in line with the head. This is the lateral plough pose.

Technique

1. Do Supta Koṇāsana (Plate 247) and come back to Halāsana.

2. Place the palms on the back of the ribs. (Plate 240)

3. Move both the legs as far as you can to the left.

4. Tighten both knees, raise the trunk up with the help of the palms and stretch the legs. (Plate 249)

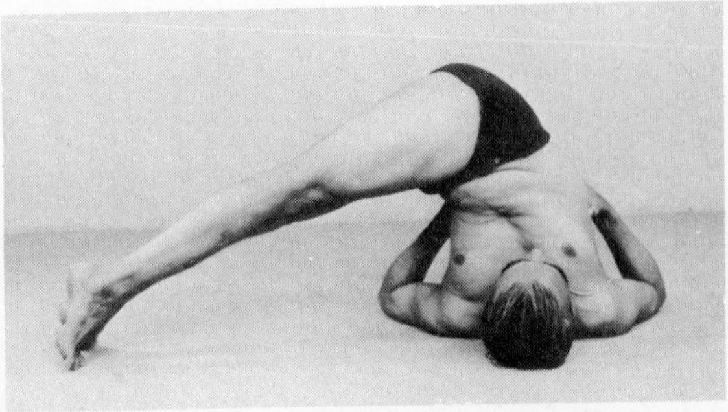

249

5. Remain in this position for half a minute with normal breathing.

6. Exhale, move the legs to the right until they are in line with the head and hold the pose for half a minute. Do not disturb the position of the chest and trunk when the legs are moved. The chest and trunk should remain as in Sarvāngāsana or Halāsana.

Effects

In this āsana, the spine moves laterally and becomes more elastic. The colon, which is inverted during the movements, is exercised properly and elimination will be complete. People suffering from acute or chronic constipation which is the mother of several diseases derive great benefit from this āsana. If rubbish is dumped outside our house we feel sick. How much more so when waste matter which creates toxins is allowed to accumulate in our own system? If this waste matter is not eliminated, diseases will enter the body like thieves and rob us of health. If the bowels do not move freely, the mind becomes dull and one feels heavy and irritable. This āsana helps us to keep the bowels free and thereby win the prize of health.

95. *Eka Pāda Sarvāngāsana* Five* (Plate 250)

Eka means one, single. Pāda means the foot. In this variation of

Sarvāṅgāsana, one leg is on the floor in Halāsana, while the other is in a vertical position along with the trunk.

Technique

1. Do Sālamba Sarvāṅgāsana I. (Plate 223)

2. Keep the left leg up in Sarvāṅgāsana. Exhale and move the right leg down to the floor to Halāsana. (Plate 250.) It should remain stiff and straight and not bend at the knee.

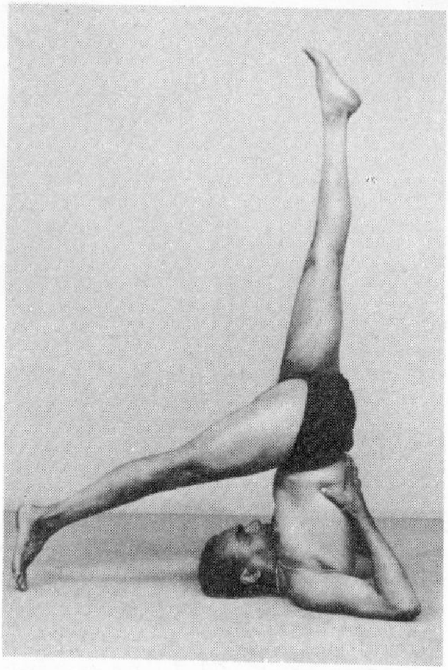

250

3. While resting the right leg on the floor, the left knee should be kept taut and not allowed to tilt sideways. The left leg should be kept straight, facing the head.

4. Stay in the pose for 20 seconds maintaining normal breathing.

5. Exhale, lift the right leg back to Sarvāṅgāsana, and then move the left leg down to the floor in Halāsana, keeping the right leg vertically up and stiff. Lifting the leg from the floor back to Sarvāṅgāsana exercises the abdominal organs more than if one brings both legs down to Halāsana.

6. Stay on this side for the same length of time.

Effects

This āsana tones the kidneys and the leg muscles.

96. *Pārśvaika Pāda Sarvāngāsana* Six* (Plate 251)

Pārśva means the side. In Eka Pāda Sarvāngāsana (Plate 250) the lower leg rests behind the head, whereas here it rests sideways in line with the trunk.

Technique

1. Perform Eka Pāda Sarvāngāsana on both sides as described above and come back to Sarvāngāsana.

2. Exhale, move the right leg down sideways to the floor until it is in line with the trunk. (Plate 251.) Keep the right leg straight and stiff and do not bend it at the knee.

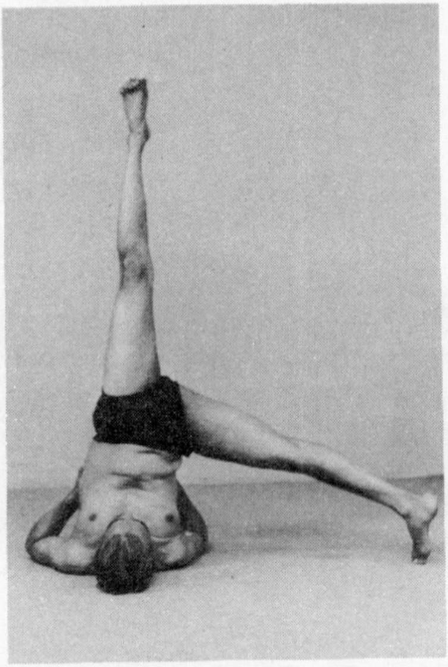

251

3. The left leg which is vertically up should be kept straight and not allowed to tilt to the right. The ribs should be lifted with the palms to expand the chest fully.

4. Remain in the pose for 20 seconds with normal breathing, exhale, and go back to Sarvāngāsana. Repeat with the other leg for the same length of time and return to Sarvāngāsana.

Effects

This pose relieves constipation and also tones the kidneys.

97. *Pārśva Sarvāngāsana* Nine* (Plate 254)

Pārśva means side or flank. This Sarvāngāsana variation is done by giving the trunk a lateral twist.

Technique

1. From Sālamba Sarvāngāsana I (Plate 223) turn the trunk and legs to the right.

2. Place the left palm on the left hip, so that the coccyx rests on the wrist. (Plate 252.) Lower the body on the left hand and bear the weight of the body on the left elbow and wrist. (Plate 253)

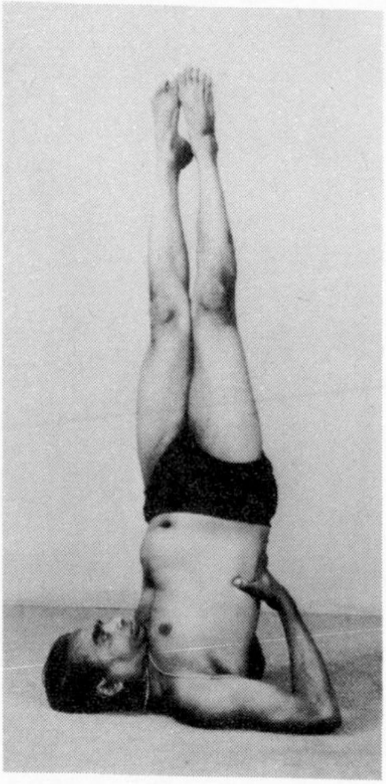

252

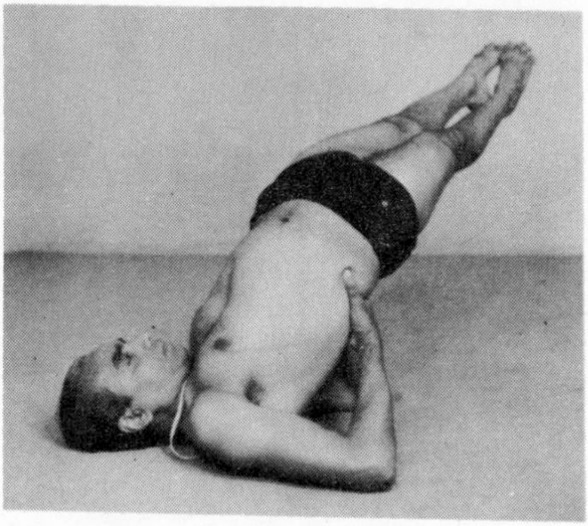

253

3. The right palm remains as in Sarvāngāsana on the back dorsal region.

4. Move the legs over the left palm at an angle (Plate 254) and stay in this position for 20 seconds breathing normally.

5. Exhale, come back to Sālamba Sarvāngāsana I and repeat on the right side for the same length of time. (Plate 255)

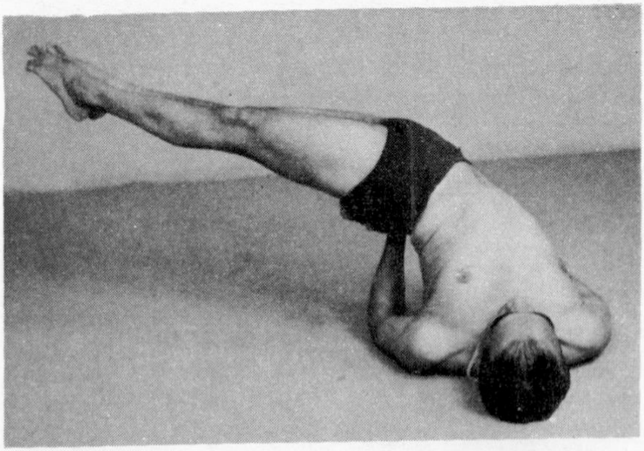

254

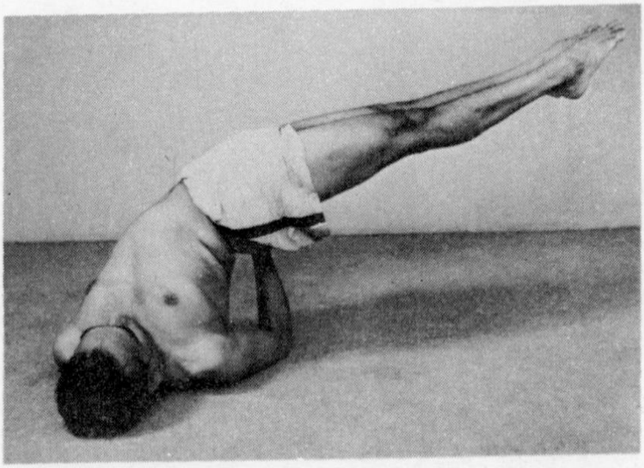

255

Effects

This āsana strengthens the wrists. It also exercises the liver, pancreas and spleen and ensures a generous blood supply to them. These organs are thereby kept in a healthy condition.

98. *Setu Bandha Sarvāngāsana* – also called *Uttāna Mayūrāsana* Ten* (Plate 259)

Setu means a bridge and Setu Bandha means the formation or construction of a bridge. In this position, the body is arched and supported on the shoulders, soles and heels. The arch is supported by the hands at the waist.

Ut means intense and tān means to stretch. This āsana resembles a stretched peacock (Mayūra), hence the name.

Technique

1. Do Sālamba Sarvāngāsana. (Plate 223)

2. Rest the palms well on the back, raise the spine up, take the legs back straight (Plate 256) or bend the knees (Plate 257) and throw the legs back over the wrists to the floor. (Plate 258.) Stretch out the legs and keep them together. (Plate 259)

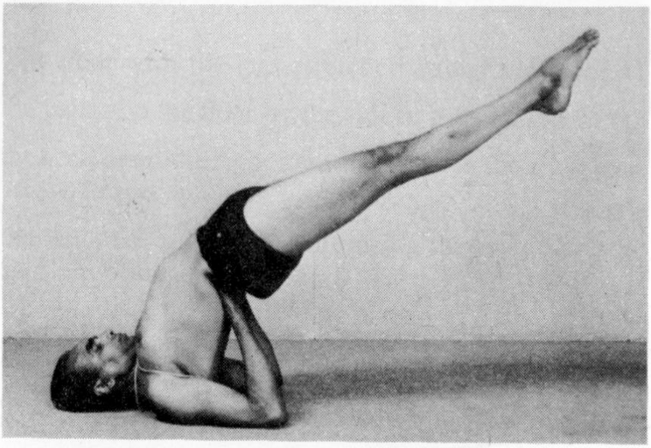

256

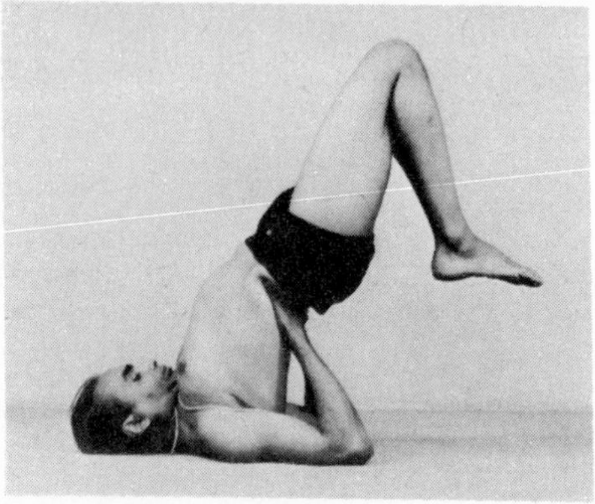

257

3. The whole body forms a bridge, the weight of which is borne by the elbows and the wrists. The only parts of the body in contact with

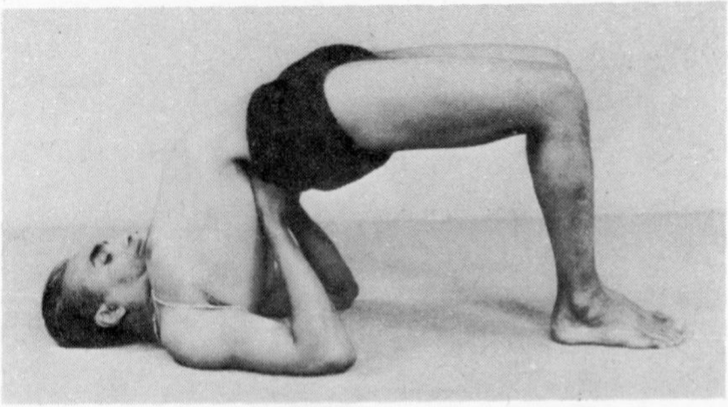

258

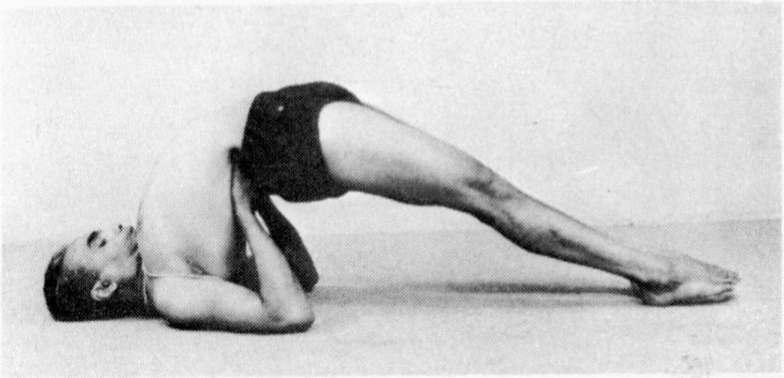

259

the ground will be the back of the head and neck, the shoulders, the elbows and the feet. Stay in the pose from half a minute to a minute with normal breathing.

4. It is possible to lessen the pressure on the elbows and the wrists by stretching the spine towards the neck, keeping the heels firmly on the ground.

99. *Eka Pāda Setu Bandha Sarvāṅgāsana*–also called *Eka Pāda Uttāna Mayūrāsana* Eleven* (Plate 260)

Eka means one and pāda means the foot. This is a variation of the previous āsana, with one leg high in the air.

Technique

1. After staying in Setu Bandha Sarvāṅgāsana (Plate 259), exhale and lift the right leg up to a perpendicular position. (Plate 260.) Stretch both the legs fully and hold this pose for 10 seconds.

2. Inhale, bring the right leg to the floor, exhale, lift the left leg to the perpendicular and stretch out both the legs fully. Stay for the same length of time. Inhale and bring the leg to the floor.

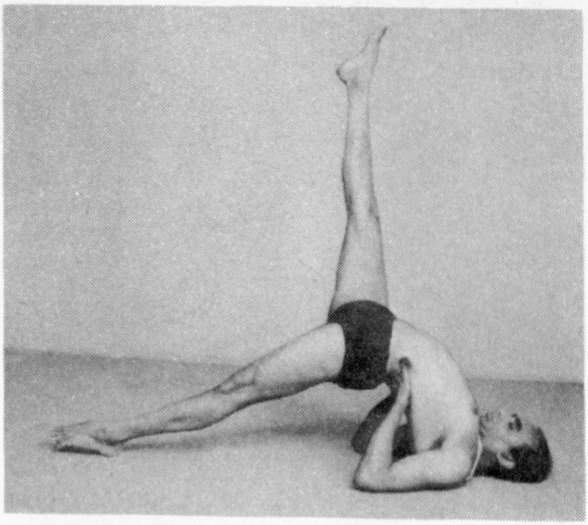

260

3. Exhale, swing the legs back to Sarvāngāsana (Plate 223), slide them gradually to the floor by removing the hands from the back and rest on the floor.

Effects of Setu Bandha Sarvāngāsana and Eka Pāda Setu Bandha Sarvāngāsana

These two āsanas give the spine a backward movement and remove the strain on the neck caused by the other various movements of Sarvāngāsana.

A healthy and flexible spine indicates a healthy nervous system. If the nerves are healthy a man is sound in mind and body.

100. *Ūrdhva Padmāsana in Sarvāngāsana* Four* (Plate 261)

Ūrdhva means above, high. Padma means a lotus. In this Sarvāngāsana variation, the legs, instead of being kept straight up, are bent at the knees and crossed so that the right foot rests on the left thigh and the left foot on the right thigh as in the lotus pose. (Plate 104)

Technique

1. From Sālamba Sarvāngāsana, bend the legs at the knees and cross them. First place the right foot over the left thigh, and then the left foot over the right thigh.

2. Stretch the crossed legs vertically up, move the knees closer to each other and the legs as far back as possible from the pelvic region. (Plate 261)

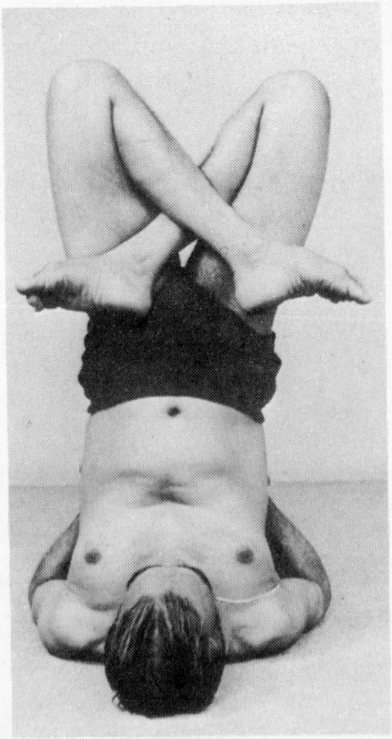

261

3. Stay in this pose from 20 to 30 seconds with deep and even breathing.

4. To increase the stretch, perform the pose by giving the trunk a lateral twist following the technique of Pārśva Sarvāṅgāsana. (Plate 254.) This is called:

101. *Pārśva Ūrdhva Padmāsana in Sarvāṅgāsana* Seven* (Plates 262 to 265)

(Pārśva means flank.)

5. Stay on each side for 10 to 15 seconds with normal breathing.

6. Exhale, come back to Ūrdhva Padmāsana and rest awhile.

7. Now, with an exhalation arch the trunk back (Plate 266) following the technique of Setu Bandha Sarvāṅgāsana. (Plate 259.) Gradually stretch the thighs back until the knees rest on the floor forming a bridge over the hands. This is called:

102. *Uttāna Padma Mayūrāsana* Twenty-five* (Plate 267)

Uttāna means an intense stretch, padma is a lotus and mayūra a peacock.

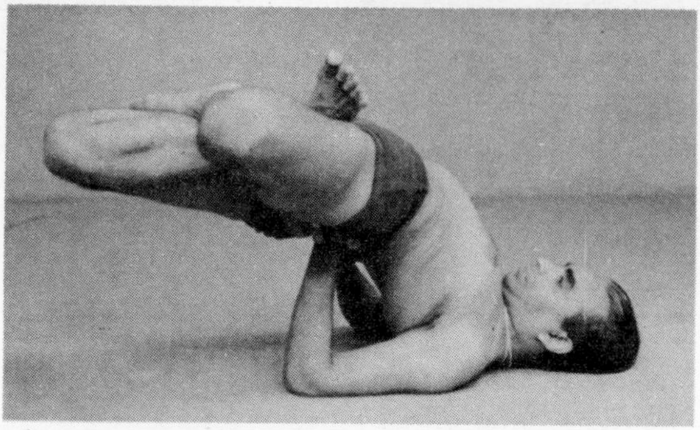
262

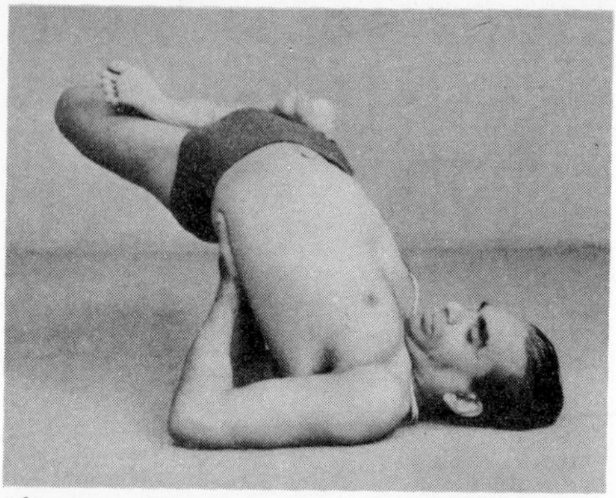
263

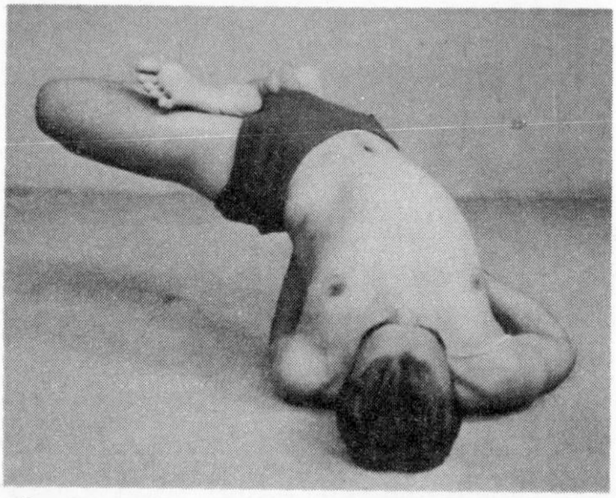
264

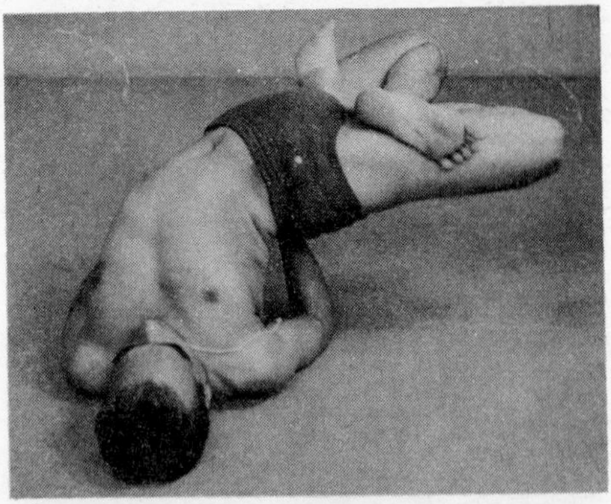

265

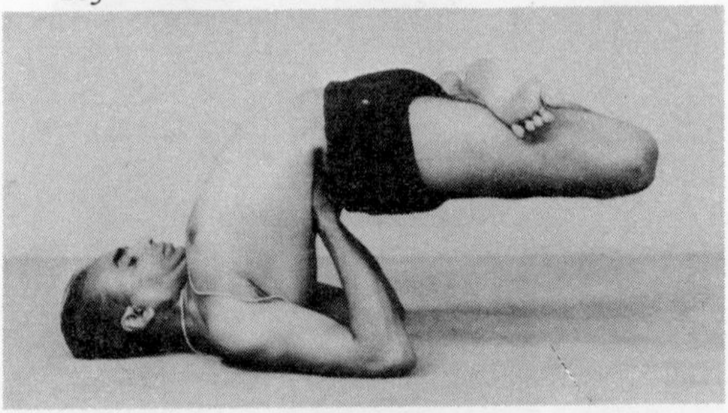

266

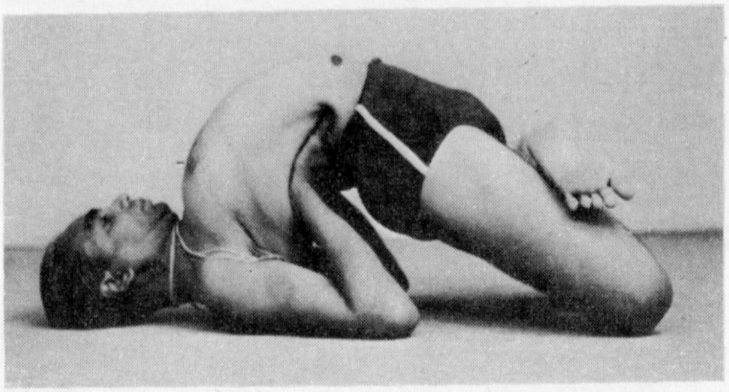

267

8. Stay in this position for 10 to 15 seconds with normal breathing.

9. Exhale, come back to Ūrdhva Padmāsana.

10. Uncross the legs, return to Sālamba Sarvāṅgāsana and repeat the pose by first placing the left foot over the right thigh and then the right

foot over the left thigh. Stay for an equal length of time in all these positions as in the earlier ones.

103. *Piṇḍāsana in Sarvāṅgāsana* Five* (Plate 269)

Piṇḍa means embryo or foetus. In this variation of Sarvāṅgāsana which is a continuation of the earlier posture, the bent crossed legs are brought down until they rest on the head. The posture resembles that of an embryo in the womb, hence the name.

Technique

1. From Ūrdhva Padmāsana in Sarvāṅgāsana (Plate 261), exhale, bend and lower the crossed legs from the hips towards the head.

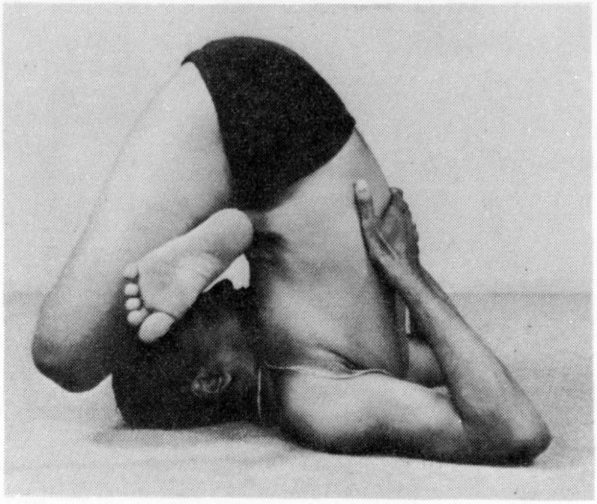

268

2. Rest the legs over the head. (Plate 268)

3. Release the hands from the back, and clasp the legs. (Plate 269.) While clasping, move the trunk nearer to the neck to rest the legs well.

4. Remain in this position from 20 to 30 seconds with normal breathing and go back to Ūrdhva Padmāsana in Sarvāṅgāsana.

104. *Pārśva Piṇḍāsana in Sarvāṅgāsana* Eight* (Plates 270 and 271)

Pārśva means the side or flank. In this Piṇḍāsana variation of the earlier pose, both the bent knees are moved sideways and placed on the floor on the same side of the trunk. This is the lateral embryo pose in Sarvāṅgāsana.

Technique

1. After releasing the handclasp from Piṇḍāsana (Plate 269) bring the hands back and place the palms at the back of the ribs. (Plate 268)

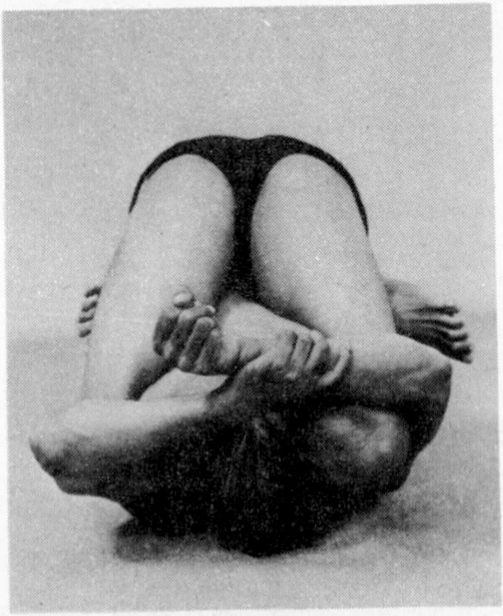

269

2. Turn the hips sideways to the right, exhale and lower both knees to the floor. The left knee should be by the side of the right ear. (Plate 270)

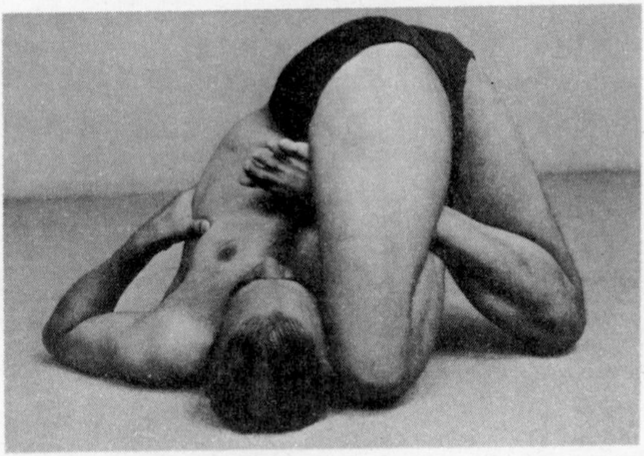

270

3. The left shoulder will be raised off the floor in the beginning. Push the shoulder against the floor and press the left hand firmly against the back. If this is not done, you will lose balance and roll over to one side.

4. Due to the lateral twist, breathing will be fast and difficult as the diaphragm is pressed in this position.

5. The knee near the ear will not rest on the floor to start with, but only after long practice.

6. Stay in this position for 20 to 30 seconds, with normal breathing.

7. Exhale, come up from the right side and move the crossed legs over to the left, so that the left foot will be near the left ear. (Plate 271.) Stay here also for the same length of time.

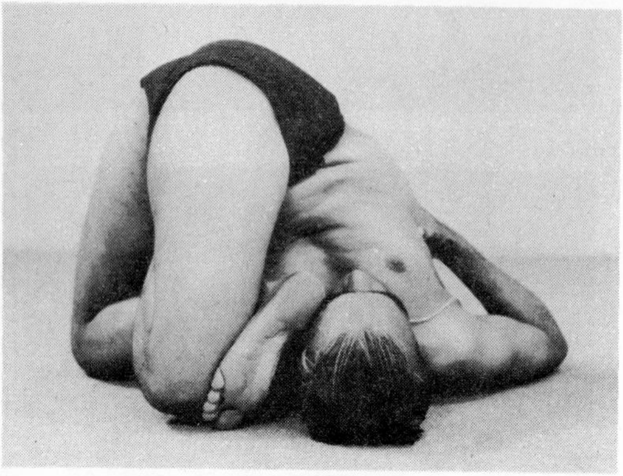

271

8. Go back to Ūrdhva Padmāsana. (Plate 261.) Release the lotus pose by uncrossing the legs and return to Sālamba Sarvāngāsana.

9. Now change the position of the crossed legs. Cross the legs again by putting the left foot over the right thigh first and then the right foot over the left thigh instead of the other way as done earlier.

10. Repeat the movements again on both the sides as described earlier.

Effects of Ūrdhva Padmāsana and Pārśva Piṇḍāsana movements in Sarvāngāsana

The change of crossing the legs brings equal pressure on both sides of the abdomen and colon and relieves constipation. For those suffering from chronic constipation a longer stay in Pārśva Piṇḍāsana is recommended, and one minute on each side will prove most efficacious. Griping pain in the stomach is relieved by these poses.

Persons with extremely flexible knees, can easily perform these positions. It is, however, difficult for many people to cross the legs in Padmāsana. For them a longer stay in Pārśva Halāsana (Plate 249)–

(there also the spine and trunk get a lateral twist but the legs remain straight) – is recommended.

In all these positions breathing at first will be fast and laboured. Try to maintain normal breathing.

Note. The spine is given the forward, lateral and backward movements in these variations of Sarvāngāsana. In Halāsana, Eka Pāda Sarvāngāsana, Karṇa Pīḍāsana and Pinḍāsana the spine moves in the forward direction. In Pārśvaika Pāda Sarvānga, Pārśva Halāsana and Pārśva Pinḍāsana the spine moves laterally, as in Pārśva Sarvāngāsana and in Pārśva Ūrdhva Padmāsana. In Setu Bandha and Uttāna Padma Mayūra it is given a backward movement. These movements tone the spine on all sides and keep it healthy.

It is related that in the Krita Age (the first Age of the Universe) a host of Dānavās (giants and demons) became invincible in battle under the leadership of Vṛtra and scattered the Devas (or Gods) in all directions. Realising that they could not regain their power until Vṛtra was destroyed, the gods appeared before their Grandsire, Brahmā, the creator. Brahmā instructed them to consult Viṣṇu who asked them to obtain the bones of a sage called Dadhīcha, from which to make a demon-slaying weapon. The gods appeared before the sage and begged the boon according to Viṣṇu's advice. The sage renounced his body for the benefit of the gods. From the spine of Dadhīcha was fashioned Vajra, the thunderbolt, which Indra the king of the gods hurled and slew Vṛtra.

The story is symbolical. The Dānavās represent the tāmasic qualities in men and diseases. The Devas represent health, harmony and peace. To destroy the tāmasic qualities and the diseases due to them and to enjoy health and happiness, we have to make our spines strong as a thunderbolt like the spine of Dadhīcha. Then we shall enjoy health, harmony and happiness in abundance.

105. *Jaṭhara Parivartanāsana* Five* (Plates 274 and 275)

Jaṭhara means the stomach, the belly. Parivartana means turning or rolling about, turning round.

Technique

1. Lie flat on the back on the floor. (Plate 219)

2. Stretch out both arms sideways in line with the shoulders, so that the body resembles a cross.

3. Exhale, raise both legs together until they are perpendicular to the floor. They should remain poker stiff, so do not bend them at the knees. (Plate 272)

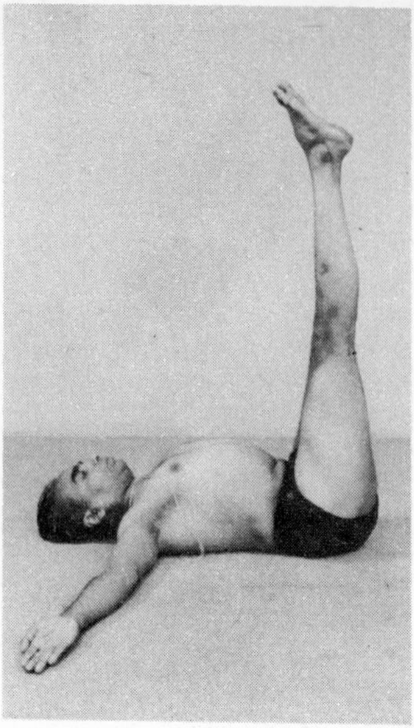

272

4. Remain in this position for a few breaths. Then exhale, and move both the legs sideways (Plate 273) down towards the floor to the left until the toes of the left foot almost touch the finger-tips of the outstretched left hand. (Plate 274.) Try and keep the back well on the floor. In the initial stages, the right shoulder will be lifted off the floor. To prevent this ask a friend to press it down, or catch hold of a heavy piece of furniture with the right hand when the legs are turned sideways to the left.

5. Both legs should go down together, the knees being kept tight throughout. As far as possible keep the lumbar portion of the back on the floor and turn the legs only from the hips. When the legs are near the outstretched left hand, move the abdomen to the right.

6. Stay in the pose for about 20 seconds, keeping the legs stiff throughout. Then move the still stiffened legs slowly back to the perpendicular with an exhalation. (Plate 272)

7. Remain with the legs perpendicular for a few breaths and then repeat the movements by lowering the legs to the right and turning the abdomen to the left. (Plate 275.) Stay here also for the same length of

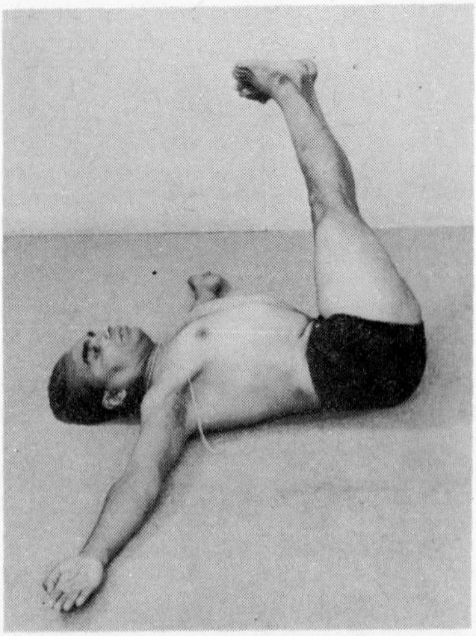

273

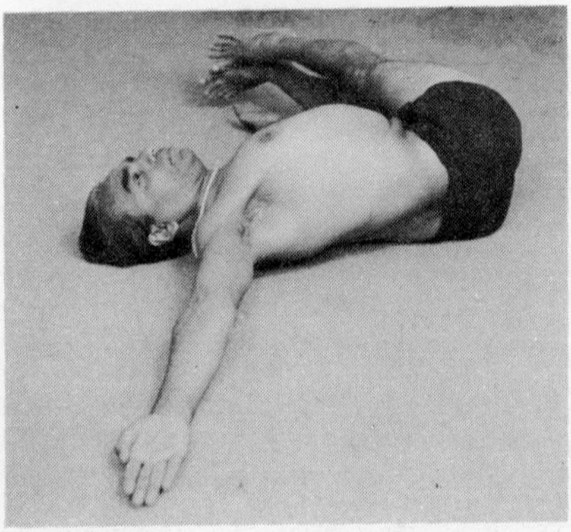

274

time and with an exhalation, come back to the perpendicular legs position (Plate 272) and then gently lower the legs to the floor (Plate 219) and relax.

Effects

This āsana is good for reducing excess fat. It tones and eradicates sluggishness of the liver, spleen and pancreas. It also cures gastritis and strengthens the intestines. By its regular practice all the abdominal

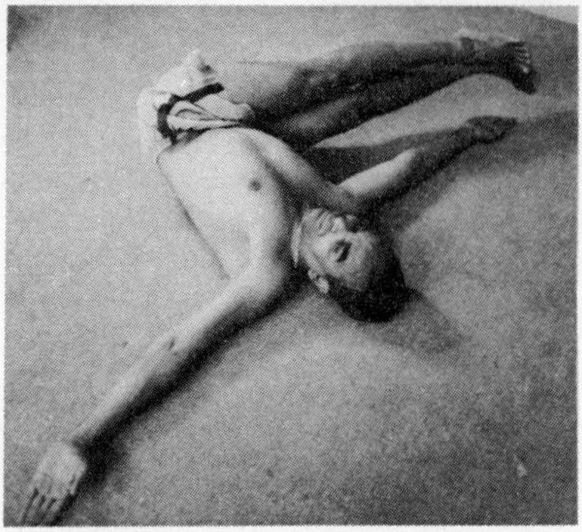

275

organs are kept in trim. It helps to relieve sprains and catches in the lower back and the hip region.

106. *Ūrdhva Prasarita Pādāsana* One* (Plates 276 to 279)

Ūrdhva means upright, above, high. Prasarita means extended, stretched out. Pāda means foot.

Technique

1. Lie flat on the back keeping the legs stretched out and tightened at the knees. Place the hands by the side of the legs. (Plate 219)

2. Exhale, move the arms over the head and stretch them out straight. (Plate 276.) Take two breaths.

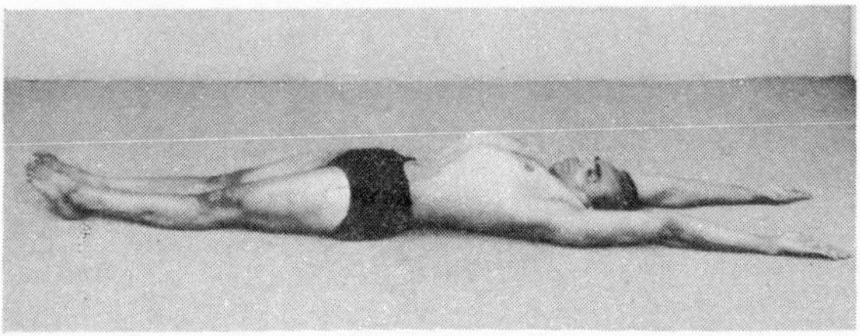

276

3. Exhale, raise the legs up through 30 degrees (Plate 277) and hold the position for 15 to 20 seconds with normal breathing.

4. Exhale, move the legs up to 60 degrees (Plate 278) and hold for 15 to 20 seconds with normal breathing.

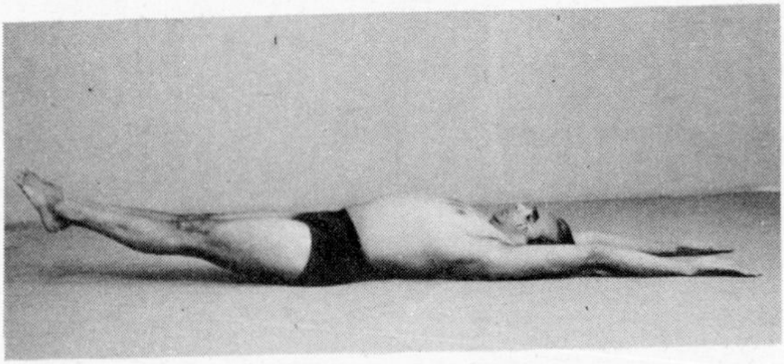

277

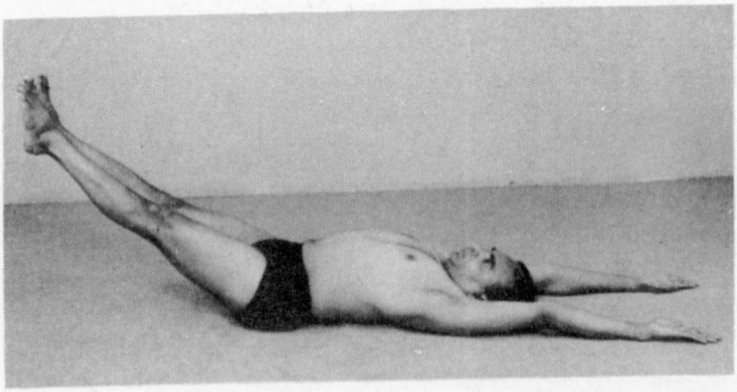

278

5. Again exhale, move the legs higher still to the perpendicular (Plate 279) and hold it for 30 to 60 seconds with normal breathing.

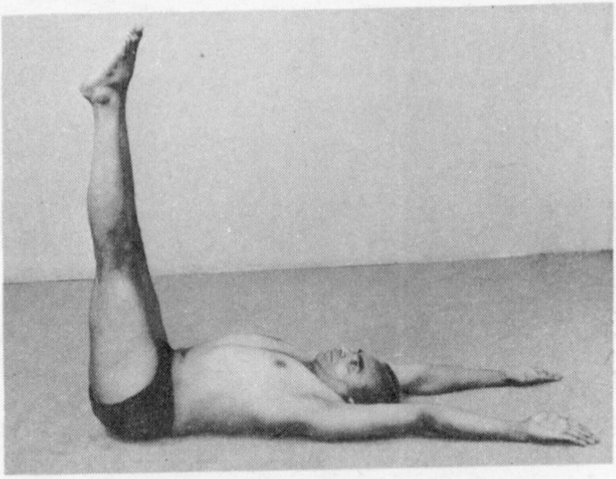

279

6. Now exhale, lower the legs slowly to the floor and relax.

7. Repeat 3 or 4 times from position 2 to 6.

Note. If you cannot do all the three positions at one stretch, do them in 3 steps, resting between each.

Effects

This āsana is a wonderful exercise for reducing fat round the abdomen. It strengthens the lumbar region of the back, tones the abdominal organs, and relieves those suffering from gastric trouble and flatulence.

107. *Chakrāsana* Four* (Plates 280 to 283)

Chakra means a wheel. In this pose, lie flat on the floor, lift both legs, raise them straight up together and bring them over the head to Halāsana. (Plate 239.) Place the hands by the ears and roll over the head. This rolling over resembles the movement of a wheel, hence the name.

Technique

1. Lie flat on the back on the floor. (Plate 219)

2. Exhale, raise both the legs together and bring them over the head and rest the toes on the floor as in Halāsana. (Plate 239.) Take 2 or 3 breaths.

3. Move the hands over the head, bend the elbows and place the palms down beside the shoulders, the fingers pointing away from the feet. (Plate 280)

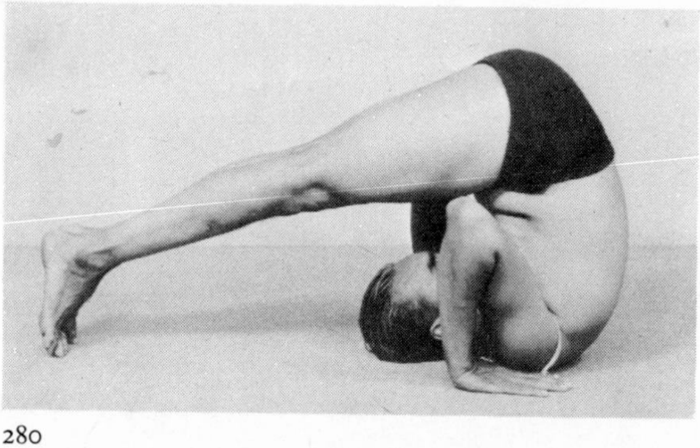

280

4. Exhale, press the palms on the floor and stretch the legs further to raise the back of the neck and roll over the head as in Plates 281, 282 and 283.

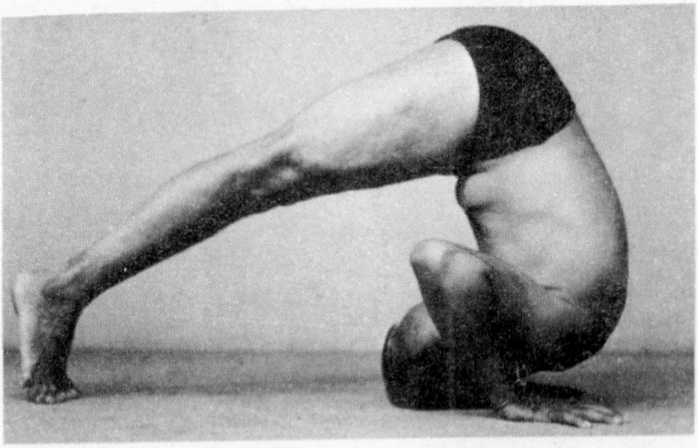

281

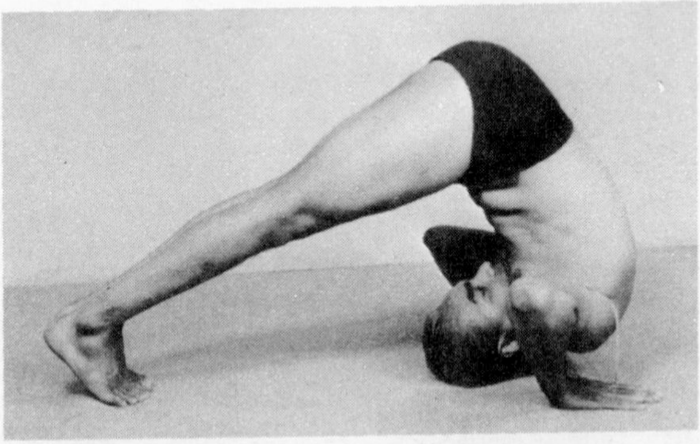

282

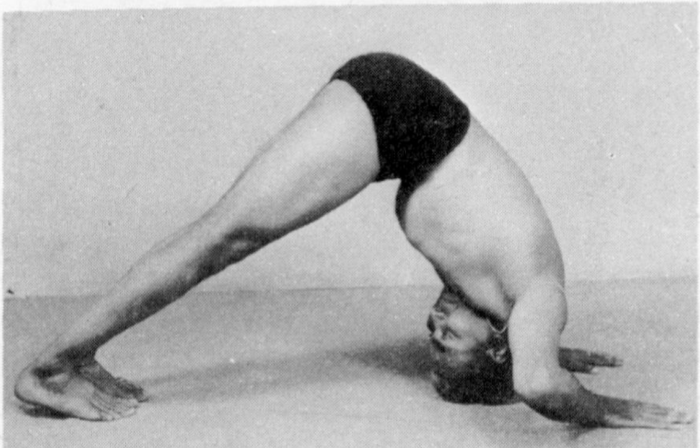

283

5. Now stretch the arms out straight and go into Adho Mukha Śvānāsana. (Plate 75)

6. Bend the elbows, lower the trunk to the floor, turn over on the back and relax.

Effects

This āsana tones the abdominal organs and the spine. Due to the wheeling movement, the blood circulates round the spinal column and rejuvenates it. It is also good for people suffering from gastric trouble and a sluggish liver.

108. *Supta Pādānguṣṭhāsana* Thirteen* (Plate 285)

Supta means lying down. Pāda is the foot. Anguṣṭha means the big toe. This āsana is done in three movements.

Technique

1. Lie flat on the back, stretch both legs and keep the knees tight. (Plate 219)

2. Inhale, raise the left leg from the floor until it is perpendicular. Keep the right leg stretched fully on the floor and rest the right hand on the right thigh.

3. Raise the left arm and catch the left big toe between the thumb and the fore and middle fingers. (Plate 284.) Take 3 or 4 deep breaths.

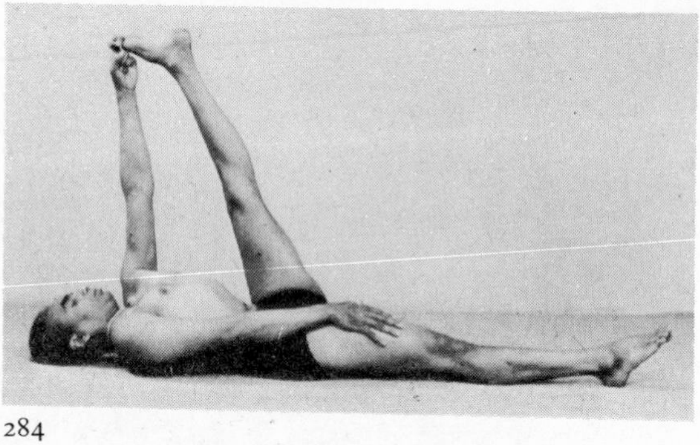

284

4. Exhale, raise the head and trunk from the floor, bend the left arm at the elbow and pull the left leg towards the head without bending it at the knee. Pull the leg down, lift the head and trunk up together and rest the chin on the left knee. (Plate 285.) Stay in this position for about 20 seconds, keeping the right leg fully stretched straight along the floor while breathing normally.

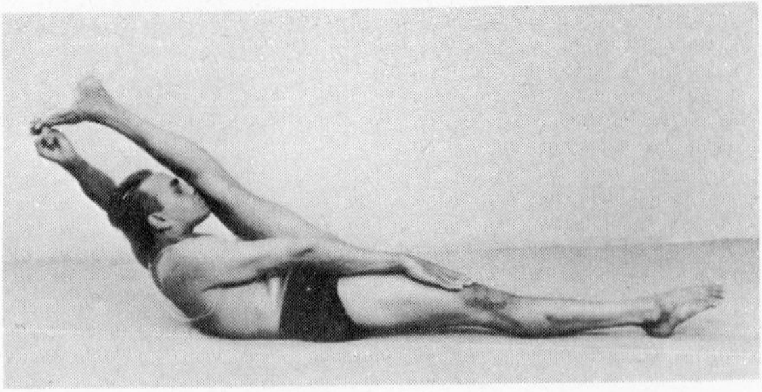

285

5. Inhale, move the head and trunk back to the floor and the left leg back to the perpendicular. (Plate 284.) This completes the first movement.

6. Exhale, hold the left big toe, bend the left knee and move the grasped toe towards the right shoulder. Bend the left elbow, stretch the left arm behind the head and move the head up into the space between the left forearm and the left shin. (Plate 286.) Take a few deep breaths.

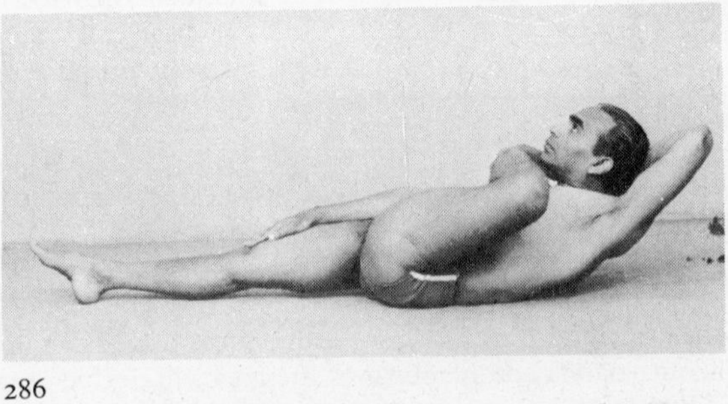

286

7. Inhale, move the head back to the floor, bring the left arm in front of the head and straighten the left arm and leg. Take the left leg back to the perpendicular, maintaining the toe hold throughout. (Plate 284.) During this movement also the right leg remains fully extended on the floor throughout and the right hand rests on the right thigh. This completes the second movement.

8. Exhale, and without disturbing the head and trunk or lifting the right leg off the floor, move the left arm and leg sideways to the left down to the floor. (Plate 287.) Do not release the toe hold but bring the left arm in level with the shoulders on the floor. Stay in this position

for about 20 seconds without bending the left leg at the knee. Breathe normally.

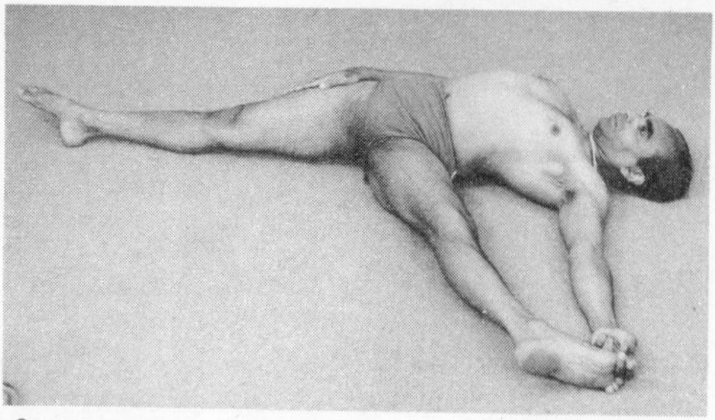

287

9. Now inhale and without bending the left leg at the knee, bring it back to the perpendicular without releasing the grip on the left big toe or disturbing the right leg stretched on the floor. (Plate 284)

10. Exhale, release the toe grip, rest the left leg on the floor beside the right one and keep the left hand on the left thigh. This completes the third movement. To start with it is difficult to keep the extended leg stretched right out on the floor throughout these three movements. Therefore, ask a friend to keep the leg down by pressing the thigh just above the knee, or press the foot against a wall.

11. After completing the three movements on the left side, take a few deep inhalations and then repeat them on the right, substituting the word 'left' for the word 'right'.

Effects

The legs will develop properly by the practice of this āsana. Persons suffering from sciatica and paralysis of the legs will derive great benefit from it. The blood is made to circulate in the legs and hips where the nerves are rejuvenated. The pose removes stiffness in the hip joints and prevents hernia. It can be practised by both men and women.

109. *Anantāsana* Nine* (Plate 290)

Ananta is a name of Viṣṇu and also of Viṣṇu's couch, the serpent Śeṣa. According to Hindu mythology, Viṣṇu sleeps in the primeval ocean on his couch Śeṣa, the thousand-headed serpent. In his sleep a lotus grows from his navel. In that lotus is born the Creator Brahmā, who fashions the world. After the creation, Viṣṇu awakens to reign in the highest heaven, Vaikuṇṭha. The pose is found in the temple dedicated to Lord Ananta Padmanābha (padma = lotus: nābha = navel) of Trivandrum in South India.

Technique

1. Lie flat on the back. (Plate 219.) Exhale, turn to the left and rest the body, keeping the side in contact with the floor.

2. Raise the head, stretch the left arm beyond the head in line with the body, bend the left elbow, raise the forearm and rest the head on the left palm which should be placed above the ear. (Plate 288.) Stay in this position for a few seconds with either normal or deep breaths.

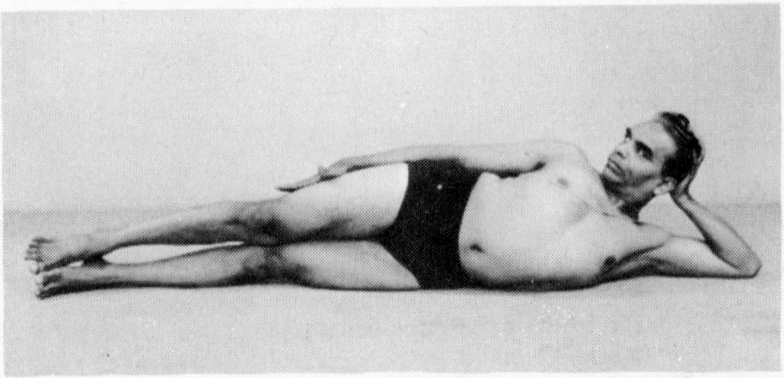

288

3. Bend the right knee and catch the right big toe with the right thumb and the fore and middle fingers. (Plate 289)

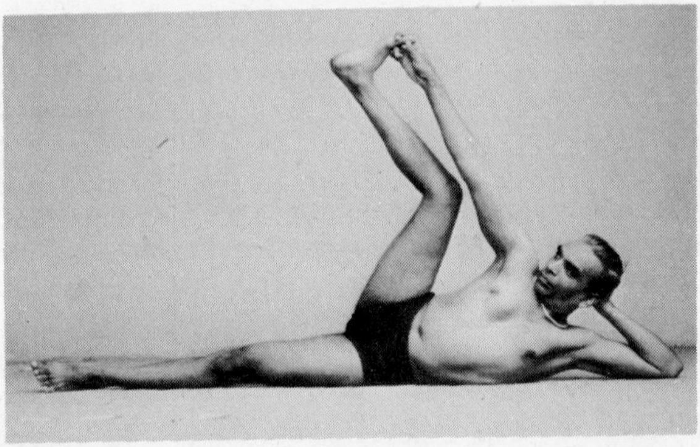

289

4. Exhale, stretch the right arm and leg up vertically together. (Plate 290.) Hold the pose from 15 to 20 seconds with normal breathing.

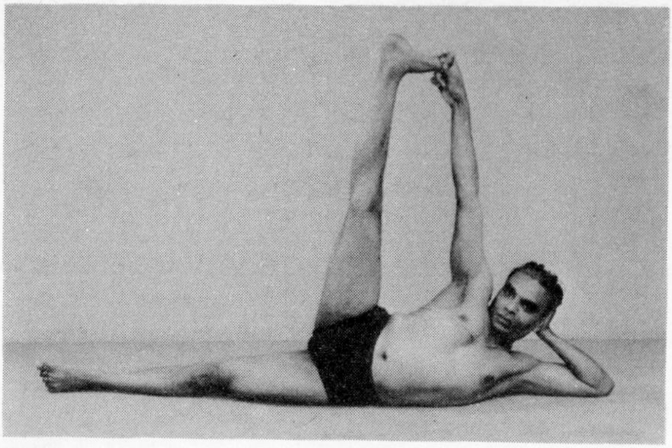

290

5. Exhale, bend the right knee and return to the position described in para. 2.

6. Lower the head from the left palm and roll over on the back. (Plate 219)

7. Repeat the pose on the other side for the same length of time and then relax.

Effects

The pelvic region benefits from this exercise and the hamstring muscles are properly toned. The āsana also relieves backaches and prevents the development of hernia.

110. *Uttāna Pādāsana* Nine* (Plate 292)

Uttāna means stretched out or lying on the back with the face up. Pāda means a leg.

Technique

1. Lie flat on the back, keeping the feet together and the knees tight. (Plate 219.) Take 3 or 4 deep breaths.

2. Exhale, raise the back off the floor and arch it up by stretching the neck and moving the head back until the crown of the head rests on the floor. (Plate 291.) If resting the crown on the floor proves difficult, bring the hands by the side of the head, raise the neck and pull the head as far back as possible by raising the dorsal and lumbar regions of the back from the floor. Then rest the arms at the side. Take 2 or 3 breaths.

3. Stretch the back and with an exhalation lift the legs up until they are

about 45 to 50 degrees from the floor. Raise the arms, join the palms and keep them parallel to the legs. (Plate 292.) The arms and the legs should be kept stiff and not bent at the elbows or knees. Keep the legs together at the thighs, knees, ankles and feet.

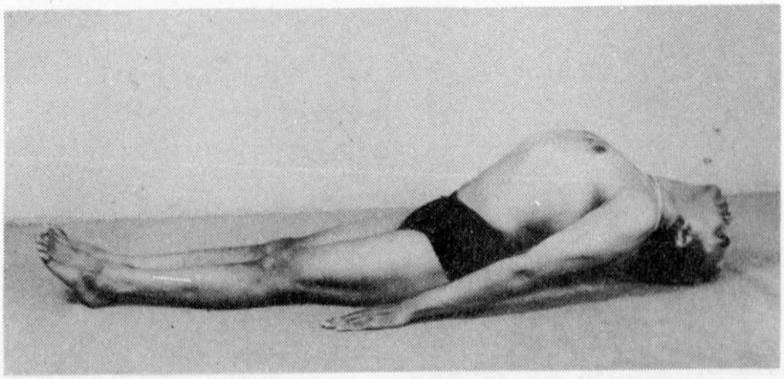

291

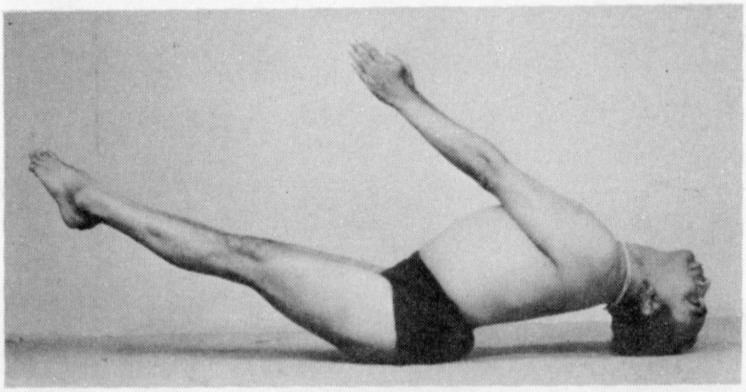

292

4. Extend the ribs fully and remain in this pose for half a minute with normal breathing. The body should be balanced only on the crown of the head and the buttocks.

5. Exhale, lower the legs and arms to the floor, straighten the neck, release the head grip, lower the trunk and relax lying flat on the back on the floor.

Effects

The āsana gives full expansion to the chestwall and keeps the dorsal portion of the spine supple and healthy. It tones the neck and back and regulates the activity of the thyroids by ensuring their supply of healthy blood. The abdominal muscles are also stretched and strengthened.

111. *Setu Bandhāsana* Fourteen* (Plate 296)

Setu means a bridge. Setu bandha means the construction of a bridge. In this posture, the whole body forms an arch and is supported at one end by the crown of the head and at the other on the feet, hence the name.

Technique

1. Lie flat on the back on the floor. (Plate 219.) Take a few deep breaths.

2. Bend the knees, widen the legs at the knees and bring the heels in towards the buttocks.

3. Keep the heels together and rest the outer sides firmly on the floor.

4. Bring the hands by the side of the head and, with an exhalation, raise the trunk and arch the body up to rest the crown of the head on the floor. (Plate 293.) Pull the head as far back as possible by stretching the neck up and lifting the dorsal and lumbar regions of the back off the floor.

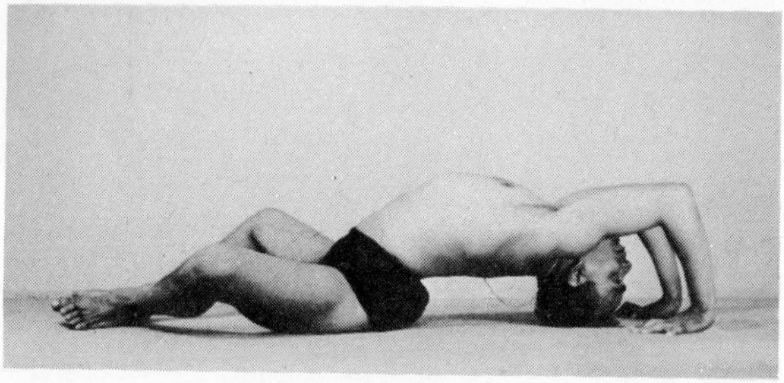

293

5. Fold the arms across the chest and hold the left elbow with the right hand and the right elbow with the left hand. (Plate 294.) Take 2 or 3 breaths.

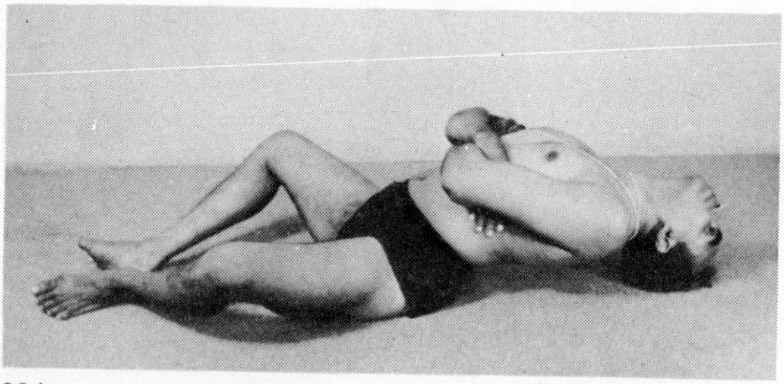

294

6. Exhale, draw the hips up (Plate 295) and stretch out the legs until they are straight. (Plate 296.) Join the feet and press them firmly to the

ground. The whole body now forms a bridge or an arch. One end of it is supported by the crown of the head and the other end on the feet.

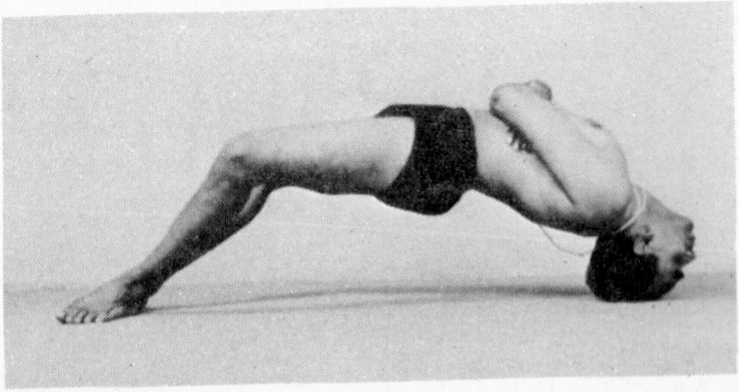

295

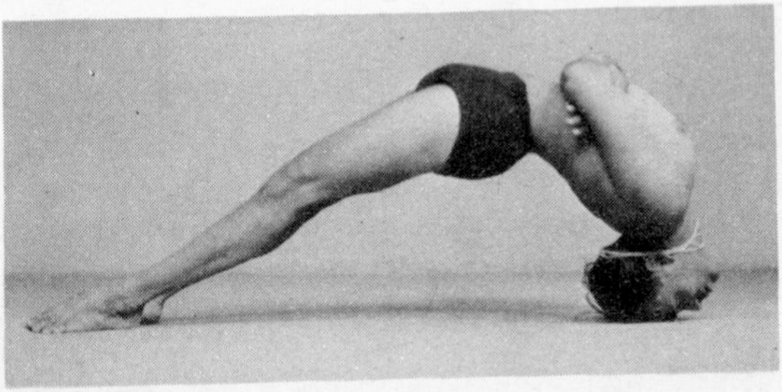

296

7. Hold this position for a few seconds with normal breathing.

8. Exhale, unfold the arms and place the hands on the floor, bend the knees, lower the legs and trunk to the floor, release the head grip, straighten the neck, lie flat on the back and relax.

Effects

The āsana strengthens the neck and tones the cervical, dorsal, lumbar and sacral regions of the spine. The extensor muscles of the back grow powerful and the hips are contracted and hardened. The pineal, pituitary, thyroid and adrenal glands are bathed in blood and function properly.

112. *Bharadvājāsana I* One* (Plates 297 and 298)

Bharadvāja was the father of Droṇa, the military preceptor of the Kauravas and Pāṇḍavas, who fought the great war described in the Mahābhārata. This āsana is dedicated to Bharadvāja.

Technique

1. Sit on the floor with the legs stretched straight in front. (Plate 77)

2. Flex the knees, move the legs back and bring both feet to the right side beside the hip.

3. Rest the buttocks on the floor, turn the trunk about 45 degrees to the left, straighten the right arm and place the right hand on the outer side of the left thigh near the left knee. Insert the right hand underneath the left knee, the palm touching the floor.

4. Exhale, turn the left arm from the shoulder behind the back, bend the left elbow and with the left hand clasp the right upper arm above the right elbow.

5. Turn the neck to the right and gaze over the right shoulder. (Plates 297 and 298)

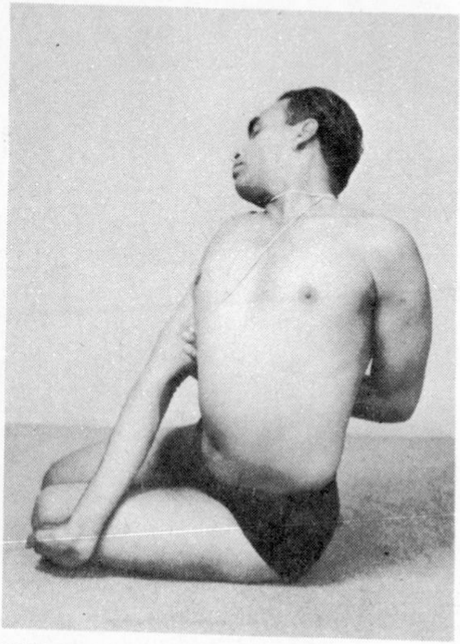

297

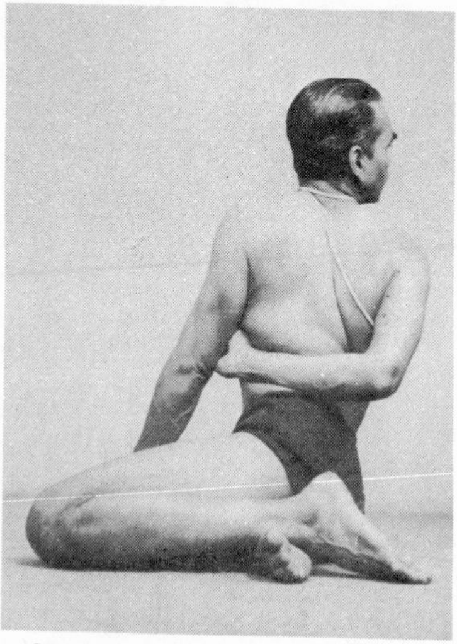

298

6. Hold the position for half a minute with deep breathing.

7. Loosen the hand grip, straighten the legs and repeat the pose on the other side. Here, bring both the feet beside the left hip, turn the trunk to the right, straighten the left arm, place the left palm underneath the right knee and catch the left upper arm near the elbow with the right hand from behind the back. Stay there for an equal length of time.

Effects

This simple āsana works on the dorsal and lumbar regions of the spine. People with very stiff backs find the other lateral twisting positions extremely difficult. This pose helps to make the back supple. People with arthritis will find it very beneficial.

113. *Bharadvājāsana II* Two* (Plates 299 and 300)

Technique

1. Sit on the floor with the legs stretched straight in front. (Plate 77)

2. Bend the left leg at the knee, hold the left foot with the hands and place it at the root of the right thigh near the pelvis so that the left heel is kept near the navel. The left leg will then be in the half lotus pose.

3. Bend the right foot at the knee and bring the right foot back and rest the right heel beside the right hip. The inner side of the right calf will touch the outer side of the right thigh. Keep both the knees on the floor near each other.

4. Exhale, turn the left arm from the shoulder behind the back, bend the left elbow, bring the left hand near the right hip and catch the left foot with the left hand.

5. Straighten the right arm, place the right hand on the outer side of the left thigh near the left knee. Insert the right hand underneath the left knee, the palm touching the floor and the fingers pointing to the right. (Plates 299 and 300)

6. Hold the left foot tight and turn the trunk to as far to the left as you can. Turn the neck in either direction and gaze over the shoulder.

7. Stay in the pose from half a minute to a minute with normal or deep breathing.

8. Then release the pose and repeat it on the other side for the same length of time. Here the right foot will be placed at the root of the left thigh and will be held from behind the back by the right hand. The left leg will be bent at the knee and the left heel will rest on the floor beside the left hip. The left hand will be placed underneath the right knee and the trunk will be twisted as far to the right as possible.

9. After completing the āsana on both the sides, stretch out the legs, straighten the arms and rest.

Effects

The knees and shoulders become flexible by the practice of this pose. It

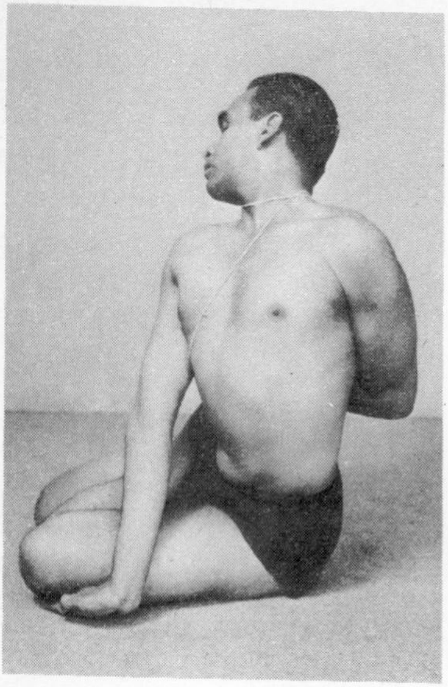

299

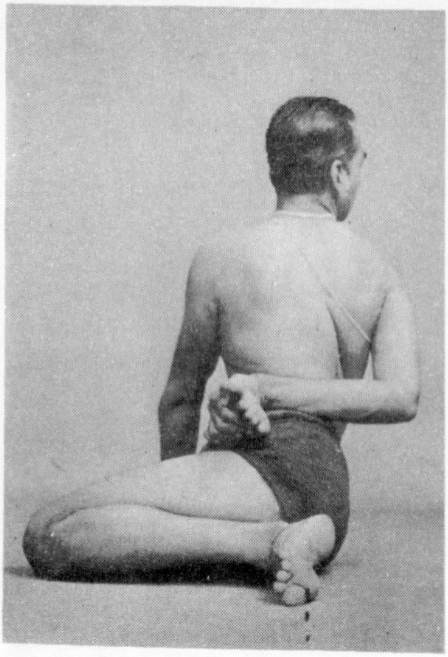

300

is not very effective for people with elastic spinal movements, but the arthritic will find the pose to be a blessing.

114. *Marīchyāsana III* Ten* (Plates 303 and 304)

This is one of the sitting lateral twisting postures.

Technique

1. Sit on the floor with the legs stretched straight in front. (Plate 77)

2. Bend the left knee, place the sole and heel of the left foot flat on the floor. The shin of the left leg should be perpendicular to the floor and the calf should touch the thigh. Place the left heel near the perineum. The inner side of the left foot should touch the inner side of the outstretched right thigh.

3. With an exhalation, turn the spine about 90 degrees to the left, so that the chest goes beyond the bent left thigh and bring the right arm over the left thigh. (Plate 301)

4. Place the right shoulder beyond the left knee and stretch the right arm out forwards by turning the spine still more to the left and stretching the region at the back of the right floating ribs. (Plate 302.) Take two breaths.

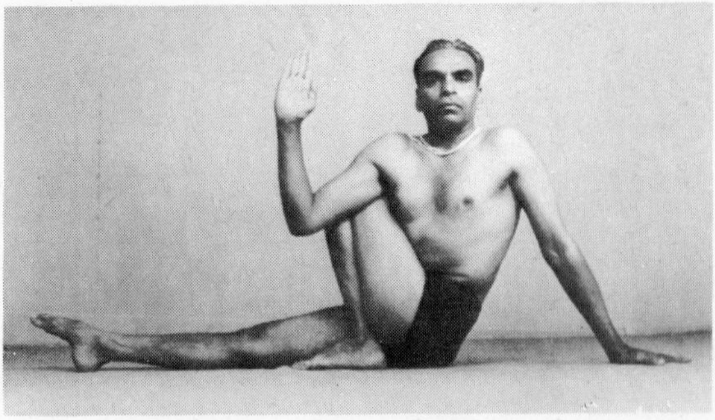

301

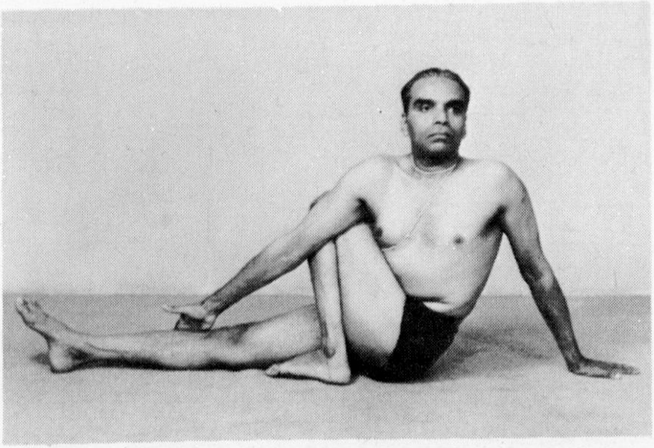

302

5. With an exhalation, twist the right arm round the left knee, flex the right elbow and place the right wrist at the back of the waist. Inhale and hold the pose.

6. Exhale deeply and turn the left arm from the shoulder behind the back. Either clasp the left hand behind the back with the right hand or vice versa. (Plates 303 and 304.) In the beginning, one finds it difficult to twist the trunk sideways, but with practice, the armpit touches the bent knee. After one has twisted the arm round the knee, one also finds it difficult to clasp the fingers of one hand with the other. Gradually one learns to clasp the fingers, then the palm and lastly to hold the hand at the wrist behind the back.

7. The right arm should lock the left bent knee tightly. There should be no space between the right armpit and the bent left knee.

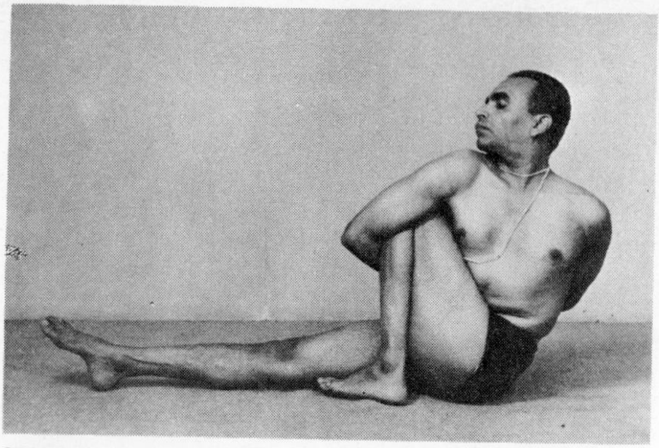

303

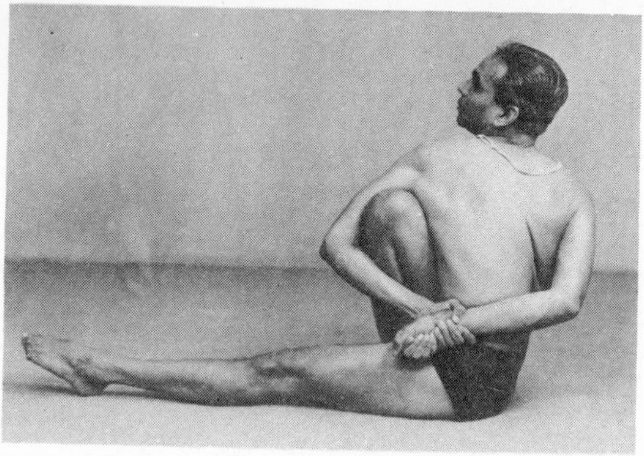

304

8. After clasping the hands at the back, turn the spine still more to the left by tugging at the clasped hands.

9. The whole of the outstretched right leg should remain straight and securely on the floor, but you will not be able to achieve this to start with. Tighten the muscles of the outstretched thigh so that the knee-cap is pulled up towards the thigh and also tighten the muscles of the calf of the outstretched leg. Then the leg will remain firm and extended on the floor.

10. Stay in this position from half a minute to a minute with normal breathing. The neck may be turned either way to gaze at the toes of the extended leg on the floor or to look over the shoulder.

11. Unclasp the hands at the back and turn the trunk back to its original position. Lower the bent leg and extend it fully on the floor.

12. Then repeat the pose on the other side. This time bend the right knee and place the right foot firmly on the floor so that the right heel touches the perineum and the inner side of the right foot touches the outstretched left thigh. Turn the trunk about 90 degrees to the right so that the left armpit touches the bent right knee. With an exhalation, twist the left arm round the right knee and bring the left hand to the back of the waist. Then throw the right arm behind the back from the shoulder and flexing the right elbow, bring the right hand to the left hand and clasp them. Turn still more to the right and gaze at either the toes of the outstretched left leg or over the right shoulder. Stay on this side also for the same length of time. Unclasp the hands, turn the trunk back to normal, stretch the right leg on the floor and relax.

Effects

By the regular practice of this āsana, splitting backaches, lumbago and pains in the hips disappear rapidly. The liver and the spleen are contracted and so are toned and cease to be sluggish. The muscles of the neck gain power. Sprains in the shoulder and displacement of the shoulder joints are relieved and the shoulder movements become free. The intestines also benefit from this āsana. Its effects will be less on lean persons, for whom there are better poses described later. It also helps to reduce the size of the abdomen.

115. *Marīchyāsana IV* Eleven* (Plate 305)

This variation combines the movements of Marīchyāsana II (Plate 146) and Marīchyāsana III. (Plate 303)

Technique

1. Sit on the floor with legs stretched straight in front. (Plate 77)

2. Bend the right leg at the knee and place the right foot at the root of the left thigh. The right heel should press against the navel and the toes should be stretched and pointing. The right leg is now in half Padmāsana.

3. Bend the left leg at the knee, place the sole and heel of the left foot flat on the floor. Keep the shin perpendicular to the floor so that the left thigh and the calf touch each other and the left heel touches the perineum.

4. With an exhalation, turn the spine about 90 degrees to the left, so that the right armpit touches the outer side of the left thigh.

5. Place the right shoulder beyond the left knee and stretch the right arm forward by turning the spine still more to the left by stretching the region at the back of the floating ribs. Take a breath.

6. Exhale, move the right arm round the left knee, bend the right elbow and place the right hand at the back of the waist. The left knee is locked tightly in the right armpit. Take a breath.

7. Now with a deep exhalation, twist the left arm from the shoulder behind the back and clasp the right hand behind the back with the left hand. Stretch the chest and pull up the spine. (Plates 305 and 306)

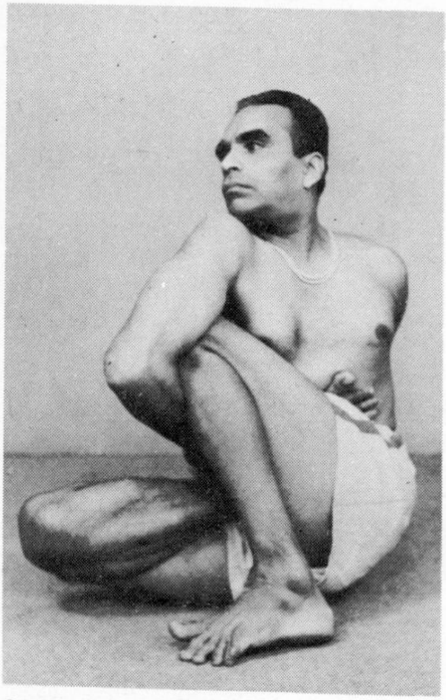

305

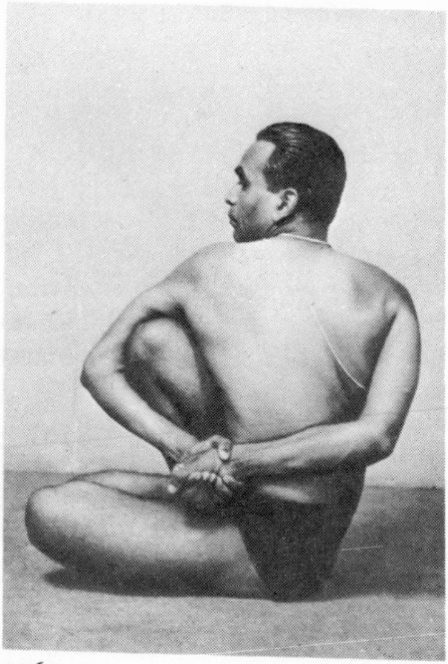

306

8. Remain in this position for 30 seconds. Breathing will be faster.

9. Release the hands and straighten the legs.

10. Then repeat the pose on the other side reading 'right' for 'left' and vice versa. Stay on both sides for the same length of time. Release the hands, straighten the legs and relax.

Effects

The pressure of the heel against the navel and the clasping of the hands behind the back rejuvenates the nerves round the navel. It tones the liver, spleen and pancreas. Calcium deposits in the shoulder joints are resolved and the pose helps free movement at the shoulders.

116. *Ardha Matsyendrāsana I* Eight* (Plates 311 and 312)

Ardha means half. In the *Haṭha Yoga Pradīpikā*, Matsyendra is mentioned as one of the founders of Haṭha Vidyā. It is related that once Lord Śiva went to a lonely island and explained to his consort Pārvati the mysteries of Yoga. A fish near the shore heard everything with concentration and remained motionless while listening. Śiva, realising that the fish had learnt Yoga, sprinkled water upon it, and immediately the fish gained divine form and became Matsyendra (Lord of the Fishes) and thereafter spread the knowledge of Yoga. Paripūrṇa Matsyendrāsana (Plates 336 and 339), where the spine is given the maximum lateral twist, is dedicated to Matsyendra. Ardha Matsyendrāsana is a milder version of that āsana.

Technique

1. Sit on the floor, with the legs stretched straight in front. (Plate 77)

2. Bend the left knee and join the thigh and calf; raise the seat from the floor, place the left foot under the buttocks and sit on the left foot so that the left heel rests under the left buttock. The foot used as the seat should be kept horizontal on the floor, the outer side of the ankle and the little toe of the foot resting on the ground. If the foot is not so placed, it will be impossible to sit on it. Balance securely in this position.

3. Then bend the right knee and lifting the right leg from the floor, place it by the outer side of the left thigh so that the outer side of the right ankle touches the outer side of the left thigh on the floor. Balance in this position, keeping the right shin perpendicular to the floor. (Plate 307)

4. Turn the trunk 90 degrees to the right until the left armpit touches the outer side of the right thigh. Bring the armpit over the right knee. (Plate 308.) Exhale, stretch the left arm from the shoulder and twist it round the right knee. Bend the left elbow and move the left wrist to the back of the waist.

5. The left arm should lock the bent right knee tightly and there should be no space between the left armpit and the bent right knee. To achieve this, exhale and move the trunk forward. Stay in this position and take 2 breaths.

6. Now exhale deeply and swing back the right arm from the shoulder, bend the right elbow, move the right hand behind the waist and either clasp it with the left hand or vice versa. At first you will be able to catch

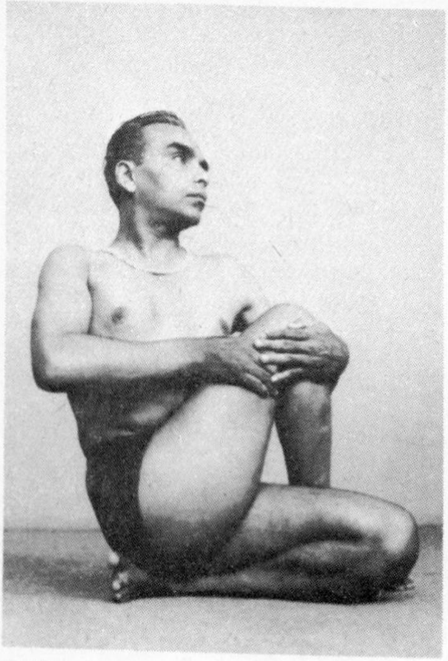
307

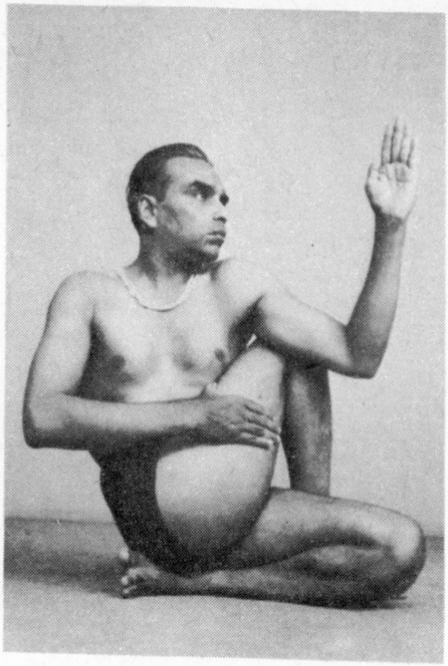
308

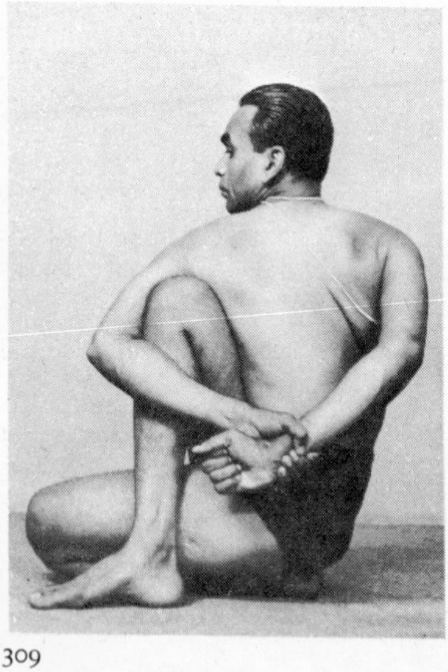
309

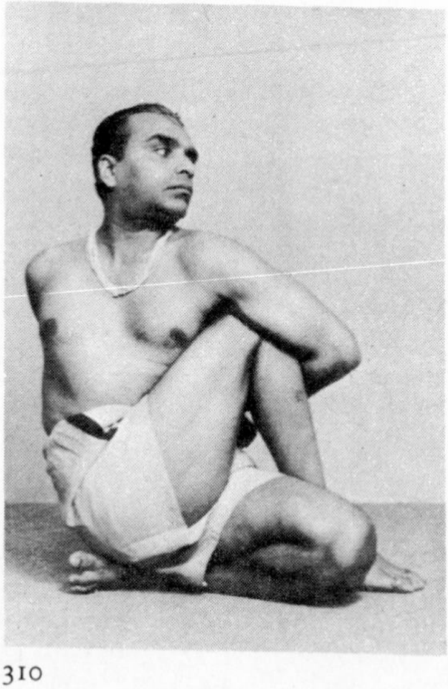
310

a finger or two. With practice it will be possible to catch the palms and then the wrists behind the back. (Plate 309)

7. The neck may be turned to the left and the gaze directed over the left shoulder (Plate 310), or to the right, and the gaze fixed at the centre of the eyebrows. (Plates 311 and 312.) The spinal twist will be greater if the neck is turned to the left than when to the right.

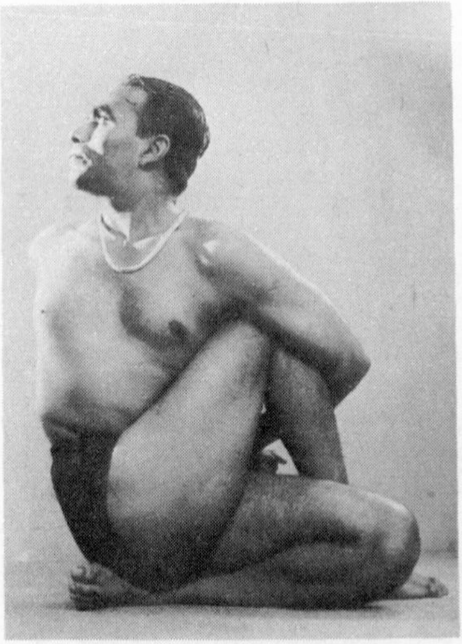

311

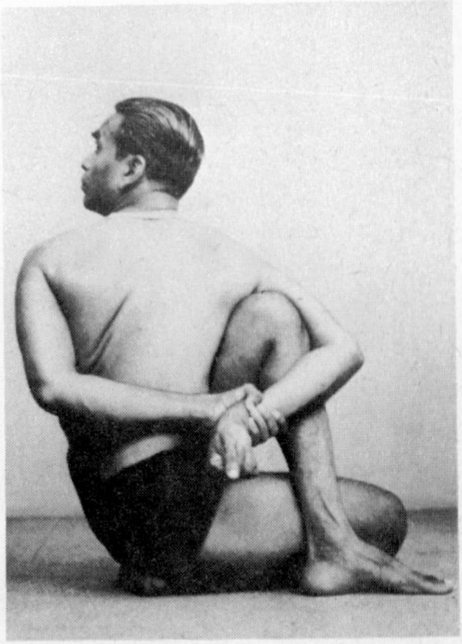

312

8. As the diaphragm is squeezed by the spinal twist, the breathing will at first become short and fast. Do not be nervous. After some practice the pose can be held from half a minute to a minute with normal breathing.

9. Release the hands, remove the right foot from the floor and straighten the right and then the left leg.

10. Repeat the pose on the other side and hold it for the same length of time. Here, bend the right leg and sit on the right foot so that the right heel is under the right buttock. Place the left leg over the right leg and rest the left foot on the floor so that the outer side of the left ankle touches the outer side of the right thigh on the floor. Turn the trunk 90 degrees to the left, placing the right armpit over the left knee and twist the right arm round the left knee. Flex the right elbow and move the right hand behind the waist. Hold the pose and take 2 breaths. Again

exhale completely and swing the left arm back from the shoulder, bend the left elbow and clasp the hands behind the back at the wrist. Then release and relax.

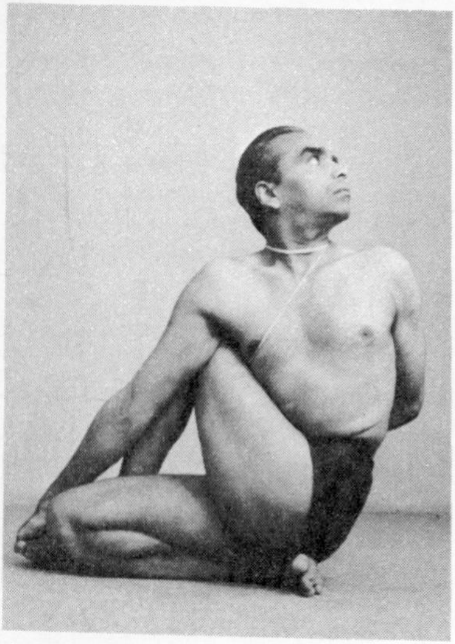

313

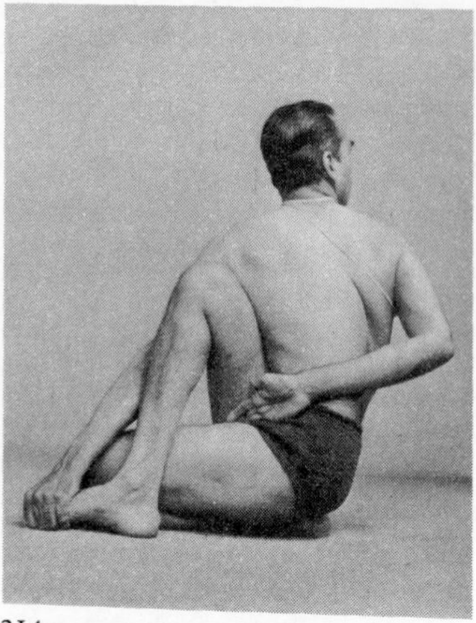

314

11. In the beginning it may not be possible to twist either arm round the opposite knee. In that case try and hold the opposite foot, keeping the arm straight at the elbow. (Plates 313 and 314.) It also takes time to clasp the hands behind the back. Gradually, the backward stretch of the arms will increase, and one will be able to catch at first the fingers, next the palms, then the wrist and as the pose is mastered even the fore-arms above the wrists. Beginners who find it difficult to sit on the foot can sit on the floor. (Plates 315 and 316)

Effects

By the practice of this āsana, one derives the benefits mentioned under Marīchyāsana III. (Posture 114 and Plate 303.) But here as the range of movement is more intensified, the effects will also be greater. In Marīchyāsana III the upper part of the abdomen is squeezed. Here the lower part of the abdomen has the benefit of the exercise. The prostate and bladder are not enlarged if one practises regularly.

117. *Mālāsana I* Eight* (Plate 321)

Mālā means a garland.

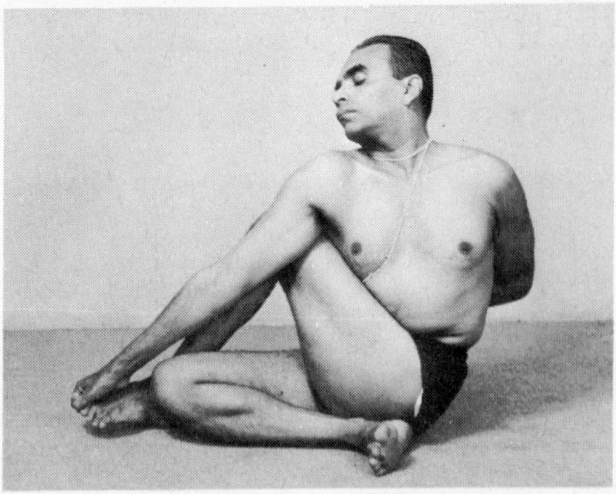

315

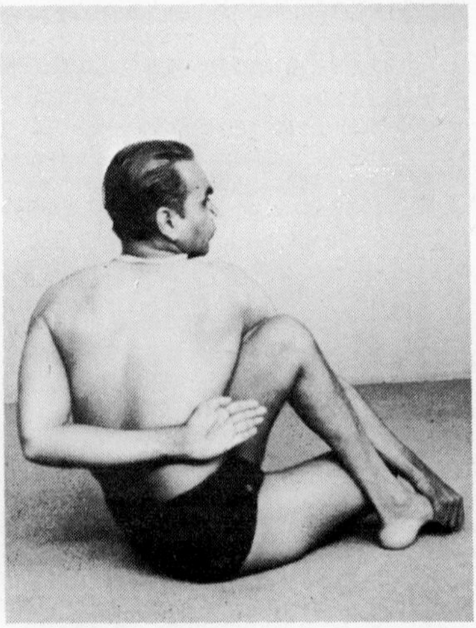

316

There are two different techniques for doing this āsana which are given below.

Technique

1. Squat on the haunches with the feet together. The soles and the heels should rest completely on the floor. Raise the seat from the floor and balance. (Plate 317)

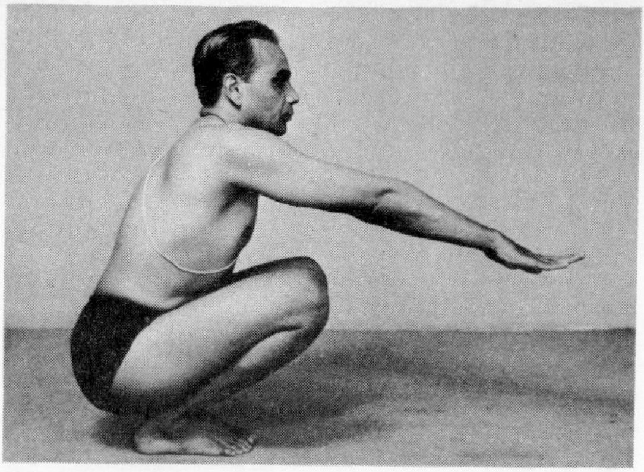

317

2. Now widen the knees and move the trunk forward.

3. Exhale, wrap the arms round the bent legs and rest the palms on the floor. (Plate 318)

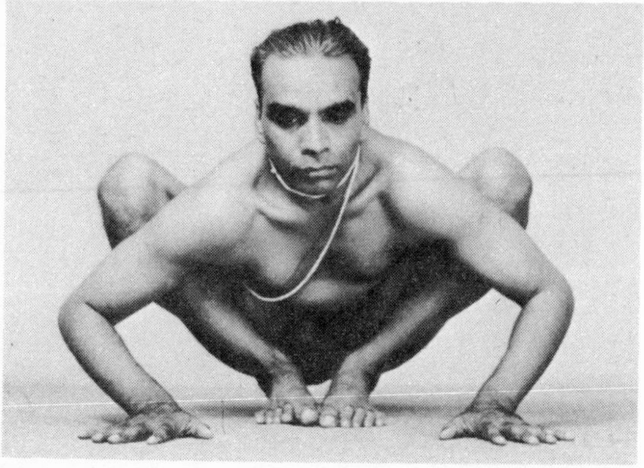

318

4. Take the hands one by one behind the back and clasp the fingers. (Plates 319 and 320)

5. Then stretch the back and neck up.

6. Remain in this position for 30 to 60 seconds breathing normally.

7. Now exhale, bend forward and rest the head on the floor. (Plate 321.) Stay in this position also for 30 to 60 seconds with normal breathing.

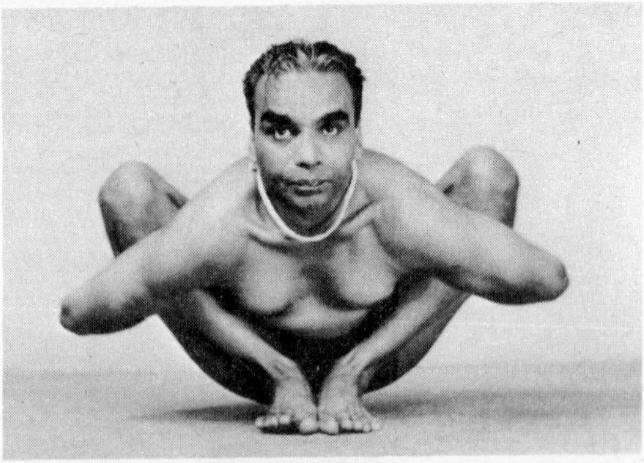

319

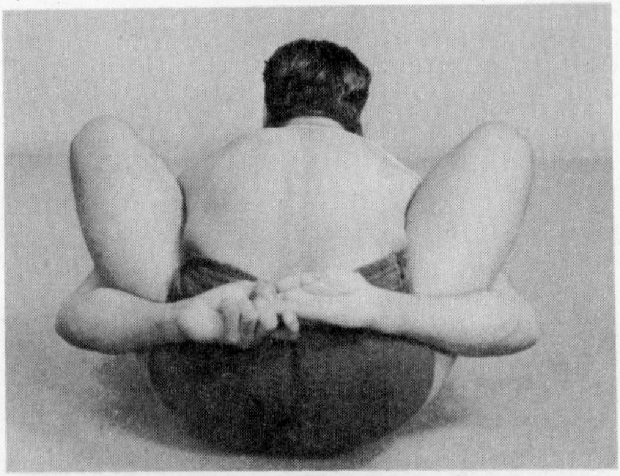

320

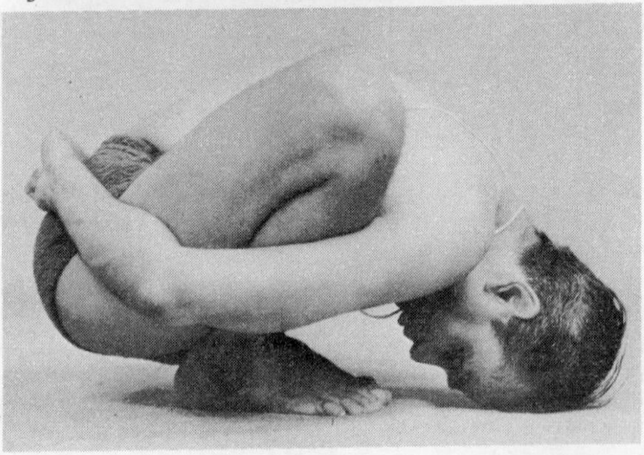

321

8. Inhale, raise the head from the floor and return to position 5.

9. Release the hands and rest on the floor.

Effects

The āsana tones the abdominal organs and relieves backaches.

118. *Mālāsana II* Two* (Plate 322)

1. Squat on the haunches with the feet together. The soles and heels should rest completely on the floor. Raise the seat from the floor and balance. (Plate 317)

2. Widen the thighs and knees and move the trunk forward until the armpits extend beyond the knees.

3. Bend forward and catch the back part of the ankles.

4. After gripping the ankles, exhale and move the head down to the toes and rest the forehead on them. (Plate 322)

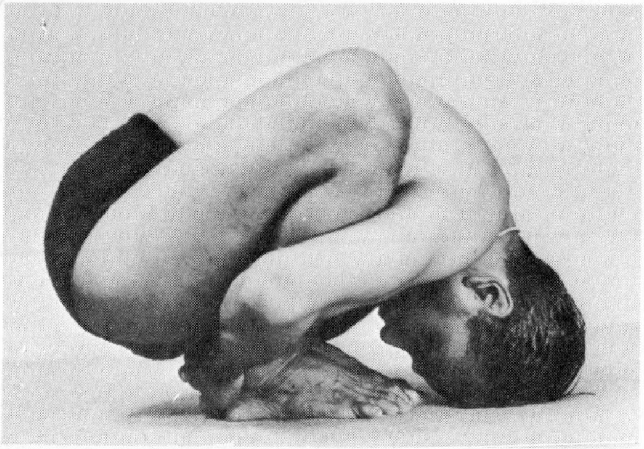

322

5. Maintain the pose for about a minute breathing normally.

6. Inhale, raise the head, release the ankle grip and relax on the floor.

Effects

By doing this posture the abdominal organs are exercised and gain strength. Ladies suffering from severe pain in the back during the menstrual period will obtain relief in this pose and the back will feel soothed.

In these two poses the arms hang from the neck like a garland, hence the name.

119. *Pāśāsana* Fifteen* (Plates 328 and 329)

Pāśā means a noose or cord. In this posture, squat on the floor, turn the trunk about 90 degrees to one side, twist one arm round both the thighs and turning the other arm from the shoulder clasp hands behind the back. The arms are used as a noose to hold the trunk to the legs, hence the name.

Technique

1. Squat on the floor with the soles and heels completely on the floor.

2. Keep the knees and feet together, raise the seat from the floor and balance. (Plate 317)

3. After securing the balance, twist the trunk about 90 degrees to the right until the left armpit is beyond the outer side of the right thigh near the right knee. (Plate 323.) To achieve the maximum twist, flex the left knee about an inch forward.

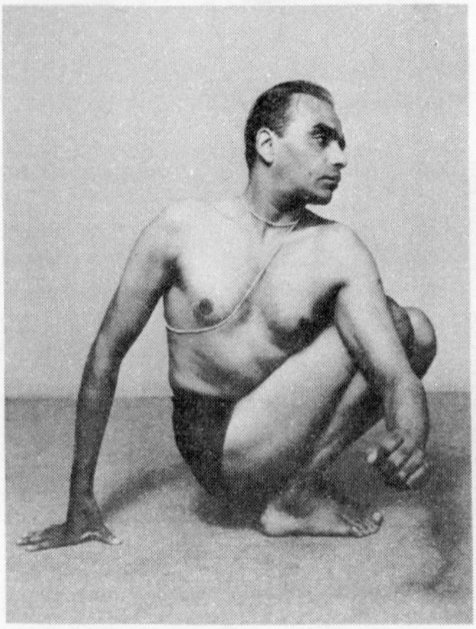

323

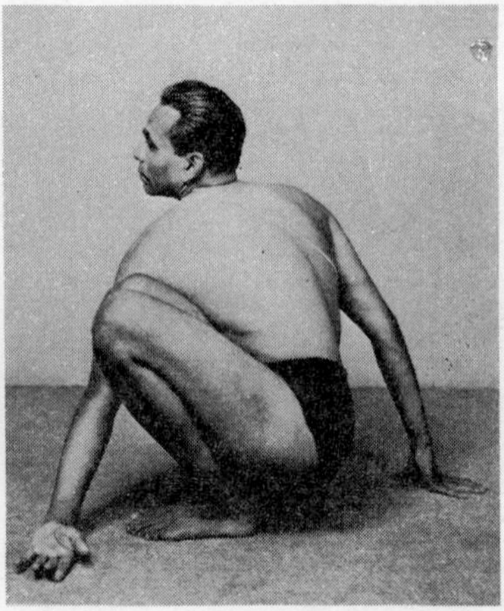

324

4. Exhale, extend the left arm from the shoulder (Plate 324), leave no space between the left armpit and the right thigh, turn the left arm round the right thigh and, bending the left elbow towards the left leg, bring the left hand near the left hip. Take a breath.

5. Exhale, twist the right arm from the shoulder behind the back, bend the right elbow and hook the fingers behind the back near the left hip. (Plate 325)

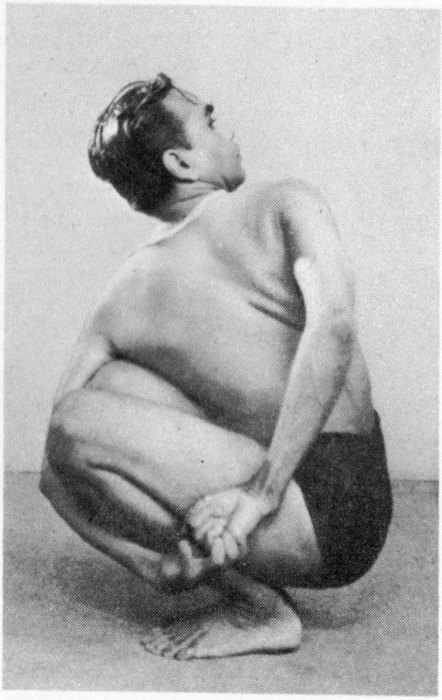

325

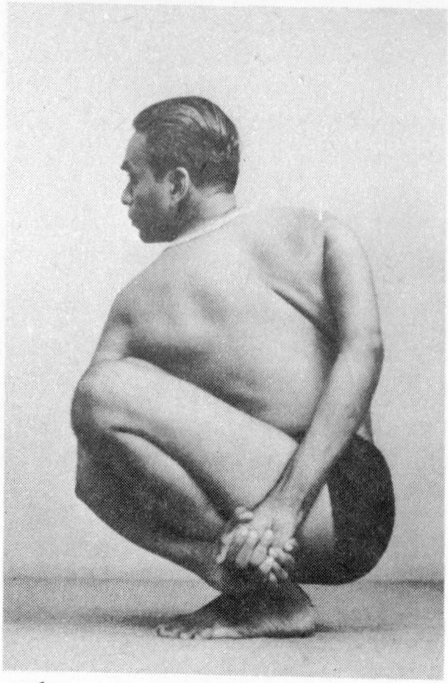

326

6. Gradually clasp the palms (Plate 326) and when this becomes easy, clasp the wrists. (Plates 327, 328 and 329)

7. Tighten the calf muscles to maintain the balance, twist the spine as far to the right as you can and stay in the pose from 30 to 60 seconds with normal breathing. Turn the neck and gaze over either shoulder.

8. Release the hand clasp and repeat the pose on the other side. Here, twist the trunk to the left, bring the right arm round the left thigh, bend the right elbow and bring the right hand near the right hip. Then with an exhalation turn the left arm back from the shoulder, bend the left elbow and clasp the right hand with the left behind the back near the right hip.

Effects

The pose gives strength and elasticity to the ankles. Persons whose work entails standing for hours will rest their feet in this position. It tones the spine and makes one agile. The shoulders move freely and grow

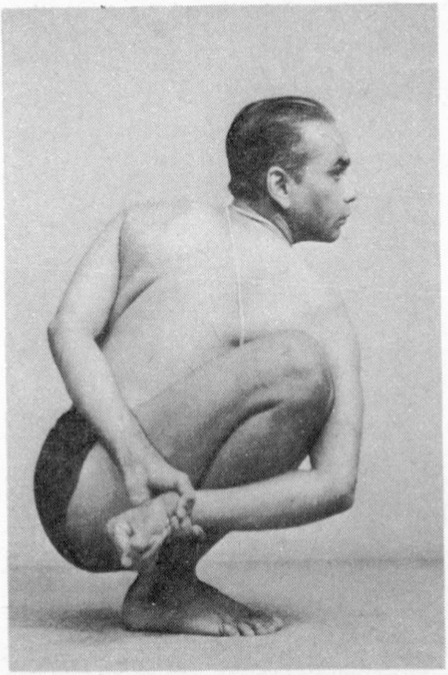

327

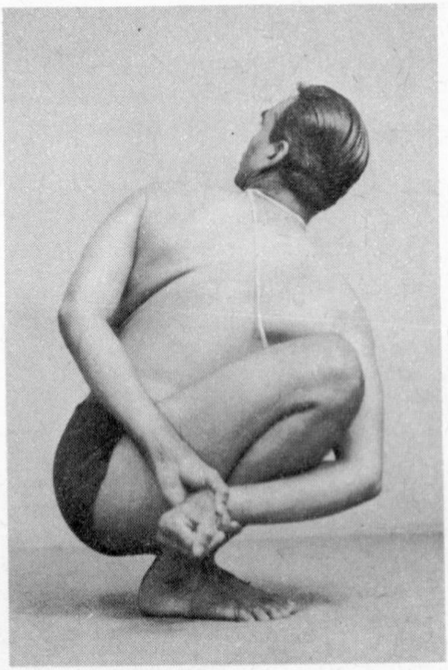

328

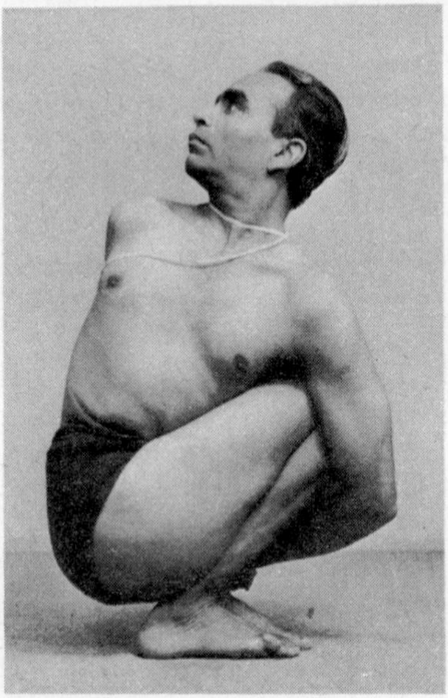

329

stronger. The pose reduces fat around the abdomen, massages the abdominal organs and at the same time expands the chest fully. It is more intense than Ardha Matsyendrāsana I and II (Plates 311 and 330) and so it gives greater benefits. It is good for curing sluggishness of the liver, spleen and pancreas and is recommended for persons suffering from diabetes. It also improves digestion.

120. *Ardha Matsyendrāsana II* Nineteen* (Plates 330 and 331)

This āsana is a variation of Ardha Matsyendrāsana I (Plate 311) and it gives a greater lateral twist to the spine.

Technique

1. Sit on the floor with the legs stretched straight in front. (Plate 77)

2. Bend the right knee and place the right foot at the root of the left thigh, pressing the heel against the navel.

3. Exhale, turn the trunk 90 degrees to the left, swing the left arm from the shoulder behind the back, bend the left elbow and with the left hand grasp the right ankle or shin.

4. The left leg should remain stretched straight on the floor throughout, and the sole of the left foot or the left big toe should be held by the right hand and the right arm should be kept straight. To start with one finds it difficult to keep the left leg stretched throughout on the floor. In that case bend the left knee, catch the left big toe with the right hand and then straighten out both the right arm and the left leg. Turn the neck to the right and gaze over the right shoulder. (Plates 330 and 331)

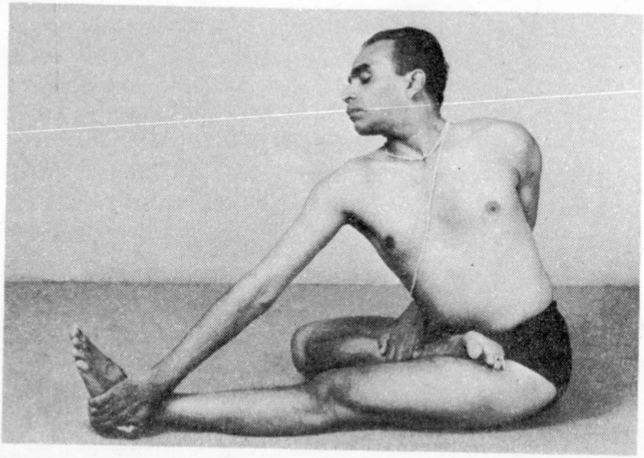

330

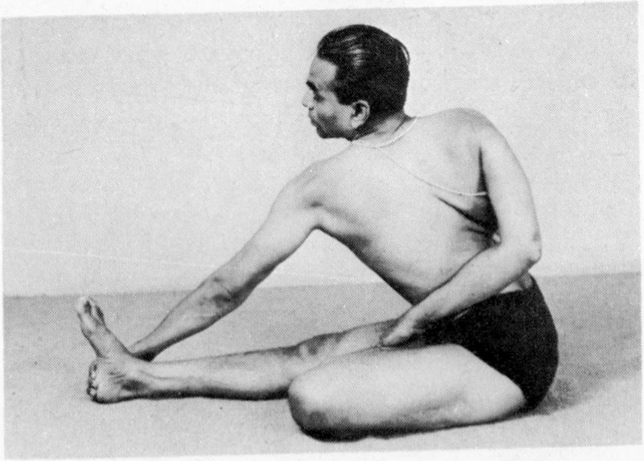

331

5. Keep the knees near each other and stay in the position from 30 to 60 seconds while trying to maintain normal breathing which at first will be fast due to the lateral twist.

6. Release the grip on the legs, straighten them and then repeat the pose on the other side, changing the word left to that for right and vice versa.

7. Stay on both sides for the same length of time and then relax.

Effects

The abdominal organs are toned by being contracted on one side and stretched on the other. Due to the lateral twist of the spine, backaches, lumbago and pain in the hip joints disappear rapidly. The neck muscles become more powerful and the shoulder movements become easier. The prostate and bladder do not become hypertrophied if one practises this āsana regularly. It helps one to achieve Paripūrṇa Matsyendrāsana (Plates 336 and 339), where the spine is given the maximum lateral twist.

121. *Ardha Matsyendrāsana III* Twenty-two* (Plates 332 and 333)

Technique

1. Sit on the floor with the legs stretched straight in front. (Plate 77)

2. Bend the left knee and place the left foot at the root of the right thigh, pressing the heel against the navel.

3. Bend the right knee, lift the right leg from the floor and place it by the outer side of the left thigh. Then the outer side of the right ankle will touch the outer side of the left thigh on the floor. Take 2 or 3 breaths.

4. Exhale, turn the trunk 90 degrees to the right and bring the left shoulder over the right knee. Do not leave any space between the left armpit and the right thigh and hold the right foot with the left hand.

5. Swing the right arm behind the back, bending it at the elbow and rest the hand at the back.

6. Turn the neck to the right, raise the chin and gaze either at the centre of the eyebrows or at the tip of the nose. (Plates 332 and 333)

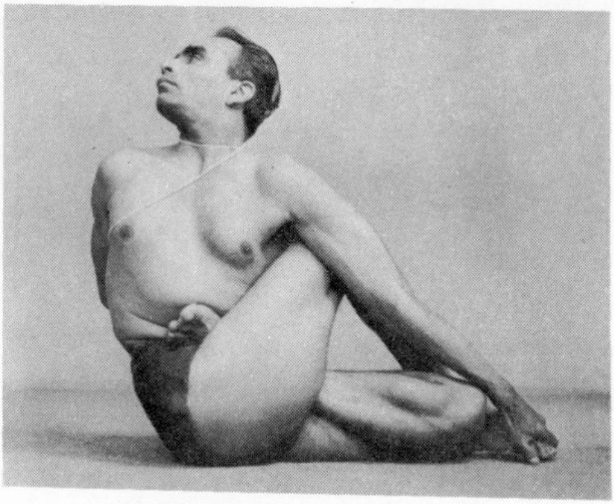

332

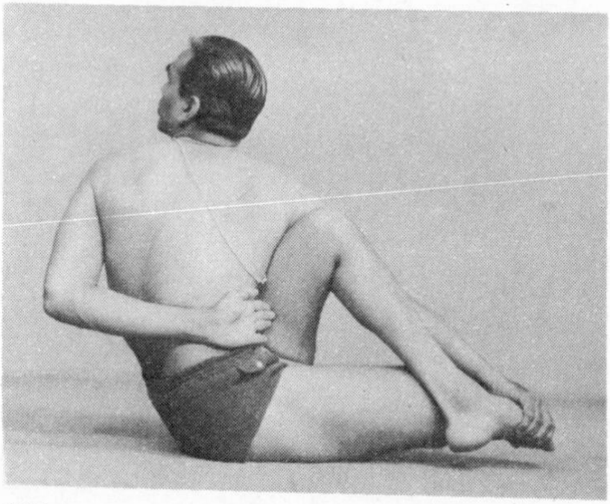

333

7. Stay in the position from 30 to 60 seconds according to capacity. Breathing will be faster but try to make it normal.

8. Release your hold on the right foot, lift it over the left thigh and stretch the right leg straight. Then release the left leg and stretch it out straight.

9. Repeat the pose on the other side for the same length of time and relax.

Effects

This exercises and massages the abdominal organs and keeps them healthy. It tones the spine and keeps it elastic. It is a preparatory pose for Paripūrṇa Matsyendrāsana. (Plates 336 and 339)

122. *Paripūrṇa Matsyendrāsana* Thirty-eight* (Plates 336 and 339)

Paripūrṇa means entire or complete. Matsyendra was one of the founders of Haṭha Vidyā.

Verse 27 of the *Haṭha Yoga Pradīpikā* states 'Matsyendrāsana increases the appetite by fanning the gastric fire and destroys terrible diseases in the body; when practised it rouses Kuṇḍalinī and makes the moon steady.'

It is said that the breath in the right nostril is hot and that in the left one is cold. Therefore, the breath in the right nostril is called the sun breath and the right nāḍi is referred to as piṅgalā (of the colour of fire) and the breath of the left nostril is called the moon breath and the left nāḍi is called iḍā. The moon travelling in iḍā sprinkles its nectar through the entire system and the sun travelling through piṅgalā dries out the whole system, for the human body is regarded as a miniature universe. It is said that the moon is located at the root of the palate, ever dropping cool ambrosial nectar that is wasted by feeding the gastric fire. Matsyendrāsana prevents this.

This āsana is dedicated to the founder of Haṭha Vidyā Matsyendra.

Technique

1. Sit on the floor with the legs stretched straight in front. (Plate 77)

2. Flex the right knee and place the right foot at the root of the left thigh, the right heel pressing against the navel. Bend the left knee up and bring it near the chest.

3. Exhale, twist the trunk to the left, and swinging the left arm from the shoulder catch the right ankle with the left hand from behind the back. (Plate 334.) Grip the ankle firmly. This is the first stage.

4. Lift the left foot over the right thigh and place it on the floor by the outer side of the right knee. (Plate 335.) Take a few breaths. This is the second stage.

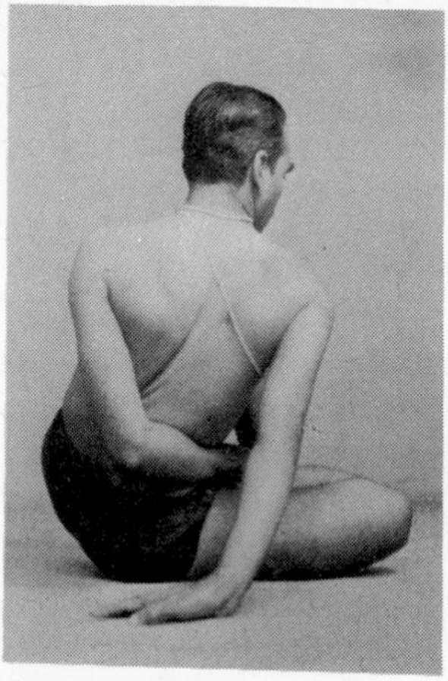

334

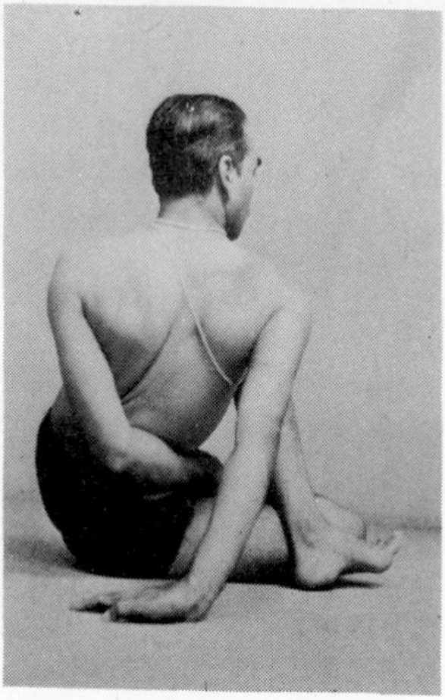

335

5. Again exhale, turn the trunk to the left to bring the right shoulder over to the left knee and hold the left foot with the right hand. Turn the neck to the left, raise the chin and gaze up. (Plate 336.) This is the final stage of the āsana. Stay in this pose from 30 to 60 seconds according to your capacity. Breathing will be faster due to the pressure on the diaphragm.

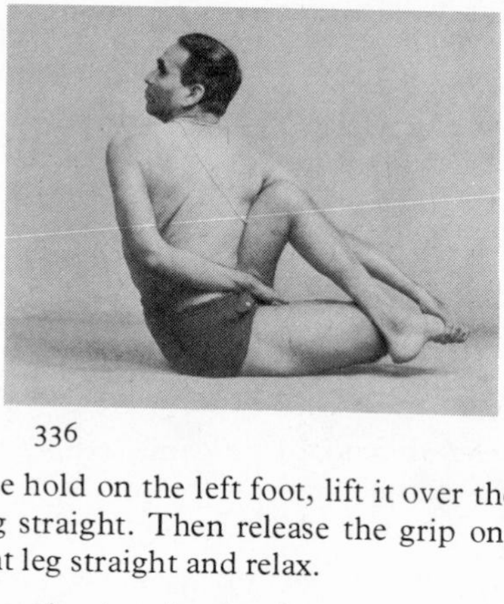

336

6. First release the hold on the left foot, lift it over the right thigh and stretch the left leg straight. Then release the grip on the right ankle, stretching the right leg straight and relax.

7. In this pose the spine is twisted to its utmost limit and so it is easier if all movements are done with exhalation.

The following technique should be employed to practise on the other side.

1. Sit on the floor with the legs stretched straight in front. Bend the left knee and place the left foot at the root of the right thigh, the left heel pressing against the navel.

2. Exhale, turn the trunk to the right, swing the right arm from the shoulder, grip the left ankle firmly with the right hand from behind the back and bend the right leg up. (Plate 337.) This is the first stage.

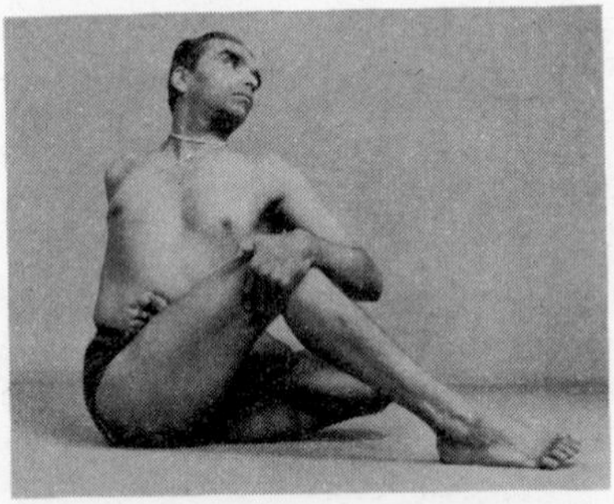

337

3. Lift the right foot over the left thigh and place it on the floor by the outer side of the left knee. (Plate 338.) Take a few breaths. This is the second stage.

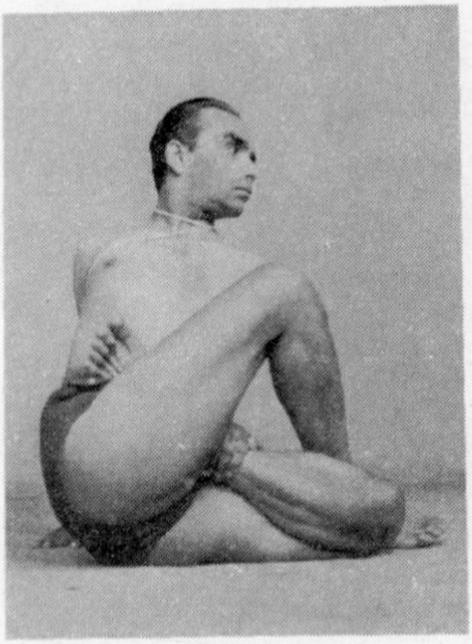

338

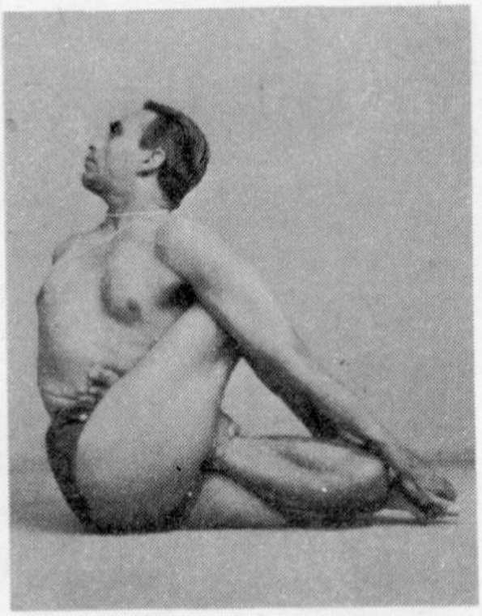

339

4. Exhale again, turn the trunk to the right to bring the left shoulder over the right knee and with the left hand hold the right foot. Turn the

neck to the right, raise the chin and gaze up. (Plate 339.) This is the final stage. Hold the pose on this side for the same length of time as on the other.

5. Release the hold on the right foot, lift it over the left thigh and straighten the right leg. Next release the grip over the left ankle, straighten the left leg and relax.

Effects

This difficult lateral movement tones the spine by supplying the spinal nerves with a copious supply of blood. It increases gastric activity, helps to digest food and eliminate toxins. The spine and the abdomen being kept healthy ensures tranquillity of body and mind. The spine is given the maximum lateral twist.

123. *Aṣṭāvakrāsana* Thirteen* (Plates 342 and 343)

This āsana is dedicated to the sage Aṣṭāvakra, the spiritual preceptor of King Janaka of Mithilā, who was the father of Sītā. It is related that when the sage was in his mother's womb, his father Kagola (or Kahola) made several mistakes while reciting the Vedas (the sacred scriptures). Hearing these the unborn sage laughed. The father became enraged and cursed his son to be born as Aṣṭāvakra. So it came to pass that he was born crooked in eight places. These crooks earned him the name Aṣṭāvakra or Eight-Crooks. The sage's father had been defeated in a philosophical debate by Vaṇḍi, the court scholar of Mithilā. While yet a boy the sage became a great scholar and avenged his father's defeat by worsting Vaṇḍi in argument and becoming the preceptor of Janaka. Then his father blessed him, his deformity vanished and he became straight.

The āsana is given in two stages.

Technique

1. Stand with the feet about 18 inches apart.

2. Bend the knees, rest the right palm on the floor between the feet and place the left palm on the floor just beyond the left foot.

3. Bring the right leg over the right arm and rest the back of the right thigh on the back of the right arm just above the elbow. Bring the left leg forward between the arms but close to the right one. (Plate 340)

4. Exhale and lift both the legs off the floor. Interlock the legs by placing the left foot upon the right at the ankle (Plate 341) and extend the legs sideways to the right. (Plate 342.) The right arm will be

gripped between the thighs and will be slightly bent at the elbow. The left arm should be straight. Balance on the hands for some time in this position with normal breathing. This is the first stage.

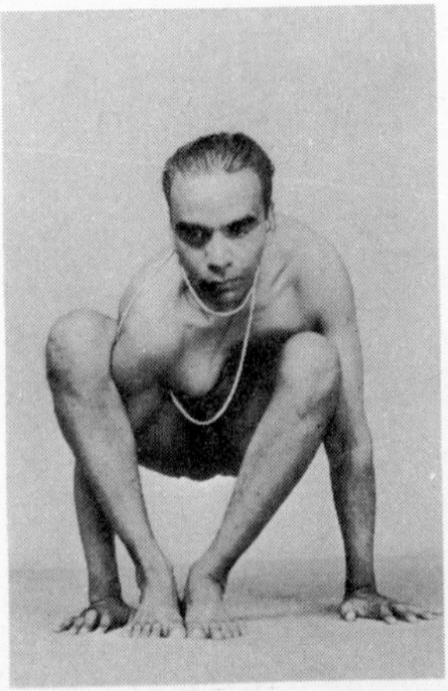

340

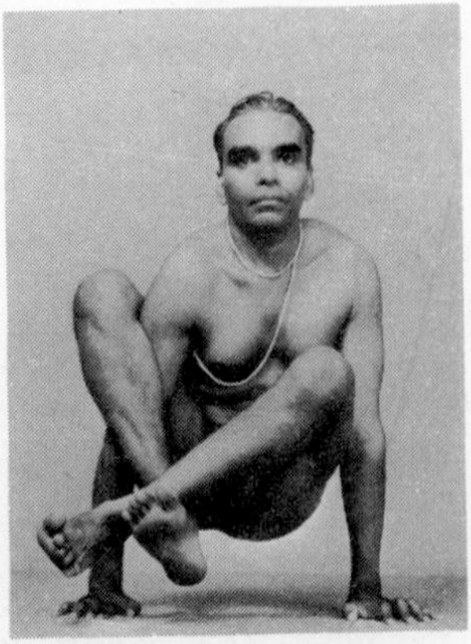

341

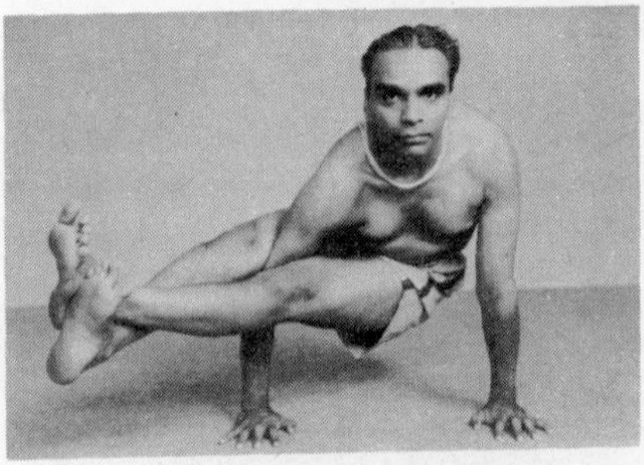

342

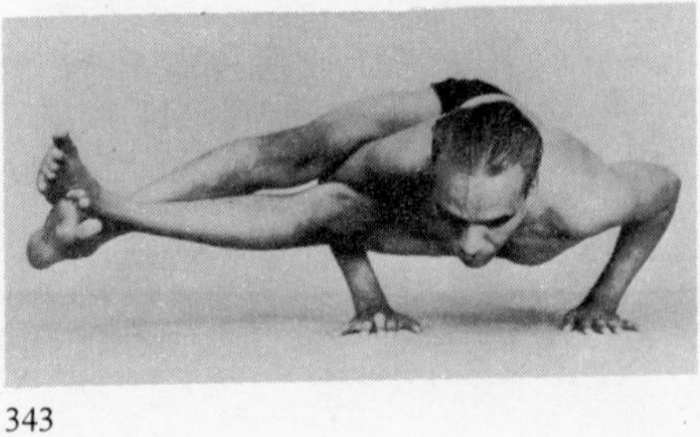

343

5. Now exhale, bend the elbows and lower the trunk and head until they are parallel to the floor. (Plate 343.) Move the head and trunk from side to side while breathing normally. This is the second stage.

6. Inhale, straighten the arms, raise the trunk (Plate 342), uncross and release the legs and lower them to the floor.

7. Repeat the pose on the other side, reading the word left for right and vice versa in positions 2 to 5 above.

Effects

This āsana strengthens the wrists and arms and also develops the muscles of the abdomen.

124. *Eka Hasta Bhujāsana* Five* (Plate 344)

Eka means one. Hasta means a hand and bhuja an arm.

Technique

1. Sit on the floor with the legs stretched straight in front. (Plate 77)

2. Exhale, bend the right leg at the knee, clasp it at the ankle with the right hand and place it on the back of the right upper arm. Now the back of the right thigh will touch the back of the upper right arm. Place it as high up as you can.

3. Place the palms on the floor and with an exhalation raise the whole body above the ground and balance. (Plate 344)

4. Stay in this position for 20 to 30 seconds with normal breathing.

5. Keep the left leg straight and parallel to the floor throughout the balance.

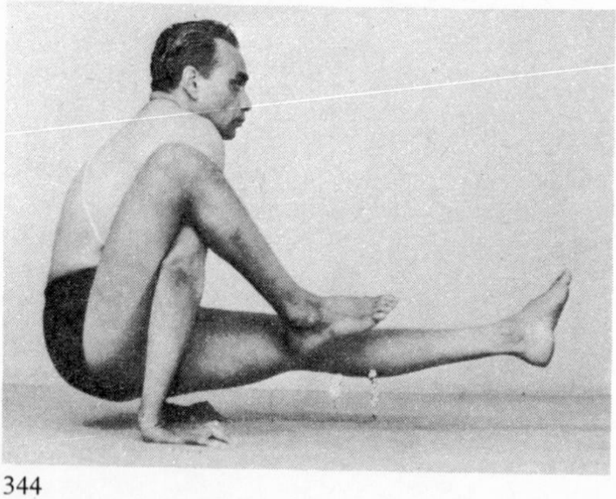

344

6. Exhale, lower the trunk to the floor, release the right leg, stretch it out straight in front and repeat on the other side for the same length of time.

Effects

This āsana strengthens the arms and exercises the abdominal organs.

125. *Dwi Hasta Bhujāsana* Four* (Plate 345)

Dwi means two or both, hasta means a hand and bhuja an arm. It is a variation of Eka Hasta Bhujāsana (Plate 344).

Technique

1. Stand with the feet 18 inches apart.

2. Bend the knees and rest the palms on the floor between the feet.

3. Bring the right leg over the right arm and rest the back of the right thigh on the back of the right upper arm. Likewise place the left thigh on the left arm.

4. Exhale, lift the feet from the floor and balance on the hands. Stretch the arms straight and keep the feet together, high up. (Plate 345)

5. Stay in the position from 20 to 30 seconds with normal breathing.

6. Exhale, bend the elbows, lower the body to the floor, release the legs, stretch them straight in front and relax.

Effects

The effects are the same as in Eka Hasta Bhujāsana.

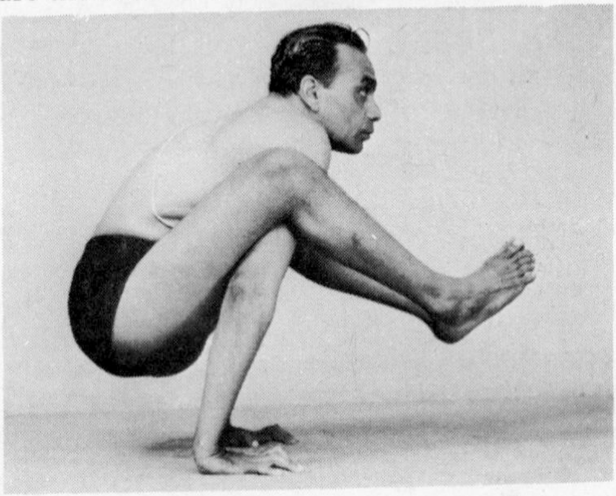

345

126. *Bhujapīḍāsana* Eight* (Plate 348)

Bhuja means an arm or shoulder. Pīda means pain or pressure. In this āsana, the body is balanced on the hands by resting the back of the knees on the shoulders, hence the name.

Technique

1. Stand in Tāḍāsana. (Plate 1.) Spread the legs till the feet are about two feet apart.

2. Stoop forward and bend the knees.

3. Place the palms on the floor about a foot and a half apart, between the legs. (Plate 346)

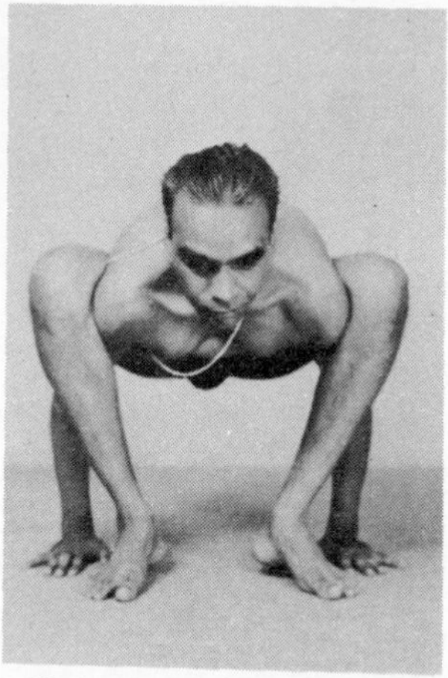

346

4. Rest the back of the thighs on the back of the upper arms. Rest the thighs on the middle of the upper arms between the shoulders and elbows.

5. While placing the thighs in this position, in the beginning raise the heels from the floor.

6. Exhale, slowly raise the toes off the floor one by one, balance on the hands (Plate 347) and then interlock the feet at the ankles. (Plate 348.) In the beginning the legs will slip down and there will be difficulty in balancing. To secure the balance try and place the back of the thighs as high up on the upper arms as you can. The arms will be slightly bent at the elbows. Try and extend the arms as far as you can and raise the head up.

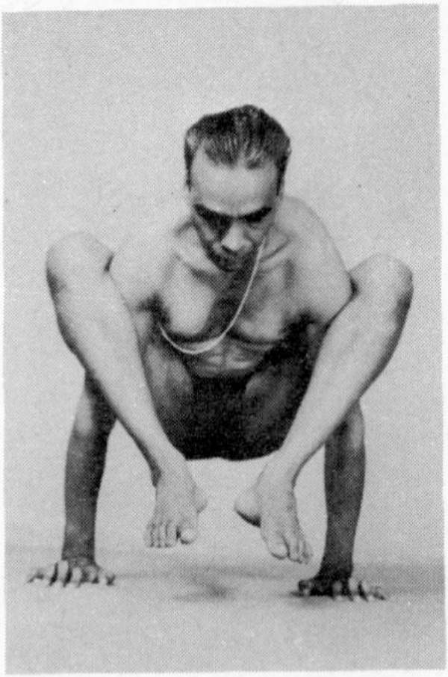

347

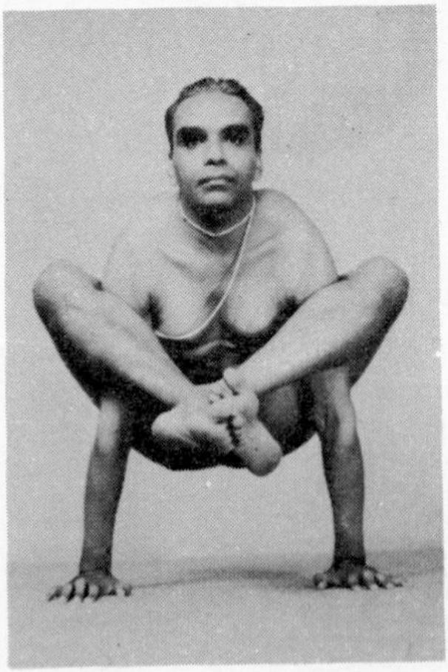

348

7. Remain in the balancing position with normal breathing as long as the wrists can bear the weight of the body. Then release the feet by taking the legs back one by one (Plates 349 and 350) and then rest them on the floor. Lift the hands from the floor and stand up in Tāḍāsana. (Plate 1)

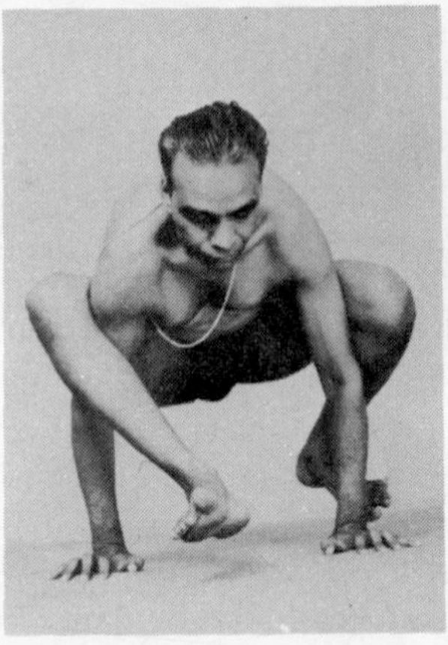

349

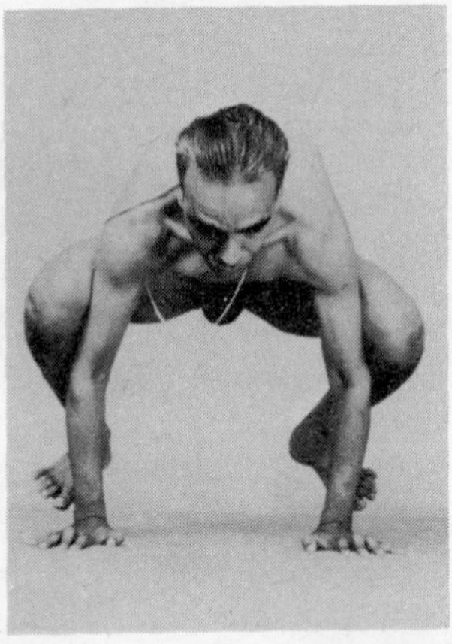

350

8. Repeat the pose by changing the position of the interlocked ankles. If, at first, the right foot is placed over the left one at the ankle, then

while repeating the pose place the left foot over the right one at the ankle.

Effects

By the practice of this āsana the hands and the wrists grow strong, as do the abdominal muscles due to contraction of the abdomen. The body will feel light. The minor muscles of the arms will be developed and toned by the practice of this pose, which requires no special apparatus or gymnasiums. The various parts of the body supply the weights and counterweights. All that is needed is strength of will.

127. *Mayūrāsana* Nine* (Plate 354)

Mayūra means a peacock.

Technique

1. Kneel on the floor with the knees slightly apart.

2. Bend forward, invert the palms and place them on the floor. The little fingers should touch and the fingers should point towards the feet. (Plate 351)

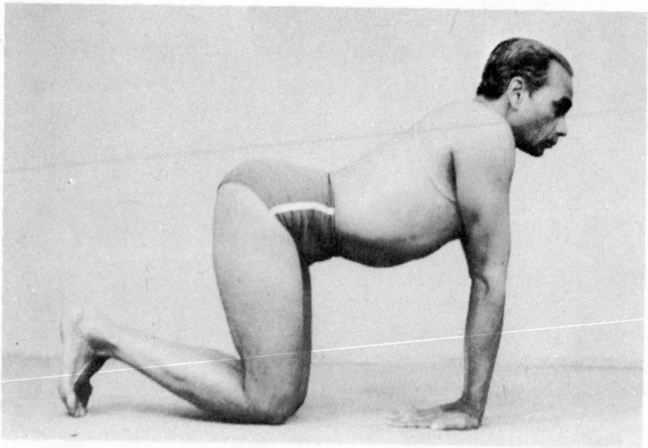

351

3. Bend the elbows and keep the forearms together. Rest the diaphragm on the elbows and the chest on the back of the upper arms. (Plate 352)

4. Stretch the legs straight one by one and keep them together and stiff. (Plate 353)

5. Exhale, bear the body weight on the wrists and hands, raise the

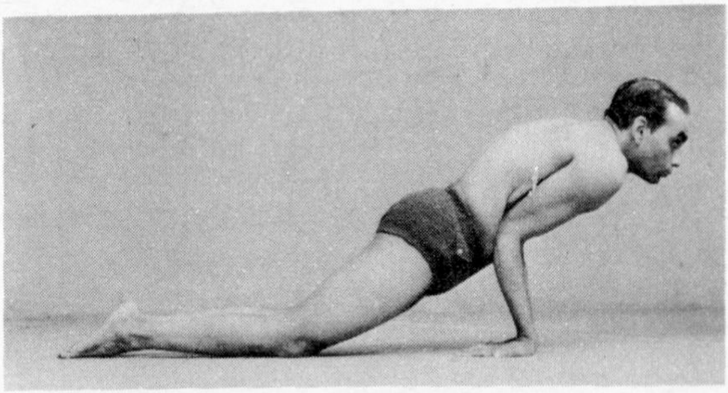

352

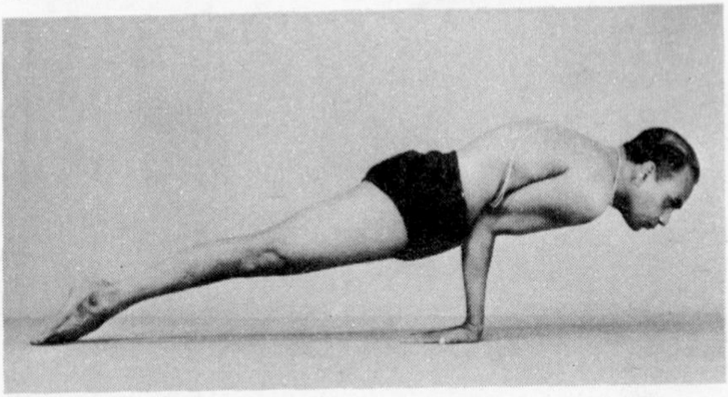

353

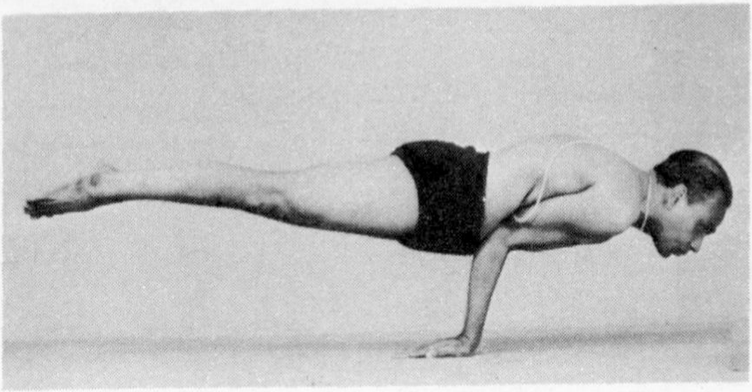

354

legs from the floor (either one by one or together) and at the same time stretch the trunk and head forward. Keep the whole body parallel to the floor with the legs stretched out straight and the feet together. (Plate 354)

6. Hold the pose as long as you can, gradually increasing the time to between 30 and 60 seconds. Do not put pressure on the ribs. The diaphragm being pressed, breathing will be laboured.

7. Lower the head to the floor and then the legs. Place the knees on the floor by the side of the hands, then lift the hands and relax.

8. After mastering this position learn to cross the legs as in Padmāsana (Plate 104) while practising the posture instead of keeping the legs stretched out straight. This variation is known as:

128. *Padma Mayūrāsana* Ten* (Plate 355)

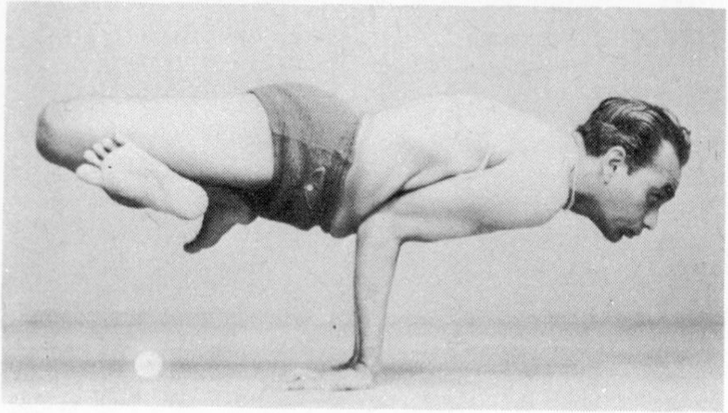

355

Effects

This āsana tones up the abdominal portion of the body wonderfully. Due to the pressure of the elbows against the abdominal aorta, blood circulates properly in the abdominal organs. This improves digestive power, cures ailments of the stomach and spleen, and prevents the accumulation of toxins due to faulty eating habits. Persons suffering from diabetes will find the pose beneficial. As a peacock destroys snakes, this āsana kills toxins in the body. It also strengthens the forearms, wrists and elbows.

129. *Haṃsāsana* Ten* (Plate 356)

Haṃsa means a swan. This posture is very similar to Mayūrāsana (Plate 354), except that the placing of the hands is different. In Mayūrāsana the little fingers touch and the fingers point to the feet, whereas in Haṃsāsana the hands are so placed that the thumbs touch and the fingers point to the head. The posture resembles the plant balance in modern gymnastics.

Technique

1. Kneel on the floor with the knees slightly apart.

2. Bend forward and place the palms on the floor. The thumbs should touch and the fingers should point forward.

3. Bend the elbows and keep the forearms together. Rest the diaphragm on the elbows and the chest on the back of the upper arms.

4. Stretch the legs straight one by one and keep them together.

5. Exhale, swing the trunk forward, bear the body weight on the wrists and hands, raise the legs from the floor and keep them stretched straight with the feet together and parallel to the floor. (Plate 356)

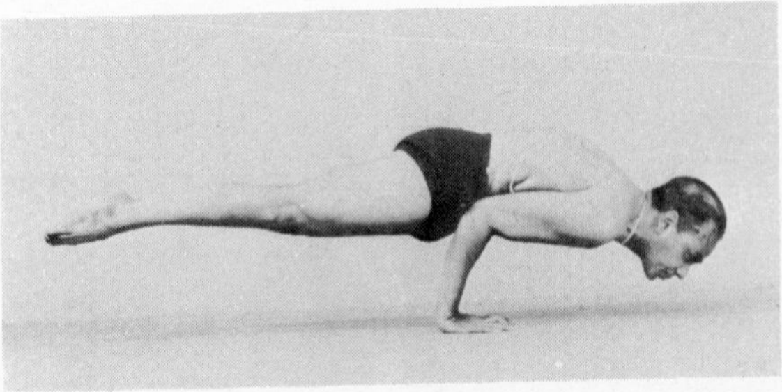

356

6. Balance in this position without holding your breath as long as you can. The forearms will not remain perpendicular to the floor due to the greater pressure on the wrists as a result of the position of the hands. It is harder to balance in Haṃsāsana than in Mayūrāsana. As the diaphragm is being pressed, breathing will be hard and laboured. The forearms do not bear the weight of the body as in Mayūrāsana.

7. Exhale and rest the head and toes on the floor. Place the knees on the floor by the side of the hands, take the weight of the body off the elbows, raise the hands and the head from the floor and relax.

Effects

This āsana tones the abdominal region of the body, because due to the pressure of the elbows against the abdominal aorta, blood circulates properly in the abdominal organs. This improves digestive power and prevents the accumulation of toxins in the system. It develops and strengthens the elbows, forearms and wrists.

130. *Pīnchā Mayūrāsana* Twelve* (Plate 357)

Pīncha means the chin or a feather. Mayūra means a peacock. At the approach of the rainy season peacocks dance. When they start they lift up their trailing tail feathers and spread them to form fans. In this posture, the trunk and legs are lifted off the floor and the body is balanced on the forearms and palms. The pose resembles that of a peacock starting his dance.

The pose is given below in two stages: in the second, the hands are lifted from the floor and the palms cupped under the chin, while the balance is maintained only on the elbows. The second stage is known as Śayanāsana. (Plate 358)

Technique

1. Kneel on the floor. Bend forward and rest the elbows, forearms and palms on the floor. The distance between the elbows should not be wider than that between the shoulders. Keep the forearms and hands parallel to each other.

2. Stretch the neck and lift the head up as high as possible.

3. Exhale, swing the legs up and try to balance without dropping the legs behind the head. (Plate 357)

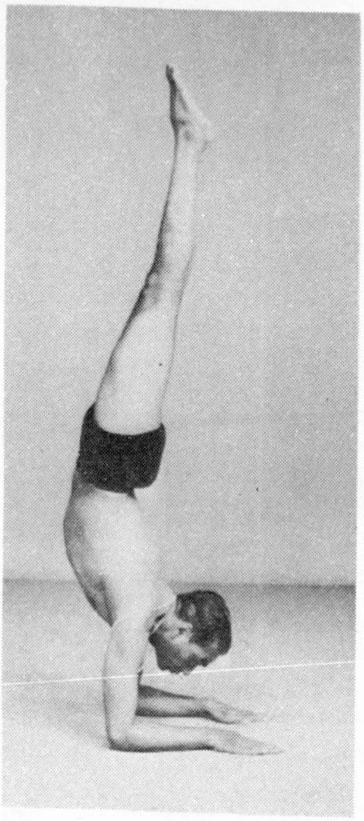

357

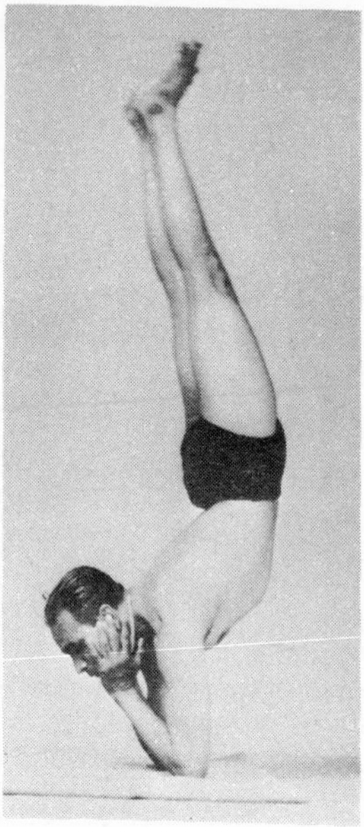

358

4. Stretch the region of the chest up vertically. Keep the legs stretched up vertically and together at the knees and ankles. The toes should point up.

5. Tighten the leg muscles at the hips and knees. While balancing, stretch the shoulders up and keep the thighs taut. Balance for a

minute. This is the first stage. In the beginning, try to get the balance by doing the pose against a wall so that you do not topple over. Gradually learn to stretch the spine and shoulders and to keep the head up and after mastering the balance do the pose in the middle of the room.

6. After perfecting the first stage, when the balance is secured lift the hands one by one from the floor, join the wrists and cupping the palms, place them under the chin. The body is balanced in this second stage of the posture only on the elbows. This is difficult, but by determined and regular practice one can achieve it. This second stage is known as the posture of repose:

131. *Sayanāsana* Fifteen* (Plate 358)

Effects

The posture develops the muscles of the shoulders and back. It tones the spine and stretches the abdominal muscles.

132. *Adho Mukha Vṛkṣāsana* Ten* (Plate 359)

Adho Mukha means having the face downwards. Vṛkṣa means a tree. The pose is the full arm balance in modern gymnastics.

Technique

1. Stand in Tāḍāsana. (Plate 1.) Bend forward and place the palms on the floor about a foot away from a wall. The distance between the palms should be the same as between the shoulders. Keep the arms fully stretched.

2. Take the legs back and bend the knees. Exhale, swing the legs up against the wall and balance. If the hands are kept far from the wall, then when the legs are supported by the wall the curvature of the spine will be great and will cause much strain. It will also be difficult to balance if the hands are kept away from the wall. Stay in the pose for a minute with normal breathing.

3. After learning to balance on the hands against the wall, take the feet away from the wall. Then try the pose in the middle of the room. Keep the legs fully stretched and the toes pointing up. Lift the head as far up as you can. (Plate 359)

Effects

The pose develops the body harmoniously. It strengthens the shoulders, arms and wrists and expands the chest fully.

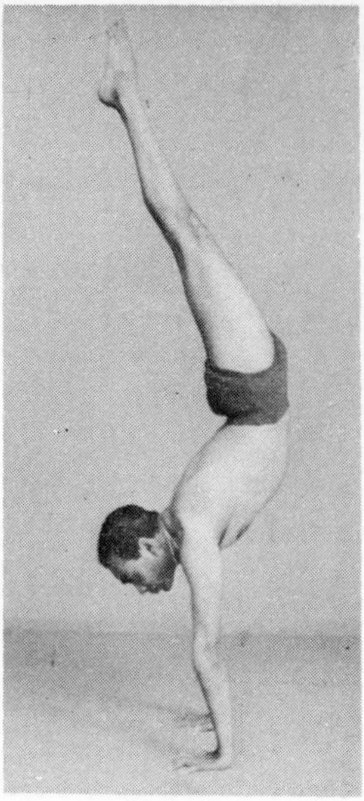

359

133. *Kūrmāsana* Fourteen* (Plates 363 and 364)

Kūrma means a tortoise. The āsana is dedicated to Kūrma the Tortoise Incarnation of Viṣṇu, the maintainer of the universe. Many divine treasures had been lost in a universal flood including amṛta (nectar) with which the gods preserved their youth. To retrieve the lost treasures the gods entered into an alliance with the demons and jointly undertook to churn the cosmic ocean. Viṣṇu became a great tortoise and dived to the bottom of the ocean. On his back was Mount Mandara for the churning stick and round the mountain was twined the divine serpent Vāsuki for the rope. The ocean was churned by the joint efforts of the gods and demons in pulling the snake and twirling the mountain. From the churned ocean emerged amṛta and various other treasures including Lakṣmī, consort of Viṣṇu and the goddess of wealth and beauty.

The pose is given in three stages. The final one resembles a tortoise with head and limbs withdrawn under its shell and is called Supta Kūrmāsana (Plate 368), the sleeping tortoise pose.

Technique

1. Sit on the floor with the legs stretched straight in front. (Plate 77.)

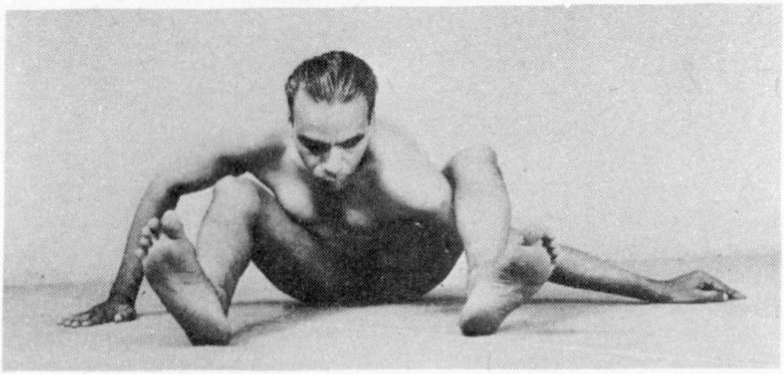

360

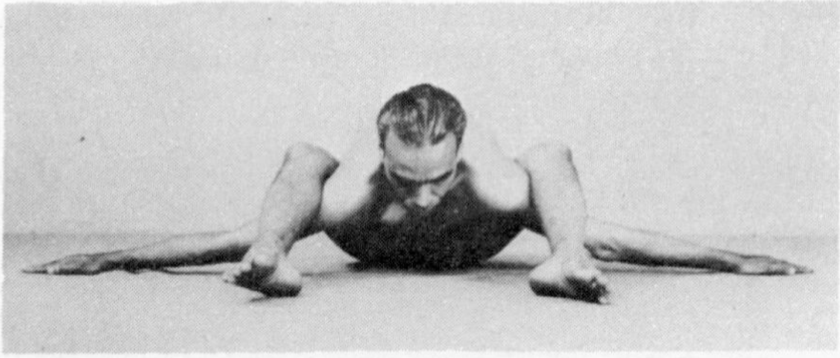

361

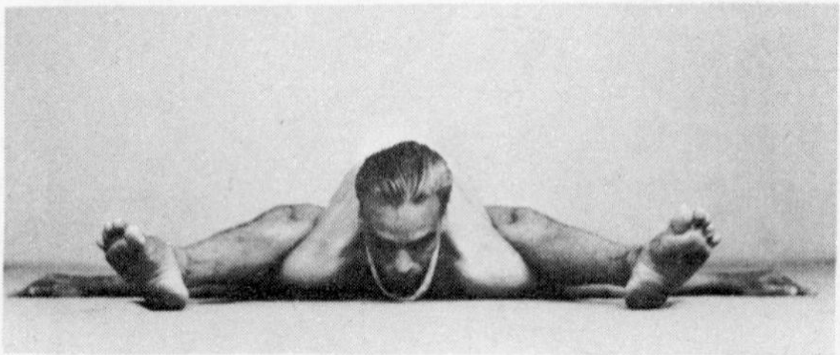

362

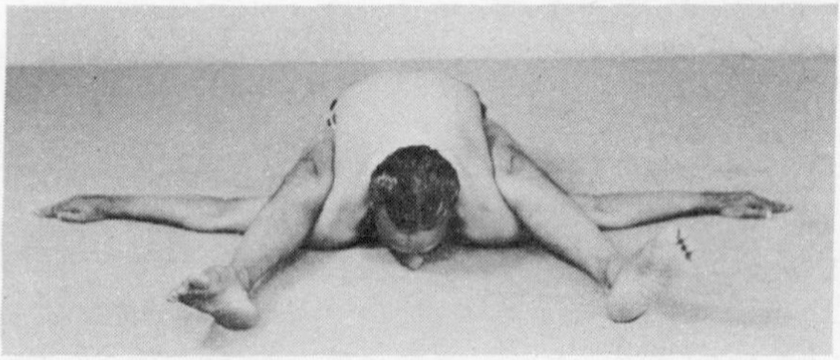

363

Widen the legs until the distance between the two knees is about a foot and a half.

2. Bend the knees and lift them up by drawing the feet towards the trunk.

3. Exhale, bend the trunk forward and insert the hands one by one under the knees. (Plates 360 and 361.) Push the arms underneath the knees and stretch them straight out sideways. Rest the shoulders on the floor and keep the palms on it. (Plate 362.) Take a breath.

4. Exhale, stretch the trunk, still more, extend the neck and bring the forehead, then the chin and lastly the chest down to the floor. Then stretch the legs straight again. (Plates 363 and 364.) The knees will then be near the armpits and the back of the knees will touch the back of the upper arms near the armpits.

5. Gradually intensify the stretch until the chin and the chest rest on the floor. Extend the legs fully also and press the heels down to the floor. This is the first stage. Hold this position from 30 to 60 seconds.

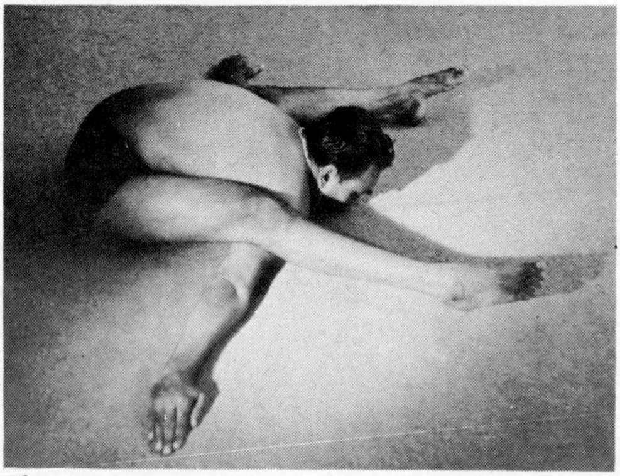

364

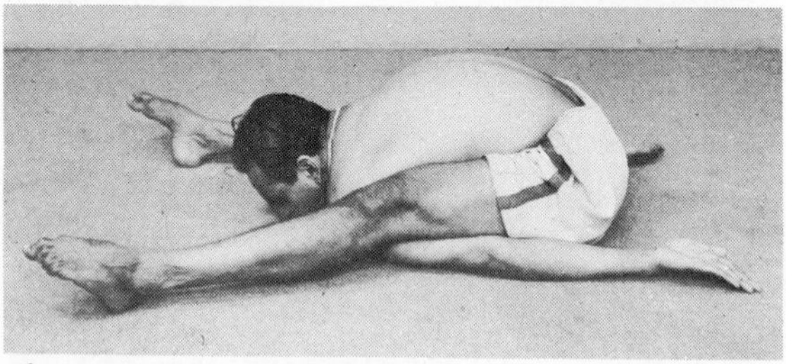

365

6. Now turn the wrists so that the palms face up, and keeping the legs, trunk and head in the same position, move the arms back from the shoulders and stretch them straight so that the forearms are near the hip joints. (Plate 365.) Stay in this position without bending the elbows for 30 to 60 seconds. This is the second stage.

7. Bend and lift up the knees. Then lift the chest slightly off the floor, move the hands behind the back by bending at the elbows and clasp them. (Plate 366)

8. Now move the feet towards the head. Interlock the feet at the ankles by placing the right foot over the left one or vice versa. (Plate 367)

9. Exhale, insert the head in between the feet and keep the forehead on the floor. The back of the head will touch the interlocked feet near the ankles. This is the final stage known as:

134. *Supta Kūrmāsana* Fourteen* (Plate 368)

Stay in this pose from one to two minutes. It is advisable to change the position of the feet while interlocking them, so that if at first the right foot is placed over the left one, when changing the position of

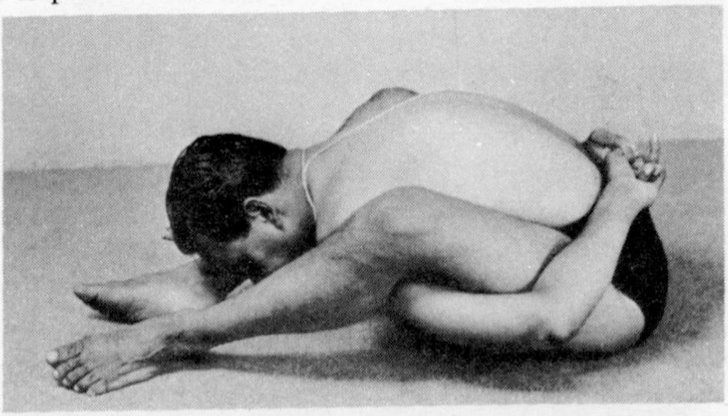

366

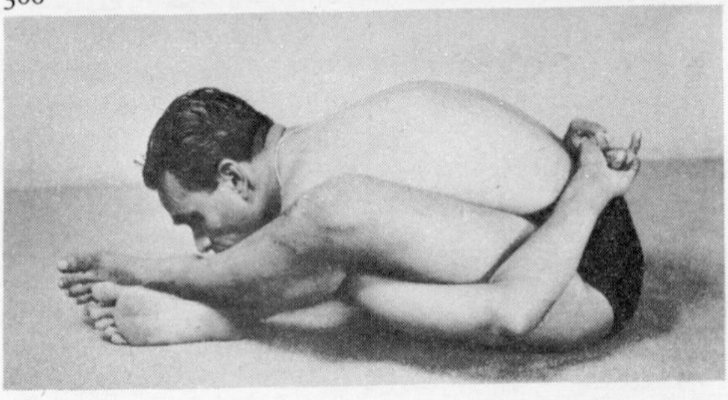

367

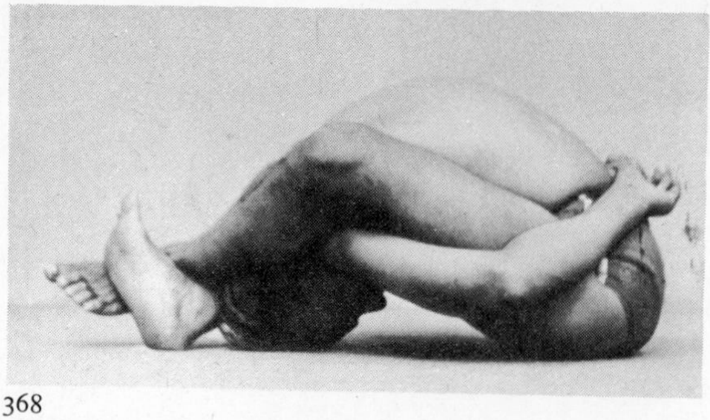

368

the feet place the left foot over the right one. This will develop the legs evenly.

10. Inhale, lift the head and release the hands and feet; stretch the legs out straight, recline on the floor and relax.

11. Breathe normally throughout the three stages described above.

Effects

This pose is sacred to a yogi. While describing the qualities of a sthita-prajñā (one who is stable of mind) to Arjuna, the Blessed Lord says: 'When, again as a tortoise draws its limbs in on all sides, he withdraws his senses from the objects of sense, and then his understanding is well-poised.' (*Bhagavad Gītā*, second discourse, verse 58.) In this pose the limbs are withdrawn and the body resembles a tortoise. The mind becomes calm and composed and one develops equanimity whether in sorrow or in joy. It will gradually become free from anxiety amid pains and indifferent amid pleasures, while the emotions of passion, fear and anger will loosen their hold upon the mind.

On the purely physical level the effects are also great. It tones the spine, activates the abdominal organs and keeps one energetic and healthy. It soothes the nerves of the brain and after completing it one feels refreshed as though one had woken up from a long undisturbed sleep.

This āsana prepares the aspirant for the fifth stage of yogic practices, namely, Pratyāhāra (withdrawal of the senses from outside objects).

135. *Eka Pāda Śīrṣāsana* Fifteen* (Plate 371)

Eka means one. Pāda means a leg or a foot. Śīrṣa means the head.

Technique

1. Sit on the floor with the legs stretched straight in front. (Plate 77)

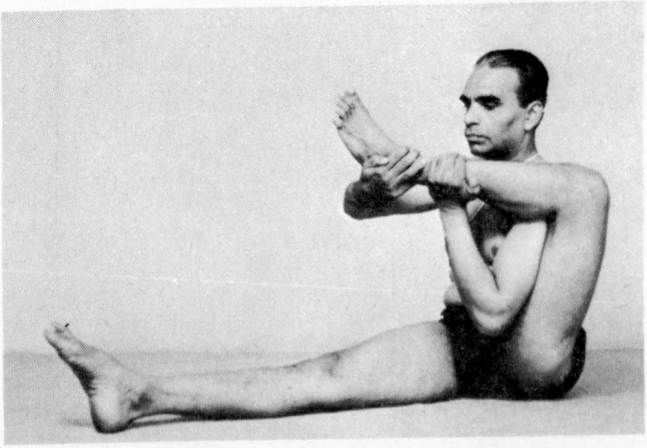

369

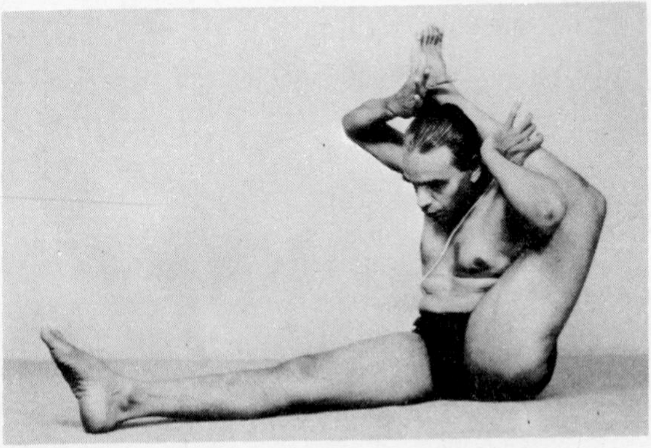

370

2. Bend the knee, lift the left foot and bring it near the trunk by holding the left ankle with both hands. (Plate 369)

3. Exhale, pull the left thigh up and back, bend the trunk a little forward and place the left leg on the back of the neck. (Plate 370.) The outer side of the lower left leg just above the ankle will touch the back of the neck.

4. Raise up the neck and head, keep the back straight, let go of the left ankle and fold the palms in front of the chest. (Plate 371.) The back of the left thigh will then touch the back of the left shoulder. If the head is not held up properly, the leg will slip off the neck. The right leg should lie straight on the floor. The back of the entire leg should touch the floor and the toes point forward.

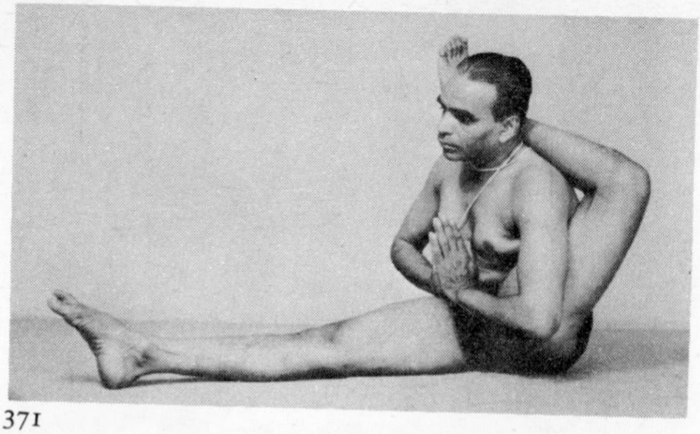

371

5. Remain in this position from 15 to 60 seconds with deep breathing.

6. Unfold the palms, hold the left ankle with both hands, lower the left leg to the ground and straighten it.

7. Repeat the pose on the right side, placing the right leg behind the neck. The left leg should lie straight on the floor. Keep the pose on both sides for the same length of time.

Effects

By the practice of this posture the neck and the back grow stronger while the thighs and the hamstring muscles are stretched fully. The abdominal muscles are contracted and the digestive power increases. Until one has practised the posture one does not realise the weight and pressure of the leg which rests on the neck.

Eka Pāda Śīrṣāsana Cycle

The āsanas given below can be done in continuation of Eka Pāda Śīrṣāsana (Plate 371) one after another at a stretch. There is no need to do them separately.

First, perform the entire cycle of āsanas doing Eka Pāda Śīrṣāsana with one leg placed on the back of the neck. Then rest for a minute or two and repeat the cycle with the other leg placed on the back of the neck. These poses are strenuous and require long practice to master.

136. *Skandāsana* Sixteen* (Plate 372)

Skanda is the name of Kārtikeya, the god of War, whose birth forms the subject matter of *Kumāra-saṁbhava*, the epic poem written by Kālidāsa. Once the gods were troubled by the demon Tāraka, who it was prophesied could only be destroyed by the son of Śiva and Pārvatī, the beautiful daughter of the mountain Himālaya. But the prospect of Śiva having a son seemed to the other gods to be very faint, because he was continually wrapped in meditation after the death of his wife Satī. Pārvatī, who was the reincarnation of Satī, was sent by the gods to wait upon Siva, but though she made many attempts to win his attention he took no notice of her. Vasanta, the god of Spring, and Kāma, the god of Love, did their best to help Pārvatī to win Śiva. Kāma shot his arrow of desire at him and disturbed him in his meditation. Śiva opened his third eye and by the flames issuing from it burnt Kāma to ashes. In order to win her husband of a former life, Pārvatī decided to follow Śiva in asceticism. She laid aside her ornaments and became a hermitess on a nearby peak, and in this guise, Śiva, who had already been smitten by Kāma's arrow, noticed and fell in love with her. Śiva and Pārvatī were married at a great ceremony, which all the gods attended. Pārvatī gave birth to the war-god Skanda, who when he grew to manhood, slew the demon Tāraka.

Technique

1. Do Eka Pāda Śīrṣāsana. (Plate 371)

2. With an exhalation, bend the trunk forward and hold the outstretched right leg with both hands as in Paschimottānāsana (Plate 160) and rest the chin on the right knee.

3. Extend the chin to prevent the leg from slipping off.

4. Stay in the pose for about 20 seconds with deep breathing.

137. *Buddhāsana* Twenty-two* (Plate 373)

Buddha means enlightened. This āsana is a continuation of Skandāsana. (Plate 372)

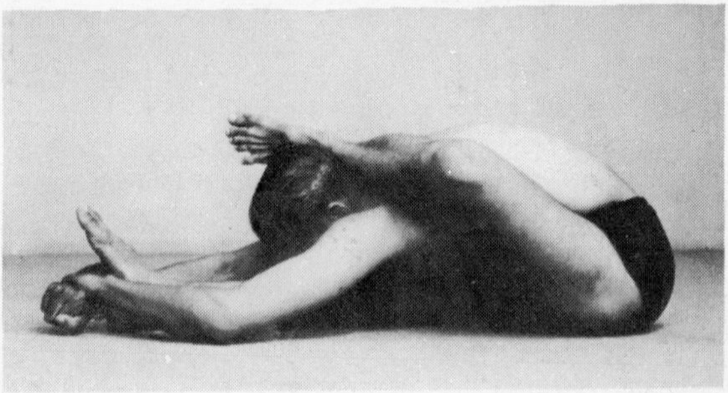

372

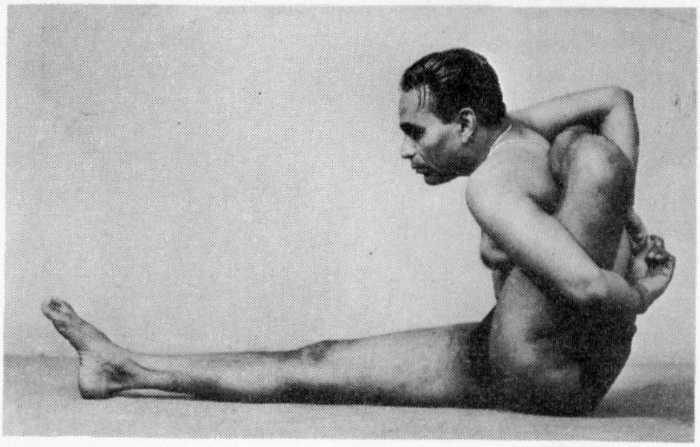

373

Technique

1. From Skandāsana (Plate 372) with the left leg placed on the back of the neck, inhale and raise the head and trunk up.

2. Hold the left ankle with the left hand and lower the leg still further.

3. Raise the right arm from the shoulder, move it sideways and turn the forearm back to bring it over the left ankle from above the left foot. (Plate 373)

4. Stay in the pose for about 15 seconds with deep breathing. Inhale, lift up the head and trunk.

138. *Kapilāsana* Twenty-two* (Plate 374)

Kapila was the name of a great sage, who is said to have been the founder of the Sankhya system of philosophy. This āsana is a continuation of Buddhāsana. (Plate 373)

Technique

1. Maintain the hand grip in Buddhāsana with the left leg placed on the back of the neck, exhale, bend the trunk forward and rest the chin on the outstretched right knee as in Paschimottānāsana. (Plate 160)

2. Stay in the pose from 10 to 15 seconds with deep breathing. Inhale, lift up the head and trunk and release the hand grip.

139. *Bhairavāsana* Sixteen* (Plate 375)

Bhairava means terrible, formidable. This is one of the eight aspects of Śiva.

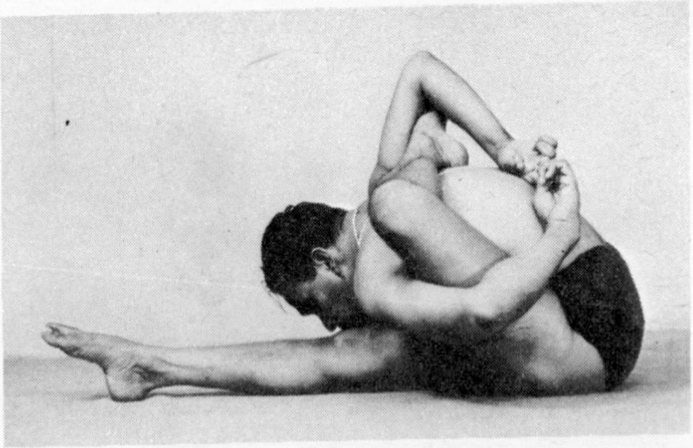

374

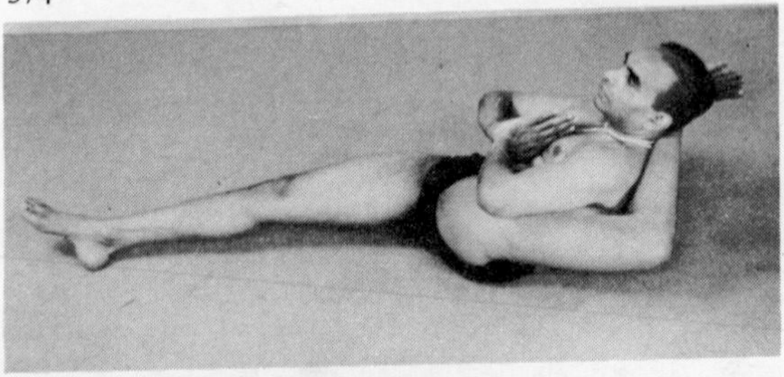

375

Technique

1. After releasing the hand grip in Kapilāsana (Plate 374), exhale and recline backwards.

2. Fold the arms across the chest. Keep the right leg stretched straight on the floor. (Plate 375)

3. Stay in the pose for about 20 seconds, with deep breathing.

140. *Kāla Bhairavāsana* Nineteen* (Plate 378)

Kāla Bhairava is Śiva in his terrible aspect as destroyer of the universe, a personification of the destructive principle.

Technique

1. After completing Bhairavāsana (Plate 375), unfold the arms from the chest, press the palms to the floor and come back to Eka Pāda Śīrṣāsana. The palms should be kept by the side of the hips.

2. Move the right leg sideways to the right.

3. Exhale, raise the body off the floor (Plate 376) and take two breaths.

4. Exhale, take the right arm off the floor, turn the trunk to the right and place the right arm along the right thigh. (Plate 377.) Take two breaths.

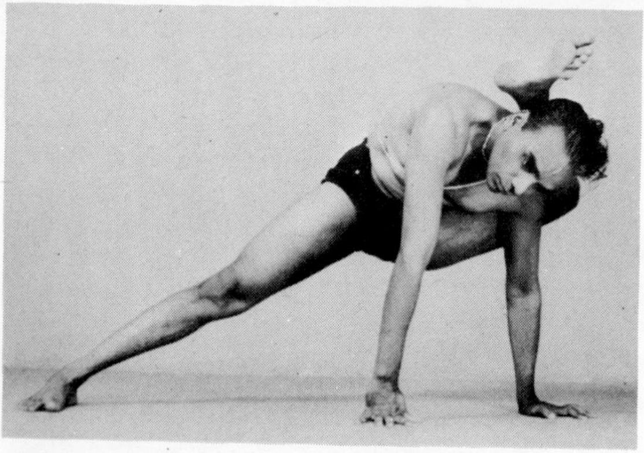

376

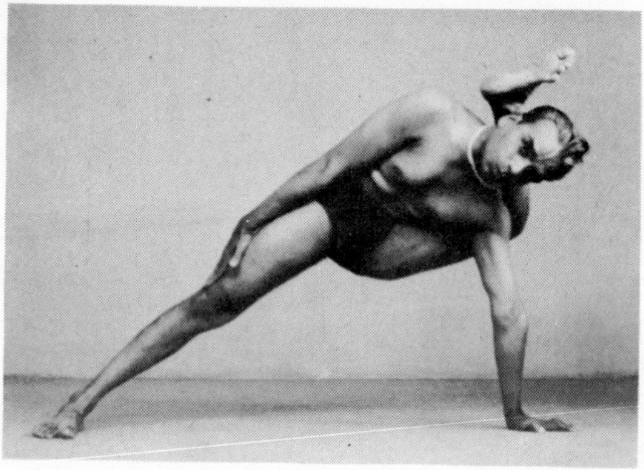

377

5. Now stretch the right arm up vertically. (Plate 378)

6. The whole body is balanced sideways on the left palm and the outer side of the right foot, the right leg forming an angle of 30 degrees from the floor.

7. Stay in the pose for about 20 seconds with deep breathing.

141. *Chakorāsana* Twenty* (Plates 379 and 380)

Chakora is a bird like a partridge, which is said to feed on moonbeams.

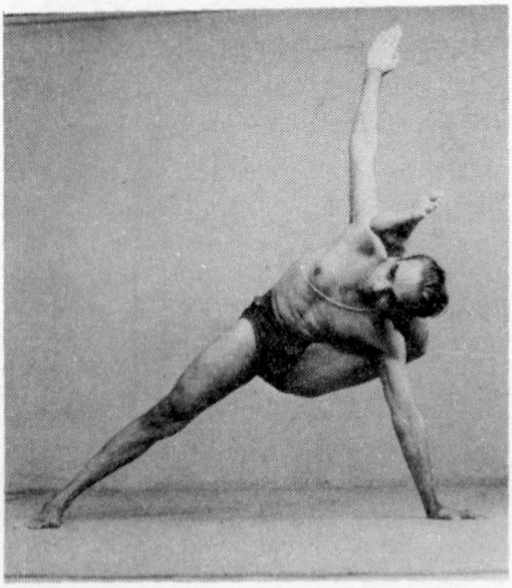

378

Technique

1. From Kāla Bhairavāsana (Plate 375), place the right palm on the floor and bending the right knee, rest on the floor with the left leg on the back of the neck, thus coming back to Eka Pāda Śīrṣāsana. (Plate 371)

2. Press the palms on the floor by the side of the hips.

3. Raise the hips off the floor and balance the body on the palms. Lift the outstretched right leg up until it forms an angle of about 60 to 75 degrees from the floor. (Plates 379 and 380.) Stay in the pose to your capacity with normal breathing.

142. *Dūrvāsāsana* Twenty-one* (Plate 383)

Dūrvāsa was the name of a very irascible sage whose anger has become proverbial.

Technique

1. From Chakorāsana (Plate 379) rest the outstretched right leg on the floor. Bend the right knee and squat by resting the palms on the floor. (Plate 381)

2. Then rest the palms on the right thigh. Exhale, press the palms on the right thigh, pull the trunk up and gradually stand up on the right leg, keeping it erect by making the muscles taut. (Plate 382)

3. Pull the waist and chest up, fold the hands in front of the chest

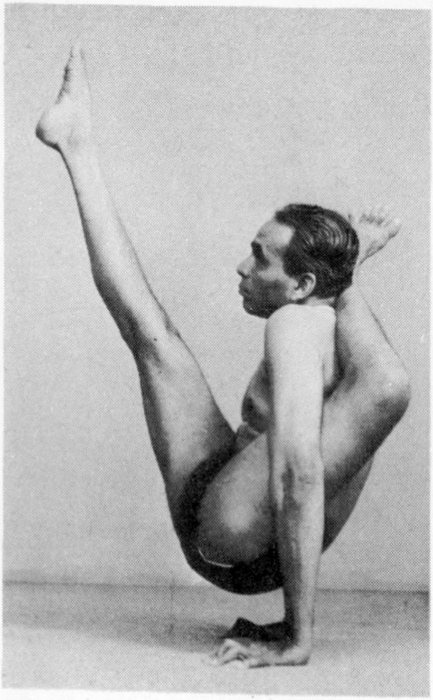
379

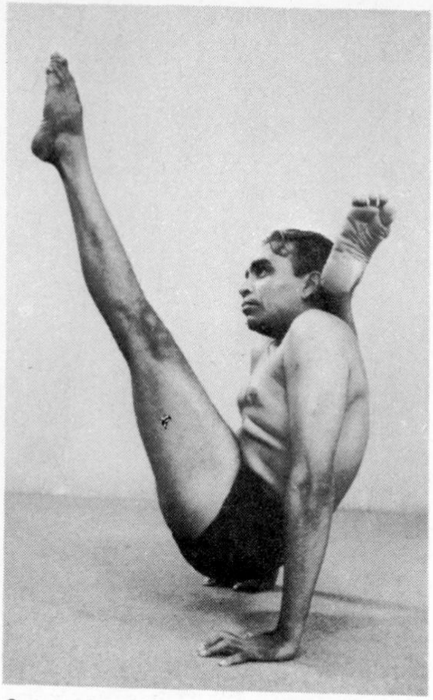
380

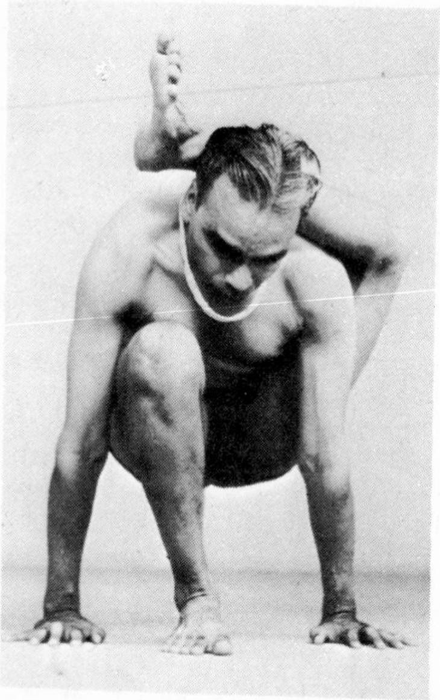
381

and balance the body on the right leg. (Plate 383.) The left leg lies across the back of the neck. Try to breathe normally.

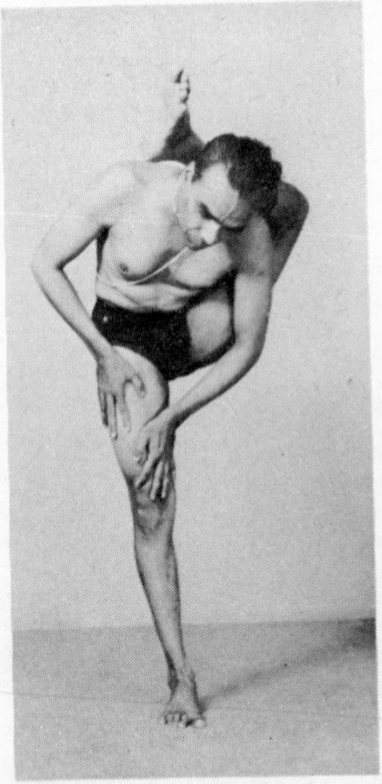

382

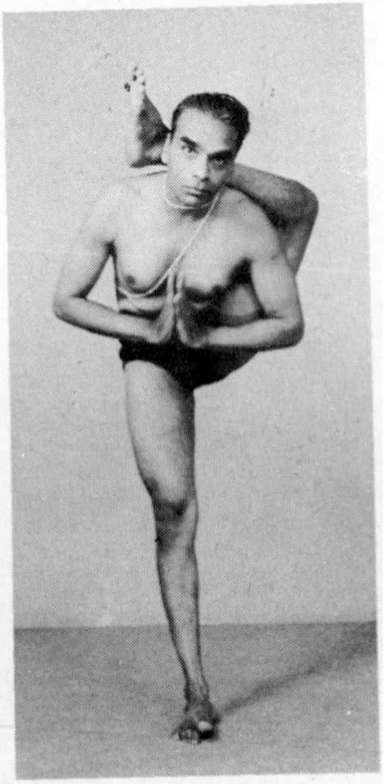

383

4. Hold the posture as long as you can. Since it is difficult to balance, use the support of a wall or a friend to start with.

143. *Ruchikāsana* Eighteen* (Plates 384 and 385)

Ruchika was the name of a sage, the grandfather of Bhagavān Paraśurāma, the sixth incarnation of Viṣṇu.

Technique

1. After completing Dūrvāsāsana (Plate 383), exhale, bend the trunk forward and rest the palms on either side of the right foot. (Plates 384 and 385)

2. Rest the head on the right knee without allowing the left leg to slip from the back of the neck. Then gradually extend the neck until the chin touches the right knee, as in Uttānāsana. (Plate 48)

3. Stay in the pose for about 15 seconds with normal breathing.

4. Bend the right knee, sit on the floor, release the left leg from the back of the neck and relax.

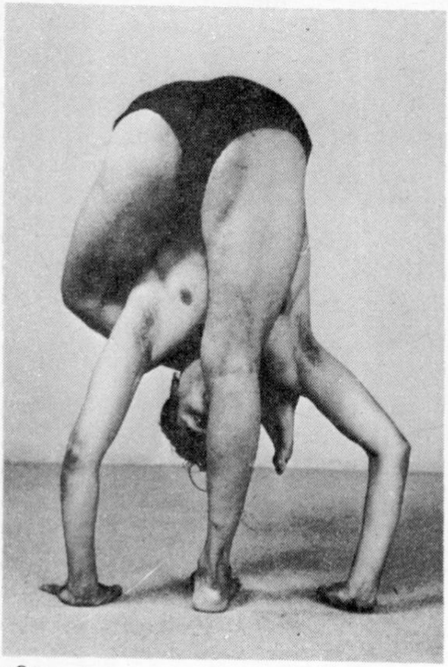
384

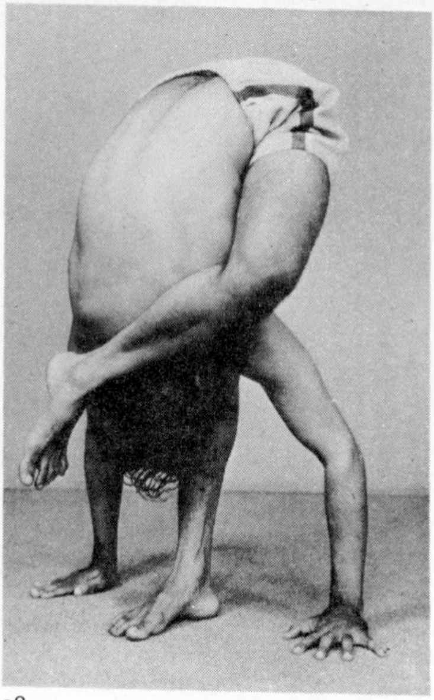
385

5. Then put the right leg behind the neck and repeat the cycle of āsanas given above, reading the word 'left' for the word 'right' and vice versa.

Effects of the āsanas in the Eka Pāda Śīrṣāsana Cycle

The various movements in this cycle of āsanas tone up the muscular, nervous and circulatory systems of the entire body. The spine receives a rich supply of blood, which increases the nervous energy in the chakras (the various nerve plexuses situated in the spine), the fly-wheels in the human body machine. These poses develop the chest and make the breathing fuller and the body firmer; they stop nervous trembling of the body and prevent the diseases which cause it; they also help to eliminate toxins by supplying pure blood to every part of the body and bringing the congested blood back to the heart and lungs for purification. By the practice of these āsanas the haemoglobin content of the blood improves, the body and mind become vigorous and the capacity for work increases.

144. *Viranchyāsana I* Nineteen* (Plates 386 and 387)

Virancha or Viranchi is one of the names of Brahmā, the supreme

Being, the first deity of the Hindu Trinity, to whom is entrusted the work of creating the world.

Technique

1. Sit on the floor with the legs stretched straight in front. (Plate 77)

2. Bend the right knee and place the right foot at the root of the left thigh in half Padmāsana.

3. Bend the left knee, bring the foot near the trunk and grasp the left ankle with both hands. Exhale, pull the left thigh up and back, bend the trunk a little forward and place the left leg on the back of the neck. The outer side of the left leg just above the ankle will touch the back of the neck.

4. Raise the head and neck up, keep the back erect and let go of the left ankle.

5. Now raise the left arm up vertically, bend it at the elbow and take it behind the back of the neck over the left leg across the neck. Lower the right arm, bend it at the elbow and raise the right forearm up behind the back till the right hand is level with and between the shoulder-blades. Clasp the hands behind the back between the shoulders. (Plates 386 and 387)

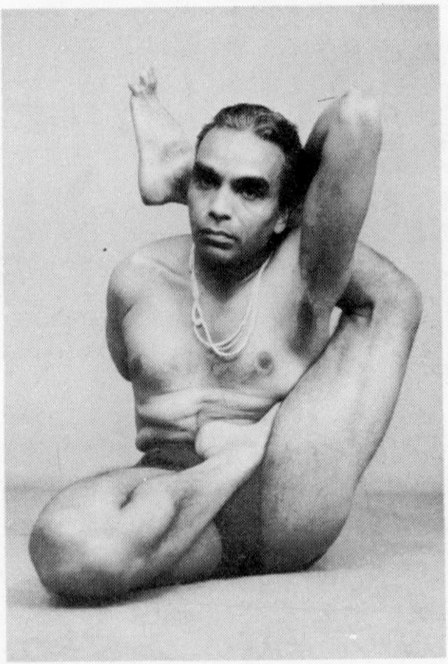

386

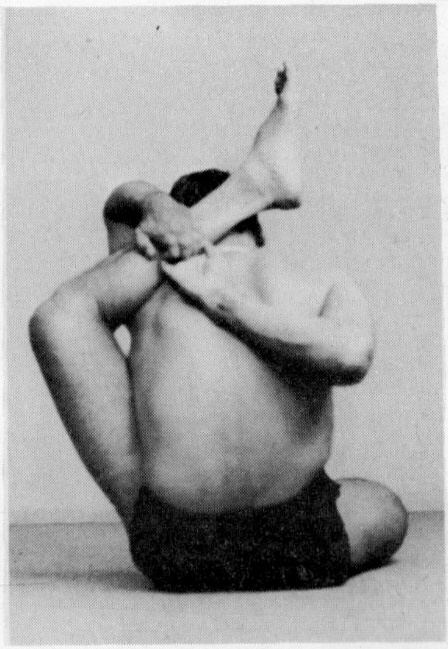

387

6. Stay in this pose from 10 to 20 seconds with normal breathing. Unclasp the hands, lower the left leg, straighten the right one and return to position 1.

7. Repeat the pose on the other side for the same length of time, reading left for right and vice versa.

145. *Viranchyāsana II* Ten* (Plate 388)

Technique

1. Sit on the floor with the legs stretched straight in front. (Plate 77)

2. Bend the left leg at the knee and move it back. Place the left foot by the hip joint, keep the toes pointing backwards and rest them on the floor. The left leg will now be in Virāsana. (Plate 89)

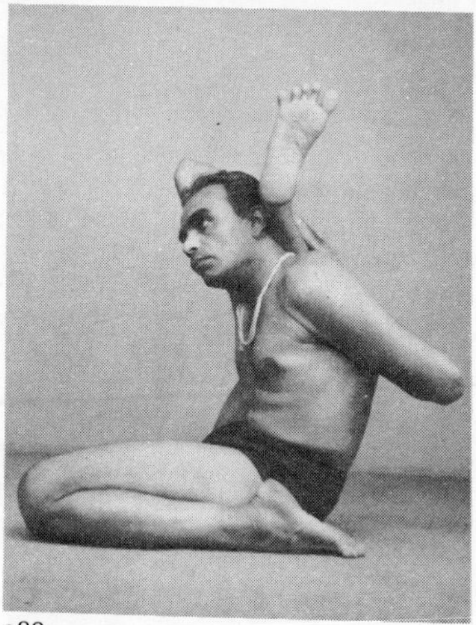

388

3. Then follow the technique stated above for Viranchyāsana I. (Plate 386)

Effects

Both these poses strengthen the back and the neck while the shoulder movements become freer. The thighs and hamstring muscles are extended fully, the abdominal muscles contract and digestive power increases.

146. *Yoganidrāsana* Eighteen* (Plate 391)

Nidrā means sleep. Yoganidrā is a state between sleep and wakefulness. It is also the name given to the sleep of Viṣṇu at the end of a Yuga, an age of the world.

In this pose the legs are interlaced behind the back of the neck and the hands are clasped behind the back which rests on the ground. The legs form the Yogi's pillow and the back is his couch. The practice of this pose warms up the body very rapidly. It is therefore used by Yogis living at high altitudes to keep warm.

Technique

1. Lie flat on the back on the floor. (Plate 219)

2. Bend both the knees and bring the legs over the head.

3. Exhale, move the right leg from behind the right shoulder by holding the right foot with both the hands and placing it well behind the back of the neck, as in Eka Pāda Śīrṣāsana. (Plate 389)

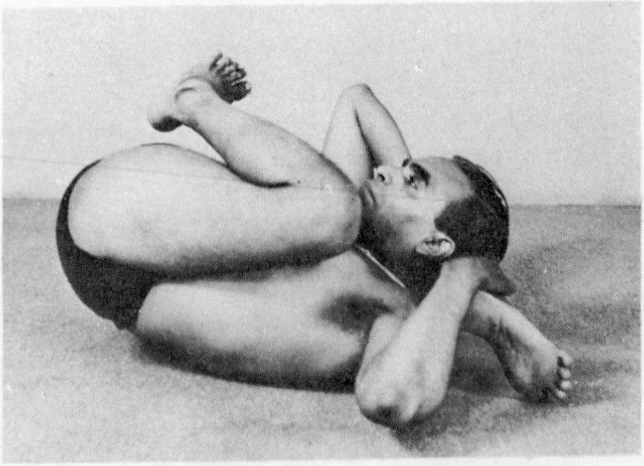

389

4. Maintain the position of the right leg, breathing in several times.

5. Exhale and with the help of the left palm move the left leg behind the left shoulder and place it under the right leg. (Plate 390.) Lock the feet at the ankles.

6. Lift the shoulders well up, move the arms behind the back and clasp the fingers. (Plate 391.) The back of the upper arms will be in contact with the back of the thighs. Take a few breaths.

7. Exhale, lift the chest well up and stretch the neck back. This is the final position (which is the reverse position of Supta Kūrmāsana, Plate 368). Stay in the pose for 30 to 60 seconds, trying to breathe normally.

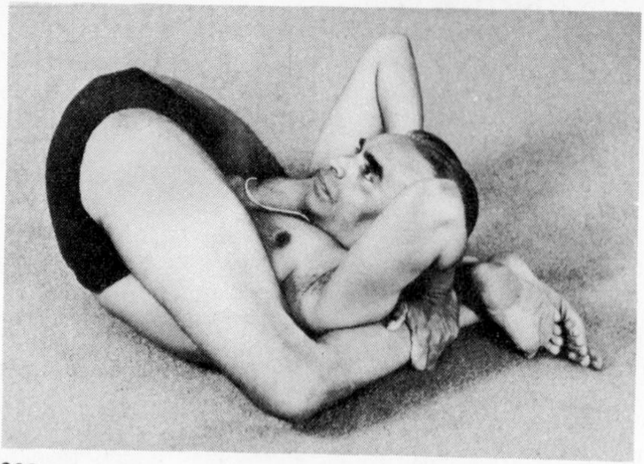

390

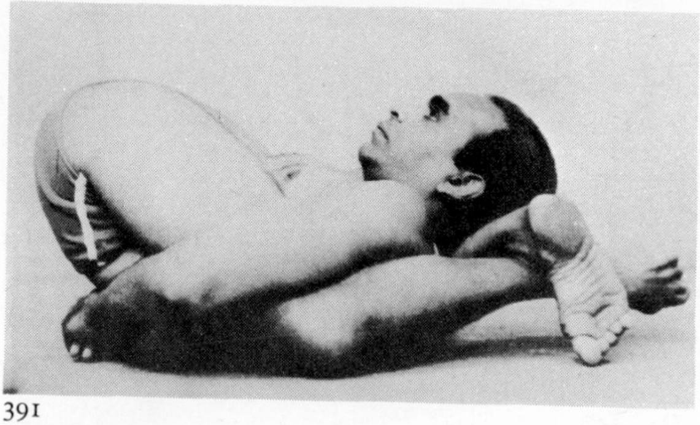

391

8. Exhale and release the hand grip behind the back and the leg grip behind the neck.

9. Relax on the floor, keeping the legs straight for some time.

10. Then repeat the pose for the same length of time, first placing the left leg behind the back of the neck with the right leg under it.

11. Loosen the hand and leg grips and relax on the floor.

12. Do not cross both legs first and then move them behind the neck. This will not give the correct feel of the āsana. Remember to bring one leg behind the back of the neck and then the other leg under the first one. Before resting the legs behind the neck, raise the neck and dorsal region and also extend the shoulders, so that the latter do not get wedged between the chest and the legs. This will ensure that the pose is correct.

Effects

In this pose the spine is given a full forward stretch and one feels a pleasing sensation in the back. It is one of the best front bending poses. Even the maximum stretch of Paschimottānāsana (Plate 160) does not give the same feeling of right exercise, comfort and rest as the correct practice of Yoganidrāsana.

In the back bending poses the lungs and the abdominal muscles are given maximum expansion. In this āsana the lungs and the abdominal muscles are contracted to the full. In a short time, the practice of the pose tones the kidneys, liver, spleen, intestines, gall bladder, prostates and the urine bladder. The abdominal organs will be free from diseases by continued practice of this pose. It also exercises the gonads and releases energy and vitality in the system. The nerves will be rested and energy will be stored in the body for better thinking and better work.

147. *Dwi Pāda Śīrṣāsana* Twenty-four* (Plate 393)

Dwi Pāda (dwi = two or both; pāda = leg or foot) means of both feet. In Eka Pāda Śīrṣāsana (Plate 371) one leg is placed behind the back of the neck. In this āsana both legs are so placed, the hands are folded in front of the chest and the body is balanced on a small section of the seat near the tail-bone. This is difficult and one is apt to fall backwards. The pose is very similar to Yoganidrāsana (Plate 391), but here the body is vertical, whereas in Yoganidrāsana the back rests on the floor.

Technique

1. Sit on the floor with the legs stretched straight in front. (Plate 77)

2. Bend both knees and bring the feet near the trunk.

3. Exhale, catch the right ankle with both hands, pull the right thigh up and back, bend the trunk a little forward and place the right leg on the back of the neck as in Eka Pāda Śīrṣāsana. The back of the right thigh will then touch the back of the right shoulder. Release the hands from the ankle and take a few breaths.

4. Exhale, catch the left ankle with the left hand, pull the left thigh up and back and place the left leg over the right one in the same manner as described above. Release the hand from the left ankle, but keep the feet locked at the ankles. Place the hands on the floor by the side of the hips and balance upright on the portion of the seat near the tail-bone. (Plate 392.) This requires practice. Try to maintain normal breathing.

5. Lift the hands off the floor, fold them in front of the chest and stay balanced in the vertical position for a few seconds or as long as you can from 10 to 30 seconds. (Plate 393.) This is the final position.

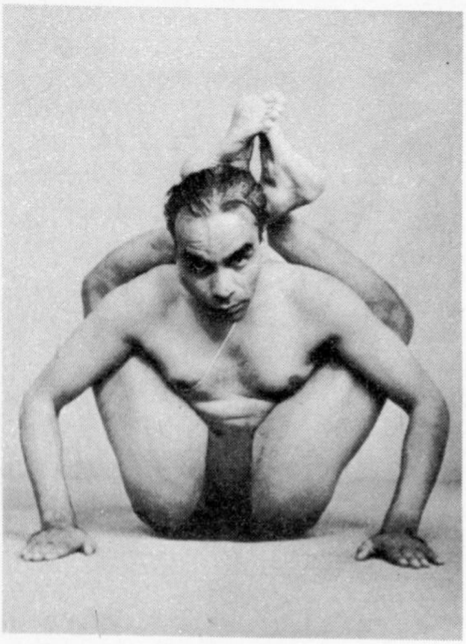

392

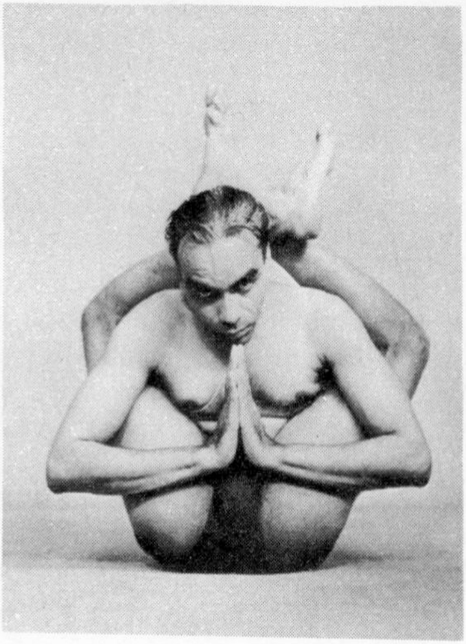

393

6. After holding this posture, place the palms on the floor by the side of the hips, exhale, straighten the arms and pull the body up by taking the weight on the hands. Do not release the ankle lock. (Plate 394.) Hold the pose from 10 to 20 seconds to your capacity.

7. Release the foot lock at the ankles, stretch the legs up vertically and balance on the hands. This is called:

148. *Tittibhāsana* Twenty-two* (Plate 395)
Tittibha is an insect like a firefly.

After staying in this position for a few seconds, bend the legs at the knees, lower the body to the floor, release the legs from the arms, stretch them straight in front and rest for a few seconds.

8. Repeat the movements for the same length of time, this time first placing the left leg on the back of the neck and then the right leg on the top of the left one. Finally relax on the floor.

Effects

In this āsana the lungs and abdominal muscles are most tightly contracted. The spine is given a full forward stretch and the abdominal organs benefit quickly from the exercise. The effect is the same as that of Yoganidrāsana (Plate 391), but in this pose the thigns are stretched

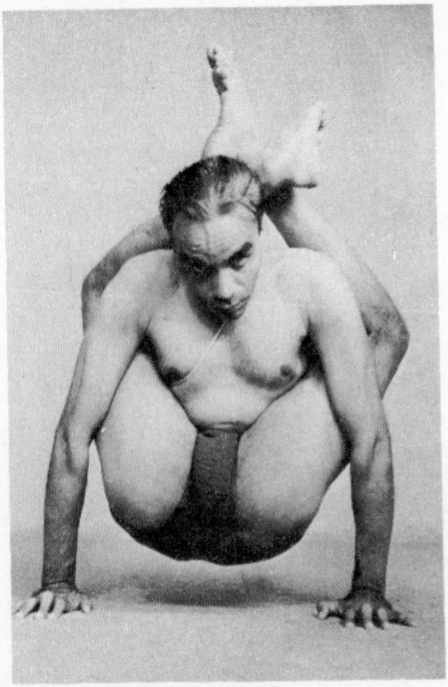

394

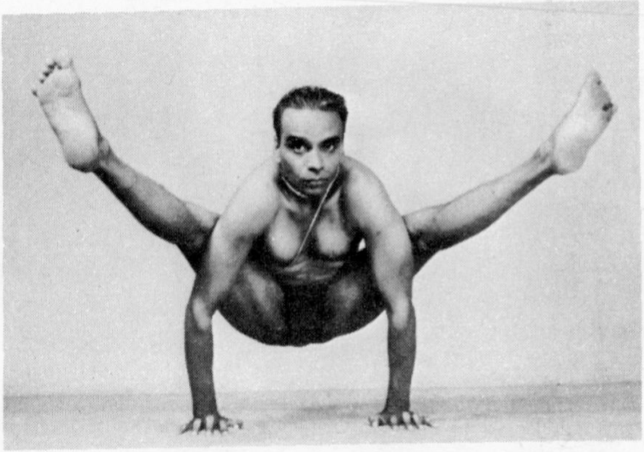

395

more and greater strain is felt on the neck, the sacrolumbar region of the spine and the abdomen.

149. *Vasiṣṭhāsana* Eighteen* (Plate 398)

Vasiṣṭha was a celebrated sage or seer, the family priest of the solar race of kings and the author of several Vedic hymns, particularly of the seventh Maṇḍala of the Ṛg Veda. He was a typical representative of the brahmanic dignity and power and is one of the seven sages who are identified with the stars of the Great Bear. The rivalry between him and the royal sage Viśvāmitra, a kṣatriya (a man of the warrior caste) who by his piety and asceticism raised himself to brahman status, forms the subject of many legends.

The āsana is dedicated to the sage Vasiṣṭha.

Technique

1. Stand in Tāḍāsana. (Plate 1.) Bend forward, rest the palms on the floor and take the legs back about 4 to 5 feet as if you are doing Adho Mukha Śvānāsana. (Plate 75)

2. Turn the whole body sideways to the right and balance on the right hand and foot only. The outer side of the right foot should rest firmly on the floor. Place the left foot over the right one, rest the left palm on the left hip and balance, keeping the body straight. (Plate 396.) In order to learn the art of balancing in this position, be close to a wall so that the inner side of the right foot rests against it.

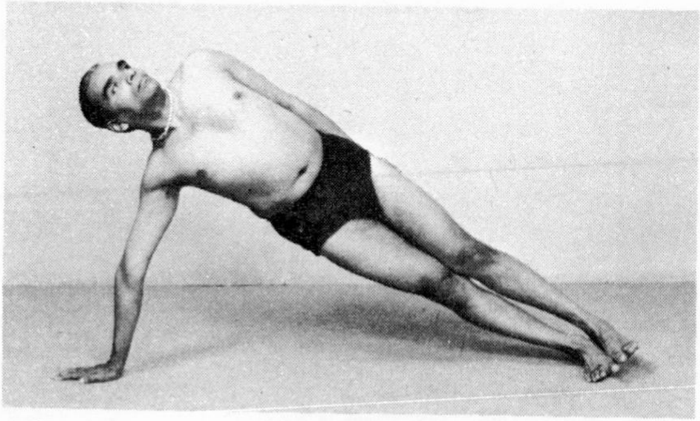

396

3. Exhale, bend the left leg at the knee, move the body slightly forward and catch the left big toe between the thumb and the index and middle fingers of the left hand. (Plate 397.) Pull the left arm and the left leg up vertically. (Plate 398.) The grip on the toe will be like that described in Supta Pādānguṣṭhāsana. (Plate 284.) Balance in this position, keeping the arms and legs rigid, with deep breathing, for about 20 to 30 seconds.

4. Release the toe grip, rest the left leg again over the right foot and lower the left hand to the hip once more.

5. Exhale, turn the body over to the left so that it balances only on the

left hand and the left foot. Repeat the pose on this side for the same length of time, following the technique stated above, reading right for left and left for right.

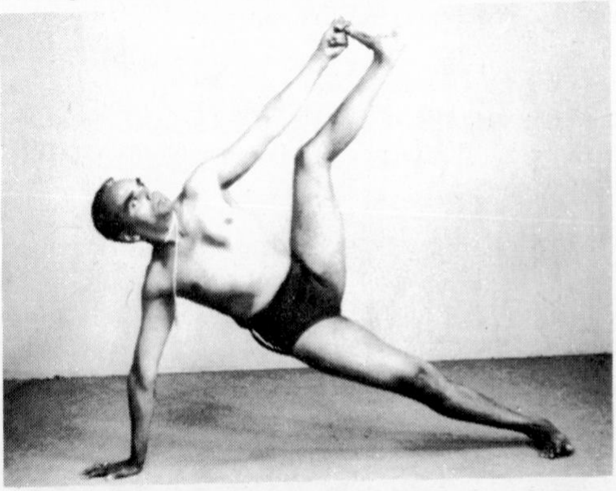

397

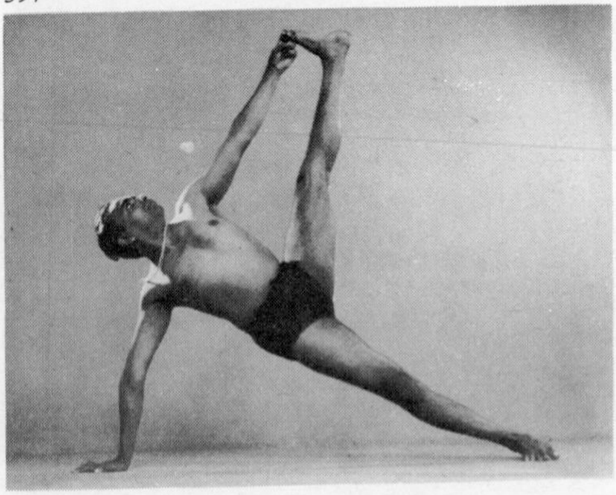

398

Effects

This pose strengthens the wrists, exercises the legs and tones the lumbar and coccyx regions of the spine.

150. *Kaśyapāsana* Nineteen* (Plates 399 and 400)

This āsana is dedicated to the sage Kaśyapa, son of the sage Marīchi, a son of Brahmā. He bore an important share in the work of creation. It is said that Kaśyapa married the thirteen daughters of Dakṣa. He begot by Aditi the twelve Adityas (the gods) and by Diti the Daityas (the demons). By his other wives he had diversified and numerous progeny such as serpents, reptiles, birds and nymphs of the lunar constellations. He was thus the father of Sūrya (the sun god) and all living beings and is often called Prajāpati (the Progenitor).

Technique

1. Stand in Tāḍāsana. (Plate 1.) Bend forward, rest the palms on the floor as in Uttānāsana (Plate 47) and take the legs back about 4 to 5 feet, in Adho Mukha Śvānāsana. (Plate 75)

2. Turn the whole body sideways to the right and balance on the right hand and foot. The outer side of the right foot should rest firmly on the floor. Place the left foot over the right foot, rest the left palm on the left hip and balance keeping the body straight. (Plate 396)

3. Exhale, bend the left knee and place the left foot at the root of the right thigh as in half Padmāsana. Swing the left arm from the shoulder behind the back and with the left hand catch the left big toe. This is the final position. (Plates 399 and 400.) Balance in it for some time with deep breathing. The entire chest and the extended right arm should be in one plane.

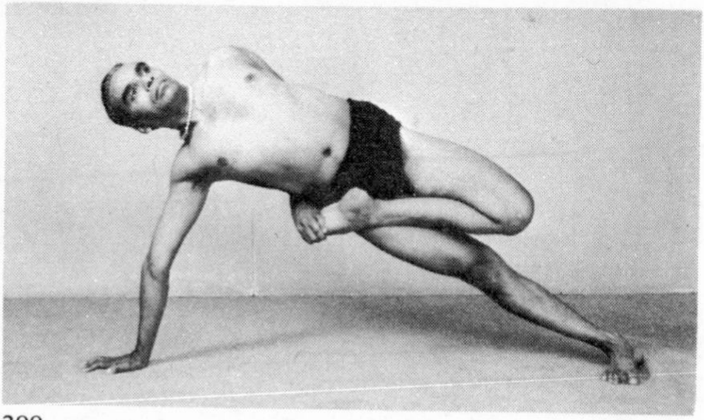

399

4. Exhale, release the left foot, place it again over the right one and put the left hand on the left thigh. (Plate 396.) Take a few deep breaths.

5. Exhale, turn the body over to the left so that it balances only on the left hand and foot. Place the right foot at the root of the left thigh in half Padmāsana and catch the right big toe from behind the back with the right hand. Balance on the both sides for an equal length of time.

6. Exhale, release the right foot and place it over the left foot and the right hand on the right thigh.

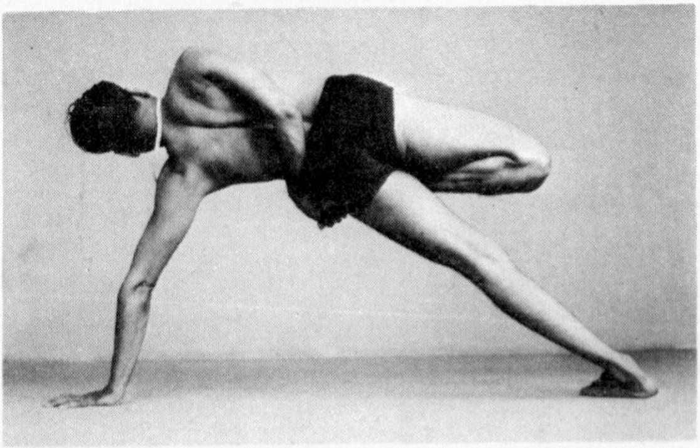

400

7. Rest the right palm on the floor and come back to Uttānāsana (Plate 47), take a few breaths and with an exhalation return to Tāḍāsana. (Plate 1)

Effects

This āsana strengthens the hands and relieves pain and stiffness in the sacral region of the spine.

151. *Viśvāmitrāsana* Twenty* (Plate 403)

Viśvāmitra was the name of a celebrated sage. He was originally a kṣatriya (a member of the warrior caste), being the king of Kanyākubja. One day while out hunting, he went to the hermitage of the sage Vasiṣṭha, and seeing there Kāmadhenu (the Cow of Plenty), offered the sage untold treasures in exchange for her. On being refused, the king tried to take her by force. A long contest ensued in which the king was defeated. Although sorely vexed, he was greatly impressed with the power inherent in Brahmanism. The king devoted himself to the most rigorous austerities until he successively achieved the status and titles of Rājarṣi (a royal sage, a saint-like prince), Riṣi (a sage or seer), Maharṣi (a great sage or patriarch of mankind) and finally Brahmarṣi (a Brahmanical sage), but he was not content until Vasiṣṭha himself called him Brahmarṣi. During his arduous penance, the heavenly nymph Menakā seduced him and conceived Śakuntalā, the heroine of Kalidasa's famous drama.

This āsana is dedicated to Viśvāmitra.

Technique

1. Stand in Tāḍāsana. (Plate 1.) Bend forward, rest the palms on the

floor and take the legs back about 4 to 5 feet, as in Adho Mukha Śvānāsana. (Plate 75)

2. Exhale, swing the right leg over the right hand and place the back of the right thigh on the back of the upper part of the right arm. (Plate 401)

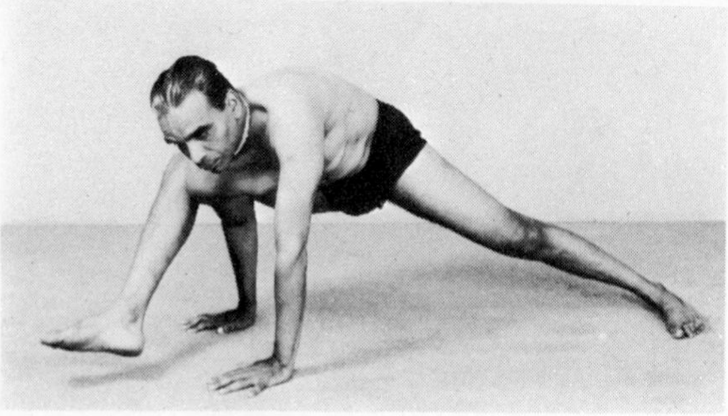

401

3. Immediately turn the body to the left, place the left arm along the left thigh and balance. (Plate 402)

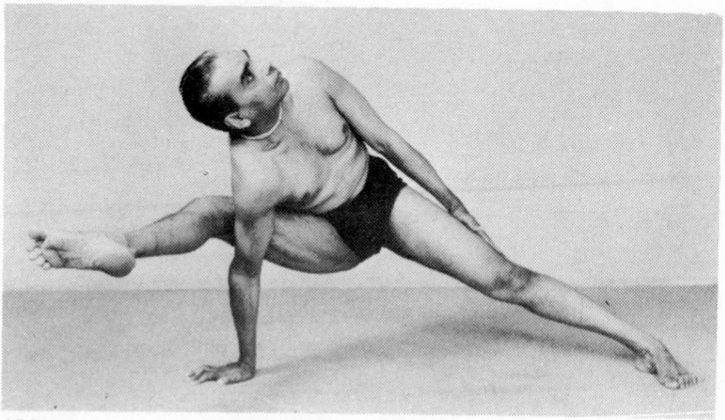

402

4. Turn the left foot sideways and press the sole and heel on the floor.

5. Stretch the right leg straight up and take two breaths.

6. Exhale, stretch the left arm up vertically from the shoulder and gaze at the outstretched left hand. (Plate 403)

7. Stay in the pose from 20 to 30 seconds with deep breathing.

8. Exhale, release the right leg and come back to position 1.

9. Repeat the pose for the same length of time on the other side, following the technique stated above, reading right for left and left for right.

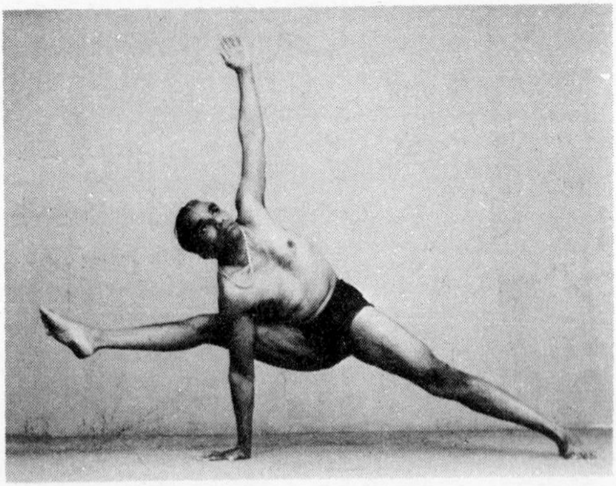

403

Effects

This pose strengthens the hands and the abdominal organs and exercises the thigh muscles.

152. *Bakāsana* Nine* (Plates 406 and 410)

Baka means a crane.
The body in this pose resembles that of a crane wading in a pool of water, hence the name.

The techniques here are given in two different ways, one for beginners and the other for advanced pupils.

Technique for beginners

1. Squat on the haunches with the feet together. The soles and heels should rest completely on the floor. Raise the seat from the floor and balance. (Plate 317)

2. Widen the knees and move the trunk forward.

3. Exhale, wrap the arms around the bent legs and rest the palms on the floor. (Plate 318)

4. Bend the elbows, raise the heels from the floor, move the trunk further forward and rest the shins on the back of the upper arms near the armpits. (Plate 404.) Take 2 or 3 breaths.

5. Exhale, swing the body forward and lift the toes off the floor. (Plate 405)

6. Stretch the arms straight and balance the entire body on the hands. (Plate 406)

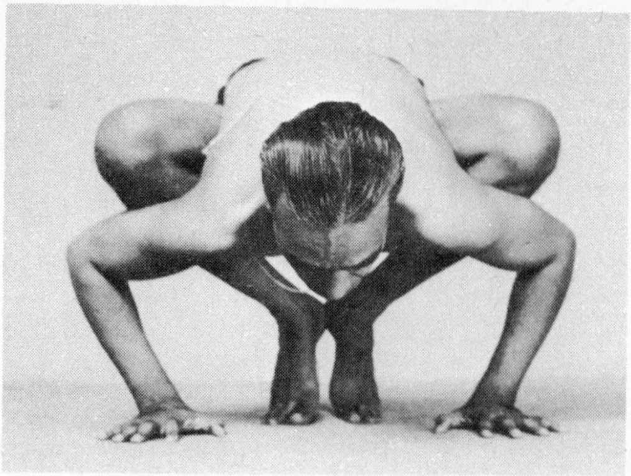

404

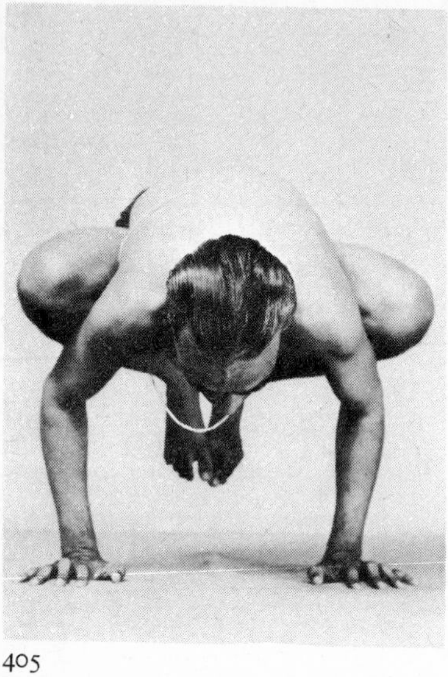

405

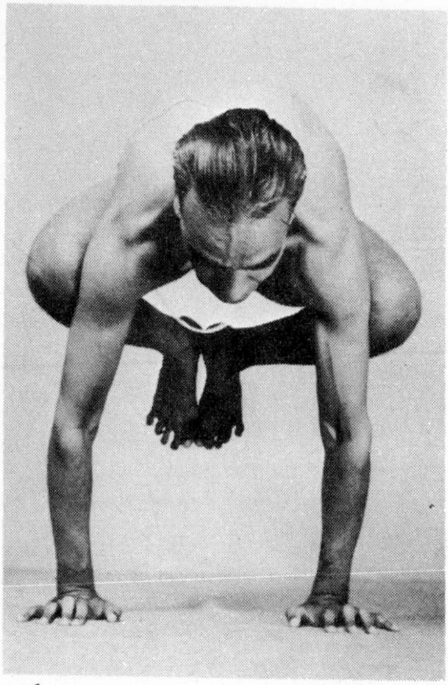

406

7. Stay in this position for 20 to 30 seconds with normal breathing.

8. Exhale, bend the elbows, lower the trunk, release the legs from the armpits, squat on the floor and relax.

Technique for advanced pupils

1. Perform Sālamba Śīrṣāsana II. (Plate 192)

2. Exhale, bend the knees and lower the legs so that the thighs touch the stomach and chest.

3. Place the right knee on the back of the upper right arm as near the armpit as possible, then the left knee similarly on the left arm. The feet should be kept together. (Plate 407.) Secure this position and balance with even breathing.

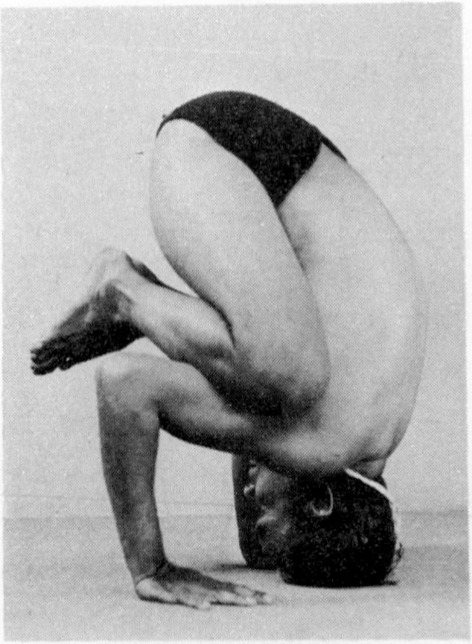

407

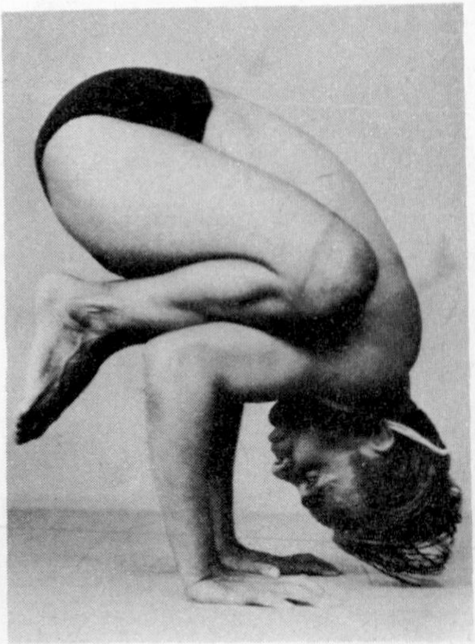

408

4. Exhale, pull the trunk up and raise the head off the floor. (Plate 408.) Stretch and straighten the arms and raise the buttocks. (Plate 409.) Extend the neck and keep the head as high as possible. (Plate 410)

5. Balance in this position on the hands for a few seconds by tightening the muscles in the region of the diaphragm. Try to breathe normally.

6. Exhale, rest the head on the floor and go back to Sālamba Śīrṣāsana II. Then lower the legs to the floor and rest. Advanced pupils may perform Ūrdhva Dhanurāsana (Plate 486) by dropping the legs back after going up in Śīrṣāsana II and then standing up straight in Tāḍāsana. (Plate 1.) After one has mastered Viparīta Chakrāsana (Plates 488 to 499) it is a soothing exercise after practising Ūrdhva Dhanurāsana.

Effects

This āsana strengthens the arms and abdominal organs since the latter are contracted.

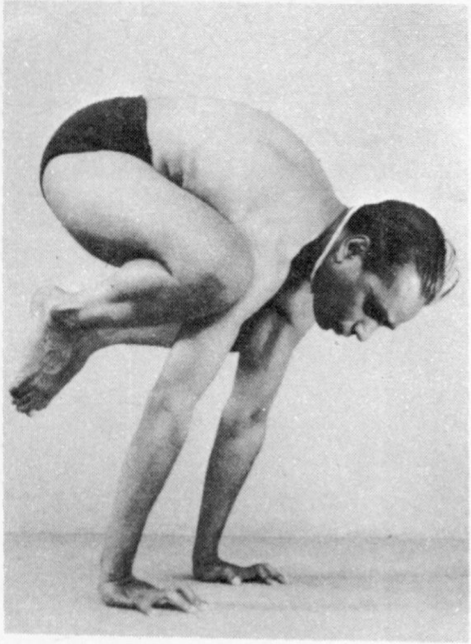

409

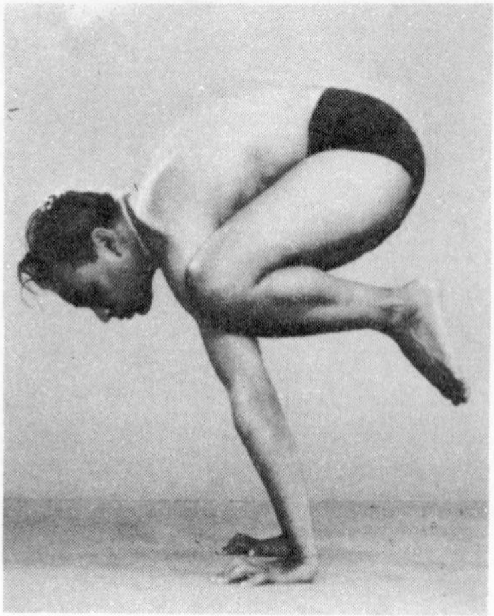

410

153. *Pārśva Bakāsana* Sixteen* (Plate 412)

Pārśva means side, flank or oblique, baka means a crane or a wading bird. Here the legs are in a lateral position.

Technique

1. Perform Sālamba Śīrṣāsana II. (Plate 192)

2. Exhale and bend the knees so that the thighs touch the stomach and chest.

3. Keep both thighs and feet together. Turn the bent legs and trunk obliquely to the right. Rest the left thigh on the back of the upper right arm as near the armpit as possible. (Plate 411.) Take a few deep breaths and balance.

4. Then with an exhalation lift the head from the floor, tighten the muscles near the diaphragm, straighten the arms and balance on the hands. (Plate 412.) Stay in this position for a few seconds with even breathing. Greater strain will be felt on the apparently free arm.

5. Bend the elbows, rest the head on the floor (Plate 411) and again go back to Sālamba Śīrṣāsana II.

6. Then bend the knees and turn the bent legs obliquely to the left.

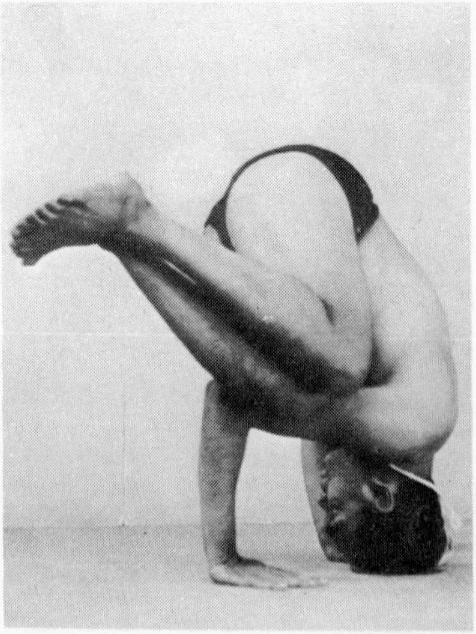

411

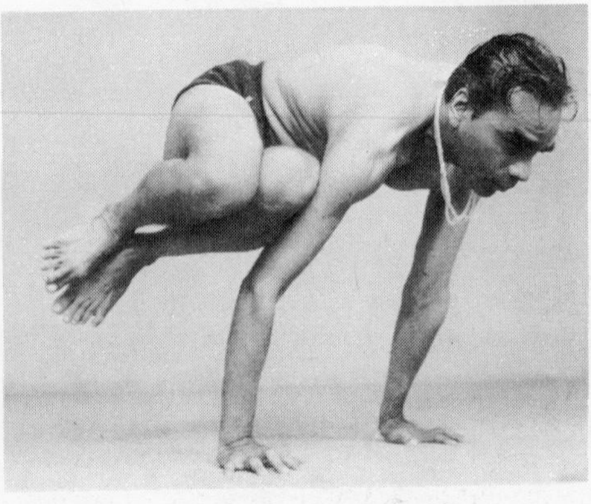

412

Rest the right thigh on the back of the upper left arm as near the armpit as possible. Exhale, lift the head off the floor and balance as in position 4.

7. Go back again to Sālamba Śīrṣāsana II after resting the head on the floor. Then either lower the legs to the floor and relax or move into Ūrdhva Dhanurāsana (Plate 486) and stand up in Tāḍāsana. (Plate 1.) When one has mastered Viparīta Chakrāsana (Plates 488 to 499), it is a soothing exercise after practising Ūrdhva Dhanurāsana.

Effects

This pose strengthens the arms. By continued practice the lateral muscles of the abdomen will develop and the intestines will grow stronger.

154. *Ūrdhva Kukkuṭāsana* Eighteen* (Plates 417, 418 and 419)

Ūrdhva means upwards. Kukkuṭa means a cock. In this posture the body resembles a strutting cock, hence the name.

Technique

1. Perform Sālamba Śīrṣāsana II. (Plate 192)

2. After securing steadiness, move into Padmāsana by placing the right foot at the root of the left thigh and the left foot at the root of the right thigh (Plate 413), then with an exhalation bend the legs and rest them on the back of the upper arms as near the armpits as possible. (Plate 414.) Secure this position and balance with even breathing.

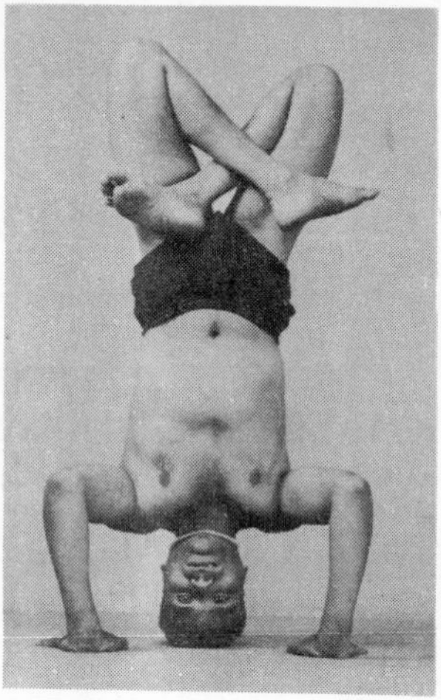

413

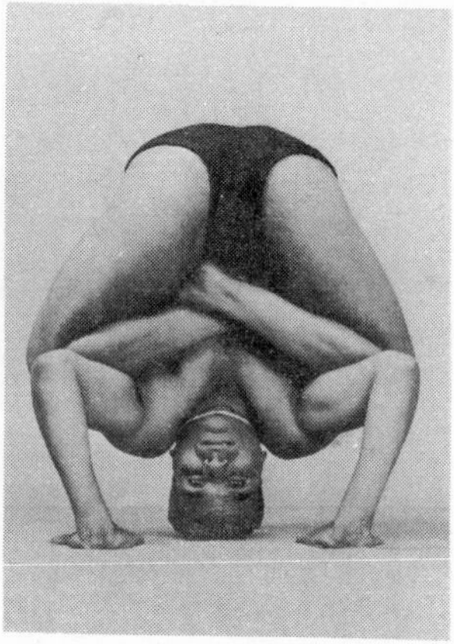

414

3. Exhale, press the palms firmly on the ground, pull the trunk up and raise the head off the floor following the stages of the movement as in Plates 415 and 416. Stretch and straighten the arms and lift up the buttocks. Extend the neck and keep the head as high as possible. (Plates 417, 418 and 419)

4. Balance in this position on the hands for a few seconds by tightening the muscles in the region of the diaphragm. Try to breathe normally.

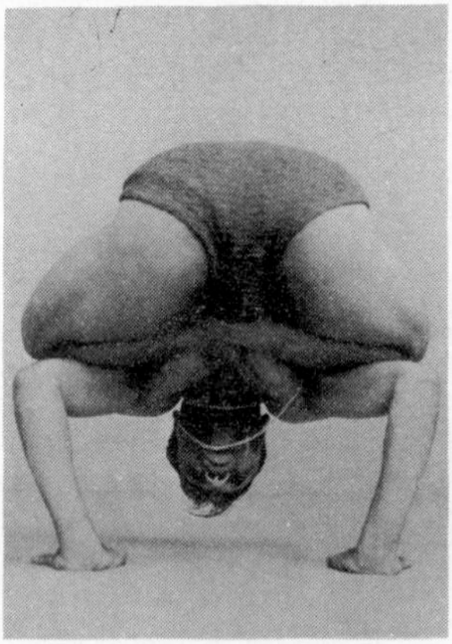

415

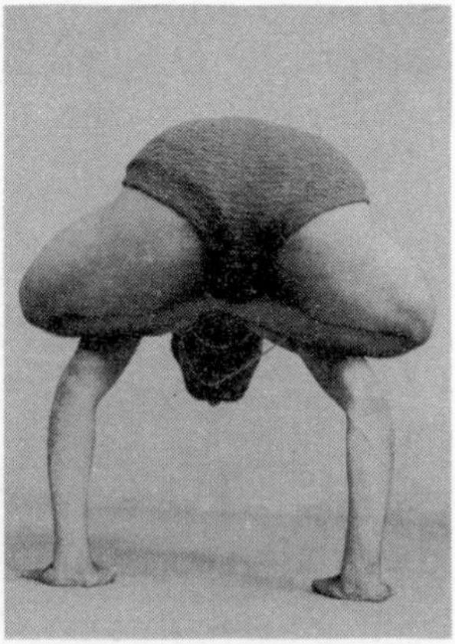

416

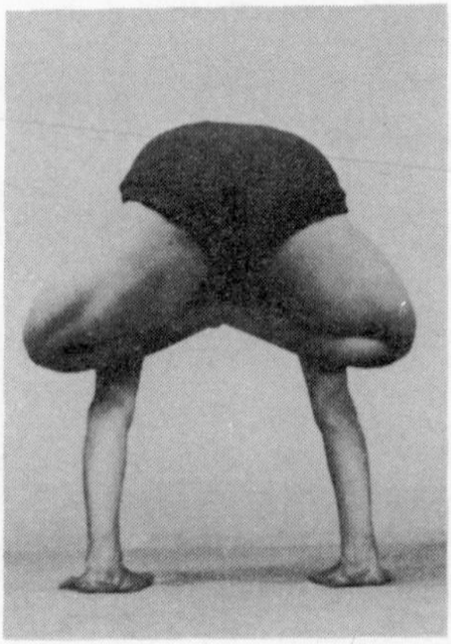

417

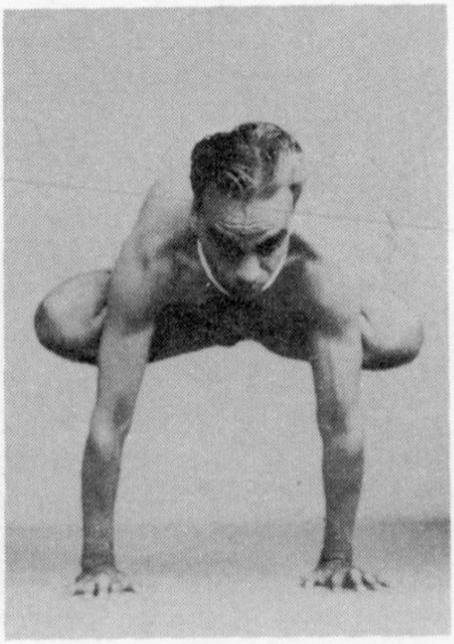

418

5. Exhale, bend the elbows, lower the head to the floor following Plates 414 and 413, and return to Sālamba Śīrṣāsana II by releasing the foot lock of Padmāsana.

6. Again perform Padmāsana, this time placing the left foot first at the root of the right thigh and the right foot at the root of the left thigh. Then repeat the āsana as stated above.

7. After staying for the same length of time on both the sides, go back to Sālamba Śīrṣāsana II, lower the legs to the floor and relax. Advanced

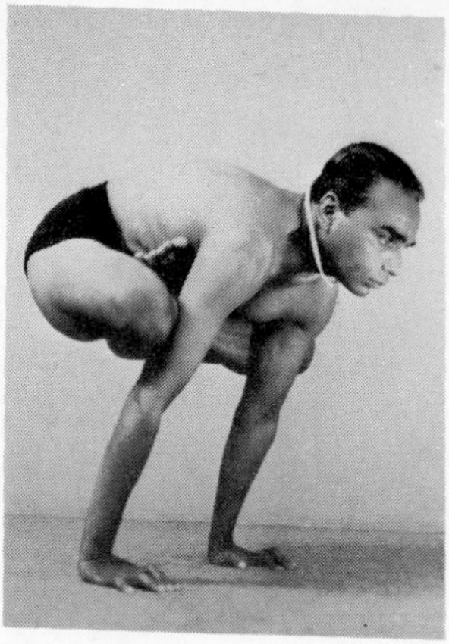

419

pupils may then move into Ūrdhva Dhanurāsana (Plate 486) by dropping the legs behind the back and extending the arms and then stand up in Tāḍāsana. (Plate 1.) When one has mastered Viparīta Chakrāsana (Plates 488 to 499), it is a soothing exercise after practising Ūrdhva Dhanurāsana.

Effects

The spine is stretched fully and the effect of Paschimottānāsana (Plate 160) is gained in a very short time. The arms and the abdominal organs will grow strong.

All these intricate and difficult positions bring results quicker than the simple ones. When the body becomes more pliable, the simple poses will have little or no effect. The wise therefore discard them and practise the intricate poses just as a scholar will not repeat the alphabet daily. But, just as dancers daily practise some basic steps and do not discard them, so also pupils of yoga should continue daily to perform Śīrṣāsana (Plates 184 to 218) and Sarvāngāsana with their cycles. (Plates 234 to 271)

155. *Pārśva Kukkuṭāsana* Twenty-four* (Plates 424 and 424a; 425 and 425a)

Pārśva means side, flank or oblique. Kukkuṭa means a cock.

Technique

1. Perform Sālamba Śīrṣāsana II. (Plate 192)

2. Move into Padmāsana by placing first the right foot on the root of

the left thigh and then the left foot at the root of the right thigh. (Plate 413.) After securing steadiness, exhale, turn the trunk to the right (Plate 420) and lower the legs so that the left thigh rests on the back of the upper right arm. (Plate 421.) Secure this position and balance for some time with even but fast breathing due to the lateral twist of the trunk.

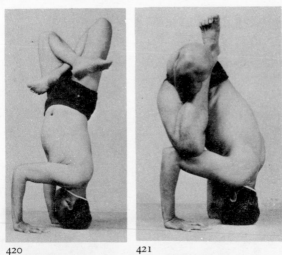

420

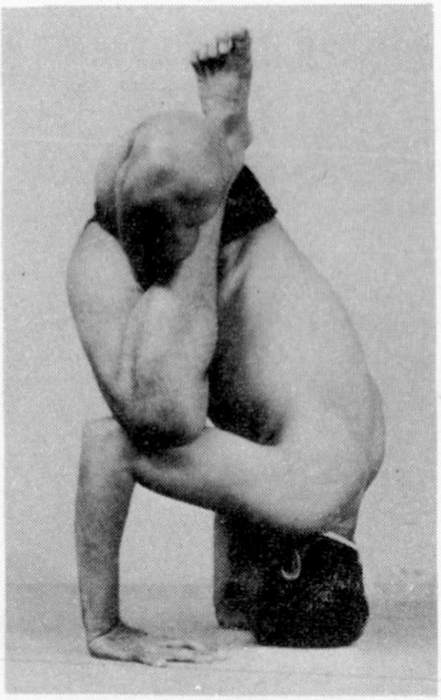

421

3. The pose is a difficult one, the hardest part being to place the thigh on the opposite hand. In the beginning one finds it difficult to balance while securing the proper placing of the thigh and one often sits down on the floor with a hard bump.

4. Exhale, press the hands firmly on the ground, raise the head from the floor (Plate 422) and pull the trunk. (Plate 423.) Stretch and straighten the arms and lift up the buttocks. Extend the neck forwards and hold the head up as high as possible. (Plate 424)

5. This is the final position. Balance the body on the hands for a few seconds as long as you can. Greater strain will be felt on the left arm which is apparently free.

6. Exhale, bend the elbows, lower the head to the floor and go up again to Śīrṣāsana II. Then release the foot lock of Padmāsana.

7. Rest for a while in Śīrṣāsana. Move into Padmāsana again, this time by placing first the left foot at the root of the right thigh and then the right foot at the root of the left thigh. Then repeat the pose on the left side. (Plate 425.) Here the right thigh will rest on the back

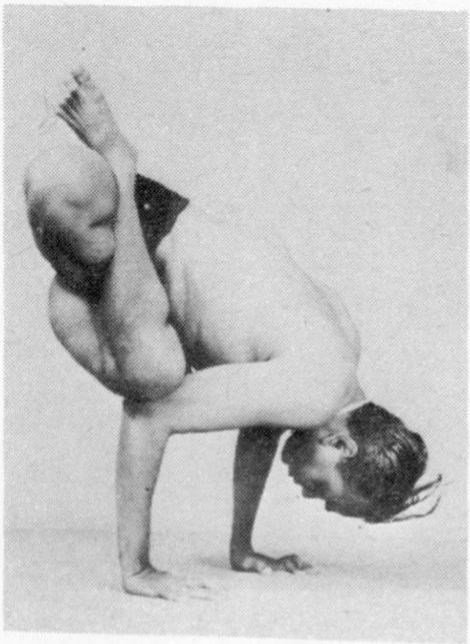

422

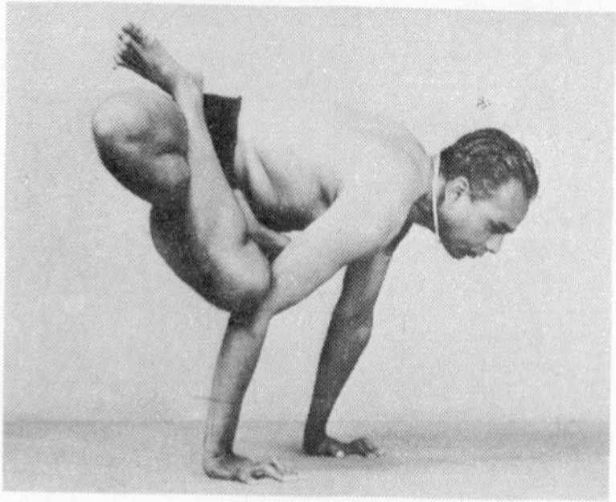

423

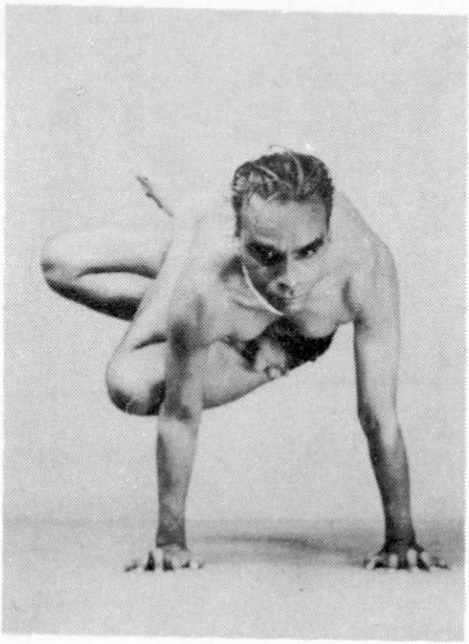

424

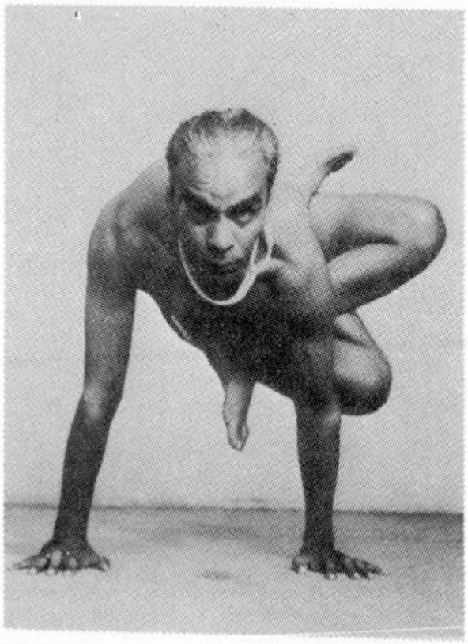

425

of the upper left arm. While balancing the body on the left side it is necessary to change the position of the legs in Padmāsana. If they are not changed, it is extremely difficult to rest the thigh on the back of the opposite upper arm.

8. Stay for the same length of time on both sides.

9. After perfecting the positions as explained above in paras 4 and 7 an attempt may be made, without releasing the foot lock in para. 6, to turn the body to the left, rest the right thigh on the upper left arm, raise the head from the floor and balance. (Plate 424a)

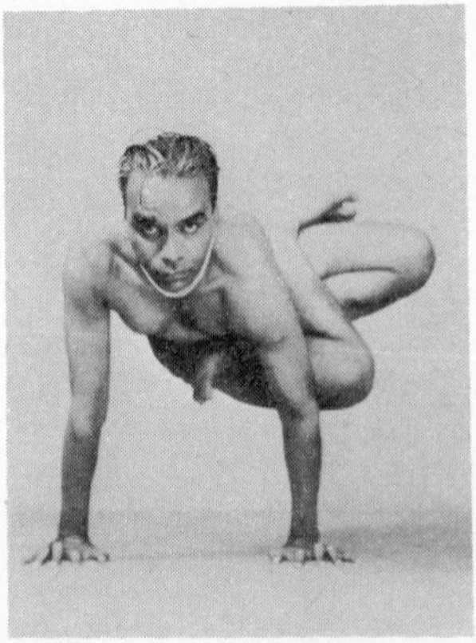

424a

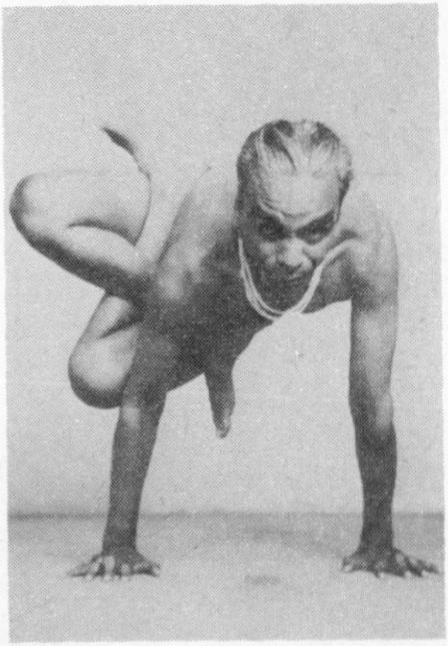

425a

10. Go back to Śīrṣāsana II. Then after completing the pose from para. 7 without changing the crossed leg by turning the body to the right, attempt to place the left thigh on the upper right arm, raise the head from the floor and balance. (Plate 425a)

11. Hold the pose for the same length of time on all occasions. Then go back to Śīrṣāsana II, lower the legs to the floor and relax. Or perform Ūrdhva Dhanurāsana (Plate 486) and then stand up in Tāḍāsana. (Plate 1.) When one has mastered Viparīta Chakrāsana (Plates 488 to 499) this is an exhilarating exercise after practising Ūrdhva Dhanurāsana.

Effects

In addition to the benefit one secures from Ūrdhva Kukkuṭāsana (Plate 419), in this variation the spine receives a lateral twist and is toned. The chest, arms and the abdominal muscles and organs become stronger and vital power increases.

156. *Gālavāsana* Sixteen* (Plates 427 and 428)

Gālava was a sage and one of Viśvāmitra's pupils. This āsana is dedicated to him.

Technique

1. Perform Sālamba Śīrṣāsana II. (Plate 192)

2. Then move into Padmāsana (by placing the right foot at the root of the left thigh, and the left foot at the root of the right thigh, Plate

413), exhale and bend the trunk so that the thighs touch the stomach and chest.

3. Take a few breaths, turn the trunk to the right and with an exhalation lower the folded legs to where the shins cross on the back of the right upper arm as near the armpit as possible. (Plate 426.) Secure the position, take a few deep breaths and balance.

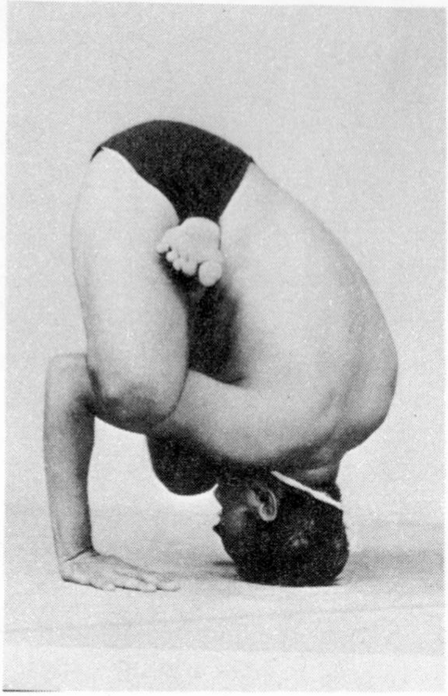

426

4. Exhale, pull the body up by raising the head from the floor, tighten the muscles near the diaphragm, straighten the arms, balance on the hands (Plate 427) and stay in this position for a few seconds up to your capacity. In this pose greater strain will be felt on the left shoulder and arm, which are apparently free.

5. Bend the elbows, rest the head on the floor and again go up to Sālamba Śīrṣāsana II without releasing the foot lock of Padmāsana.

6. Exhale, bend the trunk, rest the legs on the back of the upper left arm and balance as you did on the right. (Plate 428)

7. Bend the elbows, rest the head on the floor and go up to Sālamba Śīrṣāsana II and release the foot lock. Do Padmāsana again, this time first placing the left foot at the root of the right thigh and the right

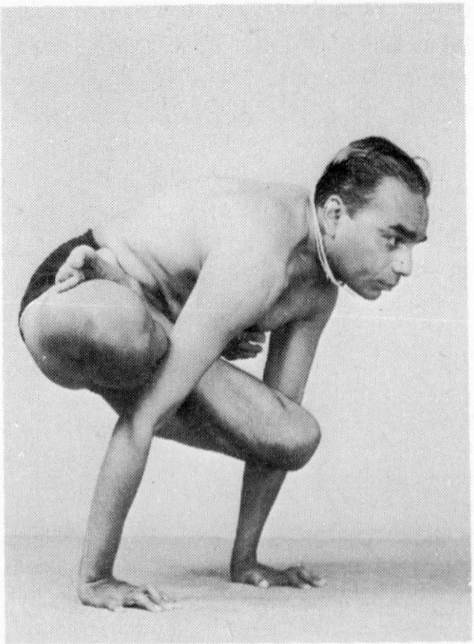

427

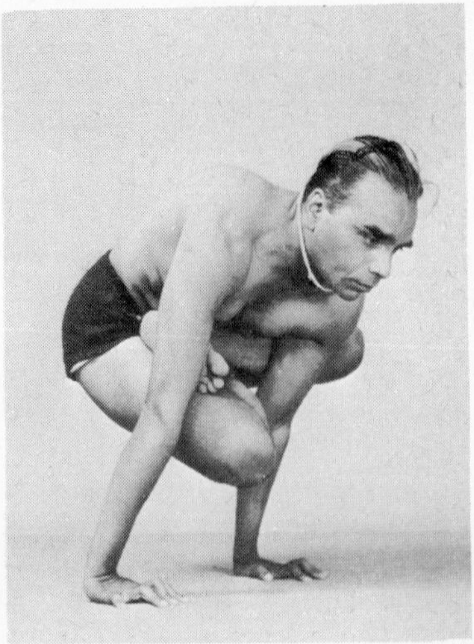

428

foot at the root of the left thigh and repeat the āsana as described above.

8. Do Sālamba Śīrṣāsana II again after resting the head on the floor. Then either lower the legs to the floor and relax or do Ūrdhva Dhanurāsana (Plate 486) and stand up in Tāḍāsana. (Plate 1.) When one has mastered Viparīta Chakrāsana (Plates 488 to 499), this exercise is soothing after practising Ūrdhva Dhanurāsana.

Effects

By continued practice of this pose, the wrists and the abdominal organs will grow stronger and the lateral muscles of the abdomen will also develop. The spine will become more elastic and the neck and shoulders will grow powerful. This pose has the combined effects of Śīrṣāsana (Plate 184), Padmāsana (Plate 104) and Paschimottānāsana (Plate 160)

157. *Eka Pāda Gālavāsana* Twenty-one* (Plates 431 and 433)

Eka means one. Pāda means a leg. Gālava is the name of a sage.

Technique

1. Perform Sālamba Śīrṣāsana II. (Plate 192)

2. Exhale, place the right foot at the root of the left thigh in half Padmāsana and bend the trunk till the legs are parallel to the floor.

3. Then bend the left leg at the knee. Take a few deep breaths. Exhale and rest the right foot on the back of the upper left arm. While placing the foot, turn it so that the toes point in the same direction as the fingers. Rest the right knee on the back of the upper right arm. (Plate 429)

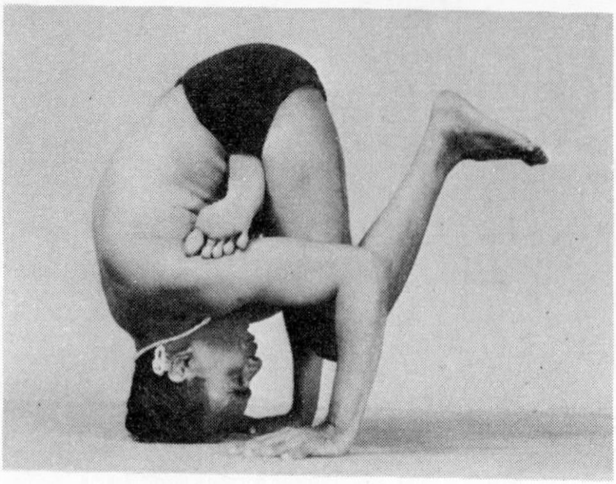

429

4. Secure the position of the right leg and take a few breaths. Stretch the left leg straight and keep it parallel to the floor. (Plate 430)

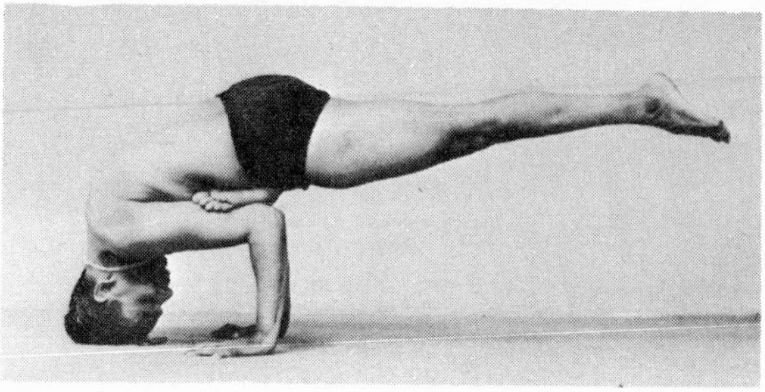

430

5. Exhale and lift the body up by raising the head off the floor. The left leg remains straight and parallel to the floor. The elbows remain bent, the upper arms stay parallel to the floor and the forearms from the wrists to the elbows remain perpendicular to it. (Plate 431)

6. Extend the neck and keep the head as high as possible. Stay in this position for a few seconds. Since the diaphragm is being pressed, breathing will be fast and laboured.

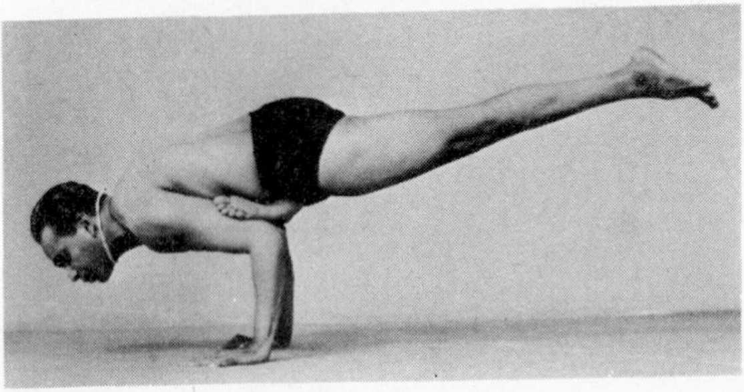

431

7. Bend the left leg at the knee, rest the head on the floor and again go up to Sālamba Śīrṣāsana II.

8. Take a few deep breaths and repeat the āsana, this time bending the left leg to half Padmāsana, placing the left foot on the back portion of the upper right arm and the left knee on the back portion of the left upper arm and raise the head off the floor. (Plates 432 and 433.) Stay for the same length of time on both sides. Return to Śīrṣāsana again.

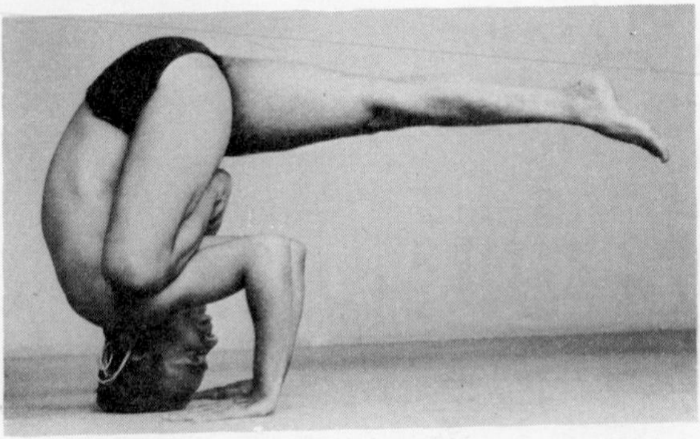

432

9. One can finish the pose by either lowering the legs to the floor or by moving into Ūrdhva Dhanurāsana (Plate 486) and then standing up in Tāḍāsana. (Plate 1.) When one has mastered Viparīta Chakrāsana (Plates 488 to 499), this exercise is exhilarating after practising Ūrdhva Dhanurāsana.

Effects

This pose strengthens the wrists. The abdominal organs are massaged by the pressure of the foot against the abdomen.

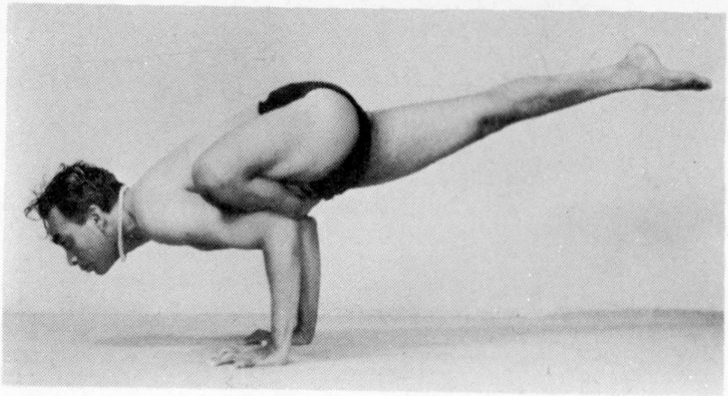

433

158. *Dwi Pāda Kouṇḍinyāsana* Twenty-two* (Plate 458)

Dwi Pāda (dwi = two or both; pāda = leg or foot) means both feet.

Kouṇḍinya was a sage belonging to the family of Vasiṣṭha and founded the Kouṇḍinya Gotra (sect). This āsana is dedicated to him.

Technique

1. Perform Sālamba Śīrṣāsana II. (Plate 192)

2. Exhale and lower the legs straight together until they are parallel to the floor. (Plate 434.) Pause here and take a few breaths.

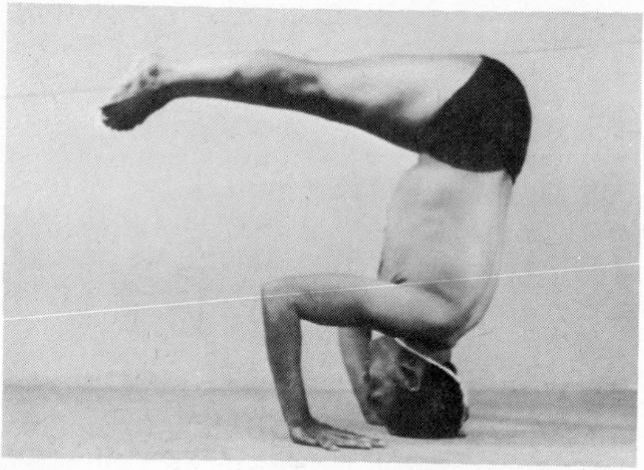

434

3. Exhale, turn the trunk slightly to the right and move both legs sideways to the right. (Plate 435.) Lower both legs together over the right arm so that the outer side of the left thigh above the knee rests on the back of the upper right arm as near the armpit as possible. (Plate 436)

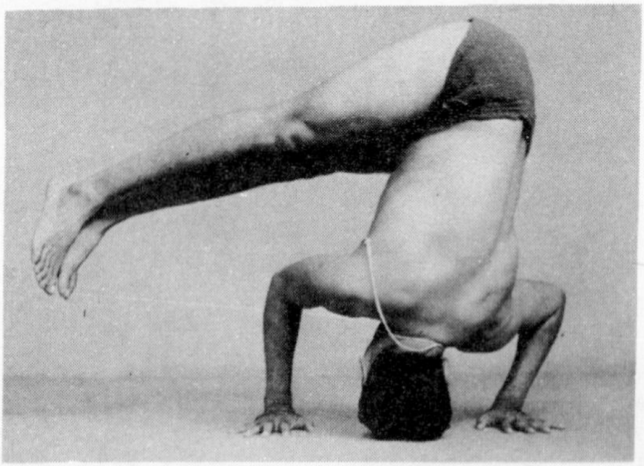
435

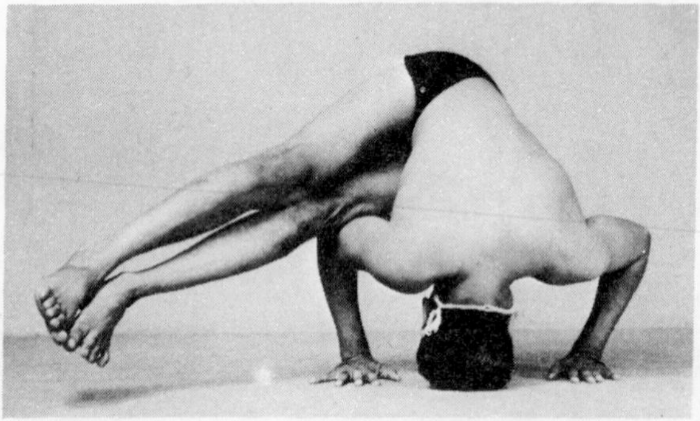
436

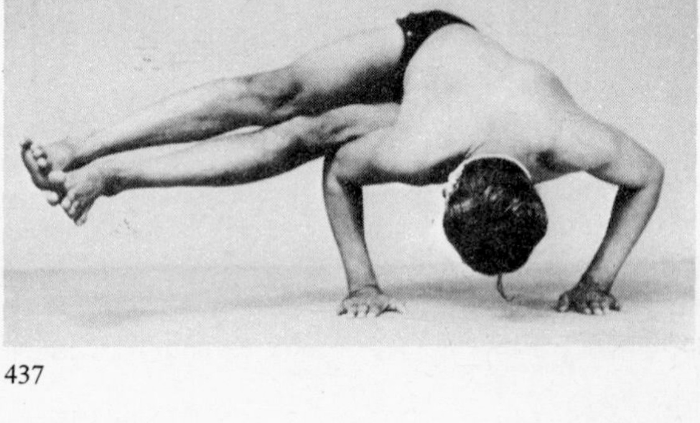
437

4. Balance and take a few breaths. Then exhale and firmly pressing down both palms to the floor, lift the head off the floor. (Plate 437.) Then raise the trunk and stretch the neck. (Plate 438.) This is the final position in which the legs will be in the air almost parallel to the floor, while due to the twist of the trunk, breathing will be fast. Balance as long as you can from 10 to 20 seconds. Greater pressure will be felt on the left shoulder and arm which are apparently free.

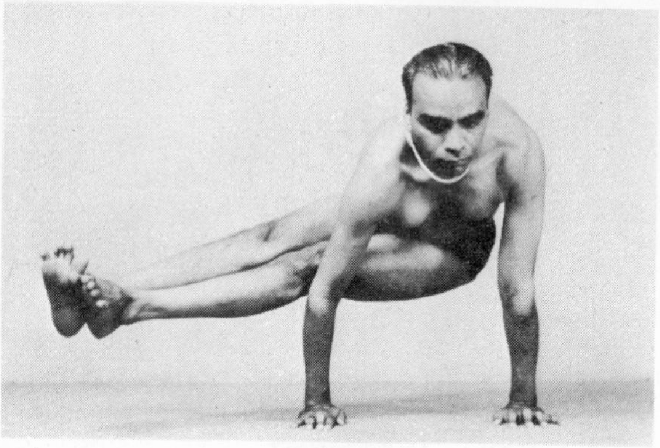

438

5. Bend the knees, rest the head on the floor and again go up to Sālamba Śīrṣāsana II. Rest here for a while and repeat the āsana on the left side as described above, reading left for right and vice versa. Here the right thigh will rest on the back of the upper left arm. Stay for the same length of time on both sides. Go up to Śīrṣāsana again.

6. To complete the pose, either lower the legs to the floor and relax or do Ūrdhva Dhanurāsana (Plate 486) and stand up in Tāḍāsana. (Plate 1.) When one has mastered Viparīta Chakrāsana (Plates 488 to 499), this exercise is exhilarating after Ūrdhva Dhanurāsana.

Effects

The pose tones the abdominal organs. The colon moves properly and toxins therein are eliminated. It requires experience to balance with the legs well stretched. The spine will become more elastic due to the lateral movement and the neck and arms will become more powerful.

159. *Eka Pāda Kouṇḍinyāsana I* Twenty-three* (Plate 441)

Eka means one. Pāda means a leg or foot. Kouṇḍinya is the name of a sage.

Technique

1. Perform Sālamba Śīrṣāsana II. (Plate 192)

2. Exhale, lower the legs straight together until they are parallel to the floor. (Plate 434.) Pause here and take a few breaths.

3. Exhale, bend the legs and move the left leg sideways to the right. Place the left leg over the back of the upper right arm so that the outer side of the left thigh above the knee rests as near the right armpit as possible. (Plate 439.) Take a few breaths and balance.

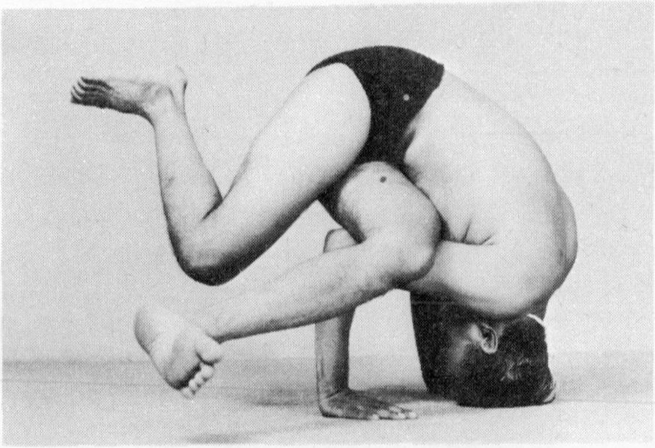

439

4. Stretch the left leg straight sideways and the right leg straight back. (Plate 440.) Take two breaths.

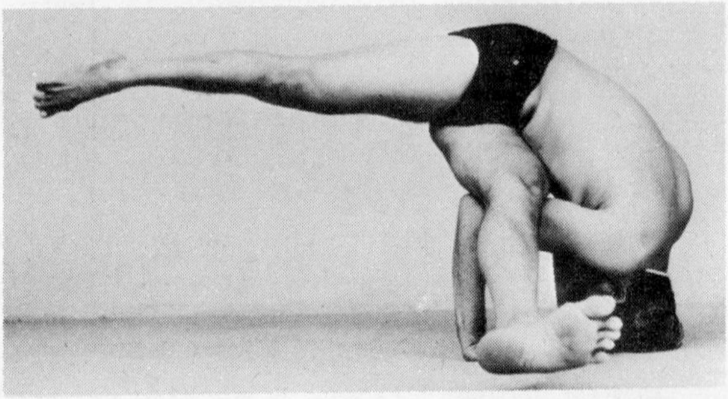

440

5. Exhale, raise the head above the floor, extend the arms and balance on the hands. Keep both legs straight and taut at the knees. (Plate 441.)

This is the final position. Remain in the pose as long as you can up to 30 seconds with normal breathing.

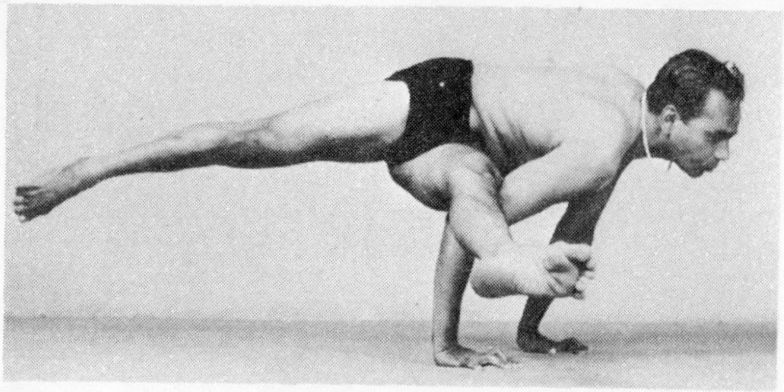

441

6. Bend both knees, exhale, rest the head on the floor and again go up to Śīrṣāsana. Rest here for some time with normal breathing.

7. Repeat the āsana on the other side for the same length of time as above, reading left for right and vice versa. Here the right thigh will rest on the back of the upper left arm and the left leg will be stretched straight back. Then again go up to Śīrṣāsana as stated in position 6.

8. To complete the pose, either lower the legs to the floor and relax, or do Ūrdhva Dhanurāsana (Plate 486) and stand up in Tāḍāsana. (Plate 1.) When one has mastered Viparīta Chakrāsana (Plates 488 to 499), this exercise is exhilarating after Ūrdhva Dhanurāsana.

Effects

The pressure of the legs on the abdomen in this pose massages the abdominal organs. The spinal twist rejuvenates and strengthens the spine. The arms and neck grow powerful.

160. *Eka Pāda Kouṇḍinyāsana II* Twenty-four* (Plates 442 and 443)

Technique

1. Perform Viśvāmitrāsana (Plate 403) with the right leg over the back of the upper right arm.

2. Exhale, place the left palm on the floor. Move the head and trunk towards the floor. Bend both the elbows, keep the body parallel to the floor, stretch both the legs straight and keep the toes off the floor. Balance the body on the hands as long as you can. The left leg will be stretched straight back while the right leg is stretched on the right side. The inner side of the right thigh rests on the back of the right upper arm. (Plates 442 and 443)

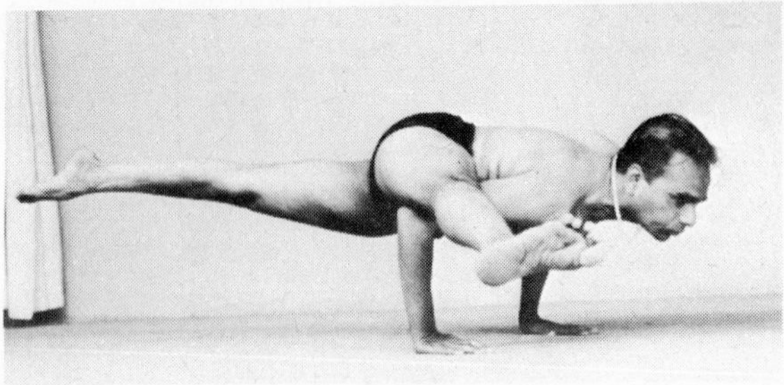

442

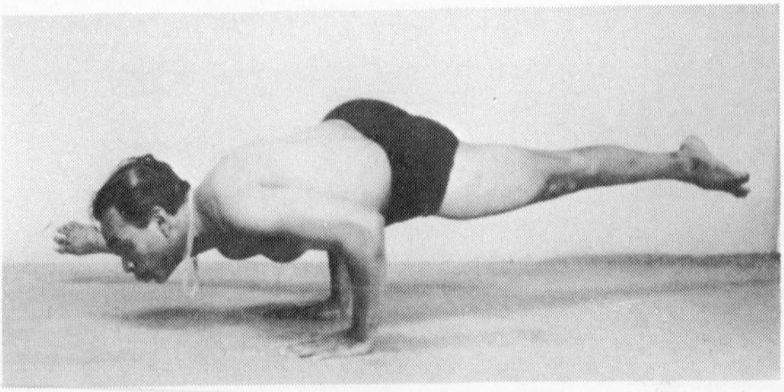

443

3. The pose is very strenuous and requires persistent effort to master. Breathing will be fast and hard. Stretch the neck and keep the head up.

4. Lower the left leg to the floor, remove the right leg from the right arm and relax for some time.

5. Repeat the pose on the other side, this time keeping the left leg on the back of the upper left arm and the right leg straight behind. Stay for the same length of time on both sides.

6. Advanced pupils may do the pose from Sālamba Śīrṣāsana II (Plate 192) by following the technique of Eka Pāda Kouṇḍinyāsana I (Plate 441), but placing one leg on the back of the upper arm of the same side as in Plate 444 and then lifting the head off the floor, keeping both legs straight and parallel to the floor.

7. Repeat the pose on the other side and then go back to Śīrṣāsana II (Plate 192), perform Ūrdhva Dhanurāsana (Plate 486) and stand in Tāḍāsana (Plate 1) or perform Viparīta Chakrāsana. (Plates 488 to 499)

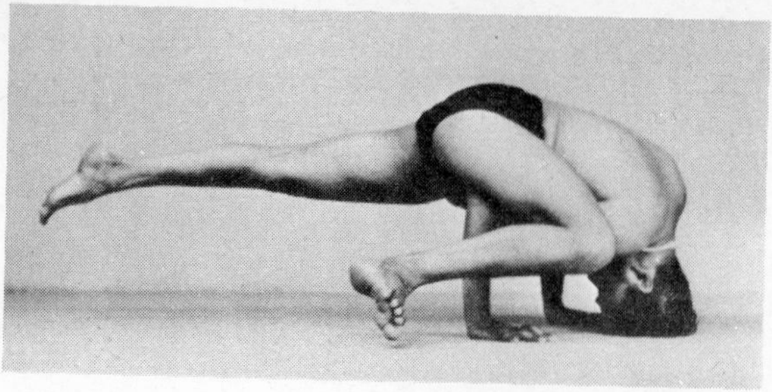

444

Effects

The pose strengthens the arms and abdominal organs and the thigh muscles.

161. *Eka Pāda Bakāsana I* Twenty-six* (Plates 446 and 447)

Eka means one. Pāda means leg or foot. Baka means a crane.

Technique

1. Perform Sālamba Śīrṣāsana II. (Plate 192)

2. Exhale, lower both legs until they are parallel to the floor. (Plate 434.) Bend the right knee and place the right shin on the back of the upper right arm as near the armpit as possible. Keep the left leg in the air parallel to the floor. (Plate 445.) Secure this position and balance with even breathing.

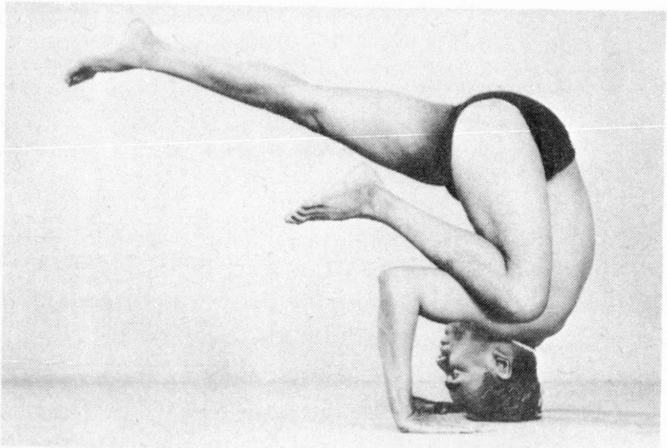

445

3. Exhale, pull the trunk up, raise the head off the floor and stretch the neck forward. Try to keep the body parallel to the floor and do not rest any part of it on the left elbow. (Plates 446 and 447)

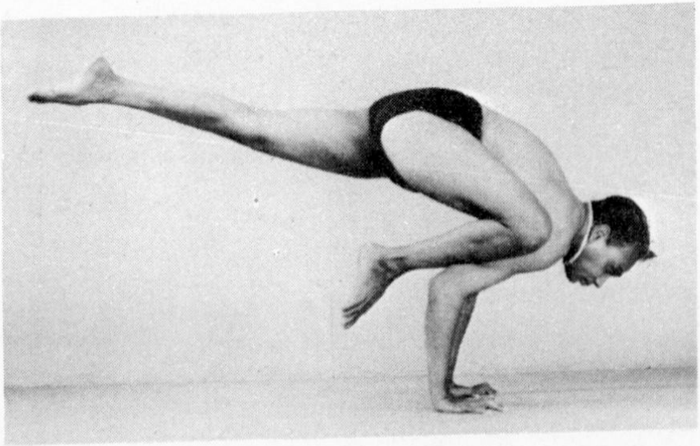

446

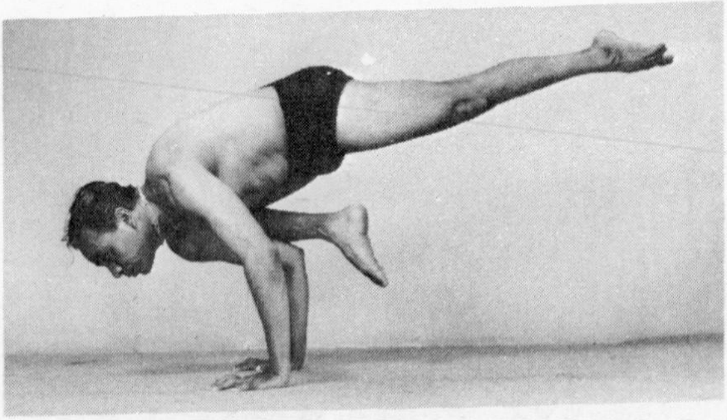

447

4. Stay in this position for 10 to 20 seconds with full extension of the spine and of the stretched left leg. Try to breathe normally. This is a difficult balancing pose.

5. Bend the left leg and rest the head on the floor. Exhale, and return to Sālamba Śīrṣāsana II.

6. Repeat the āsana on the left side for the same length of time, keeping the right leg stretched straight in the air parallel to the floor.

7. Go back to Sālamba Śīrṣāsana II, lower the legs to the floor and rest. Advanced pupils may perform Ūrdhva Dhanurāsana (Plate 486) and stand up in Tāḍāsana. (Plate 1.) When one has mastered Viparīta

Chakrāsana (Plates 488 to 499), this exercise is exhilarating after Ūrdhva Dhanurāsana.

Effects

In this pose, the organs or the abdomen are contracted on one side and stretched on the other. To balance in this pose the abdominal muscles and organs are exercised more than the arms.

162. *Eka Pāda Bakāsana II* Twenty-five* (Plates 451 and 452)

Technique

1. Perform Sālamba Śīrṣāsana II. (Plate 192)

2. Exhale, lower the legs until they are parallel to the floor. (Plate 434.) Bend the left knee and rest the left shin on the back of the upper left arm as near the armpit as possible as in Bakāsana. (Plate 410.) Move the right leg to the right until it extends beyond the right arm, so that the inner side of the right thigh touches the back of the upper right arm. (Plate 448)

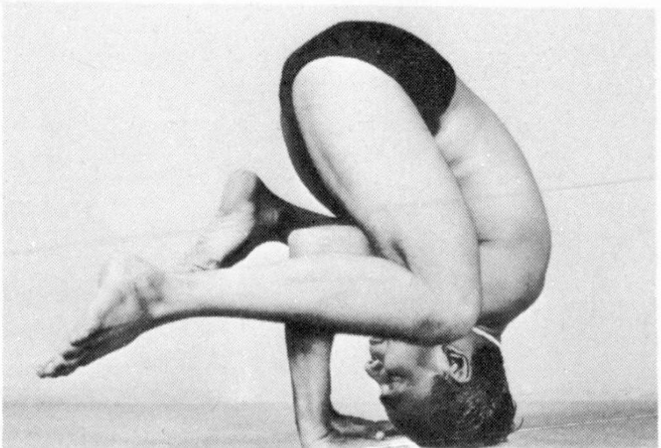

448

3. Exhale, pull the trunk up, raise the head off the floor and extend the neck forward. (Plates 449 and 450.) Now bring the right leg in front and stretch it straight without touching the floor. Stretch the arms straight and balance. (Plate 451)

4. Stay in this position for 10 to 20 seconds, with full extension of the spine and the right leg. Try to breathe normally.

5. Bend the right knee, place the head on the floor and go to Sālamba Śīrṣāsana II. (Plate 192)

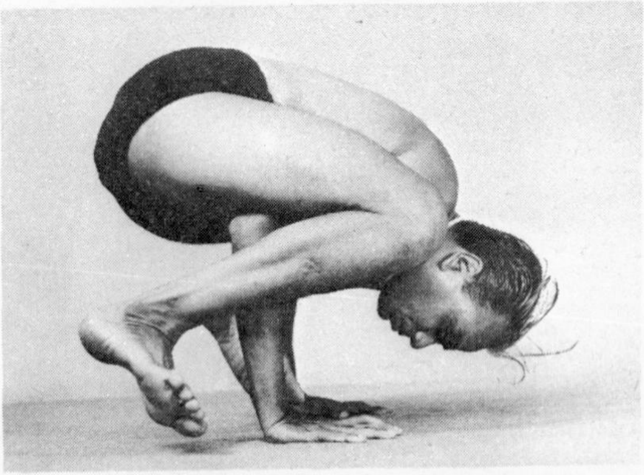

449

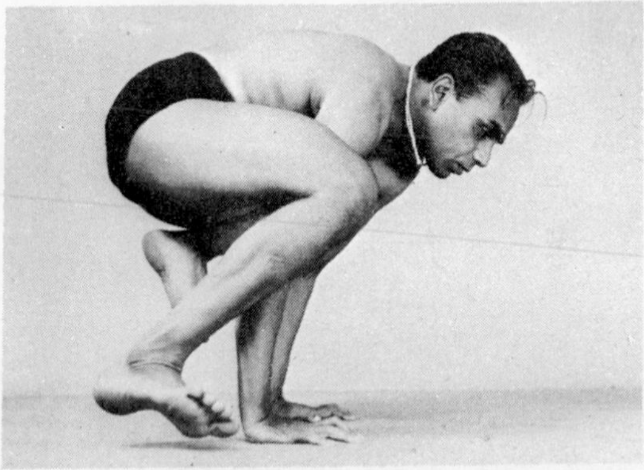

450

6. Repeat the āsana on the other side for the same length of time, keeping the left leg stretched straight in front and the bent right leg back of the upper right arm. (Plate 452)

7. There are two ways of completing the pose. You can bend the leg stretched straight in front, then go up to Śīrṣāsana and lower the legs. Once you have mastered this method you may try the other one. Here you keep the leg stretched straight in front. Then you bend the elbows, stretch the bent leg back and keep it straight and parallel to, without touching, the floor. Keep the whole body and the head off the floor. You will now be in Eka Pāda Kouṇḍinyāsana II. (Plates 442 and 443.) Then exhale, rest the head on the floor, bend both legs and go up to Śīrṣāsana II. Then move into Ūrdhva Dhanurāsana (Plate 486) followed by Viparīta Chakrāsana. (Plates 488 to 499)

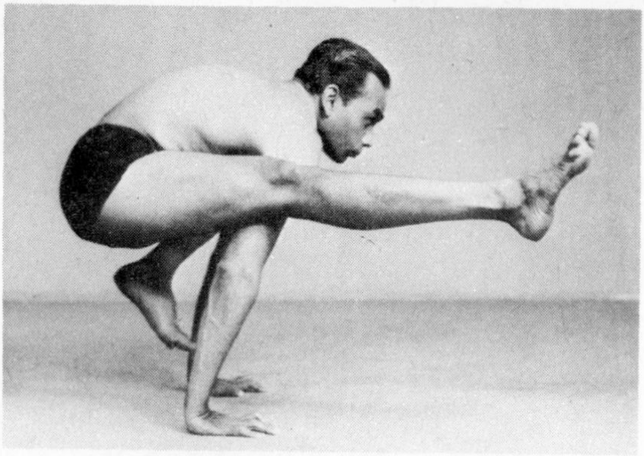

451

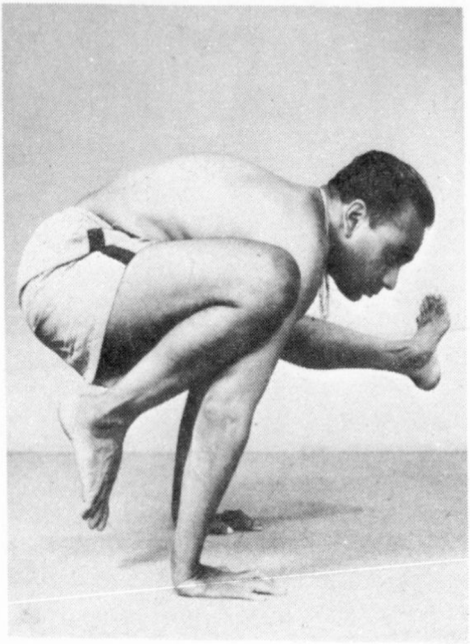

452

Effects

The abdominal organs and muscles as well as the hands, chest and back become stronger. Here our own body acts as a weight-lifting apparatus and the different directions in which it moves cause the various parts of the body to bear the weight and thereby gain strength.

163. *Yogadaṇḍāsana* Nineteen* (Plate 456)

Yogadaṇḍa means the staff of a Yogin. In this pose, the yogi sits using one leg as a crutch under the armpit, hence the name.

Technique

1. Sit on the floor with the legs stretched straight in front. (Plate 77)

2. Bend the right leg at the knee and bring the right foot beside the right hip. The right leg will now be in Vīrāsana. (Plate 86)

3. Take the left leg to the left to widen the distance between the thighs and bend it at the knee so that the left foot is near the right knee. (Plate 453)

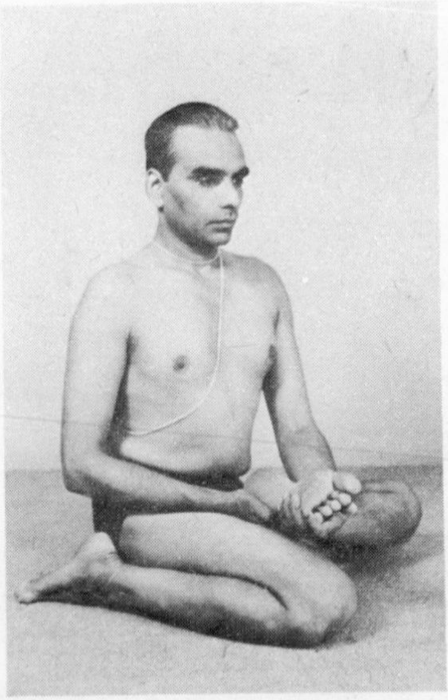

453

4. With the right hand catch the left foot. Turn the trunk to the right and with an exhalation, turn the left foot up towards the chest, keeping the left knee on the floor. Take a few breaths and with an exhalation, draw the left foot up underneath the left armpit. The left foot now rests like a crutch under the left armpit which the sole touches. (Plate 454)

5. After taking a few breaths, exhale, move the left arm from the shoulder round the left foot and bring it behind the back. (Plate 455.) Move the right arm from the shoulder behind the back and clasp the left forearm, turn the head to the left, raise the chin and gaze up. (Plate 456)

6. Stay in the pose for about 30 seconds with deep breathing.

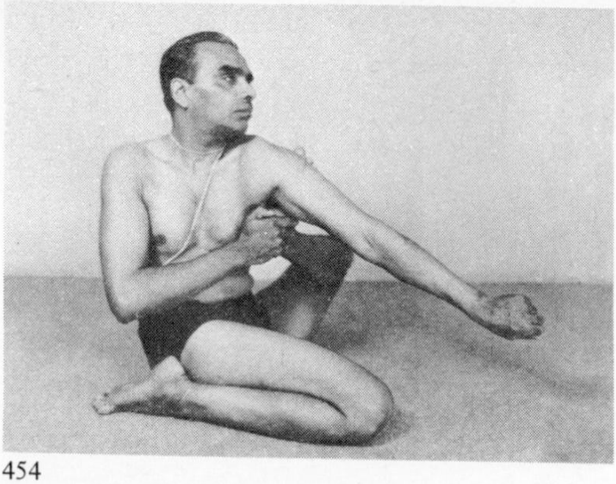

454

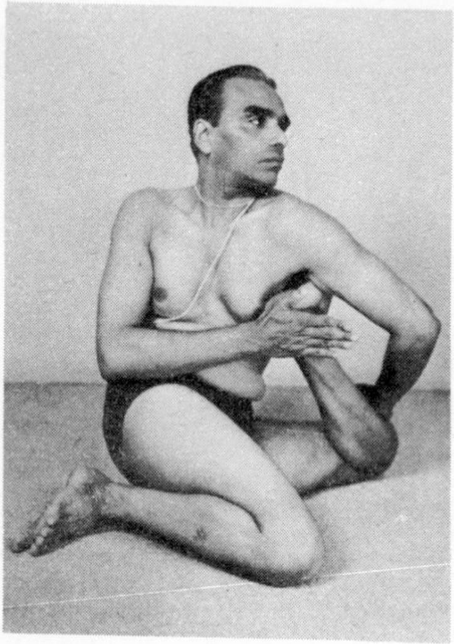

455

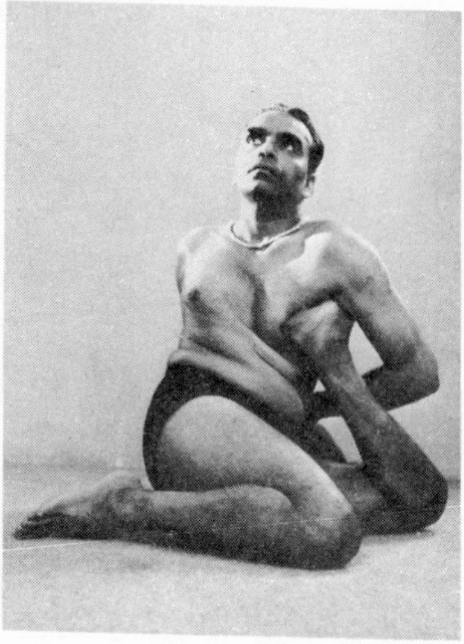

456

7. Release the hands, straighten the legs and relax.

8. Repeat the pose on the other side for the same length of time. Now, bend the left leg so that the left foot is besides the left hip and the right foot rests under the right armpit like a crutch and clasp the right forearm behind the back with the left hand.

9. It takes time and practice to be comfortable in the āsana, but when you are it is restful.

Effects

In this pose, the spine is rested and the body relaxed. It also makes the knees and ankles more elastic in movement.

164. *Supta Bhekāsana* Twenty-one* (Plate 458)

Supta means reclining. Bheka means a frog. This pose is the reverse posture of Bhekāsana. (Plate 100)

Technique

1. Sit in Vīrāsana. (Plate 86)

2. Turn the palms up and insert each hand under the respective foot. Push the feet up from the floor and recline. Take a few breaths.

3. Exhale, lift the hips off the floor (Plate 457), pull the thighs up and arch the trunk, resting the crown of the head on the floor. (Plate 458)

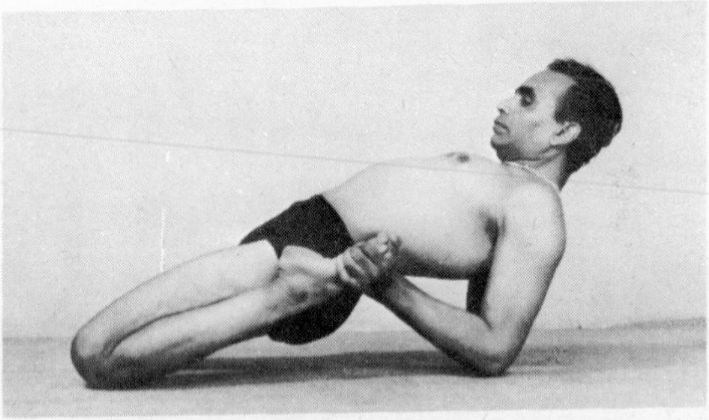

457

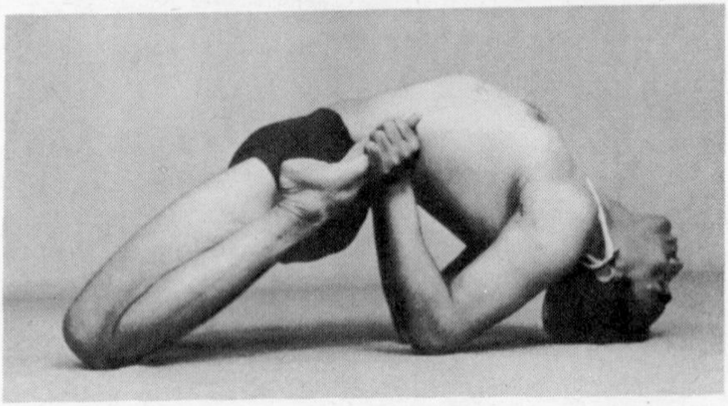

458

4. The body rests on the crown of the head, the elbows and knees. The forearms will be perpendicular to the floor and the hands will hold the outer side of the feet near the little toes. Try and raise the toes level with the hip joints.

5. Stay in the pose from 20 to 30 seconds, with normal breathing.

6. Lift the head from the floor and the hands from the feet so that the legs drop to Supta Vīrāsana. (Plate 96)

7. Sit up in Vīrāsana, straighten the legs and relax.

Effects

This āsana tones the spine. In it blood circulates well round the knees, ankles, hips and neck, and backache is relieved. It relieves any internal derangement of the knee joints. The pressure of the hands on the feet strengthens the arches and cures flat feet. Atrophy and other defects of the leg muscles are cured by its continued practice. The lungs are fully expanded and the abdominal organs benefit.

165. *Mūlabandhāsana* Thirty-two* (Plates 462 and 463)

Mūla means the root, the base, the beginning or the foundation. Bandha means a fetter, bond, or posture.

Technique

1. Sit in Baddhakoṇāsana. (Plate 101)

2. Insert the hands between the thighs and the calves and hold the feet, each with its respective hand.

3. Join the soles and heels. Raise the heels, keep the toes on the ground and drag the feet near the perineum. (Plate 459)

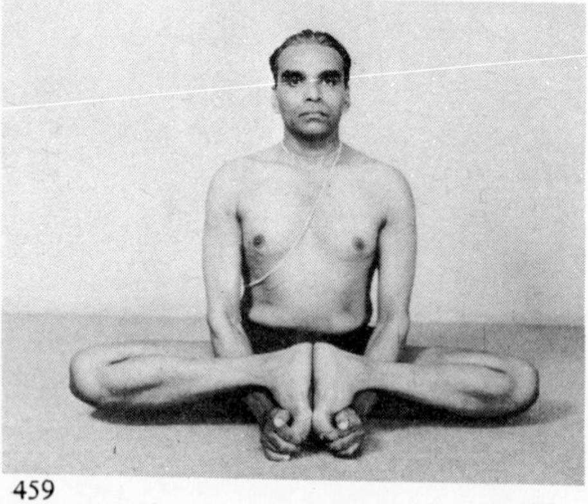

459

4. Hold this position and move the hands, so that the palms rest on the back of the hips. (Plate 460)

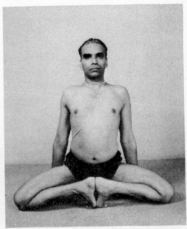

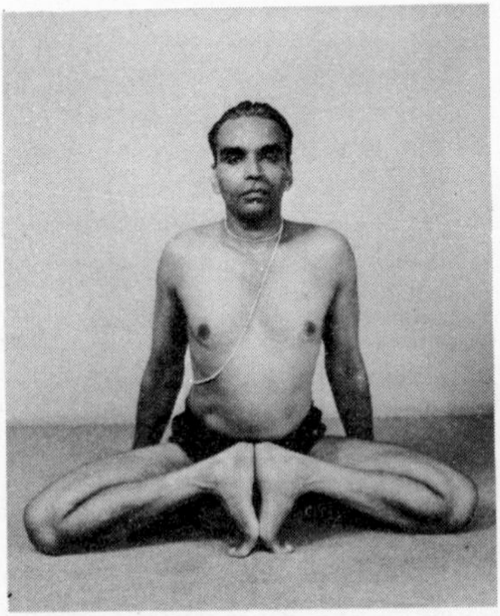

460

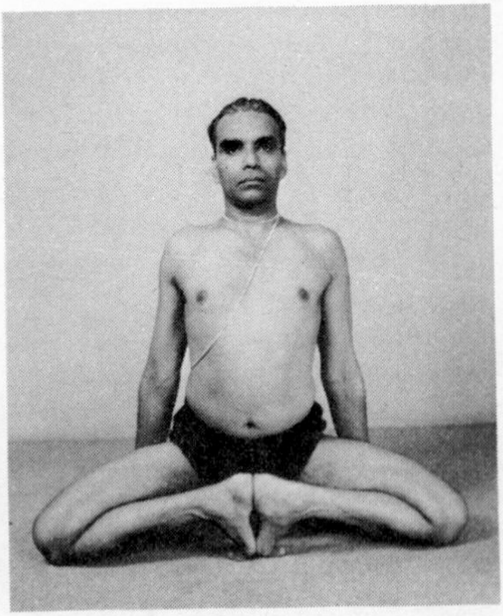

461

5. Lift the body off the floor with the help of the hands and move the hips forward (Plate 461), simultaneously turning the feet and the knees to push the heels forward without moving. (Plates 462 and 463)

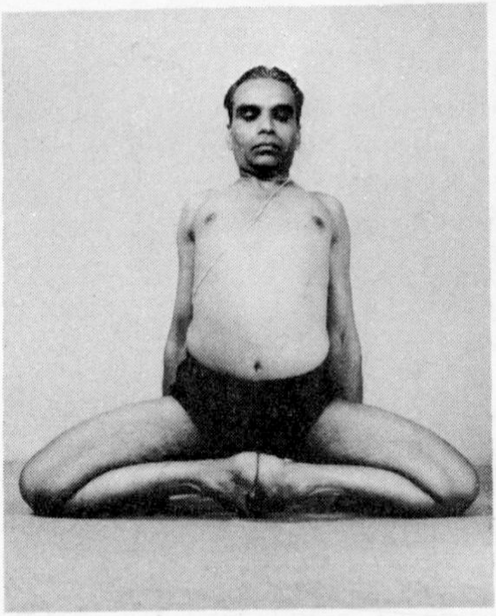

462

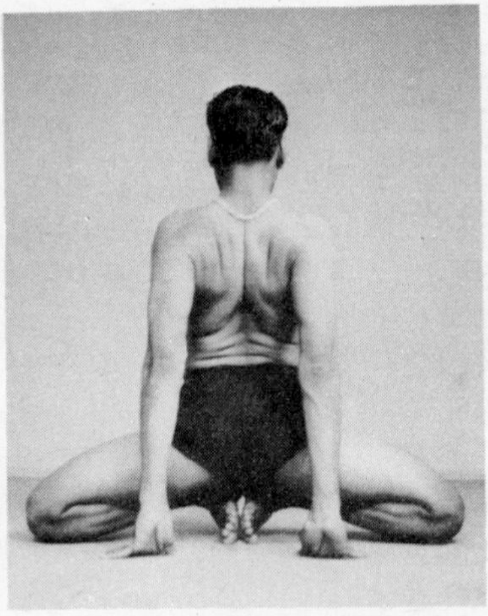

463

6. Rest the body on the toes and knees and hold the pose from 30 to 60 seconds with deep breathing.

7. To release the position move the hands in front and bear the weight on them. Lift the trunk, turn the heels and then straighten the legs. While releasing the pose do not put any weight on the legs.

Effects

This āsana exercises Mūlādhāra Chakra, the prostate gland and gonads. It also has the wonderful effect of controlling excessive sexual desire and helps to save energy. It therefore controls and stills the mind.

'The mind is the lord of the Indriyas (organs of the senses); Prāṇa is the lord of the mind; Laya or absorption is the lord of Prāṇa; and that Laya depends on Nāda (the inner sounds). When the mind is absorbed, it is called Mokṣa (emancipation); but others say that it is not: however, when the Prāṇa and Manas (the mind) have been absorbed, an undefinable joy ensues.' (*Haṭha Yoga Pradīpikā*, 4th chapter, verses 29 and 30.)

Baddhakoṇāsana (Plate 101) and Mūlabandhāsana are a great help to people with excessive sexual desire. When this desire is controlled, energy is sublimated and real joy of life is limitless.

166. *Vāmadevāsana I* Fifteen* (Plate 465)

Vāmadeva is the name of a sage, and also of Śiva, the third god of the Hindu Trinity, who is entrusted with the work of destruction.

Technique

1. Sit in Baddhakoṇāsana. (Plate 101)

2. Insert the right hand between the right thigh and calf. Keep the toes of the right foot on the ground, raise the heel and drag the foot near the perineum. Remove the hand and push the heel forward towards the floor, lift the body off the floor, move the right hip forward and put the right knee on the ground. The right foot is now in Mūlabandhāsana. (Plate 464)

3. Now place the left foot at the root of the right thigh, that is, in Padmāsana. (Plate 104)

4. Swing the left arm from the shoulder behind the back and with an exhalation catch the left big toe. With the right hand grip the front of the left foot.

5. Turn the neck to the right (Plate 465) and balance for 30 seconds with deep breathing.

6. Release the position, come back to Baddhakoṇāsana and repeat the āsana on the other side for the same length of time following the technique described above, reading left for right and vice versa.

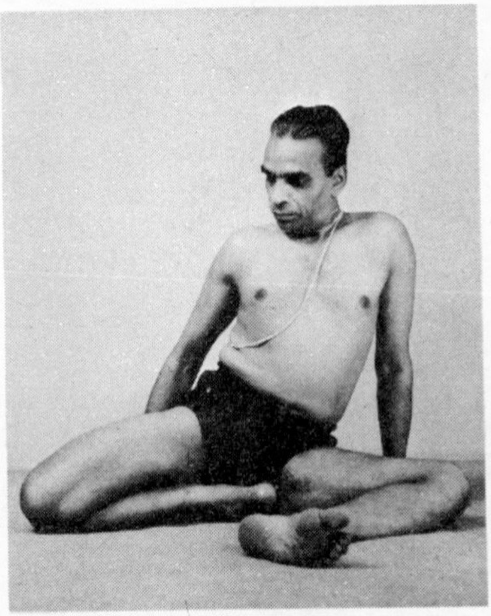

464

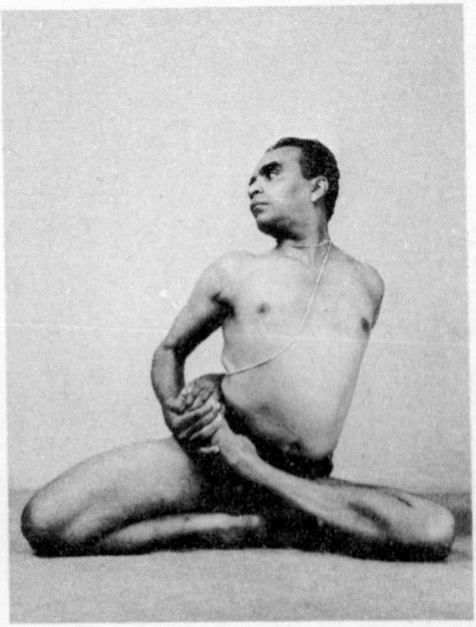

465

Effects

The pose cures stiffness of the legs and relieves pain. It keeps the genital organs healthy. It also tones the spine and aids digestion.

167. *Vāmadevāsana II* Fifteen* (Plate 466)

Technique

1. Sit on the floor and widen the thighs.

2. Bend the left knee back so that the left calf touches the back of the left thigh.

3. With the left hand lift the left foot up until the left heel touches the left hip joint. Hold the left foot with the left hand as in Bhekāsana. (Plate 100)

4. With the right hand place the right foot at the root of the left thigh as in Padmāsana. (Plate 104)

5. Using both hands press the soles of the feet together until they touch. (Plate 466)

6. The trunk will lean towards the leg in Padmāsana. Balance by gripping the hands and hold the pose for 30 seconds with deep breathing.

7. Release the hands and legs and repeat the pose on the other side,

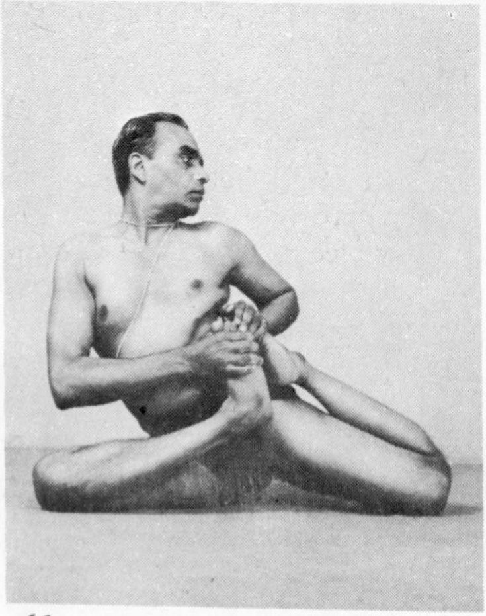

466

keeping the right foot in Bhekāsana and the left one in Padmāsana. Stay for the same length of time on both sides.

Effects

The āsana relieves pain, cures stiffness in the legs and keeps the genital organs healthy. It also tones the spine and improves digestion.

168. *Kandāsana* Thirty-nine* (Plates 470, 471, 471a and 471b)

Kanda means a bulbous root, a knot. Verses 107 and 113 in the third chapter of the *Haṭha Yoga Pradīpikā* speak of the Kanda as follows:

107. The Kuṇḍalinī sleeps above the kanda (the place near the navel where the nāḍīs unite and separate). It gives Mukti (emancipation) to the yogins and bondage to the fools. He who knows her knows Yoga.

113. The Kanda is 12 inches above the anus and extends 4 inches both ways. It has been described as round and covered as if with a soft white piece of cloth. (The word used in the text is vitasti which means a measure of length equal to 12 'angulas' (a finger's breadth), the distance between the extended thumb and little finger.)

Technique

1. Sit on the floor with the legs stretched straight in front. (Plate 77.) Bend the knees, widen the thighs, bring the feet towards the trunk until the heels are close to the perineum and keep the knees on the floor. The position is similar to Baddhakoṇāsana. (Plate 101)

2. Hold the right foot with the right palm and the left foot with the left palm.

3. With the help of the hands, draw the feet up towards the trunk, invert the ankles (Plate 467), pull the knees and thighs (Plate 468), and place the heels and the outer sides of the feet against the navel and chest. (Plate 469.) To start with the feet are likely to slip down. Practise the pose for a few weeks, holding the feet firmly against the chest.

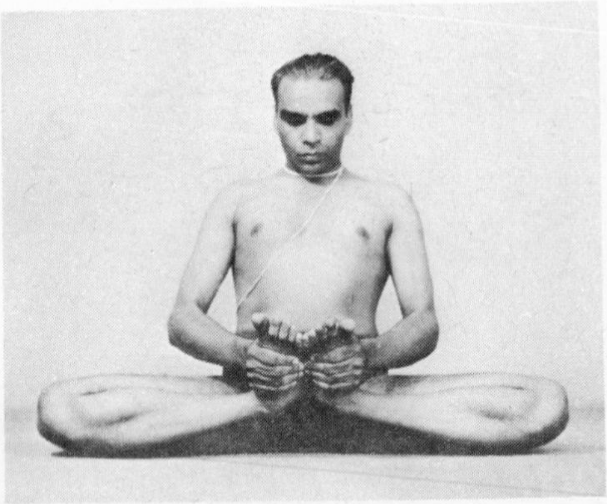

467

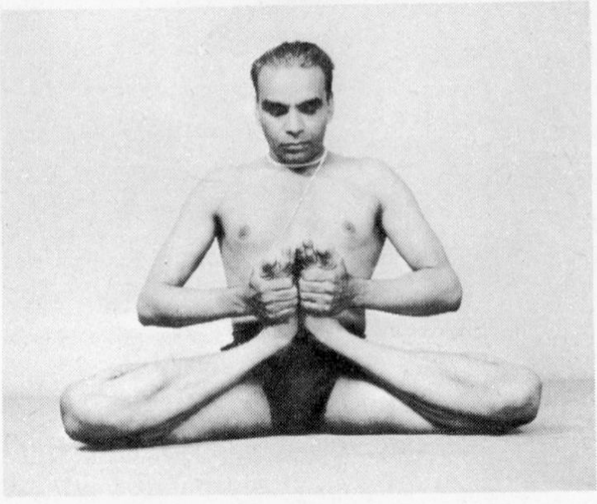

468

4. Release the hands, and either stretch the arms straight and rest the back of the hands on the knees (Plate 470) or join the palms in front of the chest. (Plate 471.) Keep the back erect and stay in the pose for about 30 seconds with deep breathing.

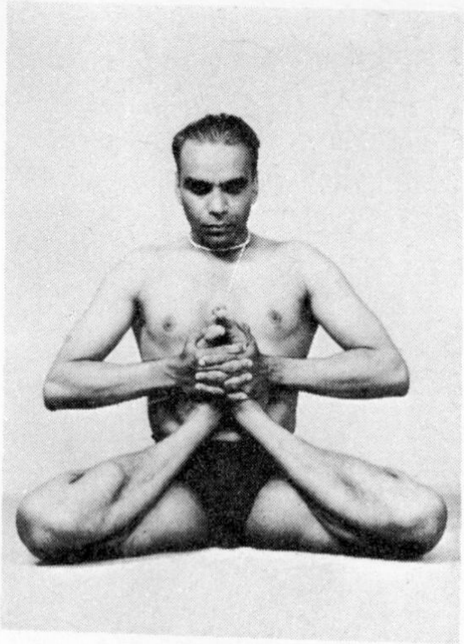

469

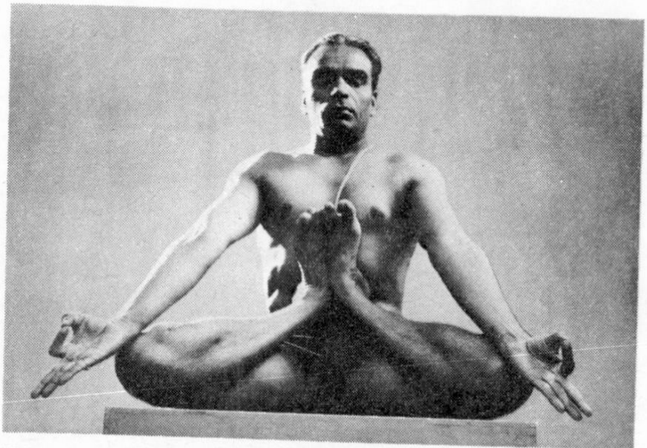

470

5. Advanced pupils may raise the hands, palms together, above the head. (Plate 471a.) Then try to join the palms behind the back and balance (Plate 471b): this is the most difficult part of the āsana.

6. Hold the feet with the hands, lower them to the floor and rest.

7. As the pelvic and other joints of the legs are rotated it takes a long time to master the pose.

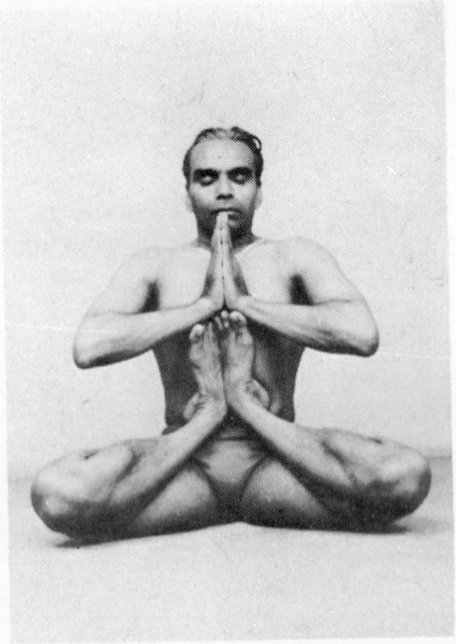

471

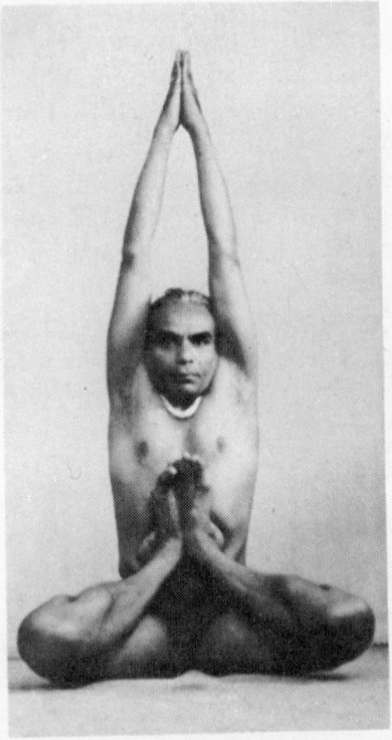

471a

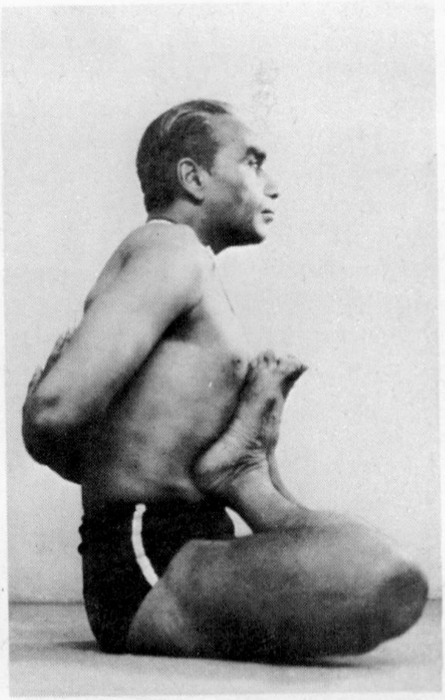

471b

Effects

Every muscle below the navel is exercised. The pose cures stiffness in the hip, knee and ankle joints. It restores sexual energy and controls sexual desires.

The āsana also exercises the Svādhiṣṭhāna Chakra (the hypogastric plexus) and the Maṇipūraka Chakra (the solar plexus), thus helping proper digestion.

169. *Hanumānāsana* Thirty-six* (Plates 475, 476 and 476a)

Hanumān was the name of a powerful monkey chief of extraordinary strength and prowess. The son of Vāyu, the god of Wind, and Anjāna, he was the friend and devoted servant of Rāma, the seventh incarnation of Viṣṇu. When Rāma, his wife Sītā and his brother Lakṣmaṇa were in exile as hermits in the Daṇḍaka forest, Rāvaṇa, the demon king of Laṅkā (Ceylon), came to their hermitage in the guise of an ascetic and seizing Sītā carried her off to Laṅkā while Rāma and Lakṣmaṇa were hunting game. The brothers searched far and wide for Sītā, and enlisted the help of Sugrīva, the king of the monkeys, and his general Hanumān. Hanumān went in search of Sītā, crossed the sea by leaping over the straits, found her in Rāvaṇa's palace, and brought the news to Rāma. With the aid of a great army of monkeys and bears Rāma built a causeway of stones across the sea to Laṅkā and after a fierce battle slew Rāvaṇa and his hosts and rescued Sītā. During the battle, Lakṣmaṇa had been struck by an arrow and lay unconscious and it was said that the only cure was the juice of a herb which grew in the Himālayās. With one prodigious leap Hanumān crossed the sea and reached the Himālayās to bring back with him the mountain top on which the life-giving plant grew and thus saved the life of Lakṣmaṇa. This āsana is dedicated to Hanumān and commemorates his fabulous leaps. It is practised by going down on the floor with the legs spread out laterally while the hands are folded in front of the chest. It resembles the splits of Western ballet.

Technique

1. Kneel on the floor. (Plate 40)

2. Rest the palms a foot apart on the floor on either side of the body.

3. Lift the knees up. Bring the right leg forward and the left leg back. (Plate 472.) Try to stretch both the legs straight with an exhalation and keep the hips up. (Plate 473.) Then press the legs and hips to the ground, and bear the weight on the hands. (Plate 474)

4. It takes a long time to master this position and to attain it one

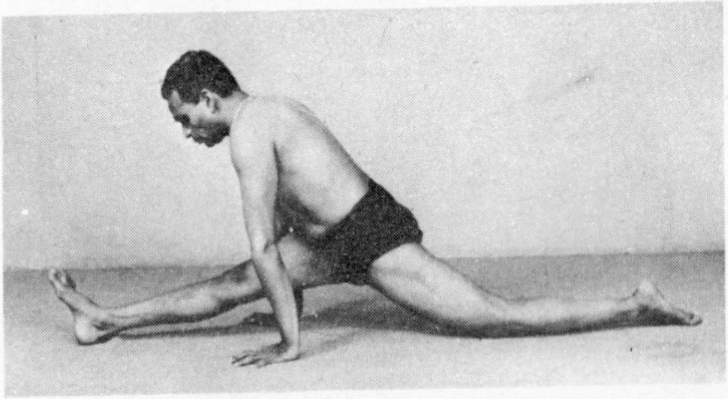

472

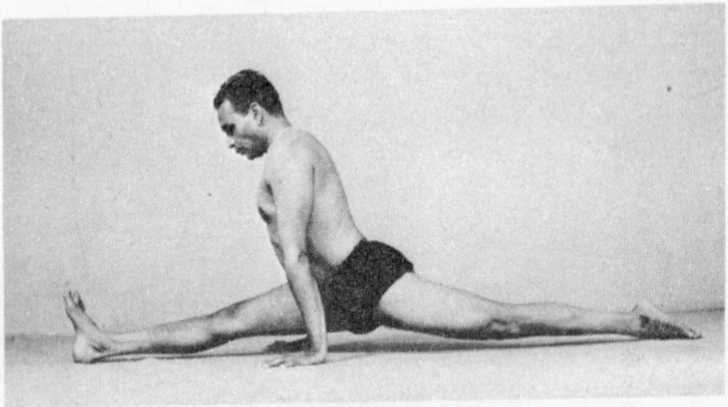

473

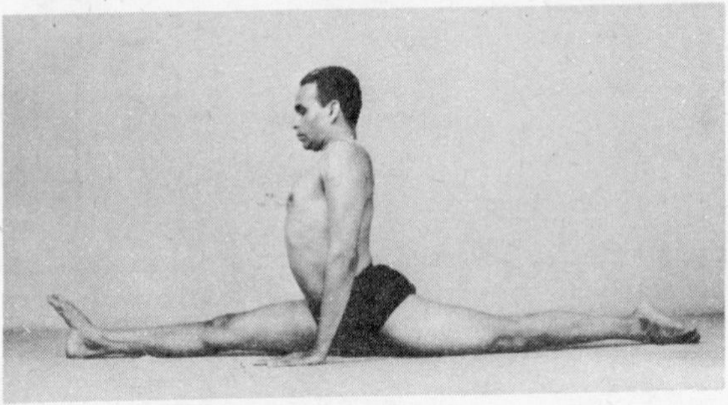

474

must make several attempts each day to rest the legs straight on the floor, with the buttocks touching the ground. The back portion of the front leg and the front portion of the rear leg should touch the floor.

5. Once the straight legs position is attained, sit on the floor, raise the hands, fold them in front of the chest and balance. (Plate 475.) Stay in the pose from 10 to 30 seconds with normal breathing.

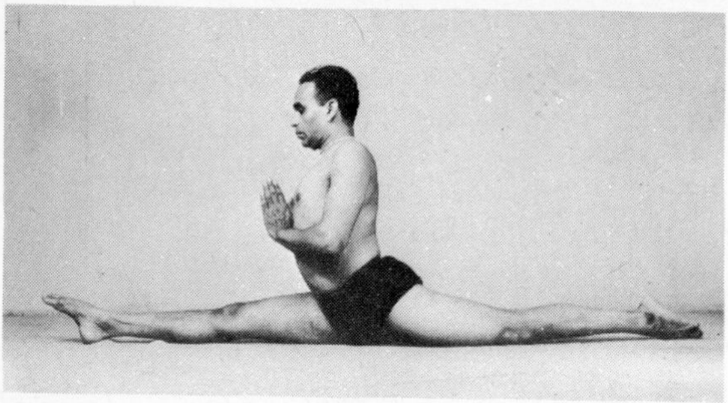

475

6. Then with the help of the hands raise the hips and repeat the pose for the same length of time, keeping the left leg in front and the right leg behind. (Plate 476)

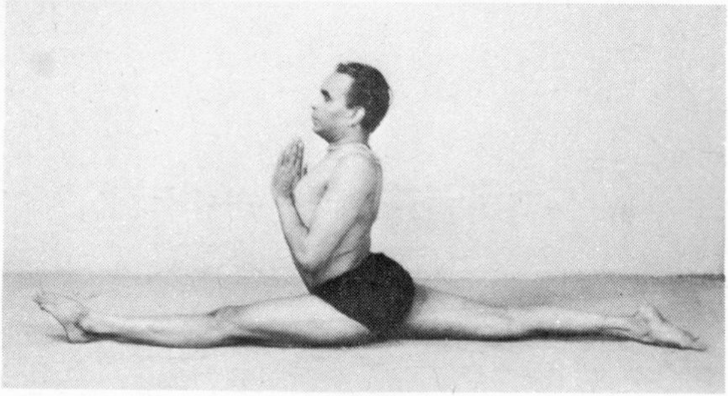

476

7. Remember that the back of the knee joint of the front leg and the knee of the back leg should touch the floor.

8. Advanced pupils may raise the hands above the head, stretch up, put the palms together and balance. (Plate 476a.) This gives an extra stretch to the legs, and relieves strain on the back.

Effects

This beautiful pose helps to cure sciatica and other defects of the legs. It tones the leg muscles, keeps the legs in condition and if practised regularly is recommended for runners and sprinters. It relaxes and strengthens the abductor muscles of the thighs.

170. *Samakoṇāsana* Thirty-eight* (Plate 477)

Sama means the same, like, even or straight. Koṇa means an angle

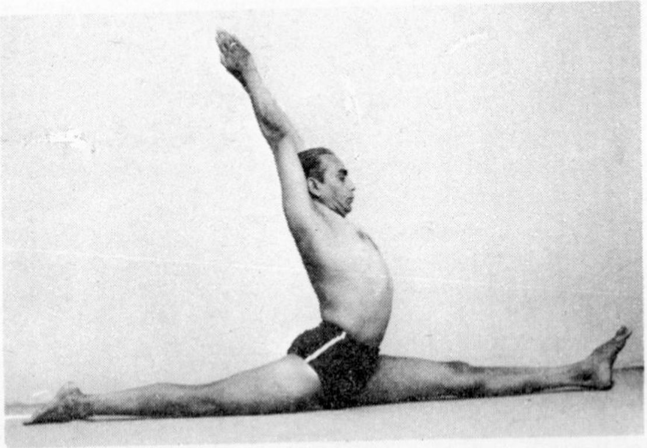

476a

and a point of a compass. In this āsana the split is performed with the legs spread apart sideways, and the hands are folded in front of the chest. It is harder to perform than Hanumānāsana. (Plate 475.) Both the legs and the pelvic region of the body are in one straight line.

Technique

1. Stand in Tāḍāsana (Plate 1), rest the hands on the hips and spread the legs apart sideways to your capacity. (Plate 29)

2. Place the palms on the floor (Plate 30) and with an exhalation stretch the legs further and further until you sit on the floor with both legs spread sideways in a straight line. The entire back of the legs, especially the back of the knees, should rest on the floor.

3. Join the palms in front of the chest (Plate 477) and stay in the pose for a few seconds.

4. Place the palms on the floor, raise the hips and bring the legs closer

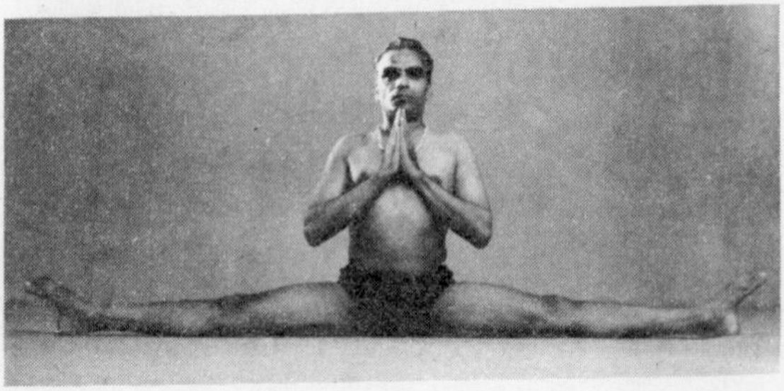

477

and closer to each other until you stand up again in Uttānāsana. (Plate 47.) Then stand in Tāḍāsana (Plate 1) and relax.

Effects

In this pose the hip joints are exercised and the legs are made to move freely in all directions. The spine is stretched and any defect in the lower part of the spine is cured. The pose, like Hanumānāsana (Plate 475), tones the leg muscles and makes the legs shapely. It prevents the development of hernia and relieves sciatic pains. It helps the blood to circulate in the pelvic region and genital organs and keeps them healthy.

171. *Supta Trivikramāsana* Thirty-nine* (Plate 478)

Supta means reclining. Trivikrama (tri = three; vikrama = a step, stride or pace) is a name of Viṣṇu. The āsana is dedicated to Vāmanāvatār, the Dwarf Incarnation of Viṣṇu. It is said that Bali, the grandson of Prahlāda, who was the king of the demons, gained control of the world. Bali practised asceticism by which his power so increased that he threatened even the gods who prayed to Viṣṇu for help. The god descended on earth and was born as the dwarf son of the Brahman sage Kaśyapa and his wife Aditi. At one of the sacrifices performed by Bali, Viṣṇu appeared before him in the form of a dwarf (Vāmana) and asked for as much earth as he could cover in three strides. Bali, who was noted for his liberality, unhesitatingly granted this boon. Thereupon, the Dwarf assumed a mighty form, and made three strides. The first covered the earth, and the second the heavens. As there was no other place for the third stride, Bali offered his own head on which the Lord planted his foot. He then sent him and all his legions to Pātāla, the nether regions, and allowed him to be its ruler. The universe was thus once more restored to the gods.

This āsana is more difficult than Hanumānāsana. (Plate 475.) Here, the pose is performed by lying on the floor on the back, then doing the splits and holding the heel of one foot near the head, while the other heel rests on the floor.

Technique

1. Lie flat on the back on the floor, keeping both legs straight. (Plate 219)

2. Raise the right leg up. Interlock the fingers, stretch the arms and hold the right heel in the cup of the hands.

3. Exhale, pull the right leg straight down behind the head and place the right big toe on the floor, without letting go of the heel. (Plate

478.) The inner side of the right calf will touch the right ear and the elbows will be widened slightly. The left leg should remain straight on the floor throughout.

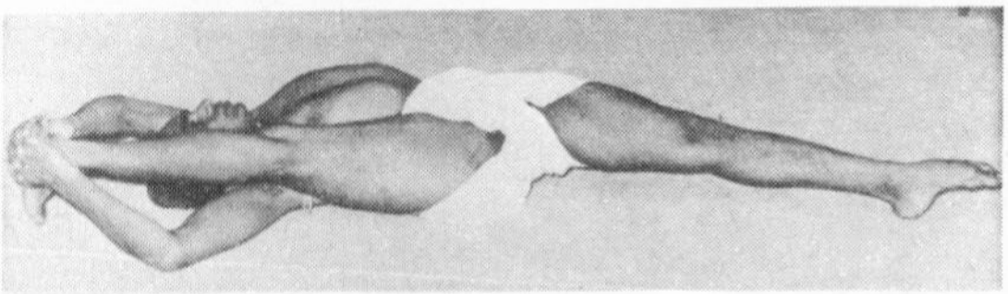

478

4. Remain in the pose as long as you conveniently can with normal breathing.

5. Release the right heel and lower the right leg beside the left one.

6. Repeat the pose for an equal length of time, now holding the left heel and keeping the right leg on the floor.

7. After finishing this strenuous pose, rest for a while and relax.

Effects

In this pose, the legs are fully stretched. It prevents and cures hernia. It also lessens sexual desire and thereby stills the mind.

172. *Ūrdhva Dhanurāsana I* Seven* (Plate 482)

Ūrdhva means upwards. Dhanu means a bow. In this posture the body is arched back and supported on the palms and soles.

Technique (This is for beginners)

1. Lie flat on the back on the floor. (Plate 219)

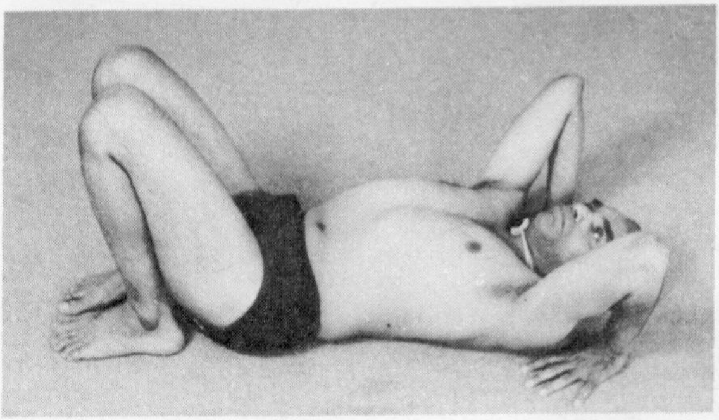

479

2. Bend and raise the elbows over the head, and place the palms under the shoulders. The distance between the palms should not be wider than the shoulders and the fingers should point towards the feet.

3. Bend and raise the knees, then bring the feet nearer until they touch the hips. (Plate 479)

4. Exhale, raise the trunk and rest the crown of the head on the floor. (Plate 480.) Take two breaths.

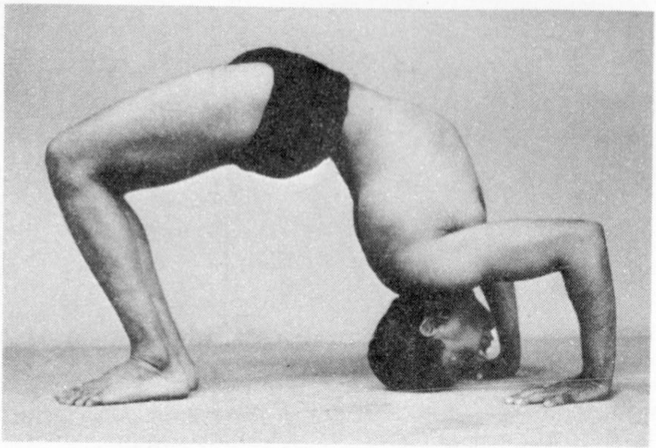

480

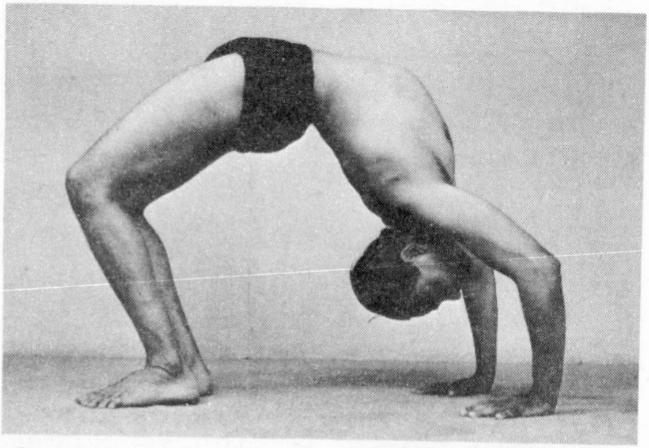

481

5. Now exhale, lift the trunk and head and arch the back so that its weight is taken on the palms and the soles. (Plate 481)

6. Stretch the arms from the shoulders until the elbows are straightened, at the same time pulling the thigh muscles up. (Plate 482)

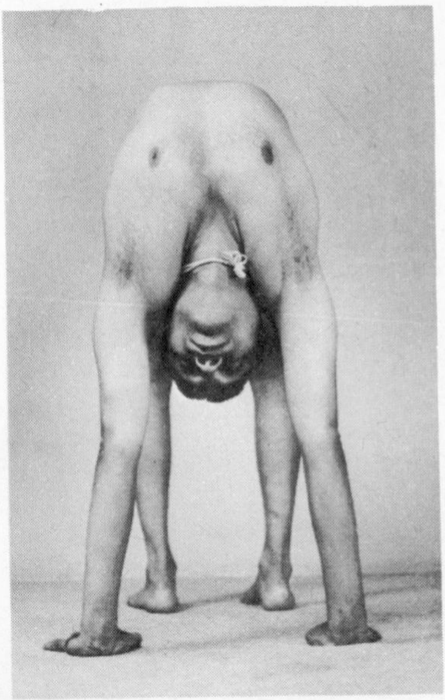

482

7. To get a better stretch, exhale and pull the thigh muscles still higher by lifting the heels off the floor. Extend the chest, stretch up the sacral region of the spine until the abdomen is taut as a drum and then lower the heels to the floor, maintaining the stretch of the spine.

8. Remain in this position from half a minute to a minute, with normal breathing.

9. With an exhalation, lower the body to the floor by bending the knees and elbows.

172a. *Ūrdhva Dhanurāsana II* Fifteen* (Plate 486)

Technique (This is for intermediate pupils)

1. Stand erect with the feet one foot apart and the palms on the hips.

2. Push the pelvic region slightly forward (Plate 483), exhale and curve the trunk back so that the weight of the body is felt on the thighs and the toes. (Plate 484)

3. Raise the arms above the head and drop the hands on to the floor. (Plate 485.) Immediately try to straighten the arms at the elbows and rest the palms on the floor. (Plate 486.) If the elbows are not stretched immediately as the palms touch the floor, one is likely to bang the head.

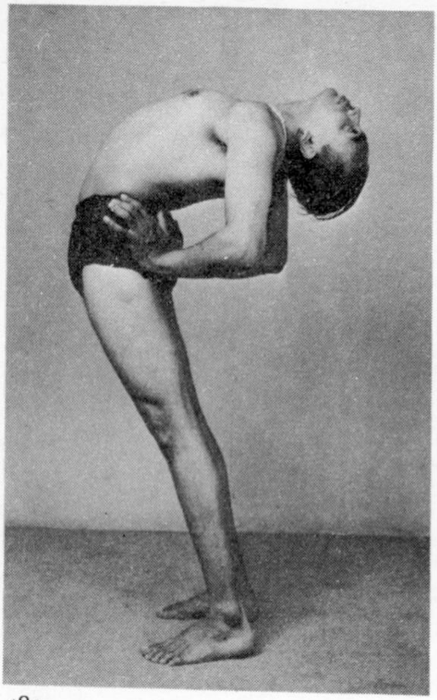
483

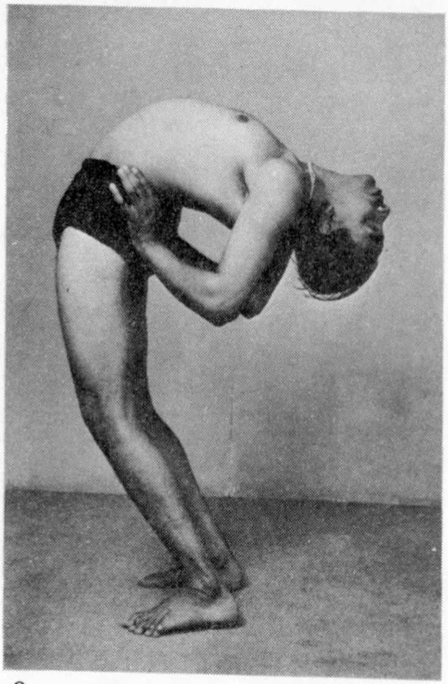
484

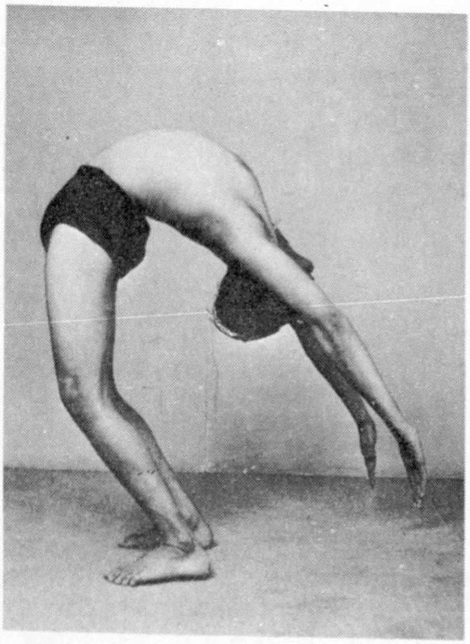
485

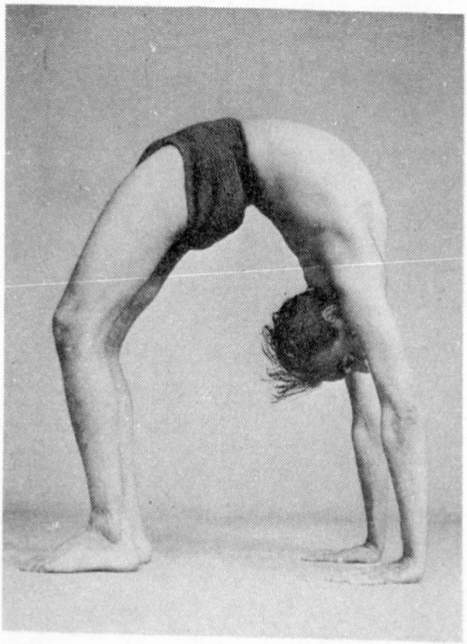
486

4. After securing the above position stretch the legs and arms straight. (Plate 487)

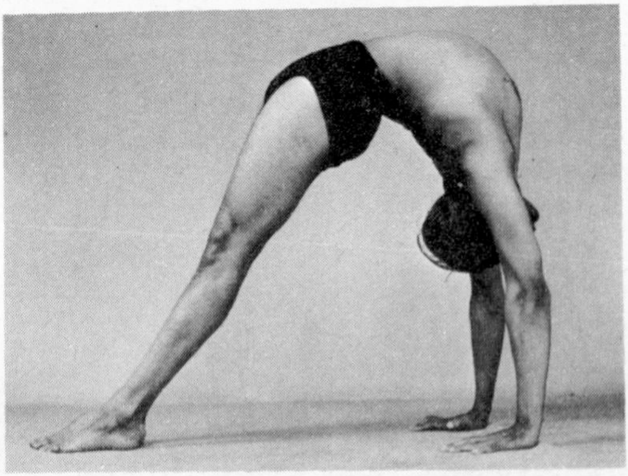

487

5. While learning the pose this way it is helpful to use a friend or a wall. Stand about three feet from a wall with your back to it. Curve the back and move the head towards the wall. Raise the arms over the head and rest the palms on the wall. Push the pelvis forward so that the body weight is felt on the thighs and move the palms down the wall until you touch the floor. Use the wall for coming up in a similar manner. After mastering this, only use the wall until you are half-way up. Then learn to do the āsana in the middle of the room.

173. *Viparīta Chakrāsana in Ūrdhva Dhanurāsana.* Twenty-six* (Plates 488 to 499)

Technique (This is for advanced pupils)

1. Stand erect. Bend forward and place the palms on the floor. Exhale and swing both legs up as though you were doing the full arm balance (Plate 359), bend the knees, arch the back and drop the legs behind the head. (Plate 486)

2. While the legs are coming down beyond and behind the head, contract the hips, extend the back up, stretch the ribs and abdomen and straighten the arms at the elbows. Unless you do this, you will sit on the floor with a bump.

3. When all this has been mastered, learn the reverse swinging movements of the leg as shown from Plates 488 to 499, so that one swings the legs up and back in a reverse somersault movement. This reverse somersault into the forward bending position is called *Viparīta*

Chakrāsana, the reversed wheel pose. (Viparīta=reverse, contrary, opposite, inverted; chakra=wheel.) Most people, however, can only learn to do it with the aid of a competent teacher.

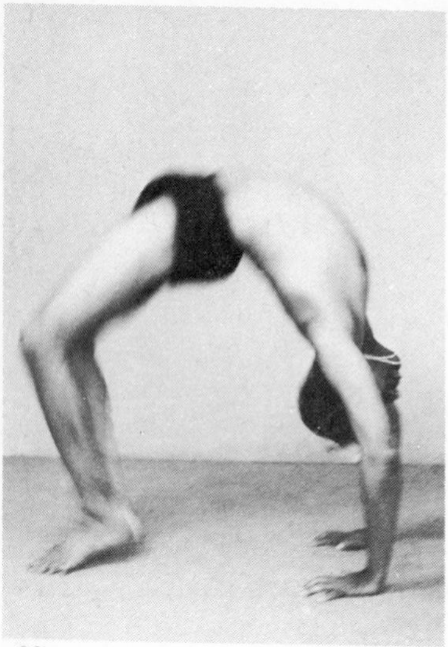
488

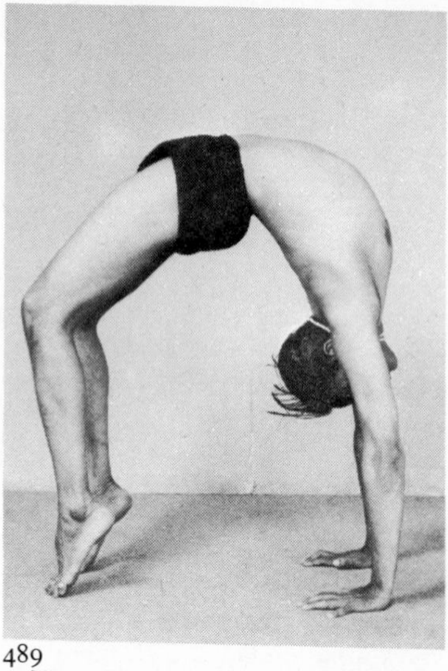
489

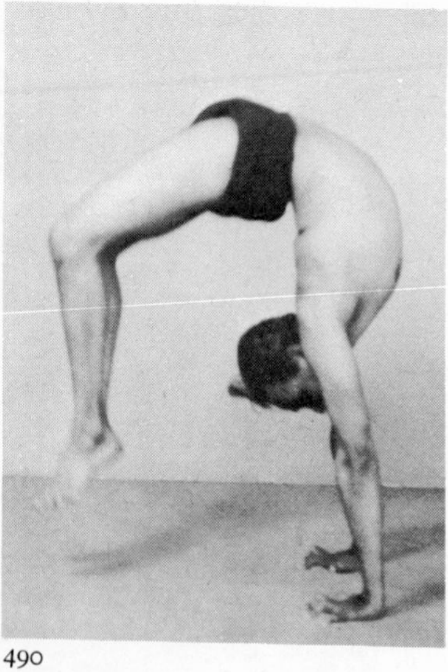
490

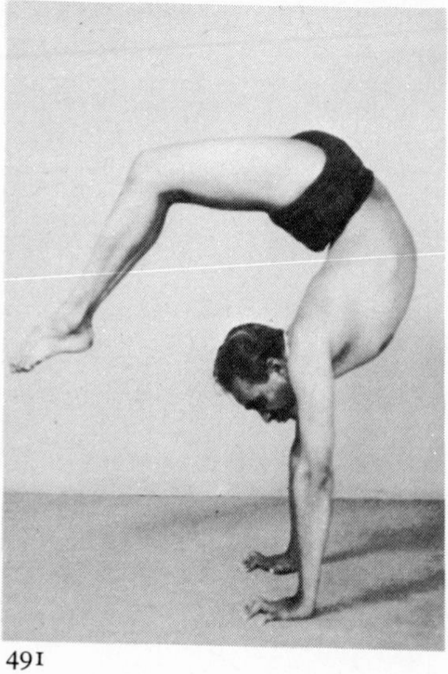
491

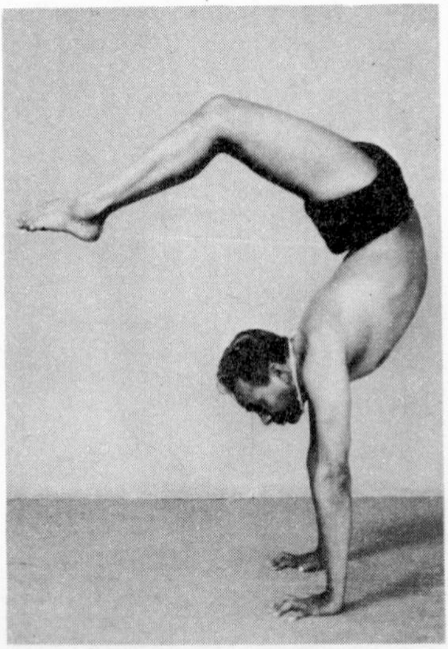
492

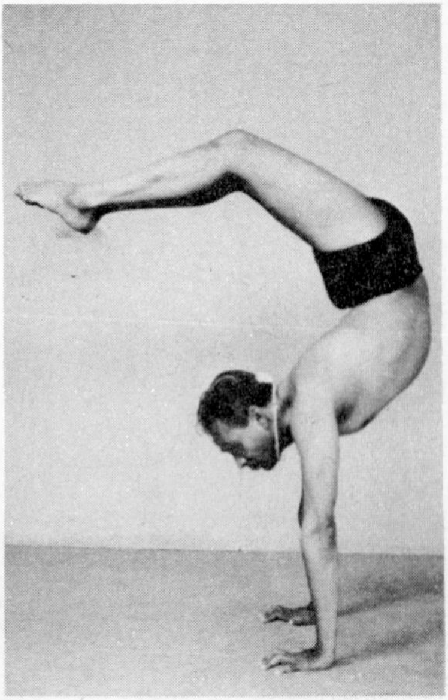
493

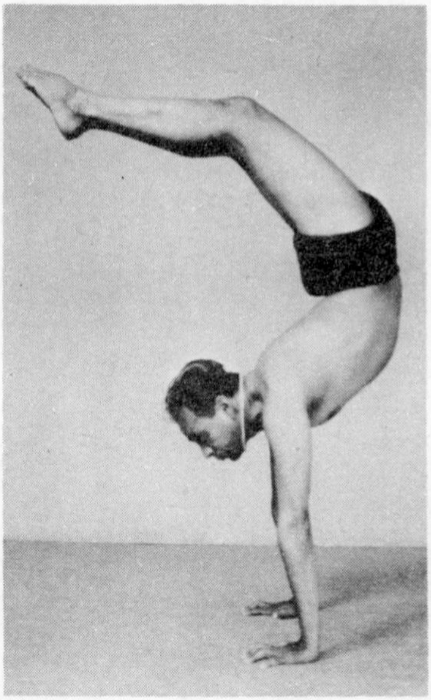
494

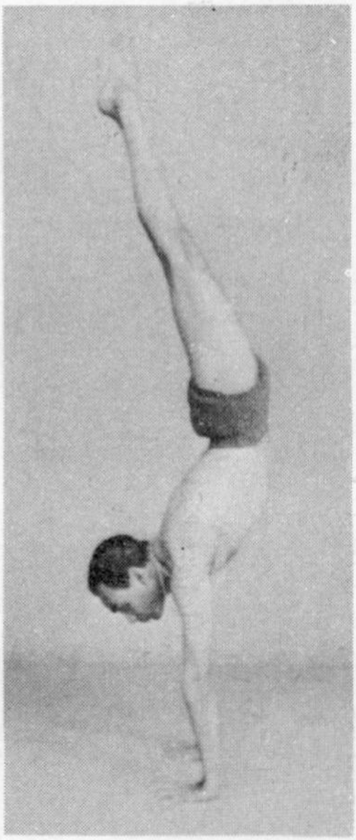
495

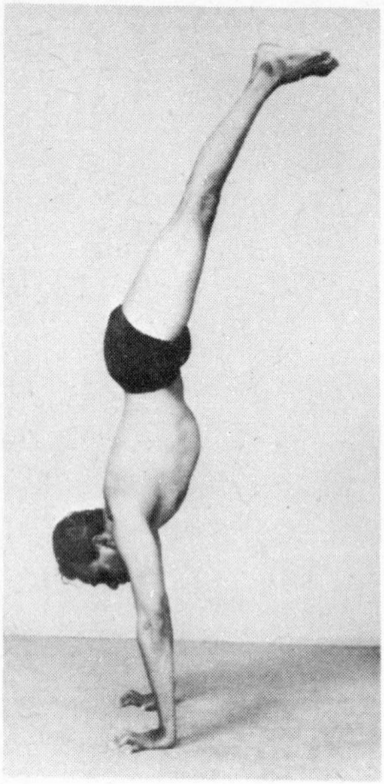
496

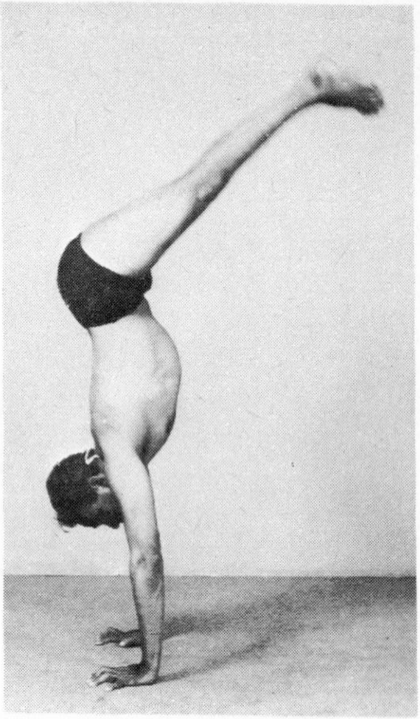
497

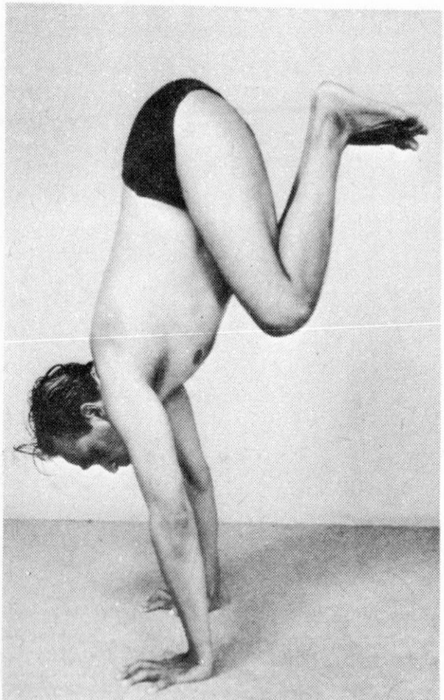
498

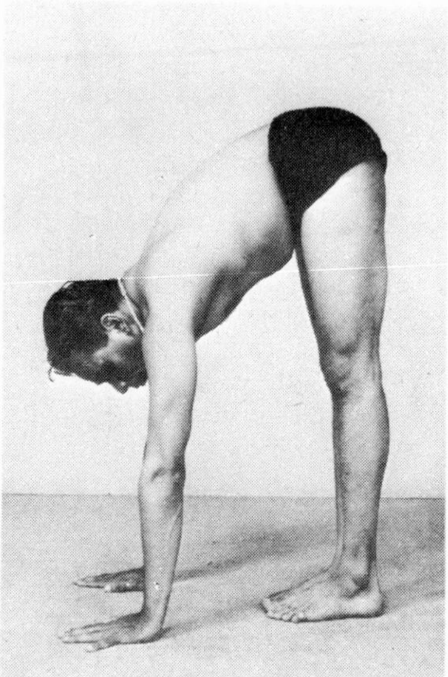
499

4. If, however, no guru is available and you have confidence in yourself, you can try to achieve the reverse somersault movement in the following manner. Do Ūrdhva Dhanurāsana near a wall so that the feet face the wall about a foot away from it. Swing the trunk with an exhalation towards the shoulders so that the weight of the body is borne on the wrists and shoulders. Then lift one leg from the floor and place the foot on the wall at the height of about two feet. Press and push against the wall with that foot, lift the other leg off the floor and with an exhalation swing the legs over the head, making a reverse somersault. After repeated attempts, you will gain confidence. You will learn to rock the body forward and backward and to swing the trunk towards the shoulders with a backward movement of the legs in the reverse somersault. When you are sure of taking the legs off the floor, then try Viparīta Chakrāsana in the middle of the room away from the wall. This is how I learnt the reverse somersault movements in Viparīta Chakrāsana.

Effects

This āsana is the beginning of the advanced and difficult back-bending poses. It tones the spine by stretching it fully and keeps the body alert and supple. The back feels strong and full of life. It strengthens the arms and wrists and has a very soothing effect on the head. Once Viparīta Chakrāsana is mastered, it can be repeated several times a day. It gives one great vitality, energy and a feeling of lightness.

174. *Eka Pāda Ūrdhva Dhanurāsana* Twelve* (Plates 501 and 502)

Eka means one. Pāda is a leg. Ūrdhva means upwards and dhanu a bow.

Technique

1. After performing Ūrdhva Dhanurāsana (Plate 486), exhale and raise the right leg off the floor.

2. Stretch the right leg straight, and keep it at an angle of about 45 degrees from the floor. (Plate 500)

3. Then lift the right hand from the floor and place it on the right thigh. (Plate 501.) The body is then balanced on the left hand and foot. Hold this position from 10 to 15 seconds, with normal breathing.

4. Exhale, lower the hands and raised leg and go back to Ūrdhva Dhanurāsana.

5. Repeat the pose by lifting the left leg and placing the left hand on the left thigh, balancing the body on the right hand and leg. (Plate 502.) Maintain the pose on this side for the same length of time.

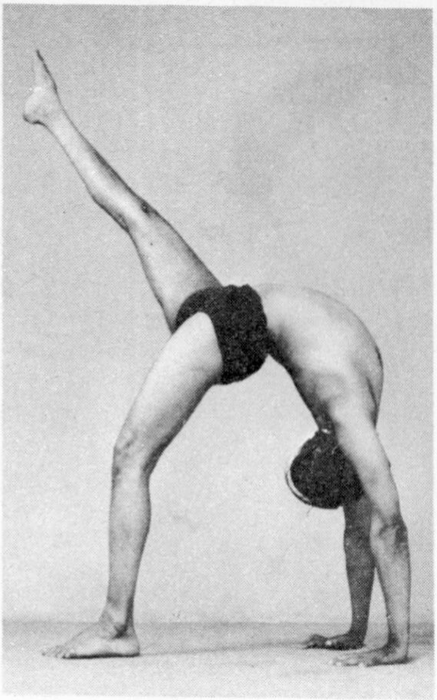

500

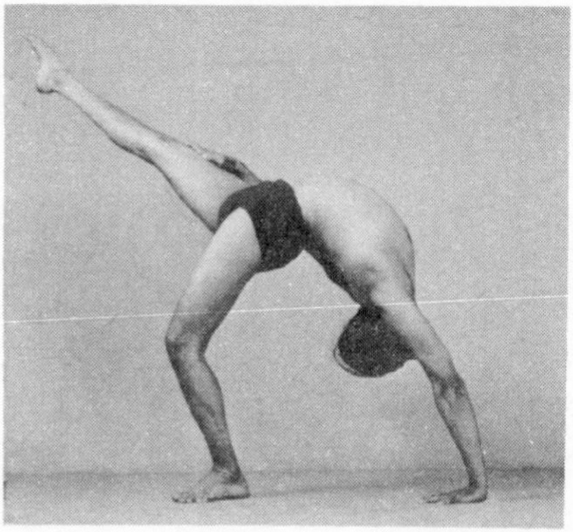

501

Effects

In addition to the benefits derived by Ūrdhva Dhanurāsana (Plate 486), this beautiful āsana develops a sense of balance and gives grace and poise.

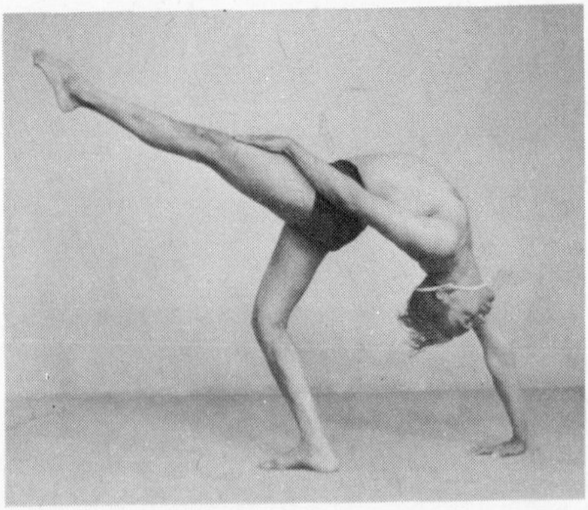

502

175. *Kapotāsana* Twenty-one* (Plates 507 and 512)

Kapota means a dove or a pigeon. In this pose the chest expands and puffs out like that of a pouter pigeon, hence the name.

Technique (For beginners)

1. Sit in Vīrāsana on a folded blanket. (Plate 90)

2. Recline back on the blanket and do Supta Vīrāsana. (Plate 95.) Stretch the arms over the head, bend the elbows and place the palms near the ears, the fingers pointing to the shoulders. (Plate 503)

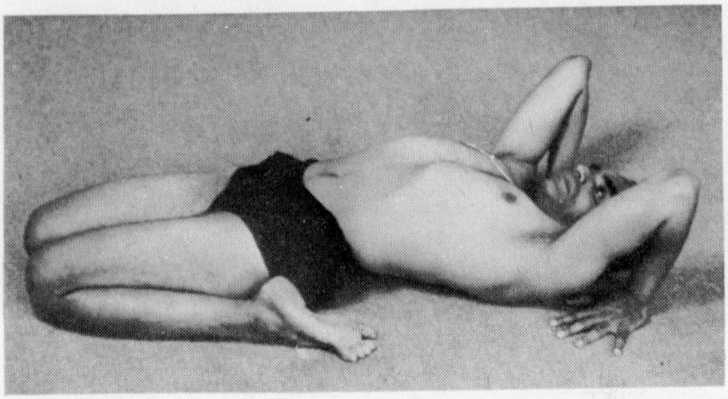

503

3. Bear the weight on the palms and exhale. Stretch the arms and raise the whole body from the knees by stretching the thighs and then join the knees. (Plate 504)

4. Contract the buttocks, stretch the entire spine, bend the elbows and hold the toes. (Plate 505.) Then rest the elbows on the floor. (Plate 506.)

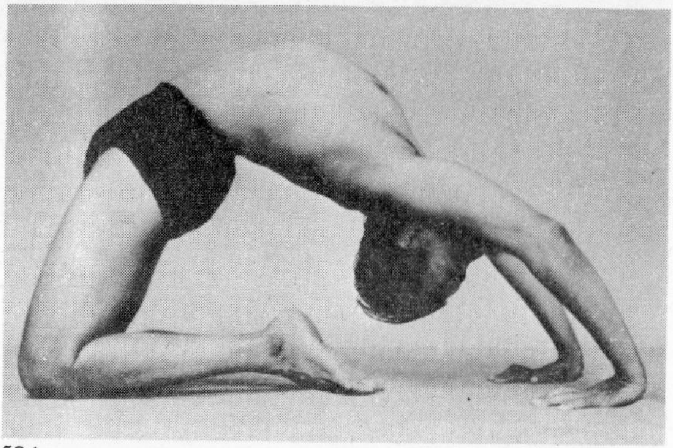

504

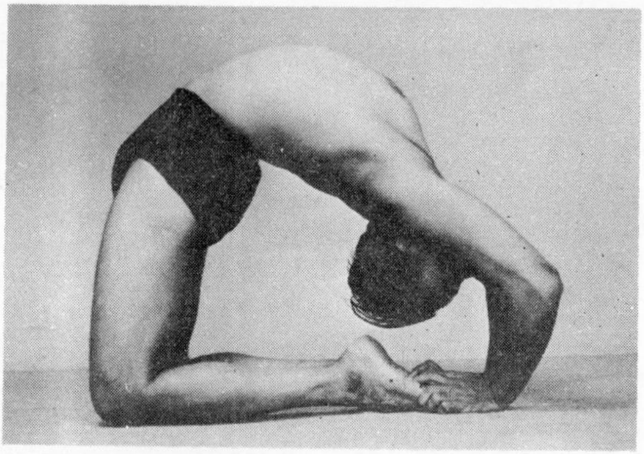

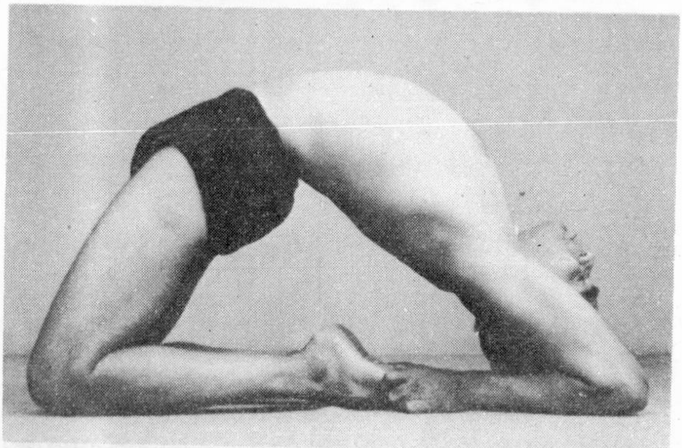

506

Breathing will be very fast and laboured as the diaphragm is fully contracted.

5. Take a few quick breaths, exhale, raise the pelvic region by tightening the muscles of the thighs. Gradually bring the hands near the heels and catch them by bringing the head towards the feet. Now place the crown of the head on the soles of the feet. (Plate 507)

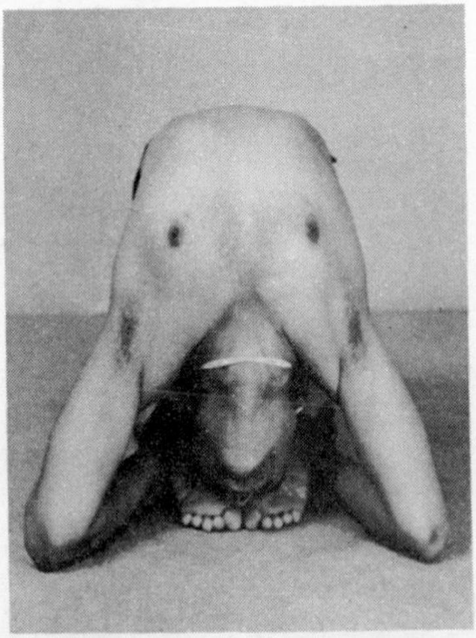

507

6. Stay in the pose for a few seconds. Gradually increase the time according to your capacity up to a minute.

7. Exhale, release the grip on the feet and lower the head and body until you are again in Supta Vīrāsana. (Plate 95.) Straighten the legs one by one and relax on the floor.

Technique (For advanced pupils)

1. Kneel on a folded blanket with the feet and knees together. Place the hands on the hips, stretch the thighs and keep them perpendicular to the floor. (Plate 40)

2. Exhale, stretch the entire spine and bend back as in Plates 508 and 509. Take the arms over the head towards the feet, place the palms on the heels and grip them. (Plate 510.) Breathing will be fast and laboured. Take a few quick breaths.

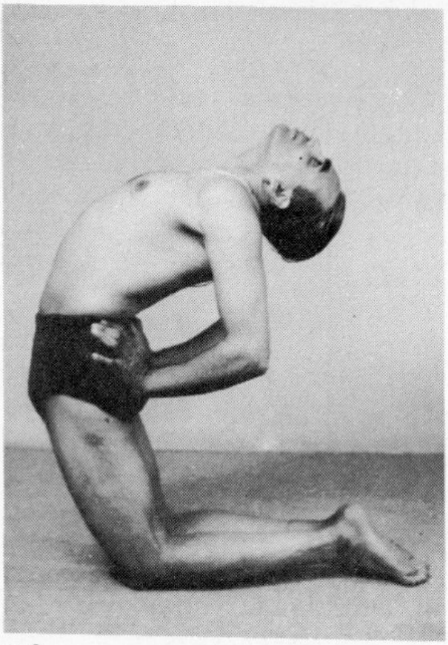

508

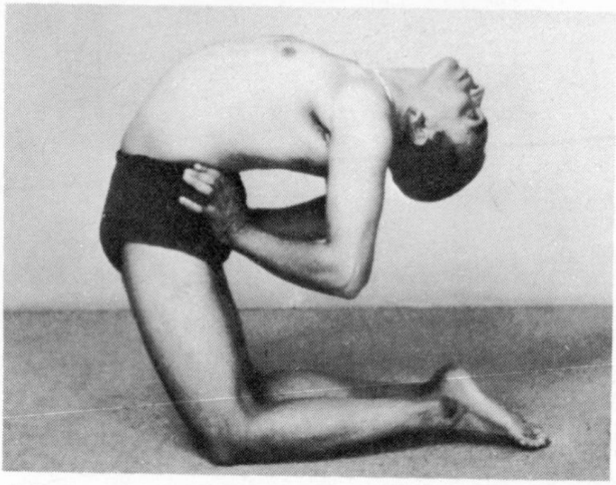

509

3. Exhale, stretch the spine still further back, bend the elbows and place them on the floor. (Plate 511)

4. Stretch the neck back and rest the crown of the head on the soles of the feet. Contract the buttocks, lift up the pelvic region, stretch the thighs and catch the ankles. (Plate 512)

5. Remain in this position as long as you can for about 60 seconds, breathing rhythmically.

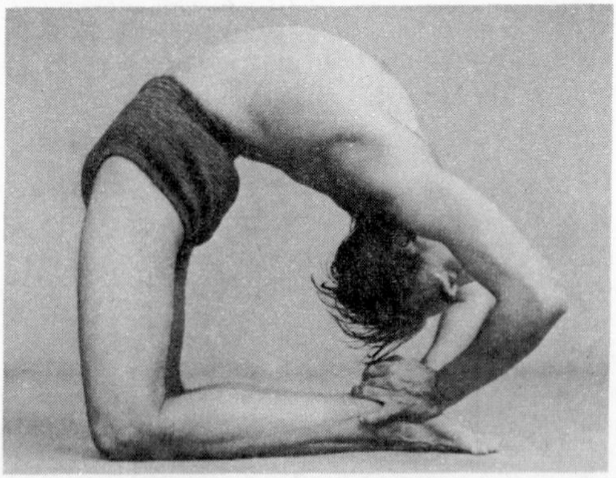
510

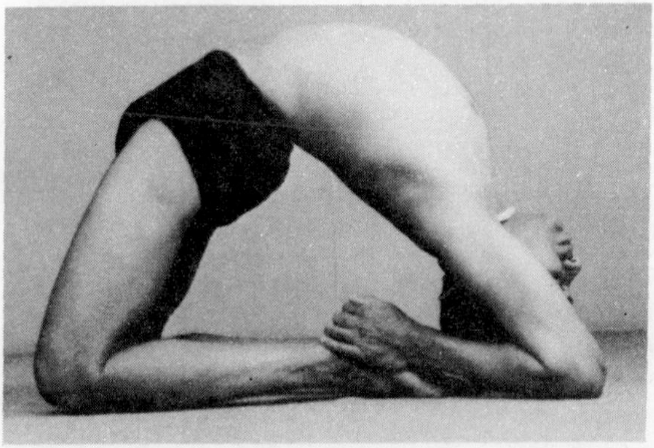
511

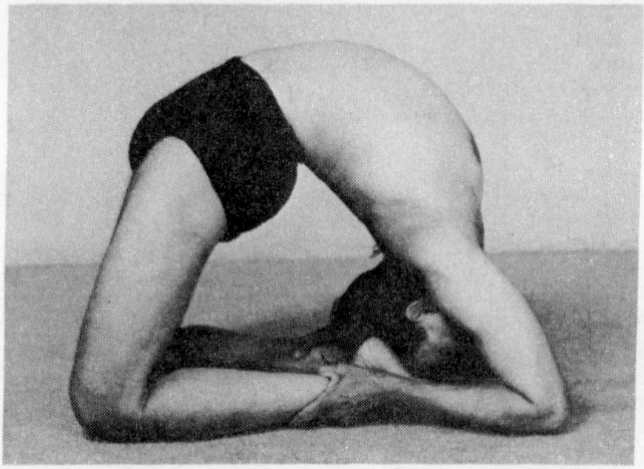
512

6. Release the grip on the feet. Extend the arms and bring the body forward until you are again standing on the knees. Then rest on the floor and relax.

Effects

The pose tones up the entire spinal region as the blood is made to circulate well round the spinal column. Since the pelvic region is stretched, the genital organs keep healthy. The diaphragm is lifted up and this massages the heart gently and helps to strengthen it. The chest expands fully. It is essential to master Kapotāsana before practising the more difficult back-bending poses, which cannot be done until you have perfected Kapotāsana and Viparīta Daṇḍāsana (Plate 516) to Maṇḍalāsana. (Plates 525 and 535)

176. *Laghu Vajrāsana* Twenty-three* (Plate 513)

Laghu means little, small, easy as well as lovely, handsome, beautiful. Vajra means a thunderbolt, the weapon of Indra, the king of gods.

Technique

1. Kneel on the floor with the knees and feet together. Rest the palms on the sides of the waist. (Plate 40)

2. Exhale, arch the spine back and at the same time tighten the muscles of the thighs. (Plates 508 and 509)

3. Push the hips forward and keep bending the spine back until the crown of the head rests on the feet. It requires great practice to achieve the necessary spinal elasticity. The weight of the body is borne only on the knees.

4. When the above position is achieved, remove the hands from the waist, stretch the arms straight from the shoulders and grip each knee with the respective hand. (Plate 513)

5. Due to the spine being stretched and the pressure against the abdomen, breathing will be fast and laboured. Try to hold the pose from 10 to 15 seconds while breathing normally.

6. Exhale, keep the knees firm, raise the head and trunk until you are kneeling again. Then sit on the floor and rest.

Effects

This āsana tones the spinal nerves and exercises the coccyx (the terminal triangular bone of the vertebral column). The pose, if practised regularly, relieves pain and disc displacements in the lower region of the spine. Due to the arch, the abdominal muscles and chest are fully extended.

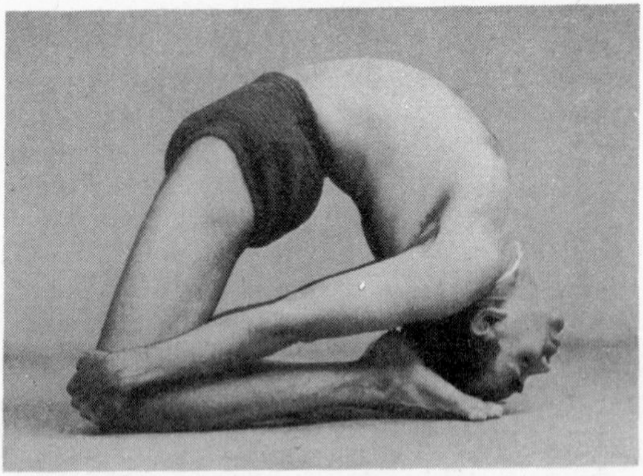

513

177. *Dwi Pāda Viparīta Daṇḍāsana* Twenty-four* (Plate 516)

Dwi Pāda means both feet. Viparīta means reverse or inverted. Daṇḍa means staff or rod, a symbol, authority or punishment as well as the body and its prostration. The Hindu devotee prostrates before the Lord lying flat upon the floor, face downwards with hands outstretched. The Yogi on the other hand prostrates himself in the graceful inverted arch described below.

Technique (For beginners)

1. Lie flat on the back. (Plate 219)

2. Extend the arms over the head, bend the elbows and place the palms underneath the shoulders, fingers pointing to the feet. Also bend and raise the knees, bring the feet near the hips and rest them on the floor. (Plate 479)

3. Exhale and at the same time lift up the head and trunk and rest the crown of the head on the floor. (Plate 480.) Take a few breaths.

4. Exhale, extend the legs, straighten them one by one bearing the weight on the hands, head and neck. (Plate 514)

5. Take the left hand off the floor and place it behind the head, resting the elbow on the floor. (Plate 515.) Take two breaths.

6. Now remove the right hand from and place the elbow on the floor, move the hand behind the head, interlock the fingers and rest the cupped hands against the back of the head. This is the final position. (Plate 516.) In it the head and the hands will be in the same position as in Sālamba Śīrṣāsana I. (Plate 190)

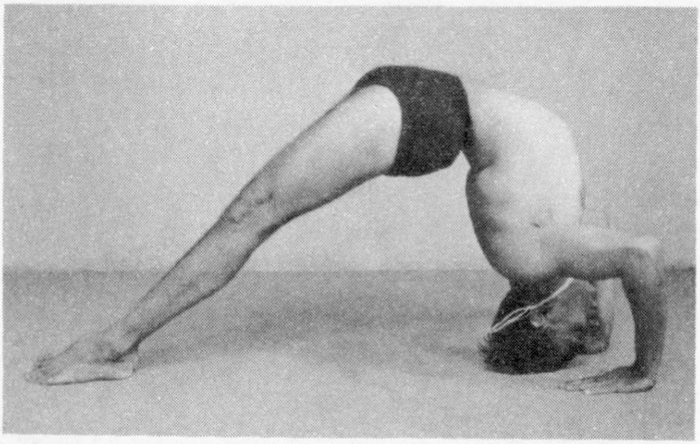

514

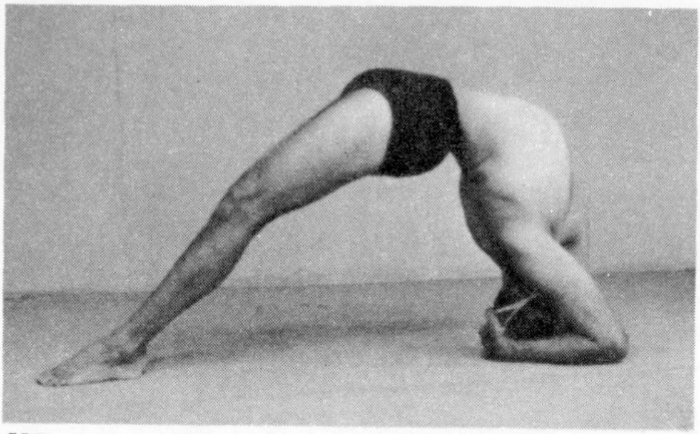

515

7. The diaphragm being contracted, breathing will be fast and short. Take a few breaths, exhale and raise the shoulders as high as you can above the floor, as also the chest, trunk, hips, thighs and calves. Stretch the legs straight from the pelvis to the ankles. Dig the heels into the floor and stay in this position to your capacity from one to two minutes.

8. Move the feet towards the head, bend the knees, release the finger-lock, raise the head from the floor, lower the trunk and relax.

9. The neck, chest and shoulders should be fully extended and the pelvic region raised as high as possible above the floor. To start with the neck will not stay perpendicular to the floor as it should and there will be a tendency for the head and forearms to slip away. So rest the feet against a wall and ask a friend to press down the elbows until the distance between the feet and the head on the floor is properly adjusted while the spine and legs are fully extended.

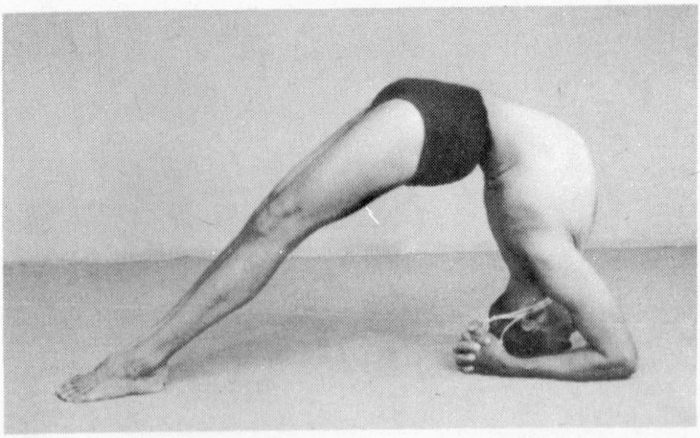

516

Technique (For advanced pupils)

1. Do Sālamba Śīrṣāsana I (Plate 190), bend the knees and drop the legs behind the back on the floor, following the various movements as in Plates 517, 518 and 519.

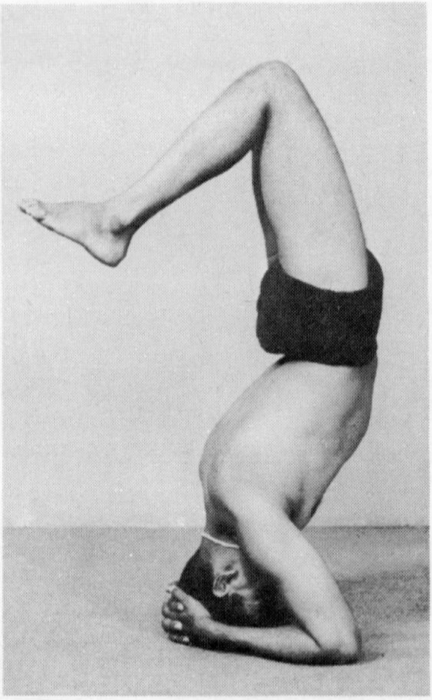

517

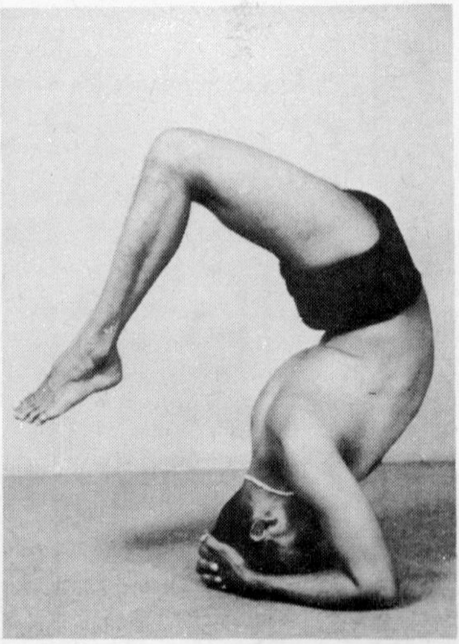

518

2. This should be done without lifting the elbows off the floor and without disturbing the position of the head on the floor.

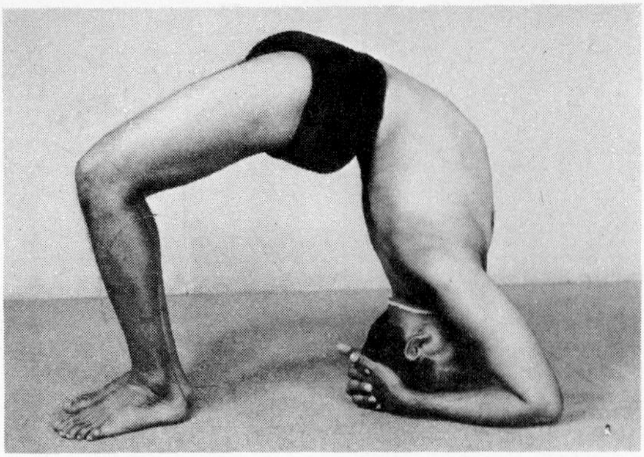

519

3. Now stretch the legs straight one by one (Plates 520 and 516) and at the same time raise and stretch the dorsal and lumbar regions of the spine. Press the heels firmly on the floor.

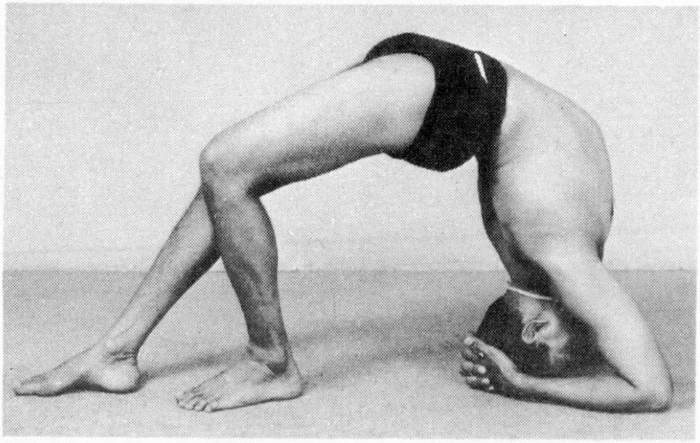

520

4. Contract the buttocks, raise the pelvic region up and tighten the knees, thighs and calves.

5. Attempt to stay in this position for a minute or two with normal breathing.

6. Then bend the knees and swing the legs up with an exhalation back to Sālamba Śīrṣāsana I. Rest there for a few seconds with deep breathing and lower the legs to the floor. Release the grip of the fingers, lift the head from the floor and relax or perform Ūrdhva Dhanurāsana (Plate 486) and stand in Tāḍāsana (Plate 1) or move into Viparīta Chakrāsana. (Plates 488 to 499)

Effects

This exhilarating pose keeps the spine sound and healthy while the chest expands fully. Along with this, one also feels the effects of Śīrṣāsana. It is recommended for relieving pain in the coccyx region of the spine.

The pose has a very soothing effect on the mind, so that the emotionally disturbed find it a great boon.

178. *Eka Pāda Viparīta Daṇḍāsana I* Twenty-six* (Plate 521)

Eka means one and Pāda a leg or foot. Viparīta means reverse or inverted. Daṇḍa is a staff or rod, a symbol of authority and punishment. It also means the body. The pose is an advanced movement of Dwi Pāda Viparīta Daṇḍāsana. (Plate 516)

Technique

1. Perform Dwi Pāda Viparīta Daṇḍāsana. (Plate 516)

2. Exhale and lift the left leg up vertically while keeping the right leg on the floor in Viparīta Daṇḍāsana. (Plate 521)

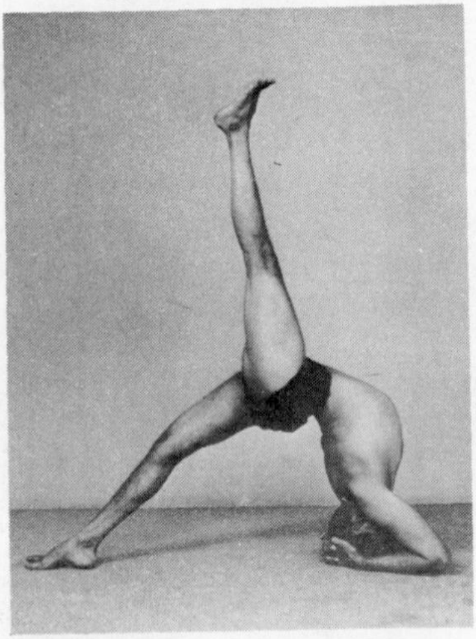

521

3. Stay in this pose with normal breathing for 10 seconds.

4. Lower the left leg and come to Viparīta Daṇḍāsana. Then with an exhalation, repeat the pose for an equal length of time, keeping the right leg perpendicular.

5. Come back to Viparīta Daṇḍāsana and then relax on the floor.

6. Advanced pupils may, with an exhalation, swing both the legs up to Sālamba Śīrṣāsana I (Plate 190), then lower them to the floor and relax or perform Ūrdhva Dhanurāsana (Plate 486) and stand up in Tāḍāsana (Plate 1) or move into Viparīta Chakrāsana. (Plates 488 to 499)

Effects

The pose tones the spine and expands the chest fully. Coupled with this are the effects of Śīrṣāsana. (Plate 190.) This exhilarating pose also soothes the mind.

179. *Eka Pāda Viparīta Daṇḍāsana II* Twenty-nine* (Plate 523)

This is a more strenuous version of the earlier āsana.

Technique

1. Perform Dwi Pāda Viparīta Daṇḍāsana. (Plate 516)

2. Move both feet towards the head.

3. Release the fingers, spread the wrists and rest the palms on the floor.

4. With an exhalation, raise the head off the floor, extend the neck towards the legs and bring the right leg nearer to the hands.

5. Catch the right ankle with both hands and keep the entire foot on the floor. (Plate 522)

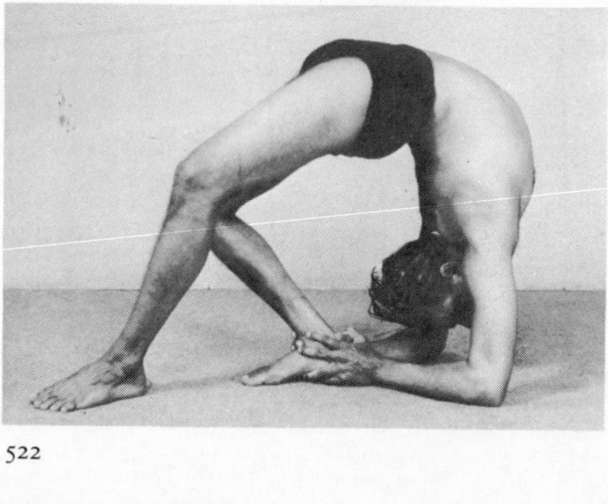

522

6. When the grip on the ankle is firm, exhale and lift the left leg up vertically by stretching the shoulders up and extending the spine. Keep the leg up taut at the knee. (Plate 523)

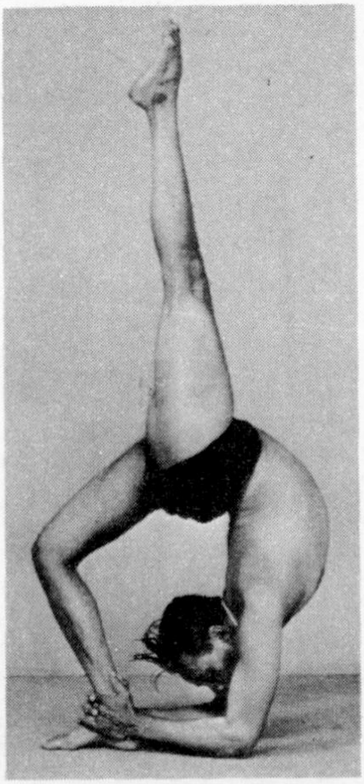

523

7. Stay in the pose from 10 to 15 seconds. Due to the contraction of the abdominal muscles, breathing will be fast and laboured.

8. Bring the left leg down to the floor.

9. Release the right ankle and catch the left one. Repeat the pose described above, now raising the right leg up vertically. Stay in the pose on the other side for the same length of time. Then lower the raised leg.

10. Release the ankle and with an exhalation swing both the legs up to Sālamba Śīrṣāsana I (Plate 190), then lower them to the floor and relax or do Ūrdhva Dhanurāsana (Plate 486) and stand up in Tāḍāsana (Plate 1) or move into Viparīta Chakrāsana. (Plates 488 to 499)

Effects

In this āsana, the abdominal muscles are exercised and the spine is toned. As the bending is more strenuous, the effect is correspondingly greater.

180. *Chakra Bandhāsana* Thirty-one* (Plate 524)

Chakra means a nerve centre, the fly-wheels in the machine, that is the human body. Bandha means a fetter or a bond. The chakras are the regions situated within the spinal column where the nāḍis cross each other. There are seven of them in the human body. They are (1) Mūlādhāra Chakra (the pelvic plexus); (2) Svādhiṣṭhāna Chakra (the hypogastric plexus); (3) Maṇipūraka Chakra (the solar plexus); (4) Anāhata Chakra (the cardiac plexus); (5) Viśuddha Chakra (the pharyngeal plexus); (6) Ājñā Chakra (the plexus of command between the two eyebrows); and (7) Sahasrāra Chakra (the thousand petalled lotus, the upper cerebral centre). The chakras are subtle and not easily cognisable. Though they are here compared to the various plexi, it should not be taken for granted that the plexi alone are the chakras.

Technique

1. Perform Dwi Pāda Viparīta Daṇḍāsana. (Plate 516)
2. Move both the feet towards the head with an exhalation.
3. Release the fingers, spread the wrists and rest the forearms on the floor, fingers pointing to the feet. Take two breaths.
4. With an exhalation raise the head off the floor and extending the neck towards the legs, bring both the feet nearer to the hands.
5. Then catch the right ankle with the right hand and the left ankle with the left hand and rest the feet on the floor. Take two breaths.
6. Grip the ankles firmly and with an exhalation, press the feet and the elbows to the floor and arch the trunk by stretching the shoulders and the thighs. (Plate 524)

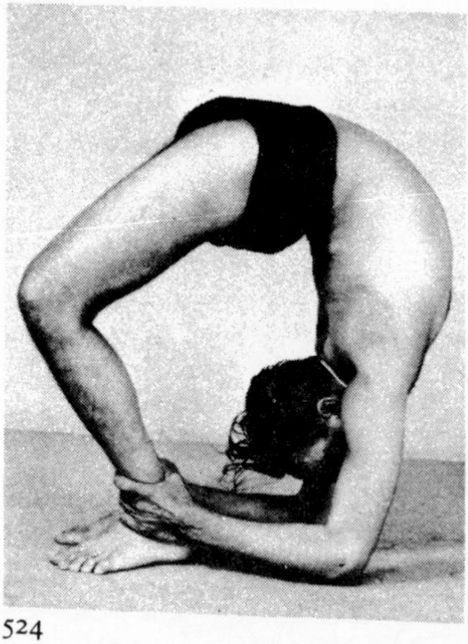

524

7. Stay in the pose from 10 to 15 seconds. Breathing will be fast.

8. Release the grip on the ankles, rest the crown of the head on the floor and interlock the fingers behind the head. Now with an exhalation swing the legs up to Sālamba Śīrṣāsana I (Plate 190) and then lower them to the floor and relax or do Ūrdhva Dhanurāsana (Plate 486) and perform Viparīta Chakrāsana (Plates 488 to 499) or stand in Tāḍāsana.

Effects

All the chakras are stimulated. The āsana helps the adrenal glands to function healthily. The rectum, kidneys, neck and eye muscles are exercised.

181. *Maṇḍalāsana* Twenty-seven* (Plates 525 to 535)

Maṇḍala means a wheel, a ring, circumference or orbit. Keeping the head and hands in Sālamba Śīrṣāsana I (Plate 190) circle round the head clockwise and then anti-clockwise. The movements of your feet will then form a circle, maṇḍala or orbit round your head which should remain stationary.

Technique

1. Perform Dwi Pāda Viparīta Daṇḍāsana. (Plate 525)

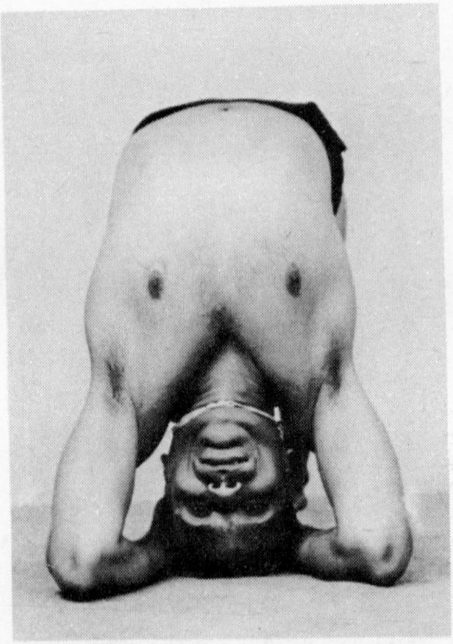

525

2. Without disturbing the head position, raise the shoulders and chest as high as possible.

3. Move the legs sideways clockwise one after the other and so circle round the head. When the legs come to the 3 o'clock and 9 o'clock positions, raise the opposite shoulder slightly, and lifting the chest up and forward, rotate the trunk as shown in the plates. (Plates 525 to 535.) The spine is given a complete circular rotation of 360 degrees.

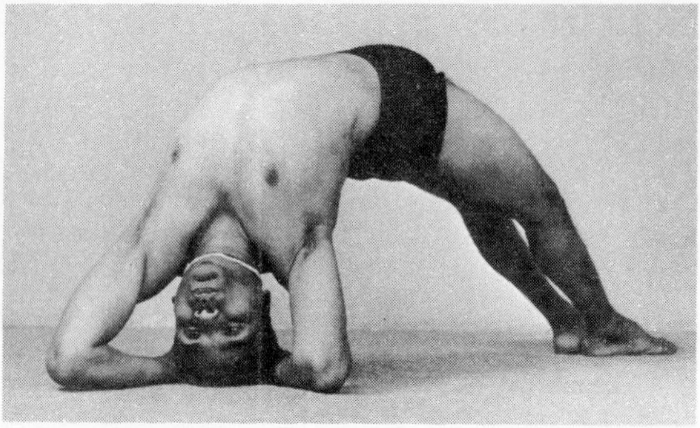

526

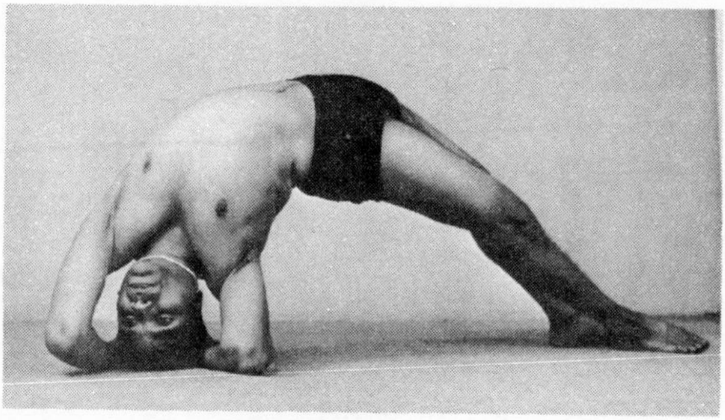

527

4. After completing the full circle clockwise, pause awhile and take a few deep breaths. Then repeat the movement anti-clockwise following the plates in the reverse order.

5. To get sufficient elasticity it is necessary first to make the spine supple by practising Viparīta Chakrāsana (Plates 488 to 499) in Ūrdhva Dhanurāsana. (Plate 486.) To start with the neck and shoulders sag towards the floor. After they have gained sufficient strength and the back has become elastic it is easier to perform this āsana.

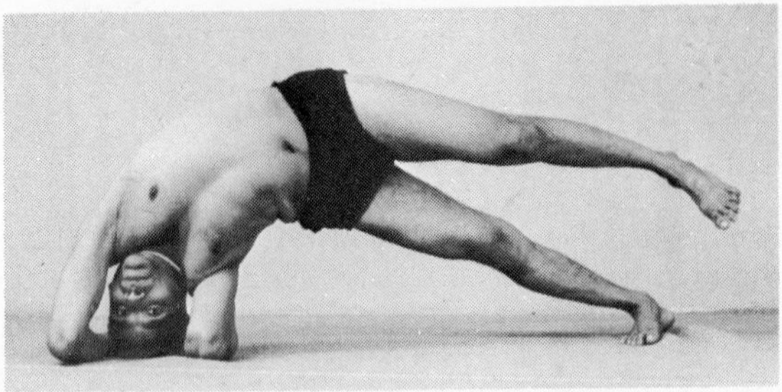

528

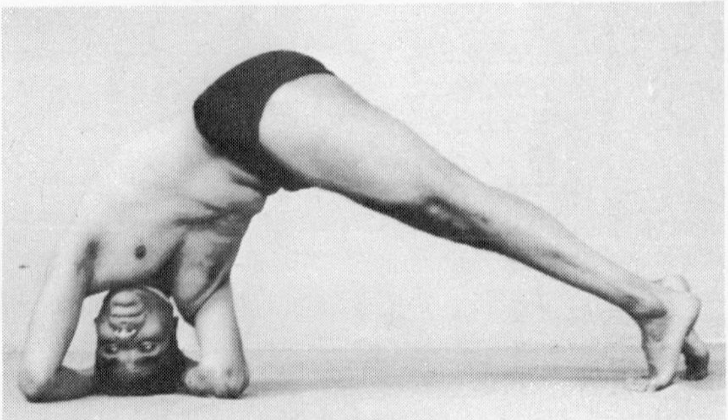

529

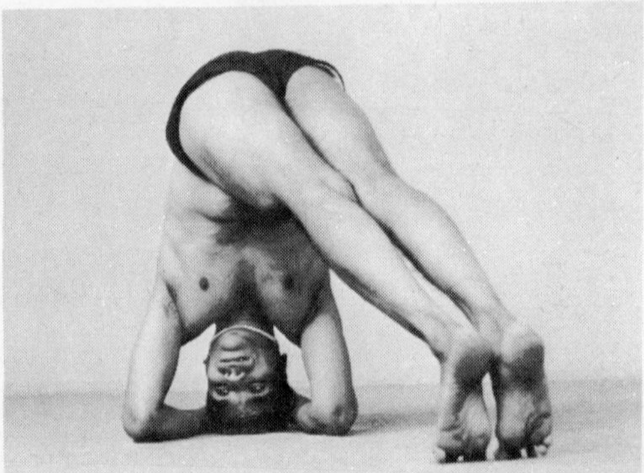

530

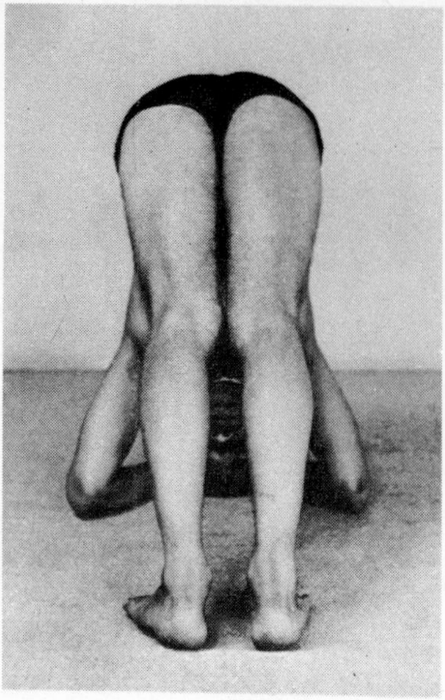

531

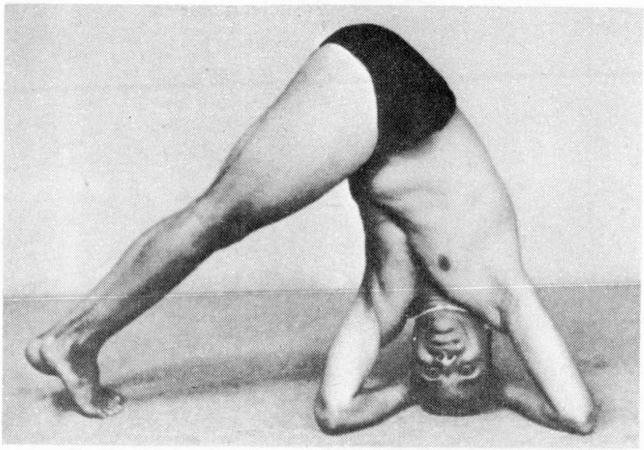

532

Effects

During the rotation, the trunk and abdomen are contracted on one side and stretched on the other side. This keeps the spine and the abdominal organs in trim and promotes health and longevity.

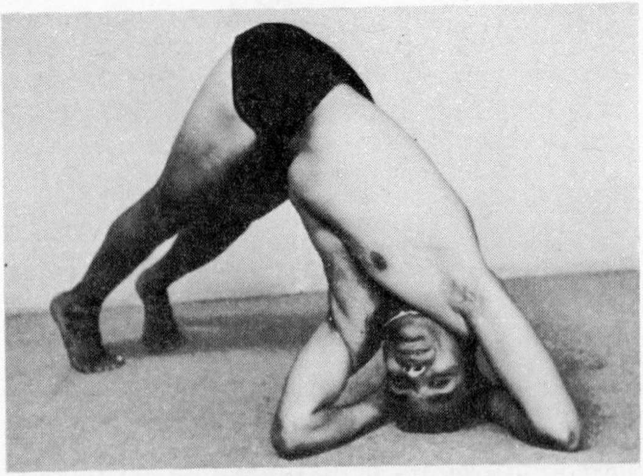
533

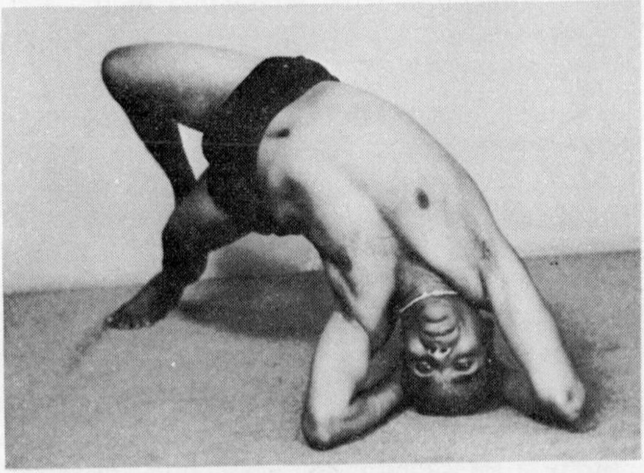
534

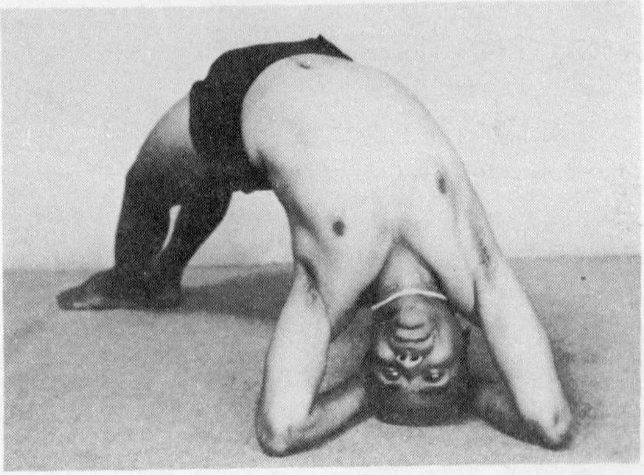
535

182. *Vṛśchikāsana I* Thirty-two* (Plates 536 and 537)

Vṛśchika means a scorpion. In order to sting its victim the scorpion arches its tail above its back and then strikes beyond its head. This posture resembles that of a striking scorpion, hence the name.

Technique

1. Kneel on the floor, bend forward and rest the elbows, forearms and palms on the floor parallel to each other. The distance between the forearms should not be wider than that between the shoulders.

2. Extend the neck and lift the head as high as you can above the floor.

3. Exhale, swing the legs and trunk up and try to balance without dropping the legs beyond the head. Stretch the region of the chest up vertically, keeping the arms from the elbows to the shoulders perpendicular to the floor. Stretch the legs up vertically and balance. This is Pīncha Mayūrāsana. (Plate 357)

4. After balancing on the forearms, exhale, bend the knees, raise the neck and head as high as you can above the floor, stretch the spine from the shoulders and lower the feet until the heels rest on the crown of the head. (Front view: Plate 536.) After you have learnt this, try to keep the knees and ankles together and the toes pointing. (Side view: Plate 537.) From the heels to the knees, the legs should be perpendicular to the head. The shins and the upper arms should be parallel to each other.

5. As the neck, shoulders, chest, spine and abdomen are all extended in this pose, breathing will be very fast and heavy. Try to breathe normally and stay in this posture as long as you can for about 30 seconds.

6. After holding the pose to your capacity, drop the legs to the floor beyond the head, lift the elbows from the floor and straighten the arms to perform Ūrdhva Dhanurāsana. (Plate 486)

7. Then, either stand up in Tāḍāsana (Plate 1) or do Viparīta Chakrāsana. (Plates 488 to 499)

8. To relieve the strain on the back caused by Vṛśchikāsana, bend forward and touch the palms on the floor without bending the knees – Uttānāsana. (Plate 48)

183. *Vṛśchikāsana II* Thirty-three* (Plate 538)

This is a harder version of the earlier one as it is practised while doing the full arm balance – Adho Mukha Vṛkṣāsana. (Plate 359)

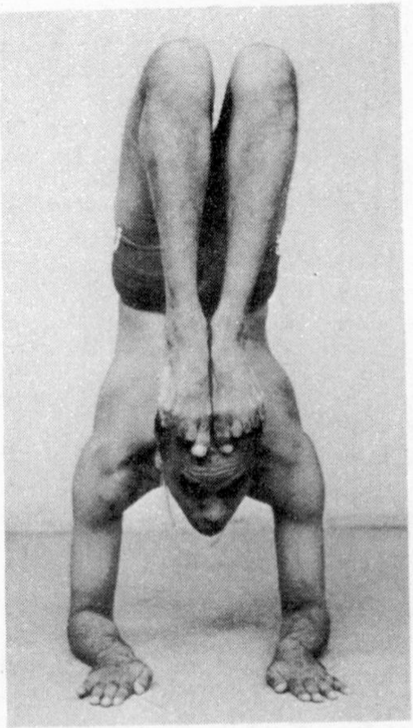

536

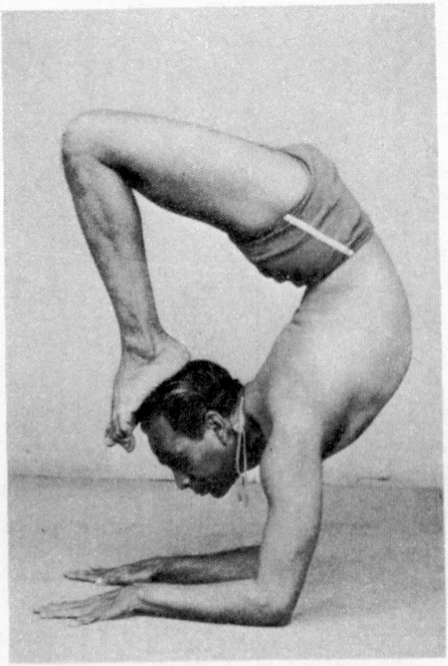

537

Technique

1. Stand in Tāḍāsana. (Plate 1.) Bend forward and place the palms on the floor. The distance between them should be the same as that between the shoulders. Keep the arms fully stretched.

2. Lift the legs and bend the knees. Exhale, swing the trunk and legs up vertically and balance on the hands. Lift the neck and head as high as possible above the floor. This is Adho Mukha Vṛkṣāsana. (Plate 359)

3. After securing the balance, exhale, bend the knees, stretch the spine and chest and lower the feet till the heels rest on the crown of the head. Keep the toes pointing. When balancing try to keep the knees and ankles joined. The shins should be perpendicular to the head and the arms to the floor. The shins and arms should be parallel to each other. (Plate 538)

4. It is extremely difficult to balance in this pose, which is much harder to perform than doing it as described earlier in Pīncha Mayūrāsana. (Plate 537)

5. It requires tremendous strength of the wrists and determined and continued effort to master this āsana. Breathing will be fast and laboured because the neck, shoulders, chest and spine are extended and the

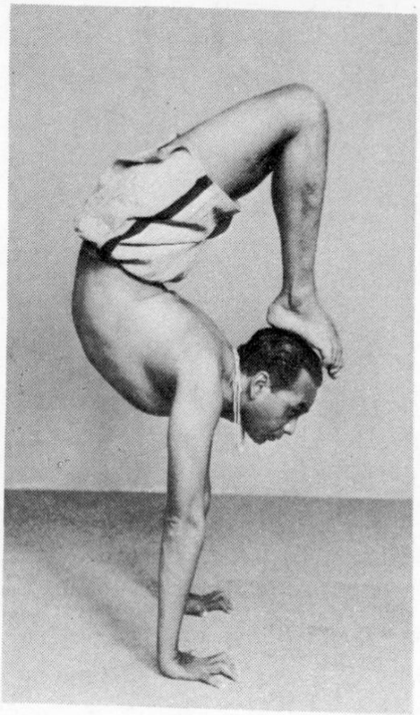

538

abdomen is contracted. Try to maintain normal breathing and stay in the pose as long as you can from 10 to 15 seconds.

6. Then drop the legs to the floor beyond the head to perform Ūrdhva Dhanurāsana (Plate 486) and either stand up in Tāḍāsana (Plate 1) or perform Viparīta Chakrāsana. (Plates 488 to 499)

7. To get relief from the strain on the back caused by Vṛśchikāsana, bend forward and touch the palms on the floor without bending the knees – Uttānāsana. (Plate 48)

Effects

The lungs expand fully while the abdominal muscles are stretched. The entire spine is vigorously toned and remains healthy. The āsana has also psychological significance. The head which is the seat of knowledge and power is also the seat of pride, anger, hatred, jealousy, intolerance and malice. These emotions are more deadly than the poison which the scorpion carries in its sting. The yogi, by stamping on his head with his feet, attempts to eradicate these self-destroying emotions and passions. By kicking his head he seeks to develop humility, calmness and tolerance and thus to be free of ego. The subjugation of the ego leads to harmony and happiness.

184. *Eka Pāda Rājakapotāsana I* Twenty-eight* (Plate 542)

Eka means one, pāda the leg or foot and kapota a dove or pigeon. Rājakapota means the king of pigeons. In this āsana, the chest is pushed forward like that of a pouter pigeon, hence the name of the pose.

Technique

1. Sit on the floor, with the legs stretched straight in front. (Plate 77)

2. Bend the right knee and place the right foot on the floor so that the right heel touches the left groin. Keep the right knee on the floor.

3. Take the left leg back and rest its entire length straight on the floor. The front of the left thigh, knee and shin and the upper part of the toes of the left foot will then touch the floor.

4. Place the palms on the waist, push the chest forward, stretch the neck, throw the head as far back as possible and balance for some time in this preparatory movement of the pose. (Plate 539)

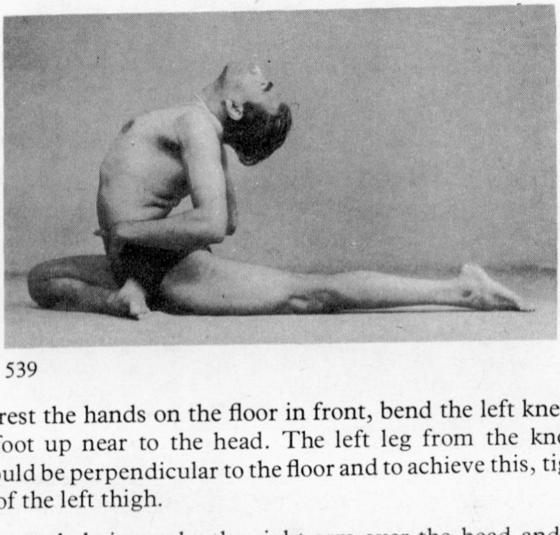

539

5. Now rest the hands on the floor in front, bend the left knee and lift the left foot up near to the head. The left leg from the knee to the ankle should be perpendicular to the floor and to achieve this, tighten the muscles of the left thigh.

6. With an exhalation, take the right arm over the head and grip the left foot with the right hand. (Plate 540.) Take a few breaths. Then exhale again and catch the left foot with the left hand. Rest the head against the left foot. (Plate 541)

7. Push the chest forward, move the hands further down, grip the ankles and lower the head so that the upper lip touches the left heel. (Plate

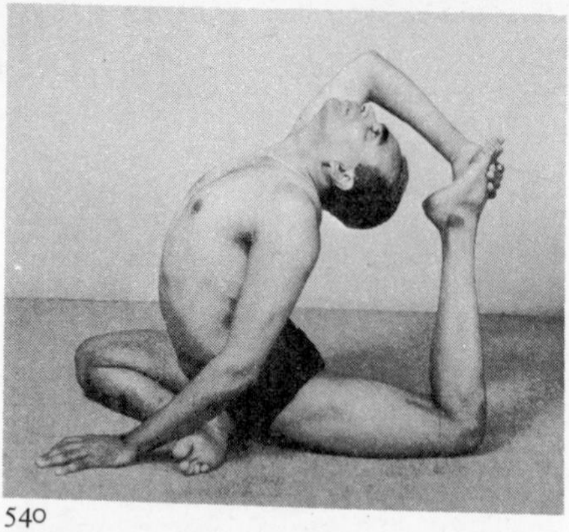

540

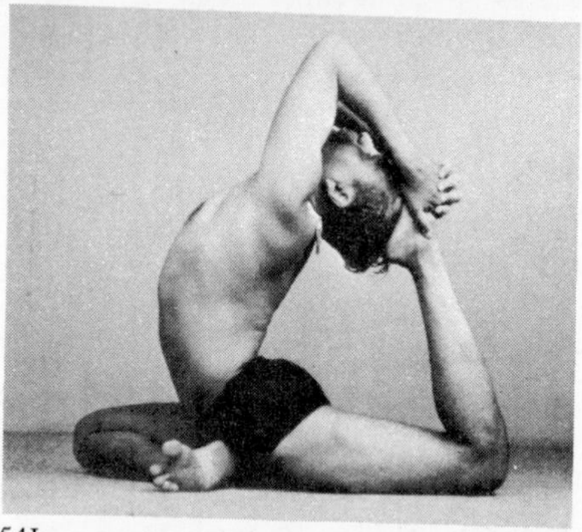

541

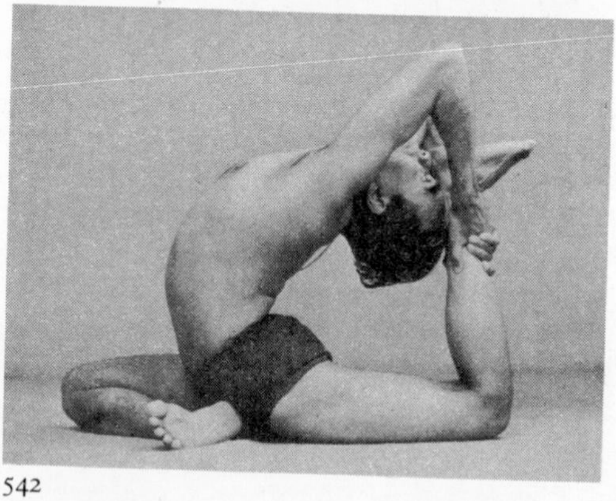

542

542.) Stay in the pose for about 10 seconds. As the chest is expanded fully while the abdomen is contracted, breathing will be fast. Try and breathe normally.

8. Release the grip of the hands on the left ankle one by one and place the palms on the floor. Straighten the left leg and bring it in front, then straighten the right leg.

9. Repeat the pose on the other side for the same length of time. This time the left foot will touch the right groin, the right leg will be stretched back and the right foot will be caught by extending both arms over the head.

185. *Vālakhilyāsana* Forty-five* (Plate 544)

The Vālakhilya were heavenly spirits the size of a thumb, produced from the Creator's body. They are said to precede the Sun's chariot and to number sixty thousand. They are referred to in Kālidāsa's epic poem *Raghuvaṁśa*. This difficult āsana is a continuation of Eka Pāda Rājakapotāsana I. (Plate 542.) (Do not attempt it until you have mastered Eka Pāda Rājakapotāsana I and can perform the latter comfortably and gracefully.)

Technique

1. Perform Eka Pāda Rājakapotāsana I. (Plate 542.) After gripping the left ankle firmly with both the hands, contract the hips and move the coccyx up. Without releasing the ankle, stretch the left leg back (Plate 543) and take a few breaths.

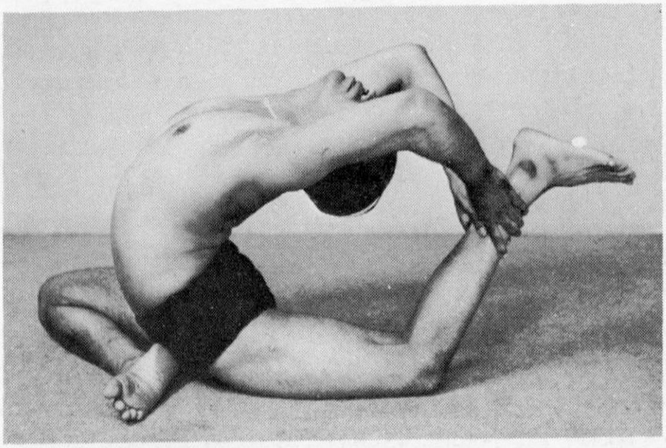

543

2. Exhale, extend the arms further and push the leg down until it lies flat on the floor. The entire front of the leg from the thigh to the toes should touch the floor. (Plate 544)

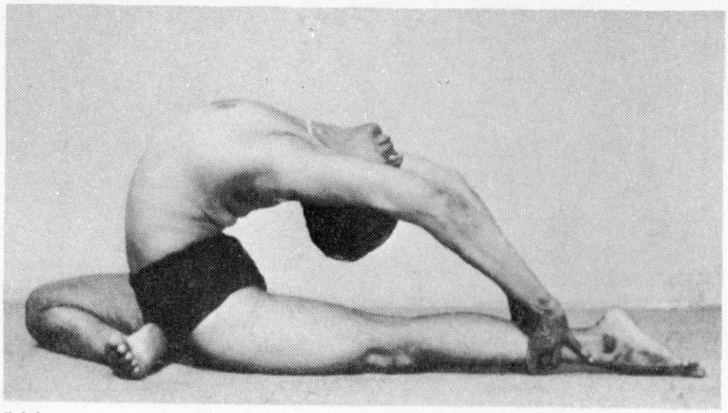

544

3. Stay in the pose for a few seconds. As the chest is fully extended while the abdominal organs are contracted, breathing will be fast and laboured.

4. Release the ankle grip, straighten the back and rest for a while.

5. Repeat the pose on the other side for the same length of time.

Effects

The pose is a counter movement of Jānu Śīrṣāsana (Plate 127) and it rejuvenates the lower region of the spine. In it more blood circulates round the pubic region, keeping it in a healthy condition. By practising this and other poses of the Rājakapotāsana cycle, disorder of the urinary system is rectified. The neck and shoulder muscles are exercised fully. The thyroids, parathyroids, adrenals and gonads receive a rich supply of blood and this increases one's vitality. This and other āsanas of the Rājakapotāsana cycle are recommended for controlling sexual desire.

186. *Eka Pāda Rājakapotāsana II* Twenty-nine* (Plate 545)

Technique

1. Sit on the floor, with legs stretched straight in front. (Plate 77)

2. Bend the right knee and place the sole and heel of the right foot flat on the floor. The shin of the right leg will then be almost perpendicular to the floor and the calf will touch the back of the thigh. Place the right heel near the perineum. The right leg will now be in Marīchyāsana I. (Plate 144)

3. Take the left leg back and rest the entire length of it on the floor.

4. Bend the left leg at the knee until the left shin is perpendicular to the floor. Balance the body on the right foot and the left knee. In order

to balance push the right knee forward until the right thigh is parallel to the floor and the shin is almost at an angle of 40 degrees to the floor.

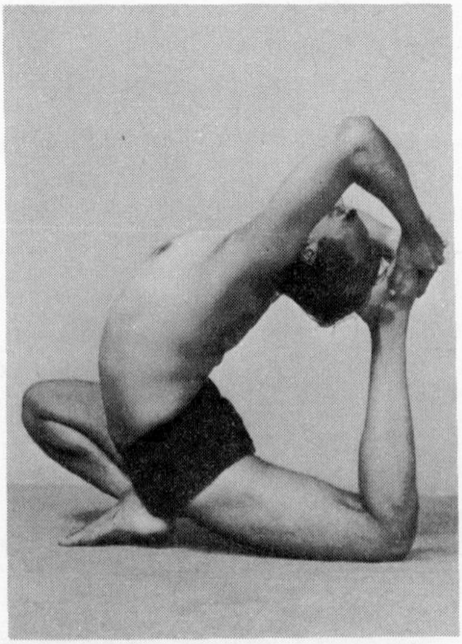

545

5. With an exhalation, take the right arm over the head and grip the left foot firmly with the right hand. Take a few breaths and after exhaling again take the left arm over the head and catch the same foot with the left hand as well. Rest the head on the foot. (Plate 545)

6. Push the chest forward and hold the pose for about 15 seconds.

7. Due to the extension of the chest and contraction of the abdomen breathing will be fast. Try to keep it normal.

8. Release the grip on the ankles and straighten the legs.

9. Repeat the pose on the other side. This time the left leg will be in Marīchyāsana I, the right foot will be caught by the hands and the balance maintained while the head rests on it. Hold the pose for the same length of time on both sides.

10. This āsana is easier than the earlier one, once the difficulty of balancing in it is overcome.

187. *Eka Pāda Rājakapotāsana III* Thirty* (Plate 546)

Technique

1. Sit on the floor, with both legs stretched straight in front. (Plate 77)

2. Bend the left leg at the knee so that the toes point back and touch the floor by the left buttock. The inner side of the left calf should touch the outer side of the left thigh and the left knee should be kept on the floor. The left leg will not be in Vīrāsana. (Plate 89)

3. Take the right leg back and rest its entire length straight on the floor.

4. Place the palms on the floor. Exhale, bend the right knee and take the right foot up near the head. The right shin from knee to ankle should be perpendicular to the floor and to get this position, tighten the muscles of the right thigh. Take a few breaths.

5. Exhale, stretch the spine and neck, throw the head back and taking the arms one by one over the head grip the right foot and rest the head on it. (Plate 546.) Balance for about 15 seconds and try to breathe normally.

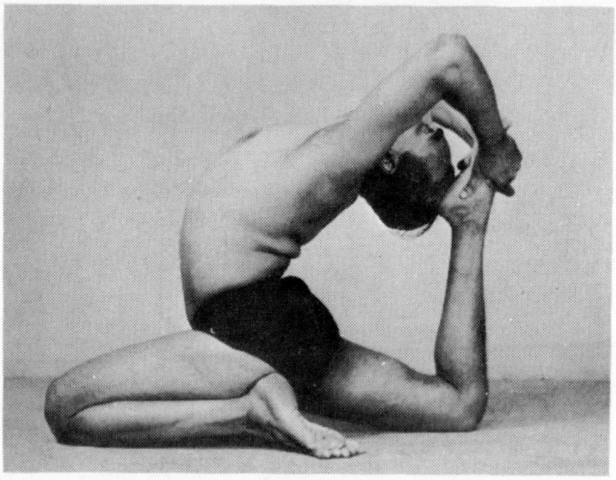

546

6. Release the grip on the right ankle and straighten the legs.

7. Repeat the pose for the same length of time on the other side. Now the right leg will be in Vīrāsana and the head will rest on the left foot which will be caught by both hands taken over the head.

188. *Eka Pāda Rājakapotāsana IV* Forty* (Plate 547)

Technique

1. Kneel on the floor and place the palms on either side of the body on the floor. Lift the knees up. Bring the right leg forward and the left leg back and stretch both legs straight with an exhalation. The back of the leg in front and the front of the leg in the rear should touch the floor.

The legs will now be in Hanumānāsana (Plate 475), which resembles the splits of Western ballet.

2. Push the chest forward, extend the neck and throw the head as far back as you can. Bend the left knee and take the left foot up near the head. The left shin from knee to ankle should be perpendicular to the floor.

3. With an exhalation, take the left arm over the head and grip the left foot with the left hand. After taking a few breaths, exhale again, take the right arm over the head and catch the left foot with the right hand. Rest the head against it. (Plate 547)

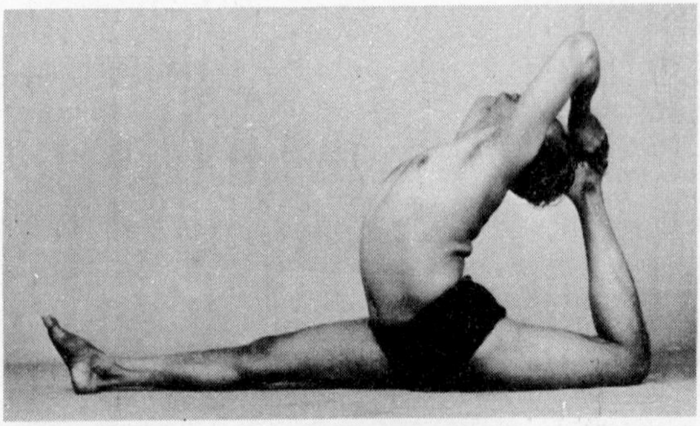

547

4. Stay in the pose for about 10 seconds. Release the grip on the left foot and come back to Hanumānāsana. (Plate 475.) Raise the hips from the floor by placing the palms on the ground.

5. Now return to Hanumānāsana, this time keeping the left leg stretched straight on the floor in front. Bend the right knee and take the right foot up near the head.

6. Repeat the pose by catching the right foot and resting the head on it. Stay for the same length of time on this side.

Effects of the Eka Pāda Rājakapotāsana Cycle

These poses rejuvenate the lumbar and dorsal regions of the spine. The neck and shoulder muscles are fully exercised and the various positions of the legs strengthen the thighs and ankles. The thyroids, parathyroids, adrenals and gonads receive a rich supply of blood and function properly, which increases vitality. In these poses more blood circulates round the pubic region, which is kept healthy. These āsanas are recommended for disorders of the urinary system and for controlling sexual desire.

189. *Bhujaṅgāsana II* Thirty-seven* (Plate 550)

Bhujaṅga means a serpent. This pose is preparatory to Rājakapotāsana (Plate 551), and resembles that of a serpent about to strike.

Technique

1. Lie flat on the floor on the stomach. Bend the elbows and place the palms on the floor on either side of the waist.

2. Exhale, lift the head and trunk up and back, by stretching the arms fully, without moving the pubic region and the legs. (Plate 73)

3. Remain in this position breathing normally for a few seconds.

4. Exhale, bend the knees and lift the feet up. The weight of the body will be felt on the pelvic region, thighs and hands. Take a few breaths.

5. Taking more pressure on the right hand, lift the left hand off the floor and with a deep exhalation swing the left arm back from the shoulder and grasp the left knee-cap. (Plate 548.) After a few breaths exhale again fast and deeply, and swinging the right arm back from the shoulder, grip the right knee-cap with the right hand. (Plate 549)

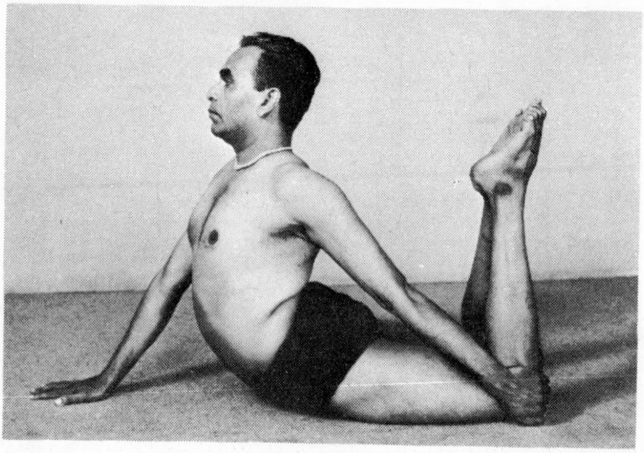

548

6. Stretch the legs straight on the floor again without loosening the grip on the knees. Stretch the neck and throw the head as far back as you can. (Plate 550.) Gradually try to bring the knees as close to each other as possible.

7. Contract the anus, tighten the thighs and hold the pose for about 15 to 20 seconds. As the spine, chest and shoulders are fully extended while the abdomen is contracted, breathing is fast and difficult.

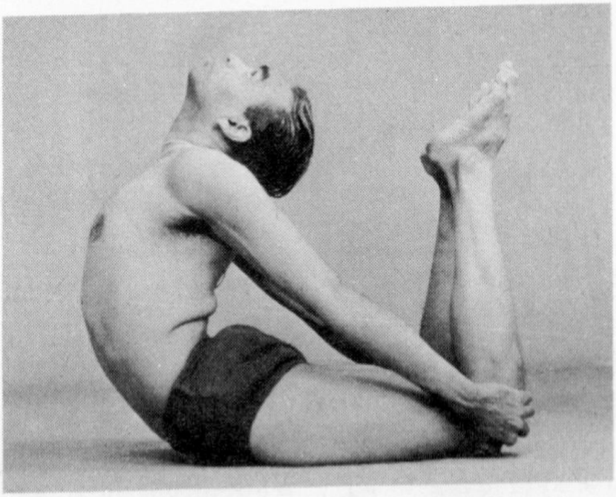

549

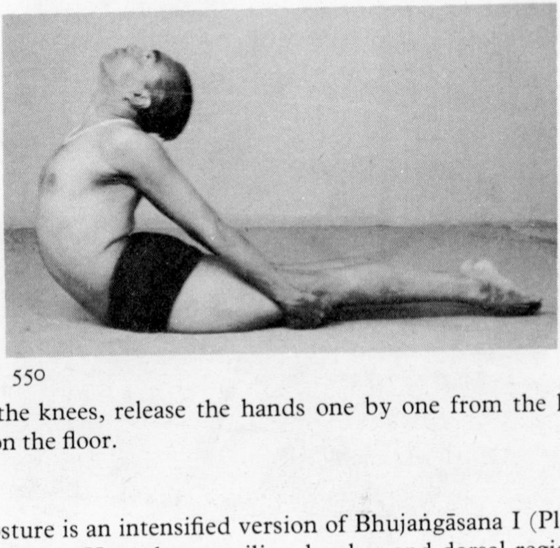

550

8. Bend the knees, release the hands one by one from the knee-caps and rest on the floor.

Effects

As the posture is an intensified version of Bhujaṅgāsana I (Plate 73) its effect is greater. Here the sacroiliac, lumbar and dorsal regions of the spine benefit along with the neck and shoulder muscles which are fully stretched. In this pose more blood circulates in the pubic region which is kept healthy. The thyroids, parathyroids, adrenals and gonads receive a copious supply of blood and this results in increased vitality. The chest is also expanded fully.

190. *Rājakapotāsana* Thirty-eight* (Plate 551)

Rājakapota means the king of pigeons. This is a very attractive but difficult pose. The chest is pushed forward like that of a strutting pigeon, hence this name.

Technique

1. Lie full length on the floor on the stomach, bend the elbows and place the palms on the floor on either side of the waist.

2. Exhale, lift the head and trunk up and back by stretching the arms fully, without moving the pubic region and the legs. Remain in this position for a few seconds, breathing normally.

3. Exhale, bend the knees and lift the feet up. The body weight will be felt by the pelvic region and the thighs. Take a few breaths.

4. Taking pressure on the right hand, lift the left hand and with a fast and deep exhalation swing the left arm back from the shoulder and catch hold of the left knee-cap. (Plate 548.) Take a few breaths. Again with a fast and deep exhalation, swing the right arm back from the shoulder and grip the right knee-cap with the right hand. (Plate 549)

5. Raise the chest and using the hold on the knees as a lever stretch the spine and neck still further back until the head rests on the soles and heels. Keep the feet together and the knees as close to each other as possible. (Plate 551)

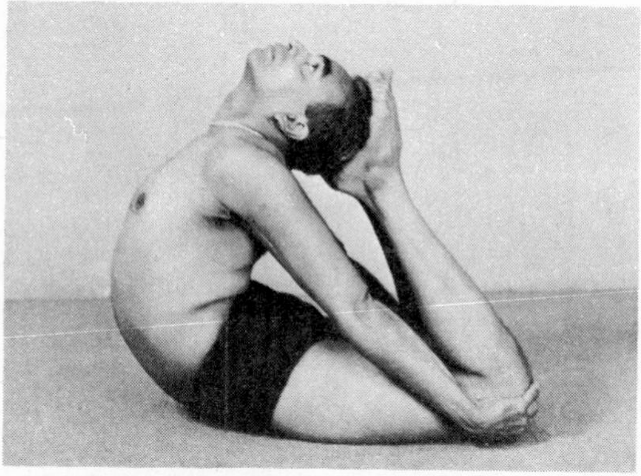

551

6. Maintain the pose as long as you can for about 15 seconds. As the spine and chest are fully extended while the abdomen is pressed against the ground, breathing will be very fast and difficult and a stay of about 15 seconds will seem like an age. The pose closely resembles Laghu Vajrāsana (Plate 513), the difference being that the body now rests on

the pelvic region and the thighs, instead of on the legs from the knees to the toes.

7. Stretch the legs straight again. Let go of the knees and bring the palms in front on the floor one by one. If both hands are released simultaneously, due to the tension of the spine one is apt to fall on the face and hurt oneself. After resting the palms one by one in front, rest the chest on the floor and relax.

8. If this is difficult, place the palms on the floor and rest the crown of the head on the feet. (Plate 552)

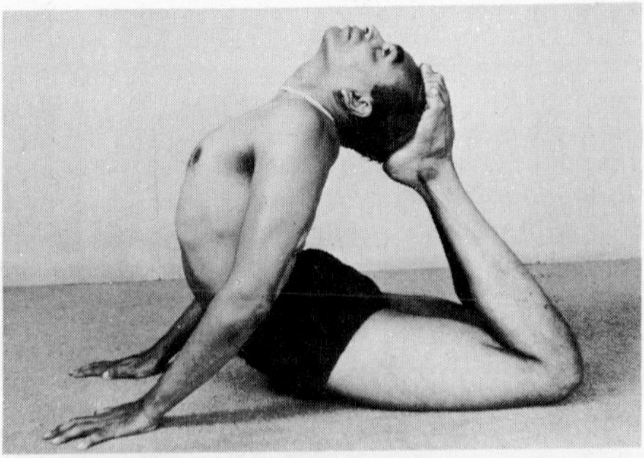

552

Effects

In Kapotāsana (Plate 512) the lumbar region of the spine feels the stretch. In Rājakapotāsana on the other hand, both the lumbar and the dorsal regions of the spine benefit by it. The neck and shoulder muscles are fully stretched and exercised. As the weight of the body falls on the pubic region, more blood circulates there so that the region is kept healthy. The abdominal organs are pressed against the floor and so are massaged. The thyroids, parathyroids, adrenals and the gonads receive a copious and rich supply of blood and this ensures increased vitality. The āsana is recommended for disorders of the urinary system. Along with Kandāsana (Plate 471) and Supta Trivikramāsana (Plate 478) Rājakapotāsana is recommended for controlling sexual desire.

191. *Pādāṅguṣṭha Dhanurāsana* Forty-three* (Plate 555)

Pāda means the foot. Aṅguṣṭha means the big toe and dhanu a bow. This is an intensified version of Dhanurāsana. (Plate 63)

The body here resembles a taut bow from the shoulders to the knees. The legs from the knees to the toes and the extended arms over the head resemble the tightly drawn bow-string.

The posture is given below in three movements.

Technique

1. Lie flat on the floor on the stomach, face downwards.

2. Put the palms on the floor on either side of the chest. Press them down and straightening the arms, raise the head and trunk off the floor as in Bhujaṅgāsana I. (Plate 73.) Bend the knees and lift the feet up. Exhale, move the feet and head closer to each other and try to touch the head with the feet. (Plate 552)

3. Place one foot over the other. Then, putting greater weight on the hand on one side, lift the other hand off the floor. With a fast and deep exhalation stretch the lifted arm from the shoulder over the head and catch the toes. (Plate 553.) Now lift the other hand off the floor with an exhalation and also grasp the toes. Maintain a firm grip on the toes and with the right hand catch the right big toe tightly and hold the left one with the left hand. (Plate 554.) Take a few breaths.

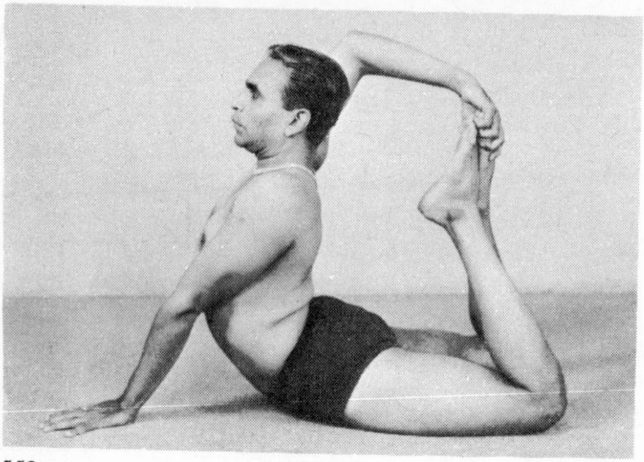

553

4. Hold the feet firmly, otherwise they will slip from the hands. Then with an exhalation stretch the arms and the legs as high as you can above the head. Try to straighten the arms at the elbows. This is the first movement. (Plate 555.) Hold the pose for about 15 seconds.

5. Maintaining the grip on the toes, now bend the elbows and pull the feet down until the heels rest on the head. Gradually increase the tension so that the heels rest first on the forehead, then on the eyes

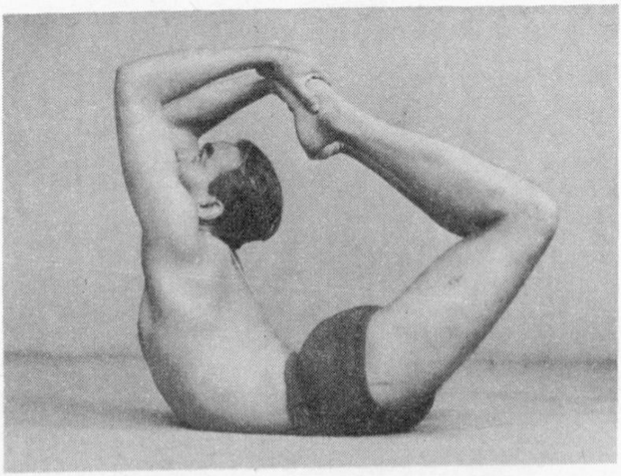

554

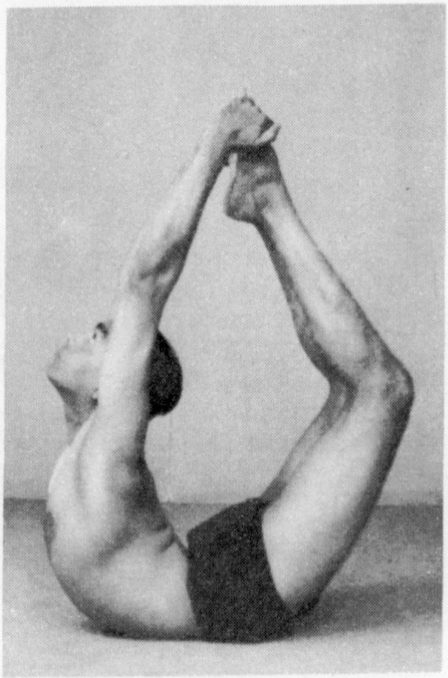

555

and lastly on the lips. (Plate 556.) This is the second movement. Stay in the pose for a few seconds.

6. Still maintaining a firm grip on the toes, lower the feet until they touch the sides of the shoulders. (Plate 557.) This is the third movement. Stay in it for a few seconds.

7. After completing the third movement, exhale and stretch the legs and

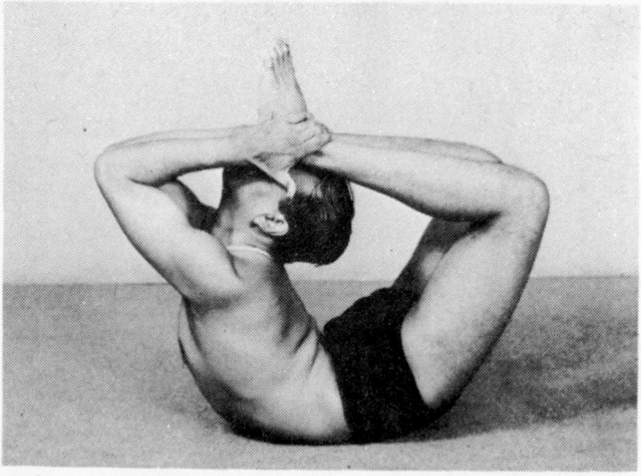

556

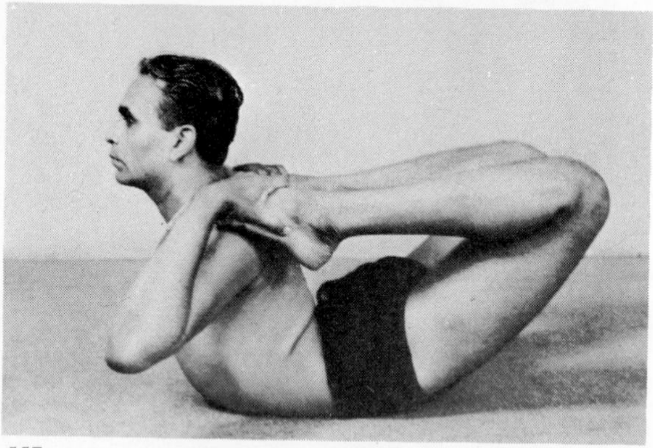

557

arms up. Release the legs one by one, putting the hands down immediately on the floor, otherwise due to the recoil of the spine, one is likely to bang the face. Then rest on the floor and relax.

8. Due to the stretch of the neck, shoulders, chest and spine as well as the pressure of the abdomen against the floor, the breathing will be very fast and laboured. Try to breathe normally during all three movements.

Effects

In this āsana, all the vertebrae benefit from the stretch. The entire body bears the strain and becomes more elastic. The whole weight falls on the abdominal area near the navel and due to the pressure on the abdominal aorta, blood circulates properly round the abdominal organs. This keeps them healthy and improves the digestion. In this posture the shoulder-blades are well stretched so that stiffness in the shoulders is relieved. The most noticeable effect, however, is that throughout the strenuous movements, the mind remains passive and still. This āsana helps to keep one trim and young in body, and fresh and alert in mind.

192. *Gheraṇḍāsana I* Forty-four* (Plates 561 and 562)

Gheraṇḍa is the name of a sage, the author of the *Gheraṇḍa Saṁhitā*, to whom the āsana is dedicated. The pose is a combination of Bhekāsana (Plate 100) and Pādāṅguṣṭha Dhanurāsana (Plate 555), the arm and leg of one side being in the position of the former āsana, while the arm and leg of the other side are in the latter āsana.

Technique

1. Lie flat on the floor on the stomach, face downwards.

2. Exhale, bend the left knee and move the left foot towards the left hip.

3. Hold the sole of the left foot with the left hand. Take a few breaths. Now rotate the left hand so that the palm touches the upper part of the left foot and the toes and fingers point to the head.

4. Exhale and push the left foot down with the left hand to bring the sole and heel closer to the ground. Lift the head and chest off the floor. The left arm and leg are now in Bhekāsana. (Plate 100.) Take a few breaths.

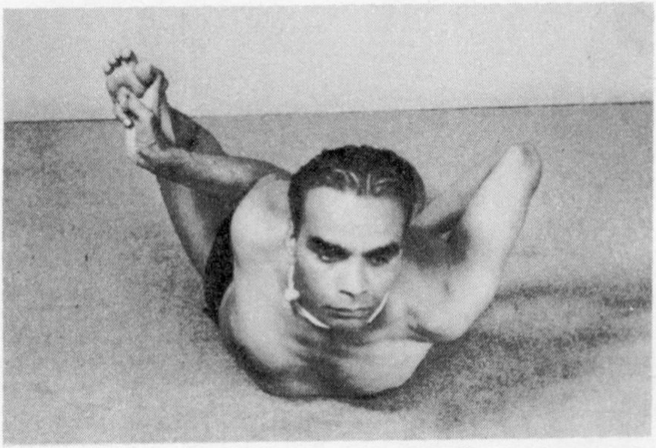

558

5. With the right hand catch the right big toe by bending the right knee. (Plate 558.) Rotate the right elbow and shoulder (Plate 559) and stretch the right arm and leg up. (Plate 560.) Take a few breaths.

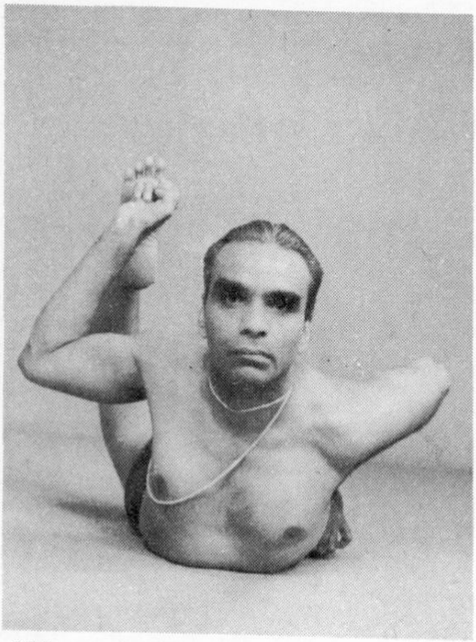

559

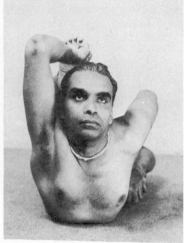

560

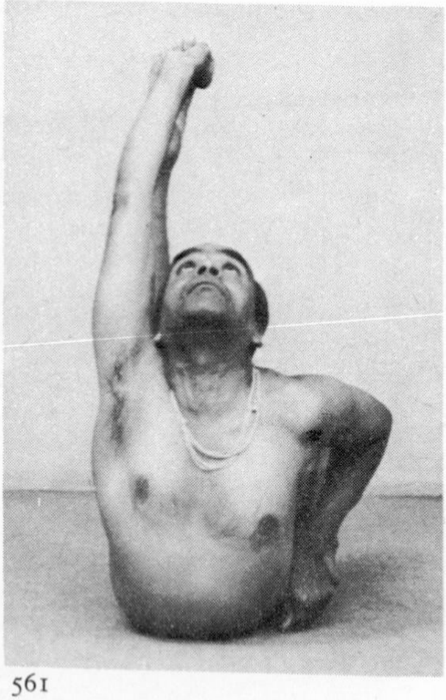

561

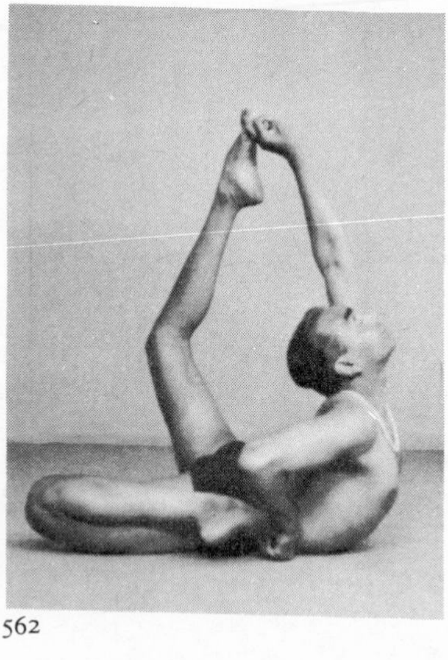

562

6. Exhale, raise the right arm and leg up vertically without releasing the grip on the right big toe. (Plates 561 and 562.) The right arm and leg are now in Pādāṅguṣṭha Dhanurāsana. (Plate 555)

7. Stay in the position from 15 to 20 seconds. Breathing will be fast due to the pressure of the abdomen on the floor.

8. Then exhale, stretch the neck and throw the head back. Bend the right elbow and knee, and pull the right leg down until the foot touches the left shoulder. (Plate 563)

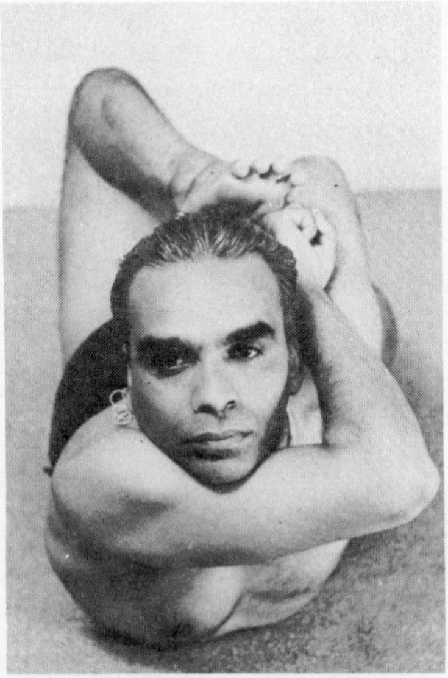

563

9. Stay in this posture for a few seconds.

10. With an exhalation come back to position 6. (Plate 561)

11. Now release the feet, stretch the legs on the floor, lower the head and chest and relax for a short time.

12. Repeat the pose, this time keeping the right arm and leg in Bhekāsana and the left arm and leg in Pādāṅguṣṭha Dhanurāsana. Stay for the same length of time in this position also. Follow the technique given above, reading left for right and vice versa.

193. *Gheraṇḍāsana II* Forty-six* (Plates 564 and 565)

In this āsana, the arm and leg of one side are in Baddha Padmāsana

(Plate 118), while the arm and leg of the other side are in Pādāṅguṣṭha Dhanurāsana. (Plate 555)

Technique

1. Sit on the floor with the legs stretched straight in front. (Plate 77.) Place the right foot at the root of the left thigh and then lie flat on the back.

2. Now roll over on the stomach without disturbing the position of the right foot. Exhale, and moving the right arm from the shoulder behind the back, catch the right big toe with the right hand. The right arm and leg are now in Baddha Padmāsana. (Plate 118.) Take a few breaths and lift the head and chest off the floor.

3. Exhale, bend the left knee and catch the left big toe with the left hand. Rotate the left arm and shoulder and without releasing the grip on the toe lift the left arm and leg up until they are in Pādāṅguṣṭha Dhanurāsana. (Plates 564 and 565)

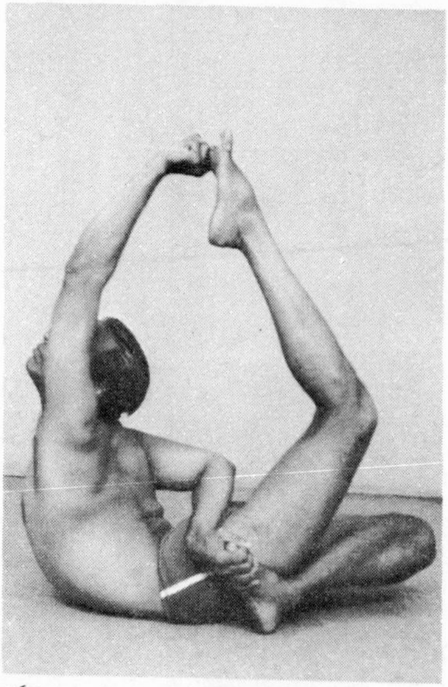

564

4. Stay in the position for 15 seconds. Breathing will be fast and laboured due to the pressure of the abdomen against the floor.

5. Then exhale, stretch the neck and throw the head back, bend the

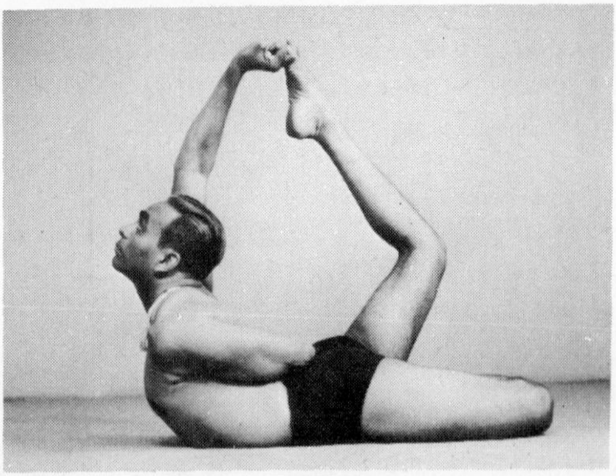

565

left elbow and knee and pull the left leg down until the foot touches the right shoulder. (Plate 566)

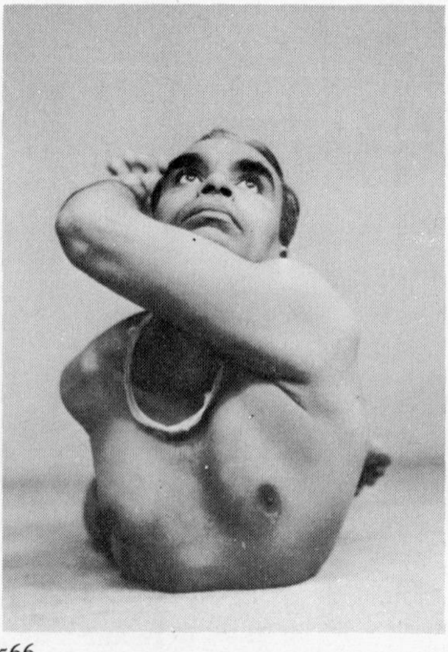

566

6. Stay in this posture for a few seconds. Due to the pressure on and contraction of the abdomen, breathing will be laboured.

7. With an exhalation come back to position 3. (Plate 564)

8. Release the hold on the feet, stretch the legs straight and lower them, the chest and head to the floor and relax for a short time.

9. Repeat the pose on the other side for the same length of time. The left arm and leg will now be in Baddha Padmāsana, while the right arm and leg will be in Pādāṅguṣṭha Dhanurāsana. Follow the technique stated above, reading left for right and vice versa.

Effects

All the vertebrae benefit from the intense stretch and the whole body becomes more supple. The abdominal area near the navel bears the weight of the body and, due to the pressure on the abdominal aorta, blood circulates properly in that region thus keeping the abdominal organs healthy. This improves the digestion. The shoulder-blades are fully extended so that stiffness in the shoulder joints is relieved. The pose makes the knees firm and relieves pain in the knee joints due to rheumatism or gout. The pressure of the hands on the feet corrects the arches and helps to cure flat feet. The pose strengthens the ankle joints, relieves pain in the heels and helps persons suffering from calcaneal spurs.

194. *Kapiñjalāsana* Forty-three* (Plate 567)

Kapiñjala is a kind of partridge, the Chātaka bird which is supposed to live only on raindrops and dew.

The pose is a combination of Vasiṣṭhānāsana (Plate 398) and Pādāṅguṣṭha Dhanurāsana (Plate 555) and is a difficult one to master.

Technique

1. Stand in Tāḍāsana. (Plate 1.) Bend forward, rest the palms on the floor and move the legs back about 4 to 5 feet as if performing Adho Mukha Svānāsana. (Plate 75)

2. Turn the whole body sideways to the right and balance it on the right palm and foot. The outer side of the right foot should rest firmly on the ground.

3. Place the left foot over the right foot, rest the left palm on the left hip and balance, without moving the body. (Plate 396.) The right side of the body is in Vasiṣṭhāsana.

4. Exhale, bend the left leg at the knees and catch the left big toe firmly between the thumb and the index and middle fingers of the left hand.

5. Rotate the left elbow and shoulder and stretch the left arm and leg behind the back to form a bow, without releasing the grip on the left big toe. (Plate 567.) The left arm and leg are now in Pādāṅguṣṭha Dhanurāsana.

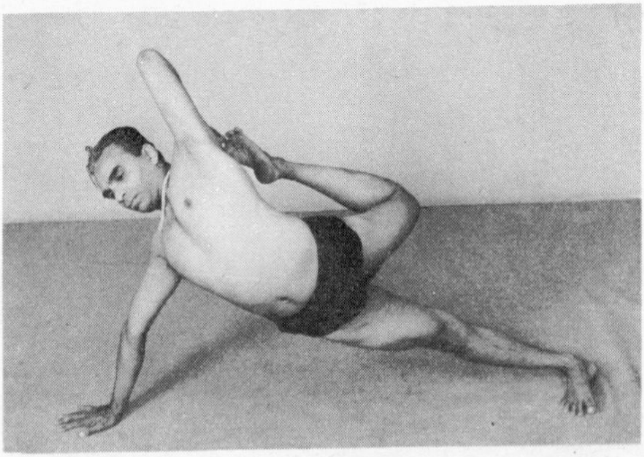

567

6. Balance for a few seconds, keeping the right arm and leg rigid and also maintaining the grip of the left hand on the left big toe. As the spine, chest, neck and shoulders are fully stretched and the abdomen is contracted, breathing will be laboured.

7. Release the grip on the left big toe, straighten the left leg and place the left foot over the right foot and the left hand on the left hip. Rest both palms and feet on the floor as in position 1 above. Then repeat the pose on the other side for the same length of time. The left side of the body will now be in Vasiṣṭhāsana (Plate 398) while the right side will be in Pādāṅguṣṭha Dhanurāsana. (Plate 555.) Follow the technique given above, reading left for right and vice versa.

Effects

In this posture the wrists are strengthened and the shoulder-blades fully exercised so that stiffness in the shoulder joints is relieved. The legs are toned and all the vertebrae benefit. The chest expands fully and the abdominal muscles become powerful. The āsana helps to keep the whole body in good condition.

195. *Śīrṣa Pādāsana* Fifty-two* (Plate 570)

Śīrṣa means the head and pāda the foot. This is the hardest of all the back-bending poses and is practised while balancing on the head in Śīrṣāsana. (Plate 190.) Here the back is arched after the head stand and the feet are brought down until the heels rest on the back of the neck and the big toes are caught by the hands and made to touch the back of the head.

Technique

1. Spread a blanket on the floor, kneel on it and perform Sālamba Śīrṣāsana I. (Plate 190)

2. Bend the knees and lower the legs behind the back. (Plates 517 and 518.) Exhale, stretch the spine, contract the buttocks, pull back and lower the thighs (Plate 568) and feet until the toes touch the back of the head. (Plate 569.) Without moving the elbows, lift the wrists slightly off the ground and catch the big toes with the hands without loosening the finger grip. (Plate 570.) Push the chest forward and stay in the pose as long as you can, for a few seconds.

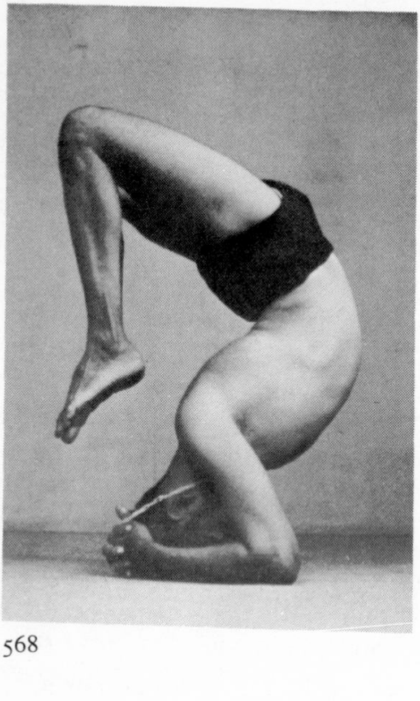

568

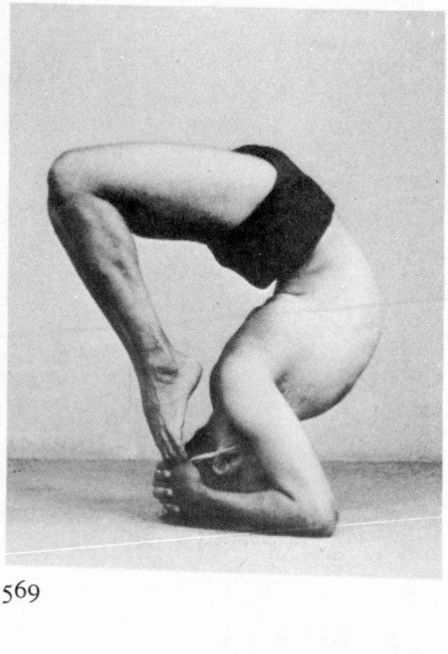

569

3. In other back-bending postures, one is able to get some help to stretch the spine. Here, however, the spine has to move independently in order to get the requisite curvature.

4. As the spine, chest, shoulders and neck are fully stretched, and the abdomen is contracted, it is difficult to breathe normally. Return to Śīrsāsana I (Plate 190), slide the legs to the floor and relax or do Ūrdhva Dhanurāsana (Plate 486) and stand up in Tāḍāsana (Plate 1), or follow on with Viparīta Chakrāsana. (Plates 488 to 499)

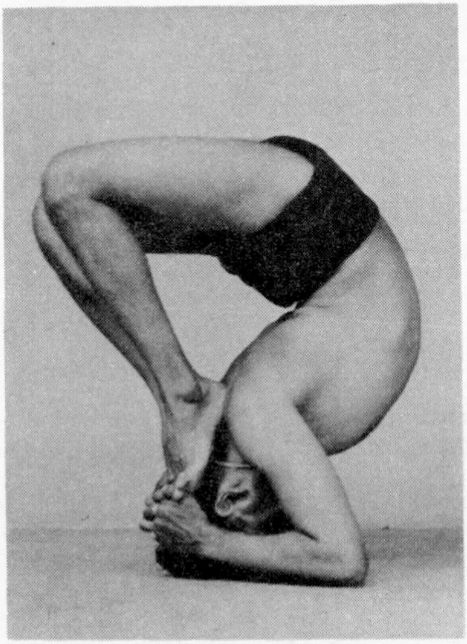

570

Effects

In addition to the effects of Śīrṣāsana I (Plate 190), all the vertebrae are exercised in this āsana. As the blood supply to the spine is increased, the nerves do not degenerate. The abdominal organs are also toned by the stretch.

196. *Gaṇḍa Bheruṇḍāsana* Fifty-six* (Plates 580 and 581)

Gaṇḍa means the cheek, the whole side of the face including the temple. Bheruṇḍa means terrible, formidable; it is also a species of bird. This difficult back-bending posture is given below in two stages.

Technique

1. Fold a blanket on the floor and lie on it full length on the stomach, face down with the hands stretched back. Stretch the neck and rest the chin firmly on the blanket, otherwise it will scrape on the floor.

2. Bend the elbows, place the hands by the chest, fingers pointing in the direction of the head. Bend the knees and move the feet towards the chest, which will be lifted slightly off the floor. (Plate 571)

3. Exhale, press the palms to the floor, kick the legs and stretch them straight. (Plate 572.) The chin, neck, arms and upper ribs are the only parts of the body touching the blanket on the floor.

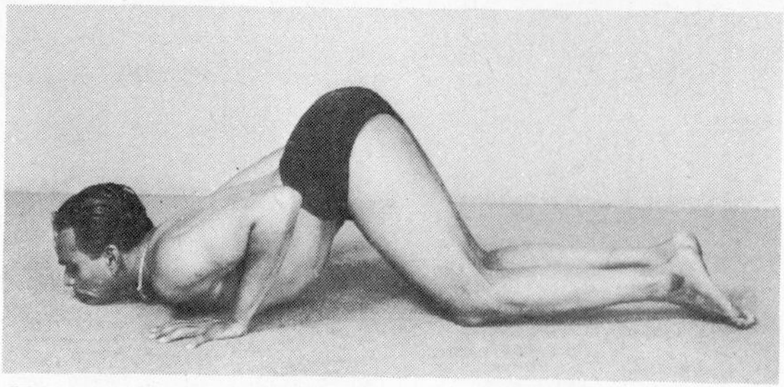

571

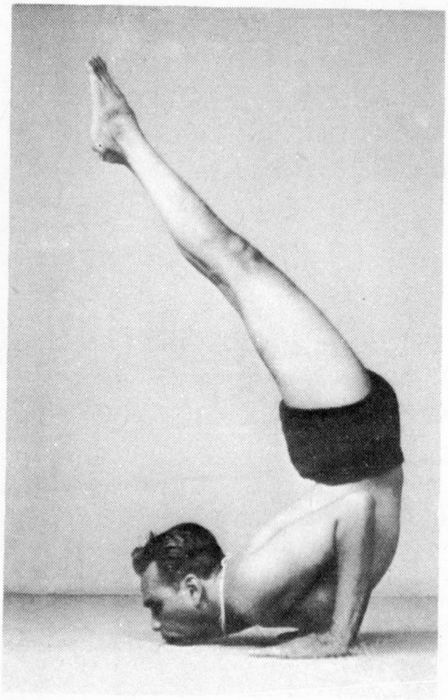

572

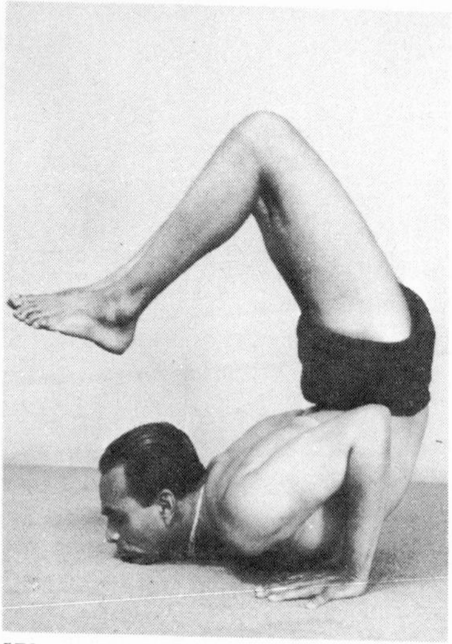

573

4. Take the pressure of the body on the neck and the chin, bend the knees (Plate 573), and lower the feet till they rest on the head. (Plate 574.) Take a few breaths.

5. Exhale, lower the legs still further and bring the feet in front of the head. (Plate 575)

6. Take the palms off the floor, widen the arms from the shoulders, bring them one by one in front of the head and clasp the feet with the hands. (Plates 576 and 577.) Take two breaths.

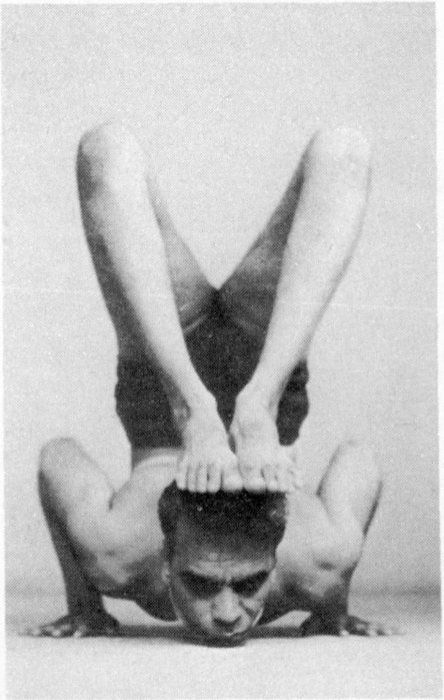

574

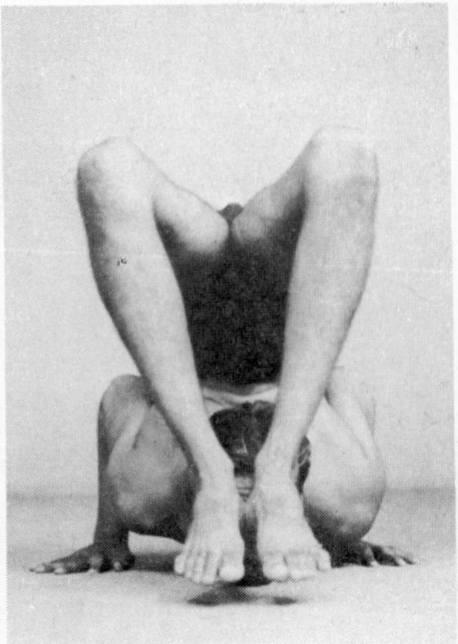

575

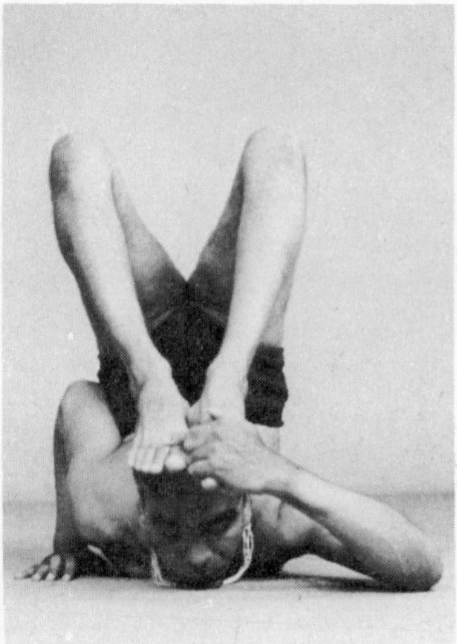

576

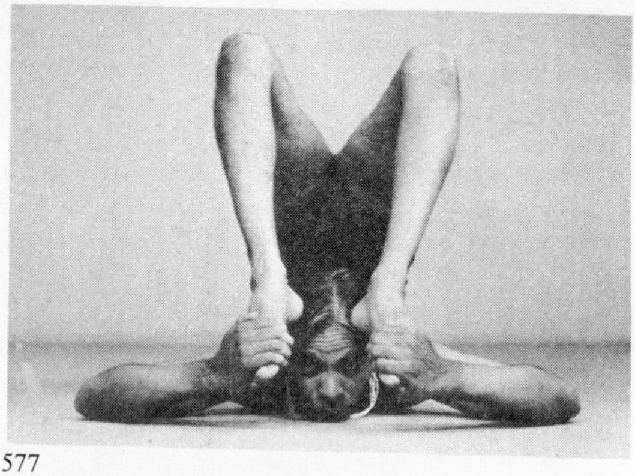

577

7. Exhale, pull the feet to the floor on each side of the face near the temples and cheeks. (Plates 578.) The heels should touch the shoulders. Now press the toes down with the wrists and forearms. (Plate 579)

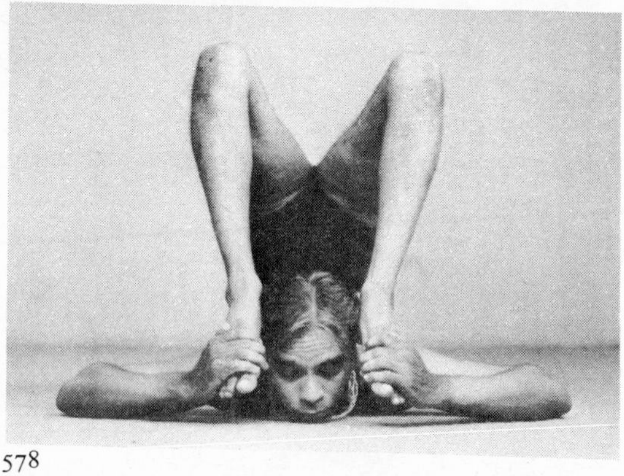

578

8. Interlock the fingers and place the palms on the floor by pressing the upper part of the feet with the wrists. (Plate 580.) This is the first stage.

9. Stay in the pose for a few seconds. Due to the intense stretch of the spine and contraction of the abdomen, breathing will be very fast and laboured. Do not hold the breath.

10. Extend the arms straight sideways like the wings of a gliding bird and balance for a few seconds. (Plate 581.) This is the second stage which is more difficult than the first one.

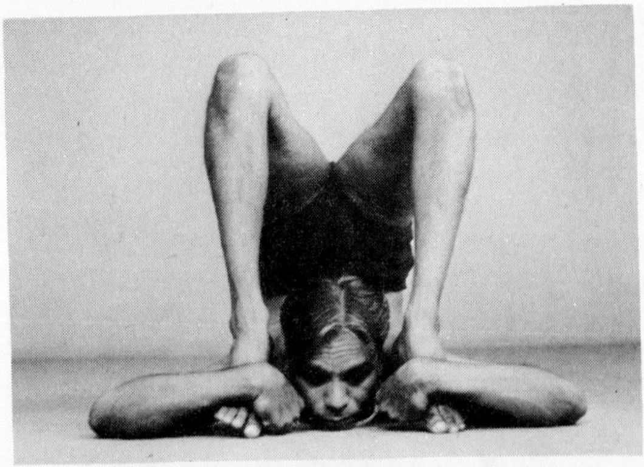

579

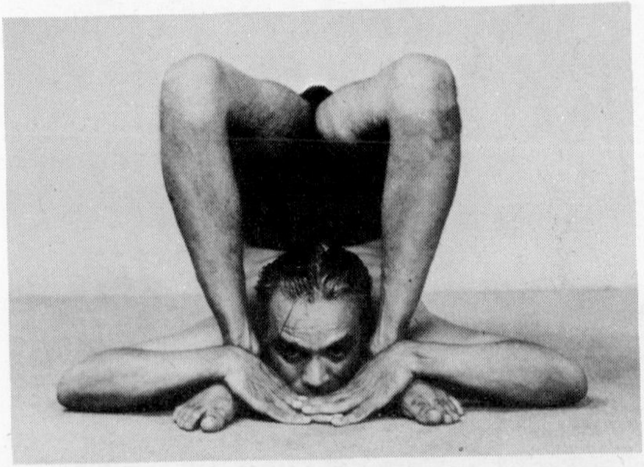

580

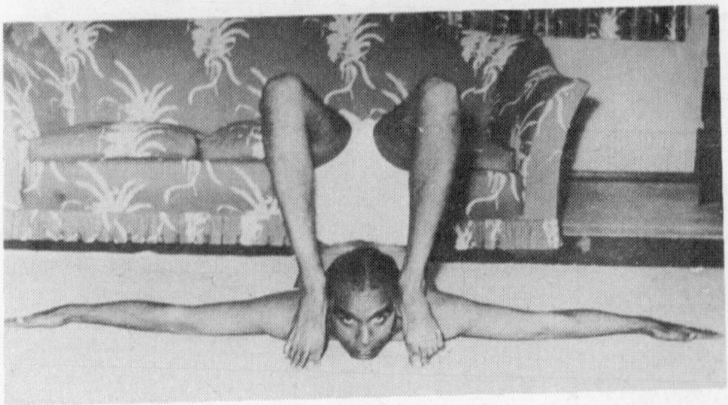

581

11. Place the palms on the floor, roll the body over the chin (Plates 582 and 583), move into Ūrdhva Dhanurāsana (Plate 486) and stand up in Tāḍāsana (Plate 1) and relax or practise Viparīta Chakrāsana. (Plates 488 to 499)

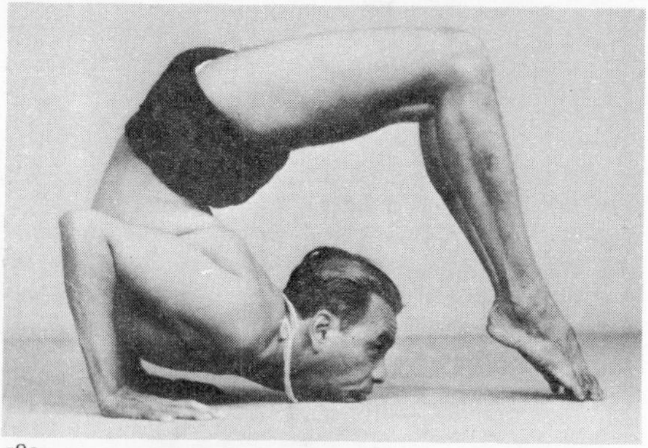

582

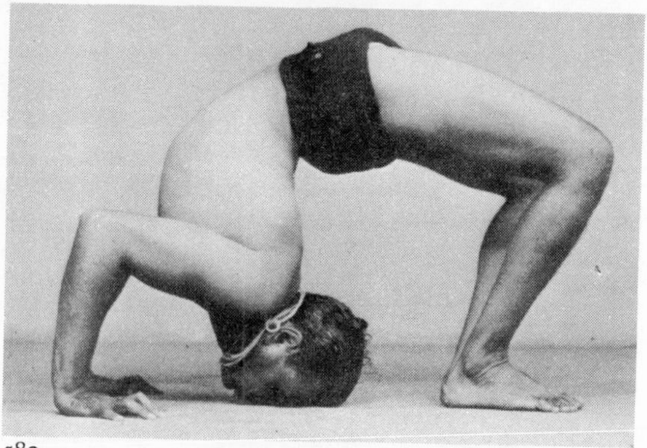

583

Effects

Apart from toning the entire spine and abdominal organs, the āsana stimulates the nerve centres in Mūlādhāra Chakra (the pelvic plexus), Svādhiṣṭhāna Chakra (the hypo-gastric plexus) and Viśuddhi Chakra (the pharyngeal plexus) and the glands situated there. Due to the copious supply of blood to these glands, their functioning improves and this leads to increased vitality.

197. *Viparīta Śalabhāsana* Fifty-eight* (Plate 584)

Viparīta means reverse, opposite or inverted. Śalabha is a locust. The stretch in this pose is more intense than in Gaṇḍa Bheruṇḍāsana (Plates 580 and 581) and the movements are converse to those in Halāsana. (Plate 241)

Technique

1. Fold a blanket on the floor and lie on it full length on the stomach, face down. Stretch the neck and rest the chin firmly on the blanket, otherwise it will scrape.

2. Bend the elbows and place the palms by the chest, fingers pointing to the head.

3. Exhale, bend, lift the knees and move the feet towards the chest, which will be lifted slightly off the floor. (Plate 571)

4. Take a few breaths and then with an exhalation, kick the legs up in the air, stretch the body up and balance (Plate 572), taking the weight of the body on the chin, neck, shoulders, elbows and wrists. Try to breathe normally.

5. Exhale, bend the knees (Plate 573), lower the legs and move the feet over and beyond the head until the toes rest on the floor. (Plate 582.) Stretch the feet as far as you can from the head and try to straighten the legs as much as possible. Stretch the arms back, palms down. (Plate 584)

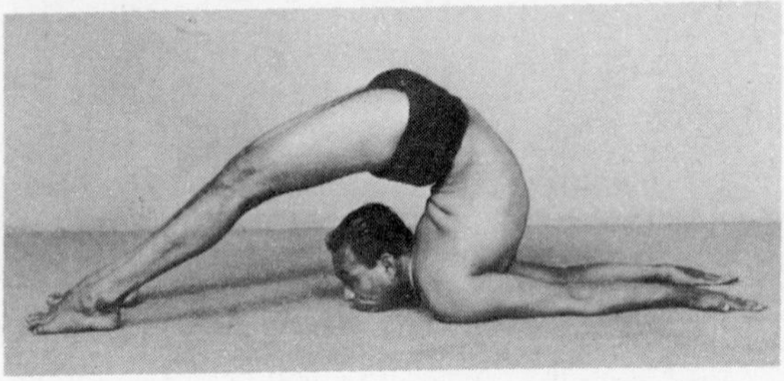

584

6. Stay for a few seconds in the āsana, which now appears to be the converse pose of Halāsana. (Plate 241.) Due to the intense stretch of the spine and pressure on the abdomen, breathing will be very fast and laboured, so do not hold the breath.

7. Bend the elbows and widen the arms. Bring the hands near the shoulders and place the palms on the floor. Bend the knees, bring the feet closer to the head (Plate 582), roll the body over the chin (Plate 583) and perform Ūrdhva Dhanurāsana. (Plate 486.) Stand up in

Tāḍāsana (Plate 1) or with an exhalation do Viparīta Chakrāsana (Plates 488 to 499) and relax.

Effects

The effects of this āsana are the same as those of Gaṇḍa Bheruṇḍ-āsana. (Plates 580 and 581.) The purpose of these two āsanas is to awaken Kuṇḍalinī the Divine Cosmic Energy in our bodies, symbolised by a coiled and sleeping serpent lying dormant in the lowest nerve centre at the base of the spine. The Yogi makes a conscious effort to arouse this latent Energy and lead it up the spine to the brain (the Sahasrāra or thousand-petalled lotus in the upper cerebral centre) and then he submerges his ego by concentrating upon the Divine Source of all energy in order to be released from worldly bondage. 'As rivers flow into the sea and so lose name and form, even so the wise man, freed from name and form, attains the Supreme Being, the Self-Luminous, the Infinite.'

198. *Tiriang Mukhottānāsana* Sixty* (Plate 586)

Tiriang means oblique, transverse, horizontal, reverse or upside down. Mukha means the face and also chief, principal or prominent. Uttāna is a deliberate or an intense stretch. In this back-bending posture the head is upside down with an intense stretch on arms, legs and the entire trunk.

Technique

1. Stand in Tāḍāsana. (Plate 1.) Spread the legs a foot apart and rest the palms on the hips.

2. Push the pelvic region slightly forward (Plate 483), exhale and curve the trunk back so that the weight of the body is felt on the thighs and feet. (Plate 484)

3. Raise the arms above the head and drop the hands to the floor. (Plate 485.) Immediately straighten the arms at the elbows and rest the palms on the floor. This is now Ūrdhva Dhanurāsana. (Plate 486)

4. Without moving the heels, widen the distance between the toes, so that the feet will be at an angle instead of parallel to each other.

5. Exhale, stretch the trunk as high as you can above the floor and bring the hands closer and closer to the feet. Stretch the head and neck as far back as possible and touch the feet with the hands. (Plate 585.) Take a few breaths which will be fast and laboured due to the intense stretch of the abdomen, chest and back.

6. With a deep exhalation, lift the hands off the floor one by one and catch the shins just above the ankles. (Plate 586.) Move the toes in and balance. This is the final position. After holding it for a few seconds according to capacity, put the hands one by one on the floor, go back to Ūrdhva Dhanurāsana (Plate 486) and then to Tāḍāsana. (Plate 1.) After mastering the technique, one can release the hands and stand up in Tāḍāsana without going back to Ūrdhva Dhanurāsana.

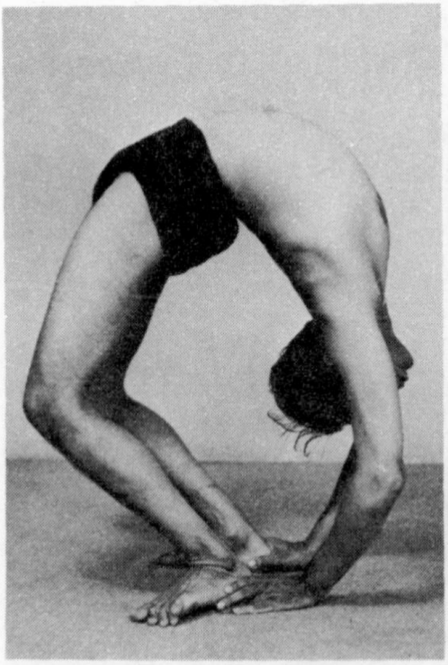

585

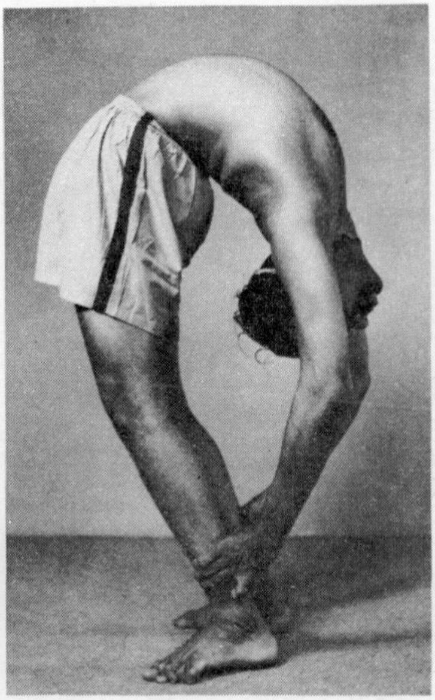

586

Effects

This difficult pose strengthens the legs and tones and vitalises the spine and abdominal organs. The chest and shoulder joints are fully stretched while the pelvic region receives an ample supply of blood and becomes healthier.

199. *Naṭarājāsana* Fifty-eight* (Plates 590, 591 and 591a)

Naṭarāja (naṭa = dancer; rāja = lord, king) is a name of Śiva, Lord of the Dance. Śiva is not only the god of mystical stillness, death and destruction, but also Lord of the Dance. In His Himālayan abode on Mount Kailāsa and in His southern home, the temple of Chidambaram, Śiva dances. The God created over a hundred dances, some calm and gentle, others fierce and terrible. The most famous of the terrible ones is the Tāṇḍava, the cosmic dance of destruction, in which Śiva, full of fury at his father-in-law Dakṣa for killing his beloved spouse Satī, surrounded by his attendants (gaṇas), beats out a wild rhythm, destroys Dakṣa and threatens the world. Śiva, as Lord of the Dance, has inspired some of the finest Indian sculptures and South Indian bronzes.

This vigorous and beautiful pose is dedicated to Śiva, Lord of the Dance, who is also the fountain and source of Yoga.

Technique

1. Stand in Tāḍāsana. (Plate 1.) Stretch the left arm out in front keeping it parallel to the floor.

2. Bend the right knee and lift up the right foot. Hold the right big toe between the thumb and the index and middle fingers of the right hand. Bend the lifted right knee and draw the leg up and back. (Plate 587)

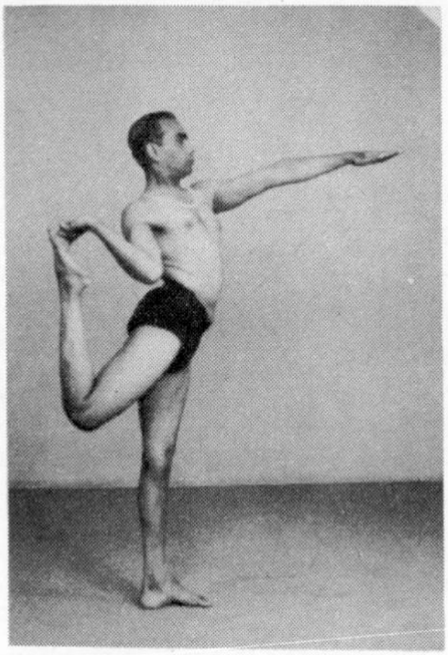

587

3. Roll the fingers and thumb of the right hand round the right big toe. Simultaneously rotate the right elbow and shoulder and stretch the right arm up behind the head, without releasing the grip on the big toe. (Plate 588.) Again pull the right arm and leg up so that they form a bow behind the back. (Plate 589.) The right thigh will be parallel to the floor and the right shin perpendicular to it. (Plates 590 and 591)

4. Bring the left arm straight in front level with the shoulder, keeping the fingers pointing forward.

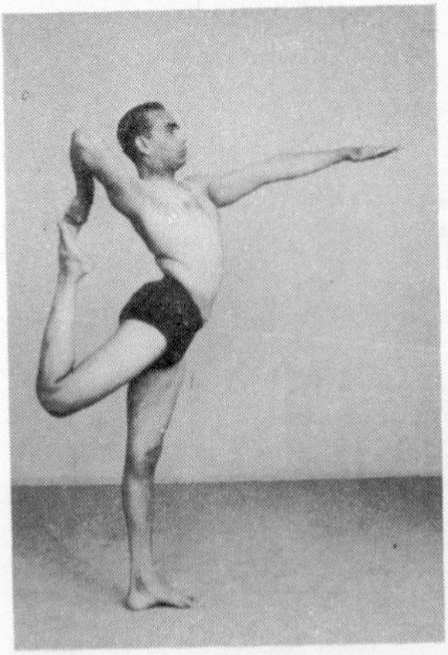

588

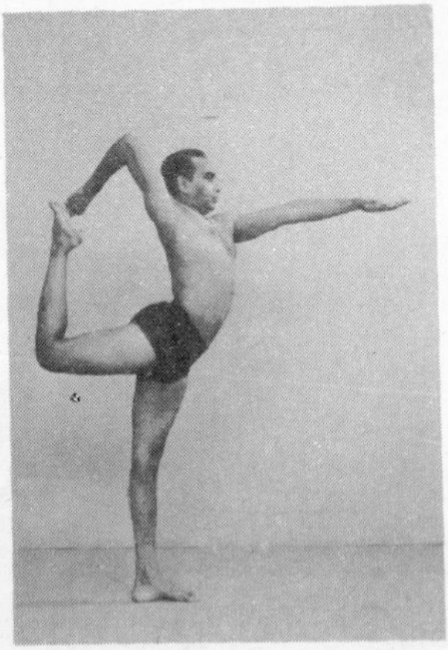

589

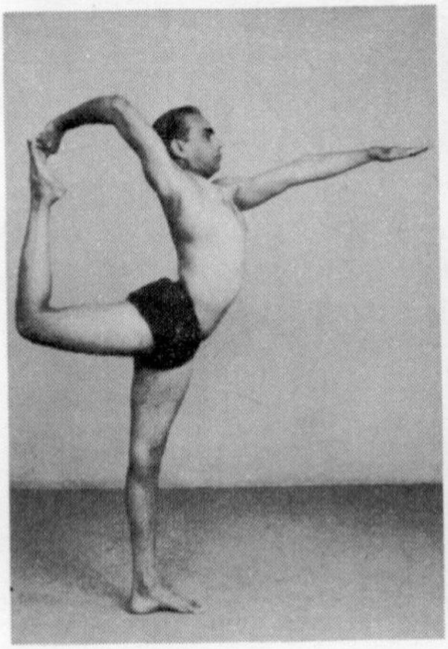

590

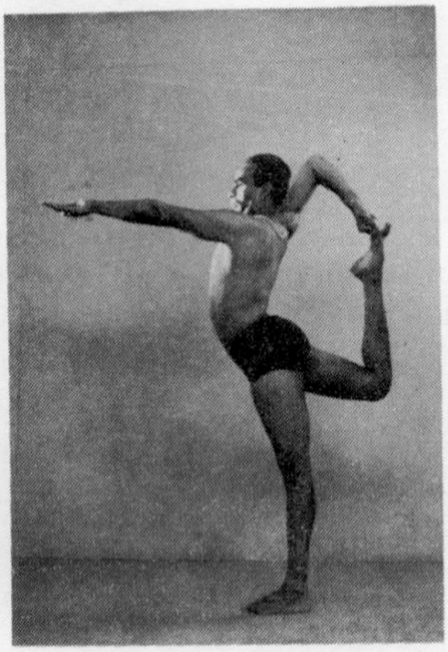

591

5. Pull the knee-cap up and keep the left leg poker stiff and perpendicular to the floor.

6. Balance firmly from 10 to 15 seconds with deep and even breathing.

7. Release the grip on the right foot, lower both arms and stand again in Tāḍāsana. (Plate 1.) Repeat the pose for the same length of time on the other side. This time, balance on the right leg, catch the left big toe behind the back with the left hand and stretch the right arm straight out in front.

8. Advanced pupils may hold the foot with both hands, rest it on the head and balance. (Plate 591a)

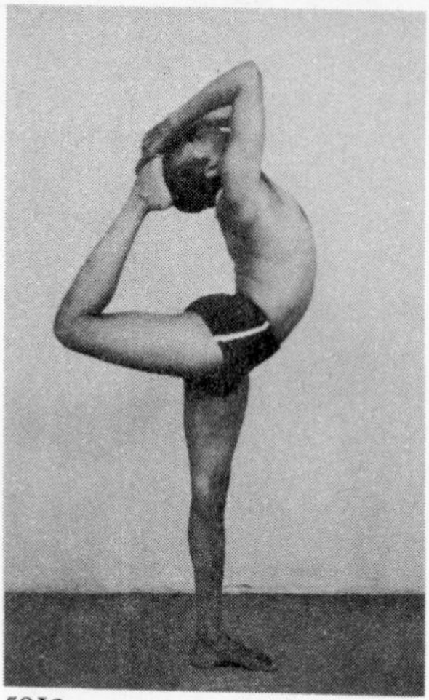

591a

Effects

This difficult balancing āsana develops poise and a graceful carriage. It tones and strengthens the leg muscles. The shoulder-blades get full movement and the chest expands fully. All the vertebral joints benefit from the exercise in this pose.

200. *Śavāsana* (Also called Mṛtāsana) (Plate 592)

Śava or Mṛta means a corpse. In this āsana the object is to imitate a corpse. Once life has departed, the body remains still and no movements are possible. By remaining motionless for some time and keeping the mind still while you are fully conscious, you learn to relax. This conscious relaxation invigorates and refreshes both body and mind. But it is much harder to keep the mind than the body still. Therefore, this apparently easy posture is one of the most difficult to master.

Technique

1. Lie flat on the back full length like a corpse. Keep the hands a little away from the thighs, with the palms up.

2. Close the eyes. If possible place a black cloth folded four times over the eyes. Keep the heels together and the toes apart.

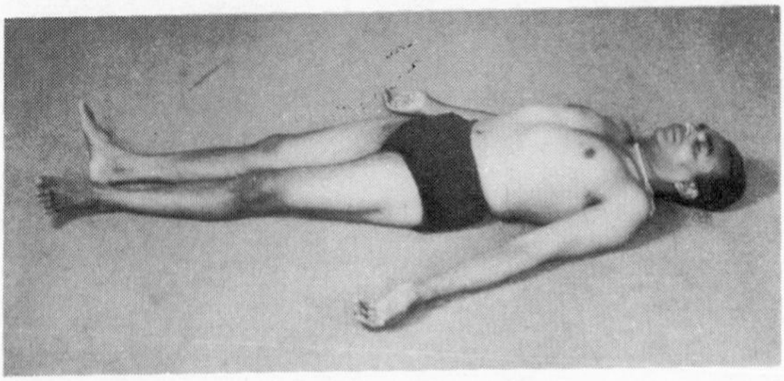

592

3. To start with breathe deeply. Later the breathing should be fine and slow, with no jerky movements to disturb the spine or the body.

4. Concentrate on deep and fine exhalations, in which the nostrils do not feel the warmth of breath.

5. The lower jaw should hang loose and not be clenched. The tongue should not be disturbed, and even the pupils of the eyes should be kept completely passive.

6. Relax completely and breathe out slowly.

7. If the mind wanders, pause without any strain after each slow exhalation.

8. Stay in the pose from 15 to 20 minutes.

9. One is apt to fall asleep in the beginning. Gradually, when the nerves become passive, one feels completely relaxed and refreshed.

In good relaxation one feels energy flow from the back of the head towards the heels and not the other way round. One also feels as if the body is elongated.

Effects

Verse 32 of the First Chapter of the *Haṭha Yoga Pradīpikā* states: 'Lying upon one's back on the ground at full length like a corpse is called Śavāsana. This removes the fatigue caused by the other āsanas and induces calmness of mind.'

Mṛtāsana is thus described in verse 11 of the Second Chapter of the *Gheraṇḍa Saṁhitā*: 'Lying flat on the ground (on one's back) like a corpse is called Mṛtāsana. This posture destroys fatigue, and quiets the agitation of the mind.'

'The mind is the lord of the Indriyas (the organs of senses); the Prana (the Breath of Life) is the lord of the mind.' 'When the mind is absorbed it is called Mokṣa (final emancipation, liberation of the soul); when Prāṇa and Manas (the mind) have been absorbed, an undefinable joy ensues.' Verses 29 and 30, chapter IV, *Haṭha Yoga Pradīpikā.*

To tame Prāṇa depends upon the nerves. Steady, smooth, fine and deep breathing without any jerky movements of the body soothes the nerves and calms the mind. The stresses of modern civilisation are a strain on the nerves for which Śavāsana is the best antidote.

Bandha and Kriyā

201. *Uḍḍīyāna Bandha* Twelve* (Plates 593 and 594)

Uḍḍīyāna means flying up. Strictly speaking it is not an āsana, but a bandha, that is a restraint. As condensers, fuses and switches control the flow of electricity, so bandhas regulate the flow of prāṇa (energy). In this bandha the prāṇa or energy is made to move from the lower abdomen towards the head. For a detailed discussion on bandha and prāṇa, see Part Three on Prāṇāyāma.

Technique

1. Stand in Tāḍāsana. (Plate 1)

2. Spread the legs a foot apart.

3. Stoop slightly forward, bending the knees slightly and place the hands with the fingers spread wide on the middle of the thighs.

4. Lower the hands until the chin rests in the notch between the collar-bones on top of the breast-bone.

5. Inhale deeply and then exhale quickly so that all the air is forced from the lungs in a rush.

6. Hold the breath (without any inhalation). Pull the whole abdominal region back towards the spine. Contract the abdominal region and lift it up towards the breast-bone, pressing the hands against the thighs. (Plate 593)

7. Maintaining the abdominal grip, lift the hands from the thighs and rest them on the hips.

8. Straighten both legs and the back without loosening the abdominal grip or raising the chin from the breast-bone. (Plate 594)

9. Relax the abdominal muscles but without moving the chin and head. If the latter move, strain is at once felt in the region of the heart.

10. Inhale slowly and deeply.

11. Throughout positions 6 to 9 above, do not inhale. Do not hold the pose for more than 5 to 10 seconds depending on your endurance.

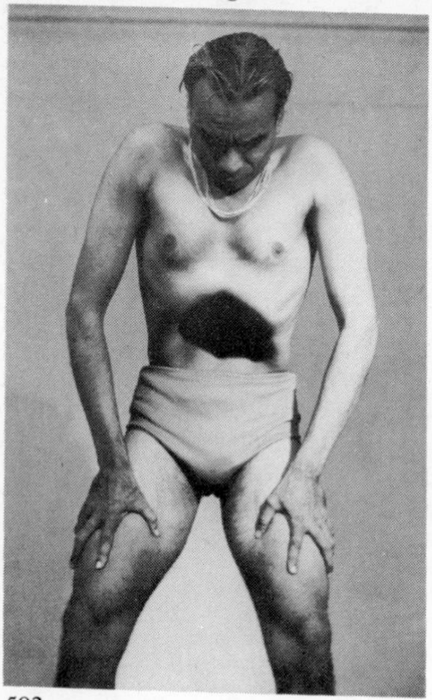

593

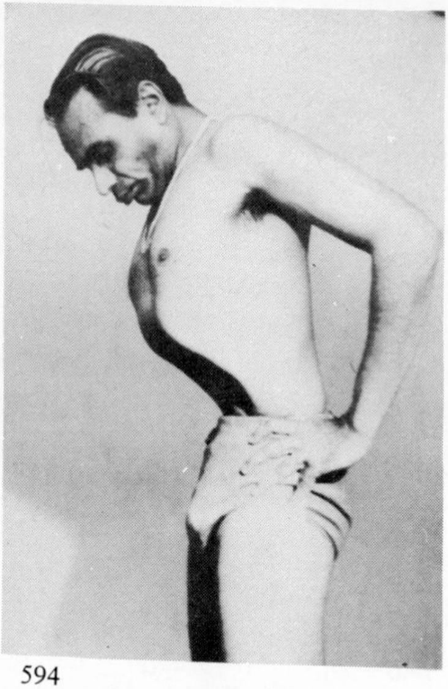

594

12. Take a few breaths, then repeat the cycle stated in paras 1 to 10 above. Do not, however, repeat it more than six to eight times at a stretch in 24 hours. Only increase the duration of the pose or the number of cycles under the personal supervision of an experienced Guru.

13. The cycles should be done only once a day at a stretch.

14. Practise on an empty stomach after evacuating both the bladder and bowels.

15. First learn Uḍḍīyāna Bandha in the standing position, then in the sitting position as a preliminary step for the practice of Prāṇāyāma.

16. It should be done during exhalation (rechaka) and retention of breath (kumbhaka) in the various types of Prāṇāyāma described in Part Three.

Effects

It tones the abdominal organs, increases the gastric fire and eliminates toxins in the digestive tract.

202. *Nauli* Sixteen* (Plates 595 and 596)

The word Nauli is not found in standard dictionaries. Ullola meaning a large wave or surge, conveys some idea of the process of Nauli where the abdominal muscles and organs are made to move laterally and vertically in a surging motion. Nau means a boat and li to cling to, lie on, hide or cover. The pitching of a boat on a stormy sea conveys some idea of the process of Nauli.

Nauli is a kriyā or process and not an āsana. Care should be observed in its performance, otherwise the process leads to numerous diseases. It is not, therefore, recommended for the average practitioner. First master Uḍḍīyāna Bandha before attempting Nauli, which is described in the *Gheruṇḍa Saṃhita* under the name Lauliki.

Technique

1. Stand in Tāḍāsana. (Plate 1)

2. Spread the legs a foot apart, bend slightly at the knees and stoop forward.

3. Place the hands with the fingers spread wide on the thighs just above the knees.

4. Lower the head until the chin rests in the notch between the collar-bones on the top of the breast-bone.

5. Inhale deeply, then exhale quickly so that all the air is forced from the lungs in a rush.

6. Hold the breath (without any inhalation). Pull the whole abdominal region back towards the spine.

7. The area between the pelvic rim and the floating ribs on both sides of the abdomen should be made passive to create hollowness there. At the same time push the abdominal recti forward. (Plate 595 front view; and Plate 596 side view)

8. Maintain this position from 5 to 10 seconds, according to your capacity.

9. Relax the grip on the recti and go back to the position described in para. 6 above.

10. Relax the abdomen and inhale slowly.

11. Take a few deep breaths. Repeat the cycle in paras 1 to 10 above, six to eight times at a stretch only once every 24 hours.

12. Practise Nauli on an empty stomach after evacuating the bladder and bowels.

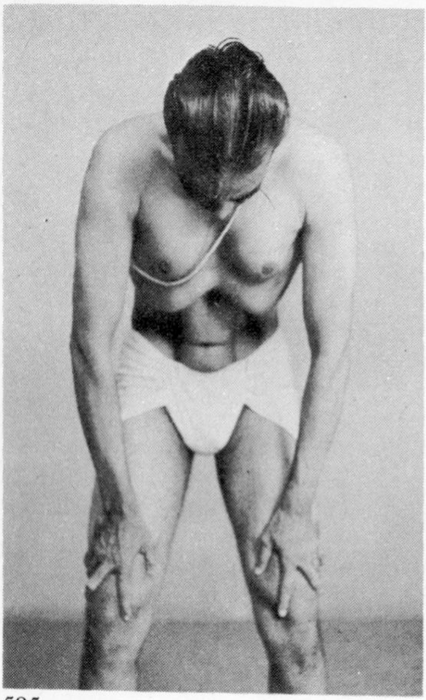

595

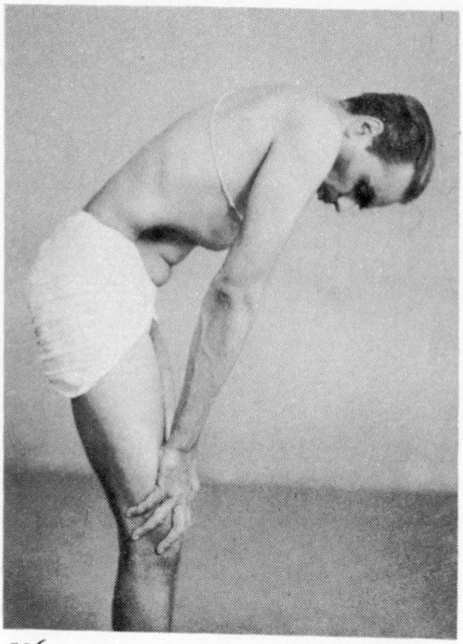

596

Effects

The abdominal recti are strengthened. The other effects of Nauli are the same as those of Uḍḍīyāna Bandha.

Part III

Prāṇāyāma

Hints and Cautions

Read and digest thoroughly the following hints and cautions before attempting the prāṇāyāma techniques mentioned later.

Qualifications for fitness

1. Just as post-graduate training depends upon the ability and discipline acquired in mastering the subject in which one graduated, so prāṇāyāma training demands mastery of āsanas and the strength and discipline arising therefrom.

2. The fitness of the aspirant for training and advancement in Prāṇāyāma is to be gauged by an experienced Guru or teacher and his personal supervision is essential.

3. Pneumatic tools can cut through the hardest rock. In Prāṇāyāma the yogi uses his lungs as pneumatic tools. If they are not used properly, they destroy both the tool and the person using it. The same is true of prāṇāyāma.

Cleanliness and Food

4. One does not enter a temple with a dirty body or mind. Before entering the temple of his own body, the yogi observes the rules of cleanliness.

5. Before starting prāṇāyāma practices the bowels should be evacuated and the bladder emptied. This leads to comfort in the bandhas.

6. Preferably prāṇāyāma should be practised on an empty stomach, but if this is difficult, a cup of milk, tea, coffee or cocoa may be taken. Allow at least six hours to elapse after a meal before practising prāṇāyāma.

7. Light food may be taken half an hour after finishing prāṇāyāma practices.

Time and Place

8. The best time for practice is in the early morning (preferably before sunrise) and after sunset. According to the *Haṭha Yoga Pradīpikā*, prāṇāyāma should be practised four times a day, in the early morning,

noon, evening and midnight, with 80 cycles at a time (chapter II, verse 11). This is hardly possible in the fast modern age. What is therefore recommended is to practise at least 15 minutes a day, but the 80 cycles are for intensely devoted practitioners, and not for the average householder.

9. The best seasons in which to start the practice are spring and autumn when the climate is equable.

10. Prāṇāyāma should be done in a clean airy place, free from insects. Since noise creates restlessness practise during quiet hours.

11. Prāṇāyāma should be practised with determination and regularity at the same time and place and in the same posture. Variation is permissible only in the type of prāṇāyāma practised, that is to say, if Sūrya Bhedana Prāṇāyāma is done one day, Śitalī may be done the next day and Bhastrikā be done on the third day. Nāḍī Shodhana Prāṇāyāma, however, should be practised daily.

Posture

12. Breathing in prāṇāyāma practices is done through the nose only, except in Śitalī and Śitakāri.

13. Prāṇāyāma is best done sitting on the floor on a folded blanket. The postures suitable are Siddhāsana, Vīrāsana, Padmāsana and Baddhakoṇāsana. Any other sitting posture may be taken provided the back is kept absolutely erect from the base of the spine to the neck and perpendicular to the floor. Some types, however, may be done in a reclining position as detailed later.

14. During practice no strain should be felt in the facial muscles, eyes and ears, or in the neck muscles, shoulders, arms, thighs and feet. The thighs and arms should be relaxed deliberately since they are unconsciously tensed during prāṇāyāma.

15. Keep the tongue passive or saliva will accumulate in the mouth. If it does, swallow it before exhalation (rechaka) and not while holding the breath (kumbhaka).

16. During inhalation and retention the rib cage should expand both forwards and sideways, but the area below the shoulder-blades and armpits should only expand forwards.

17. To start with there will be perspiration and trembling which will disappear in course of time.

18. In all the prāṇāyāma practices done in a sitting posture, the head should hang down from the nape of the neck, the chin resting in the

notch between the collar-bones on the top of the breast-bone. This chinlock or Jālandhara Bandha should be used except where specifically stated in the techniques hereafter given.

19. Keep the eyes closed throughout as otherwise the mind will wander after outside objects and be distracted. The eyes, if kept open, will feel a burning sensation, and irritability.

20. No pressure should be felt inside the ear during the practice of prāṇāyāma.

21. The left arm is kept straight, the back of the wrist resting on the left knee. The forefinger is bent towards the thumb, its tip touching the tip of the thumb. This is the Jñāna Mudrā described later in the technique.

22. The right arm is bent at the elbow and the hand is kept on the nose to regulate the even flow of breath and to gauge its subtlety. This is felt through the tips of the ring and little fingers which control the left nostril and through the tip of the thumb which controls the right nostril. Details of the right hand position are discussed in the technique. In some methods of prāṇāyāma both the hands rest on the knees in the Jñāna Mudrā.

23. When a baby learns to walk by itself, the mother remains passive bodily, but alert mentally. In an emergency, as when the child stumbles, her body springs into action to save it from a fall. So also, in the practice of prāṇāyāma the brain is kept passive but alert. Whenever the organs of the body fail to work properly, the watchful brain sends messages of warning. The ear is told to listen for the proper sound of the breath (which is described below). The hand and nose are told to observe the sensitivity of the breath flowing through the nasal passages.

24. It may be asked that if the brain is required to send warnings to the senses, how can one concentrate on prāṇāyāma? A painter absorbed in his work notes various details like perspective and composition, the colour tones and shades, the foreground and background and the strokes of the paint-brush all at once. A musician playing a melody watches his finger movements and sound patterns, the tuning of the instrument and its pitch. Though the artist and the musician are both observing and correcting the details, they are concentrating on their work. So also the yogi observes details like time, posture and an even breath rhythm, and is alert and sensitive to the flow of prāṇa within him.

25. As a careful mother teaches her child to walk carefree, so the careful mind of the yogi teaches the senses to be carefree. By continued practice of prāṇāyāma the senses become free of obsession for the things they once pined for.

26. Each should measure his own capacity when doing prāṇāyāma and not exceed it. This may be gauged as follows: suppose one can with comfort inhale and exhale for 10 seconds each in rhythmic cycles for a given length of time, say 5 minutes. If there is any change in the rhythm in which the period of inhalation or of exhalation decreases, to say 7 or 8 seconds, one has reached one's capacity. To go beyond this point, strains the lungs unduly and brings in its wake a host of respiratory diseases.

27. Faulty practice puts undue stress on the lungs and diaphragm. The respiratory system suffers and the nervous system is adversely affected. The very foundation of a healthy body and a sound mind is shaken by faulty practice of prāṇāyāma. Forceful and strained inhalation or exhalation is wrong, except in Bhastrikā Prāṇāyāma.

28. Evenness of breathing leads to healthy nerves and so to evenness of mind and temper.

29. Āsanas should never be practised immediately after prāṇāyāma. If prāṇāyāma is done first, allow an hour to elapse before starting āsanas, for the nerves which are soothed in prāṇāyāma are liable to be ruffled by the bodily movement of the āsanas.

30. Prāṇāyāma, however, may be done not less than 15 minutes after mild practice of āsanas.

31. Strenuous āsanas cause fatigue. When exhausted do not practise prāṇāyāma in any sitting posture, as the back cannot stay erect, the body trembles and the mind becomes disturbed. Deep breathing as in Ujjāyī done in a reclining position relieves fatigue.

32. When deep, steady and long breathing cannot be maintained rhythmically, stop. Do not proceed further. The rhythm should be gauged from the nasal sound produced in inhalation ('ssssssa' which sounds like a leak in a cycle tube) and exhalation (the aspirate 'huuuuuuuuum' sound). If the volume of the sound is reduced, stop.

33. Try to achieve an even ratio in inhalation (puraka) and exhalation (rechaka). For example, if one is for 5 seconds during a given continuous cycle, the other should be for the same time.

34. The Ujjāyī and Nāḍī Śodhana types of prāṇāyāma are the most

beneficial ones which can be practised by pregnant women, preferably in Baddhakoṇāsana. During pregnancy, however, the breath should never be held without the guidance of an experienced teacher.

35. After completing any prāṇāyāma practice always lie down on the back like a corpse in Śavāsana (Plate 592) for at least 5 or 10 minutes in silence. The mind should be completely switched off and every limb and sense organ completely passive as if dead. Śavāsana after prāṇāyāma refreshes both the body and the mind.

Kumbhakas

36. All the three Bandhas, namely Jālandhara, Uḍḍīyāna and Mūla, should be observed in kumbhaka (retention of breath after full inhalation or restraint following complete exhalation) as mentioned later. The bandhas are like safety-valves which should be kept shut during the practice of kumbhakas.

37. Thorough mastery of inhalation (puraka) and exhalation (rechaka) is essential before any attempt is made to learn antara kumbhaka (retention following inhalation).

38. Bāhya kumbhaka (restraint following exhalation) should not be tried until antara kumbhaka has become natural.

39. During the practice of kumbhaka there is a tendency to draw in air as well as to tighten and loosen the diaphragm and abdominal organs for the sake of increasing the period of retention. This is unconscious and unintentional. Care should be taken to avoid it.

40. If it is found difficult to hold the breath (khumbaka) after each inhalation or exhalation, do some cycles of deep breathing and then practise kumbhakas. For instance, 3 cycles of deep breathing may be followed by one cycle of kumbhaka. Then there should be another 3 cycles of deep breathing followed by a second cycle of kumbhaka, and so on.

41. If the rhythm of inhalation or exhalation is disturbed by holding the breath, lessen the duration of kumbhaka.

42. Persons suffering from eye or ear trouble (like glaucoma and pus in the ear) should not attempt to hold the breath.

43. Sometimes constipation occurs in the initial stages following upon the introduction of kumbhaka. This is temporary and will disappear in due course.

44. The normal rate of breaths per minute is 15. This rate increases

when the body is upset by indigestion, fever, cold and cough, or by emotions like fear, anger or lust. The normal rate of breathing is 21,600 breaths inhaled and exhaled every 24 hours. The yogi measures his span of life not by the number of days, but of breaths. Since breathing is lengthened in prāṇāyāma, its practice leads to longevity.

45. Continuous practice of prāṇāyāma will change the mental outlook of the practitioner and reduce considerably the craving of his senses for worldly pleasures like smoking, drinking and sexual indulgence.

46. In the practice of prāṇāyāma the senses are drawn inwards and in the silence of the kumbhaka the aspirant hears his inner voice calling: 'Look within! The source of all happiness is within!' This also prepares him for the next stage of yoga, pratyāhāra, which leads to freedom from the domination and tyranny of the senses.

47. Since the eyes are kept closed throughout the practice of prāṇāyāma, the passage of time is noted by the mental repetition (japa) of a sacred word or name. This repetition of the sacred words or names is the seed (bīja) planted in the yogi's mind. This seed grows and makes him fit for dhyāna or concentration, the sixth stage of Yoga. Ultimately it produces the fruit of samādhi, where there is experience of full consciousness and supreme joy, where the yogi merges with the Maker of the Universe and feels what he can never express—yet cannot entirely conceal. Words fail to convey the experience adequately, for the mind cannot find words with which to describe it. It is a feeling of that peace which passeth all understanding.

BANDHAS, NĀḌIS AND CHAKRAS

In order to follow the techniques of prāṇāyāma it is necessary to know something about bandhas, nāḍis and chakras.

Bandha means bondage, joining together, fettering or catching hold of. It is also a posture in which certain organs or parts of the body are contracted and controlled.

Nāḍi is a tubular channel in the body through which energy flows.

Chakras are wheels or circles. Those in the body are the fly-wheels in the body machinery.

When electricity is generated, it is necessary to have transformers, conductors, fuses, switches and insulated wires to carry the power to its destination, as without these the electricity generated would be lethal. When prāṇa is made to flow in the yogi's body by the practice of prāṇāyāma it is equally necessary for him to employ bandhas to prevent the dissipation of energy and to carry it to the right quarters without causing damage elsewhere. Without the bandhas, prāṇa is lethal.

The three main bandhas, which are important for prāṇāyāma, are: (1) Jalandhara Bandha, (2) Uḍḍīyāna Bandha and (3) Mūla Bandha.

The first one which the yogi should master is Jālandhara. Jāla means a net, a web, a lattice or a mesh. In Jālandhara the neck and throat are contracted and the chin is made to rest on the chest in the notch between the collar-bones and at the top of the breast-bone. It is mastered while doing Sarvāṅgāsana (see pp. 205–20) and its cycles, for here also the chin is pressed against the sternum. The Jālandhara Bandha regulates the flow of blood and prāṇa to the heart, the glands in the neck and the head together with the brain. If prāṇāyāma is performed without Jālandhara Bandha pressure is immediately felt on the heart, behind the eyeballs and in the ear cavity and the head feels dizzy. Jālandhara Bandha is essential in the three processes of prāṇāyāma, namely, pūraka (inhalation), rechaka (exhalation) and kumbhaka (retention).

Uḍḍīyāna means flying up. The process in Uḍḍīyāna Bandha is to lift the diaphragm high up the thorax and to pull in the abdominal organs against the back towards the spine. It is said that through Uḍḍīyāna Bandha, the great bird prāṇa is forced to fly up through the suṣumṇā nāḍi, the main channel for the flow of nervous energy, which is situated inside the meru-daṇḍa or the spinal column. It is said that Uḍḍīyāna is the best of bandhas and he who constantly practises it as taught by his Guru or master becomes young again. It is said to be the lion that kills the elephant named Death. It should be performed only during bāhya kumbhaka following rechaka, that is, during the interval between complete exhalation and fresh inhalation when breathing is suspended. It exercises the diaphragm and abdominal organs. The cavity created by the lift of the diaphragm gives a gentle massage to the muscles of the heart, thereby toning it. Uḍḍīyāna Bandha should never be attempted during antara kumbhaka, that is the interval between complete inhalation and the start of exhalation when breath is retained, otherwise it will strain the heart and diaphragm and the eyes will puff out.

Mūla means root, source, origin or cause, basis or foundation. Mūla Bandha is the region between the anus and the scrotum. By contracting this region, Apāna Vāyu (the prāṇa in the lower abdomen), whose course is downwards, is made to flow up to unite with the Prāṇa Vāyu, which has its seat in the region of the chest.

Mūla Bandha should be attempted first in antara kumbhaka (retention after inhalation). The region of the lower abdomen between the navel and the anus is contracted towards the spine and pulled up towards the diaphragm. In Uḍḍīyāna Bandha the entire region from the anus to the diaphragm up to the sternum is pulled back towards the spine and lifted up. But in Mūla Bandha the whole lower abdominal area between the anus and the navel is contracted, pulled back to the spine and lifted up towards the diaphragm.

The practice of contracting the anal sphincter muscles (the Aśvinī Mudrā) helps one to master Mūla Bandha. Aśva means a horse. This mudrā (a sealing posture) is so called because it suggests the staling of a horse. It should be learnt while doing various āsanas, especially Tāḍāsana, Śīrṣāsana, Sarvāṅgāsana, Ūrdhva Dhanurāsana, Uṣṭrāsana and Paśchimottanāsana.

It is said that by the practice of these bandhas the sixteen ādharas are closed. Ādhāra (from the root ('dhṛ' = to support) means a support, a vital part. The sixteen vital parts are: the thumbs, ankles, knees, thighs, prepuce, organs of generation, navel, heart, neck, throat, palate, nose, the middle of the eyebrows, forehead, head and Brahmarandhra (the aperture in the crown of the head through which the soul is said to escape on leaving the body).

There is a grave danger in attempting to learn the Uḍḍīyāna and Mūla Bandhas by oneself, without the personal supervision of an experienced Guru or teacher. Improper performance of the Uḍḍīyāna Bandha will cause involuntary discharge of semen and loss of vitality, while that of Mūla Bandha will seriously weaken the practitioner who will lack virility. Even the correct performance of Mūla Bandha has its own dangers. It increases sexual retentive power, thereby tempting the practitioner to abuse that power. If he succumbs to that temptation, he is lost. All his dormant desires are aroused and become lethal like a sleeping serpent struck with a stick. With the mastery of the three bandhas, the yogi is at the cross-roads of his destiny. One road leads to bhoga or the enjoyment of worldly pleasures; the other leads to Yoga or union with the Supreme Soul. The attraction of worldly pleasures is great. The yogi, however, feels greater attraction for their Creator. The senses open outwards and consequently they are attracted to objects and follow the path of bhoga. If the direction of the senses is changed so that they turn inwards, then they follow the path of Yoga. The yogi's senses invert to meet the Creator, the source of all creation. It is when the aspirant has mastered the three bandhas that the guidance of a Guru is most essential, for under proper guidance this increased power is sublimated for higher and nobler pursuits. The practitioner then becomes an ūrdhvaretus (ūrdhva = upwards; retus = semen) or one who lives a life of celibacy and does not dissipate his virility. He will then acquire moral and spiritual power. The power within him will shine forth like the sun.

While practising Mūla Bandha, the yogi attempts to reach the true source or mūla of all creation. His goal is the complete restraint or bandha of the chitta which includes the mind (manas), the intellect (buddhi) and the ego (ahaṁkāra).

The human body is a miniature universe in itself. Haṭha is composed of the syllables ha and ṭha which mean the sun and the moon respectively. The solar and the lunar energy is said to flow through the two main nāḍis, Piṅgala and Iḍā, which start from the right and the left nostrils respectively and move down to the base of the spine. Piṅgala is the nāḍi of the sun, while the Iḍā is the nāḍi of the moon. In between them is the Suṣumṇā, the nāḍi of fire. As stated earlier, Suṣumṇā Nāḍi is the main channel for the flow of nervous energy, and it is situated inside the meru-daṇḍa or spinal column. Piṅgalā and Iḍā intersect each other and also Suṣumṇā at various places. These junctions are called chakras or wheels and regulate the body mechanism as fly-wheels regulate an engine.

The main chakras are: Mūlādhāra Chakra which is situated in the pelvic region above the anus (mūla = root, cause, source: ādhāra = support, or vital part); Svādhiṣṭhāna Chakra above the organs of generation (sva = vital force, soul: adhiṣṭhāna = seat or abode); Maṇipūraka Chakra is the navel (maṇipūra = navel); the Manas and the Sūrya Chakras between the navel and the heart (manas = mind: sūrya = sun); Anāhata Chakra in the cardiac region (anāhata = heart); Viśuddha Chakra in the pharyngeal region (viśuddha = pure); Ājñā Chakra between the eyebrows (ājñā = command); the Sahasrāra Chakra, which is called the thousand-petalled lotus, in the cerebral cavity; and Lalāṭa Chakra which is at the top of the forehead (lalāṭa = forehead).

It may be that these chakras correspond to the endocrine glands, which supply hormones and other internal secretions to the system. The Mūlādhara and the Svādhiṣṭhāna Chakras perhaps correspond to the gonads (the testicles, penis and prostate in males and the ovaries, uterus and vagina in females). In between these two chakras is the seat of the genitals, known as Kāmarūpa after Kāma the god of passion and love. The abdominal organs like the stomach, spleen, liver and pancreas perhaps correspond to the Maṇipūraka Chakra. The two adrenals may stand for the Sūrya and Manas Chakras. The Anāhata Chakra is the heart and the main blood vessels around it. The Viśuddha Chakra may be the thyroid, parathyroid and the thymus. The Ājñā, Sahasrāra and Lalāṭa Chakras may be the brain matter and the pitutiary and pineal glands.

According to the Tantric texts the object of Prāṇāyāma is to arouse Kuṇḍalinī, the divine cosmic force in our bodies. Kuṇḍalinī is symbolised as a coiled and sleeping serpent lying dormant in the lowest nerve centre at the base of the spinal column, the Mūlādhāra Chakra. This latent energy has to be aroused and made to go up the spinal column piercing the chakras up to the Sahasrāra (the thousand-petalled lotus in the head, the network of nerves in the brain) and there to unite with the Supreme Soul. This is perhaps an allegorical way of describing the tremendous vitality, especially sexual, which is obtained by the practice of Uḍḍīyāna and Mūla Bandhas described above. The arousing of Kuṇḍalinī and forcing it up is perhaps a symbolic way of describing the sublimation of sexual energy.

Technique and Effects of Prāṇāyāma

203. *Ujjāyī Prāṇāyāma* (Plate 597)

The prefix ud attached to verbs and nouns, means upwards or superiority in rank. It also means blowing or expanding. It conveys the sense of pre-eminence and power.

Jaya means conquest, victory, triumph or success. Looked at from another viewpoint it implies restraint or curbing.

Ujjāyi is the process in which the lungs are fully expanded and the chest puffed out like that of a proud conqueror.

Technique

1. Sit in any comfortable position like Padmāsana (Plate 104), Siddhāsana (Plate 84) or Vīrāsana (Plate 89).

2. Keep the back erect and rigid. Lower the head to the trunk. Rest the chin in the notch between the collar-bones just above the breast-bone. (This is the Jālandhara Bandha.)

3. Stretch the arms out straight and rest the back of the wrists on the knees. Join the tips of the index fingers to the tips of the thumbs, keeping the other fingers extended. (This position or gesture of the hand is known as the Jñāna Mudrā, the symbol or seal of knowledge. The index finger symbolises the individual soul and the thumb the Universal Soul. The union of the two symbolises knowledge.)

4. Close the eyes and look inwards. (Plate 597)

5. Exhale completely.

6. Now the Ujjāyi method of breathing begins.

7. Take a slow, deep steady breath through both nostrils. The passage of the incoming air is felt on the roof of the palate and makes a sibilant sound (sa). This sound should be heard.

8. Fill the lungs up to the brim. Care should be taken not to bloat the abdomen in the process of inhalation. (Observe this in all the types of Prāṇāyāma.) This filling up is called puraka (inhalation).

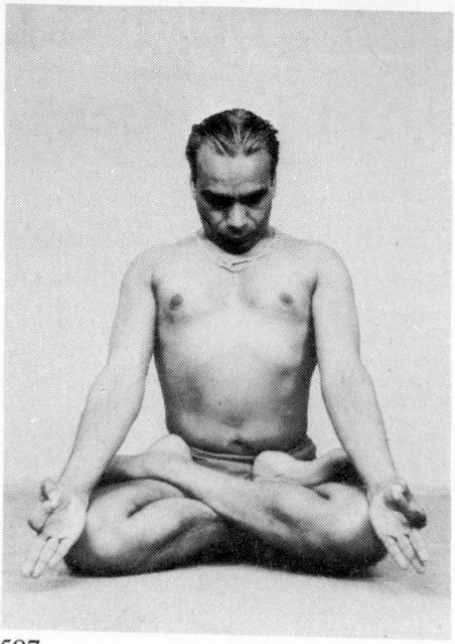

597

9. The entire abdominal area from the pubes up to the breast-bone should be pulled back towards the spine.

10. Hold the breath for a second or two. This internal retention is called antara kumbhaka. Observe Mūla Bandha as described on p. 437.

11. Exhale slowly, deeply and steadily, until the lungs are completely empty. As you begin to exhale, keep your grip on the abdomen. After two or three seconds of exhalation, relax the diaphragm gradually and slowly. While exhaling the passage of the outgoing air should be felt on the roof of the palate. The brushing of the air on the palate should make an aspirate sound (ha). This exhalation is called rechaka.

12. Wait for a second before drawing a fresh breath. This waiting period is called bāhya kumbhaka.

13. The process described from para. 7 to para. 12 completes one cycle of Ujjāyi Prāṇāyāma.

14. Repeat the cycles for five to ten minutes keeping the eyes closed throughout.

15. Lie on the floor in Śavāsana. (Plate 592)

16. Ujjāyi Prāṇāyāma may be done without the Jālandhara Bandha even while walking or lying down. This is the only prāṇāyāma which can be done at all times of the day and night.

Effects

This type of prāṇāyāma aerates the lungs, removes phlegm, gives endurance, soothes the nerves and tones the entire system. Ujjāyi without kumbhaka, done in a reclining position, is ideal for persons suffering from high blood pressure or coronary troubles.

204. *Sūrya Bhedana Prāṇāyāma* (Plate 599)

Sūrya is the sun. Bhedana is derived from the root bhid meaning to pierce, to break or pass through.

In Sūrya Bhedana Prāṇāyāma, the breath is inhaled through the right nostril. In other words the prāṇa passes through the Piṅgalā or Sūrya nādī. A kumbhaka is then performed and the breath is then exhaled through the left nostril which is the path of the Idā nāḍī.

Technique

1. Sit in any comfortable position like Padmāsana (Plate 104), Siddhāsana (Plate 84) or Vīrāsana (Plate 89).

2. Keep the back erect and rigid. Lower the head to the trunk. Rest the chin in the notch between the collar-bones just above the breast-bone. (This is Jālandhara Bandha.)

3. Stretch the left arm. Rest the back of the left wrist on the left knee. Perform Jñāna Mudrā with the left hand (as stated in stage 3 of the technique of Ujjāyi).

4. Bend the right arm at the elbow. Bend the index and middle fingers towards the palm, keeping them passive. Bring the ring and little fingers towards the thumb. (Plate 598)

5. Place the right thumb on the right side of the nose just below the nasal bone, the ring and little fingers on the left side of the nose just below the nasal bone, just above the curve of the fatty tissue of the nostrils above the upper jaw.

6. Press the ring and the little finger to block the left side of the nose completely.

7. With the right thumb, press the fatty tissue on the right side so as to make the outer edge of the right nostril parallel to the lower edge of the cartilage of the septum.

8. The right thumb is bent at the top joint and the tip of the thumb is placed at a right angle to the septum. (Plate 599)

9. Now inhale slowly and deeply controlling the aperture of the right

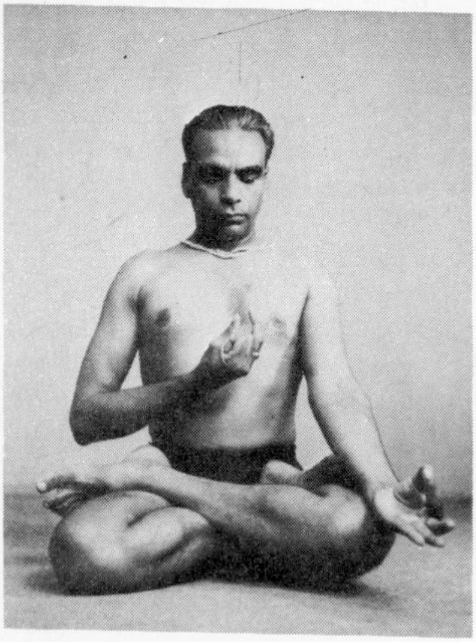

598

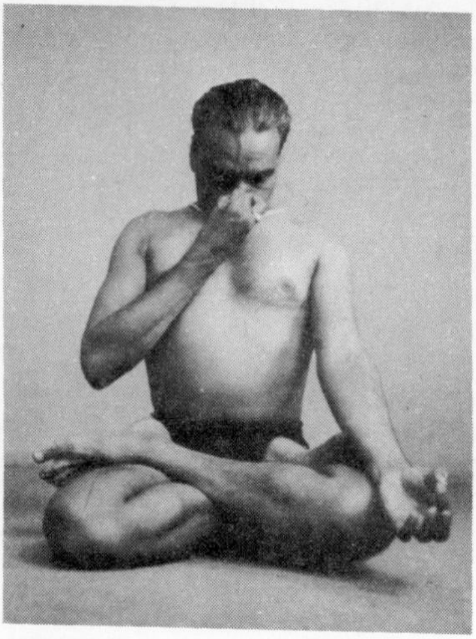

599

nostril with the tip of the thumb nearer the nail. Fill the lungs to the brim (puraka).

10. Then block the right nostril so that both are now blocked.

11. Hold the breath for about 5 seconds (antara kumbhaka) while practising Mūla Bandha (see p. 437).

12. Keeping the right nostril completely blocked, open the left nostril partially and exhale through it slowly and deeply (rechaka).

13. During the exhalation regulate the rhythmic flow of air from the left nostril by adjusting pressure with the ring and little fingers, so that the outer edge of the left nostril is kept parallel to the septum. The pressure should be exerted from the inner sides of the tips of the fingers (away from the nails).

14. This completes one cycle of Sūrya Bhedana Prāṇāyāma. Continue with more cycles at a stretch from 5 to 10 minutes, according to capacity.

15. All the inhalations in Sūrya Bhedana are from the right nostril and all the exhalations from the left nostril.

16. Throughout the process, the passage of air is felt at the tips of the fingers and the thumbs and in the nasal membranes where pressure is applied. The passage of air makes a sound similar to air escaping from a cycle tube. This sound should be maintained constant throughout by varying pressure on the nostrils.

17. The eyes, temples, eyebrows and the skin on the forehead should remain completely passive and show no sign of strain.

18. The mind should be absorbed completely in listening to the proper sound of the passage of air and in maintaining a proper rhythm in breathing.

19. Each inhalation and exhalation should last for the same length of time.

20. The inhalation and the exhalation should not be forced. An even and slow rhythm should be maintained throughout.

21. Lie down in Śavāsana after completing prāṇāyāma. (Plate 592)

Effects

By reason of the pressure on the nostrils, in this Prāṇāyāma the lungs have to work more than in the case of Ujjāyi. In Sūrya Bhedana they are filled more slowly, steadily, and fuller than in Ujjāyi. Sūrya Bhedana increases digestive power, soothes and invigorates the nerves, and cleans the sinuses.

Note. – It often happens that the passages of both the nostrils are not of the same width, one being bigger than the other. In that case the pressure of the fingers has to be adjusted. In some cases the right nostril is completely blocked while the left one is clear. In that case, inhalation may be done only through the left nostril, while exhalation is done only through the right nostril. In course of time due to the manipulation of the fingers the right nostril clears and inhalation through it becomes possible.

Caution. – Persons suffering from low blood pressure will derive benefit but those with high blood pressure or heart trouble should not hold their breath after inhalation (antara kumbhaka) whilst practising this prāṇāyāma.

205. *Nāḍī Śodhana Prāṇāyāma*

Nāḍī is a tubular organ of the body like an artery or a vein for the passage of prāṇa or energy. A nāḍī has three layers like an insulated electric wire. The innermost layer is called sirā, the middle layer damanī and the entire organ as well as the outer layer is called nāḍī.

Śodhana meaning purifying or cleansing, so the object of Nāḍī Śodhana Prāṇāyāma is the purification of the nerves. A little obstruction in a water pipe can cut off the supply completely. A little obstruction in the nerves can cause great discomfort and paralyse a limb or organ.

Technique

1. Follow the technique given in paras 1 to 8 of Sūrya Bhedana Prāṇāyāma. (Plate 599)

2. Empty the lungs completely through the right nostril. Control the aperture of the right nostril with the inner side of the right thumb, away from the nail.

3. Now inhale slowly, steadily and deeply through the right nostril, controlling the aperture with the tip of the right thumb near the nail. Fill the lungs to the brim (puraka). During this inhalation the left nostril is completely blocked by the ring and little fingers.

4. After full inhalation, block the right nostril completely with the pressure of the thumb and release the pressure of the ring and little fingers on the left nostril. Readjust them on the outer edge of the left nostril and keep it parallel to the septum. Exhale slowly, steadily and deeply through the left nostril. Empty the lungs completely. The pressure should be exerted from the inner sides of the tips of the ring and little fingers (away from the nails) (rechaka).

5. After full exhalation through the left nostril, change the pressure on it by adjusting the fingers. In the changed position, the tips of the ring and little fingers nearer the nails exert the pressure.

6. Now inhale through the left nostril slowly, steadily and deeply, filling the lungs to the brim (puraka).

7. After full inhalation through the left nostril, block it and exhale through the right nostril, adjusting the pressure of the right thumb on the right nostril as stated in para. 2 above (rechaka).

8. This completes one cycle of Nāḍī Śodhana Prāṇāyāma. Here the rhythm of breathing is as follows:

(a) Exhale through the right nostril.
(b) Inhale through the right nostril.
(c) Exhale through the left nostril.
(d) Inhale through the left nostril.
(e) Exhale through the right nostril.
(f) Inhale through the right nostril.
(g) Exhale through the left nostril.
(h) Inhale through the left nostril.
(i) Exhale through the right nostril.
(j) Inhale through the right nostril . . . and so on.

Stage (a) above is the preparatory one. The first real Nāḍī Śodhana Prāṇāyāma cycle starts at stage (b) and ends at stage (e). The second cycle starts at stage (f) and ends at stage (i). Stage (j) is the safety measure to be observed after the completion of the cycles in order to prevent gasping, breathlessness and strain on the heart.

9. Do 8 to 10 cycles at a stretch as described above. This may take 6 or 8 minutes.

10. Inhalation and exhalation from each side should take the same time. In the beginning the duration will be unequal. Persevere until equality is achieved.

11. After achieving mastery over the equal duration and precision over inhalation and exhalation on either side an attempt may be made to retain breath (antara kumbhaka) after inhaling.

12. This precision is only achieved after long practice.

13. Retention should not disturb the rhythm and equality of inhalation and exhalation. If either are disturbed curtail the period of retention or hold the breath on alternate cycles.

14. During retention after inhalation practise Mūla Bandha (see p. 437).

15. Do not attempt to hold the breath after exhalation (bāhya kumbhaka, Plate 600) until you have mastered retention after inhalation (antara kumbhaka). Then during bāhya kumbhaka practise Uḍḍiyānā (Plates 593, 594) with Mūla Bandha (see p. 437).

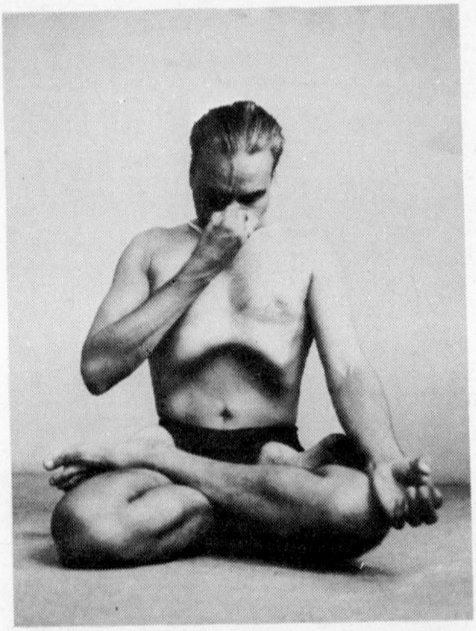

600

16. Retention and the lengthening of inhalation and exhalation should only be attempted with the help and under the guidance of an experienced Guru.

17. Always conclude by lying down in Śavāsana. (Plate 592)

Effects

The blood receives a larger supply of oxygen in Nāḍī Śodhana than in normal breathing, so that one feels refreshed and the nerves are calmed and purified. The mind becomes still and lucid.

Note. – In the beginning the body perspires and shakes, while the thigh and arm muscles become tense. Such tension should be avoided.

Caution

1. Persons suffering from high blood pressure or heart trouble should never attempt to hold their breath (kumbhaka). They can practise Nāḍī Śodhana Prāṇāyāma without retention (kumbhaka) with beneficial effect.

2. Persons suffering from low blood pressure can do this prāṇāyāma with retention after inhalation (antara kumbhaka) *only*, with beneficial effects.

Prāṇāyāmas

206. *Bhastrikā Prāṇāyāma*

Bhastrikā means a bellows used in a furnace. Here the air is forcibly drawn in and out as in a blacksmith's bellows. Hence the name. The technique is given in two stages here.

Technique Stage I

1. Follow the technique in paras 1 and 2 of Ujjāyi.

2. Take a fast, vigorous breath and exhale fast and forcefully. One inhalation and one exhalation completes a cycle of Bhastrikā. The sound made resembles air rushing through bellows.

3. Complete at a stretch 10 to 12 cycles. Then take a slow deep breath as in Ujjāyi. Retain the breath with Mūla Bandha for 2 to 3 seconds, then exhale slowly and deeply as in Ujjāyi.

4. This Ujjāyi type of breathing rests the lungs and the diaphragm and prepares them for fresh cycles of Bhastrikā.

5. Repeat the cycles of Bhastrikā three to four times with Ujjāyi breathing in between.

6. If the sound of the air lessens, and the vigour diminishes, then reduce their number.

7. After completion lie down in Śavāsana. (Plate 592)

Stage II

1. Follow the technique in paras 1 and 2 of Ujjāyi.

2. Adjust the thumb and finger pressure on the nostrils as explained in the technique of Sūrya Bhedana.

3. Close the left nostril completely but keep the right nostril partially open.

4. Inhale and exhale vigorously only through the right nostril for 10 to 12 cycles of Bhastrikā as in Stage I above.

5. Close the right nostril. Open the left nostril partially and repeat Bhastrikā for an equal number of cycles.

6. Release the fingers from the nostrils.

7. Take a few deep breaths as in Ujjāyi.

8. Repeat the cycles on both sides three or four times, doing Ujjāyi in between.

9. After completion lie down in Śavāsana. (Plate 592)

207. *Kapālabhāti Prāṇāyāma*

The process or kriyā of *Kapālabhāti* (kapāla = skull; bhāti = light, lustre) is a milder form of Bhastrikā Prāṇāyāma. In Kapālabhāti, the inhalation is slow but the exhalation is vigorous. There is a split second of retention after each exhalation. Do a few cycles of Kapālabhāti instead of Bhastrikā if the latter breathing proves too strenuous. Lie down in Śavāsana after finishing Kapālabhāti. (Plate 592)

Effects

Both Bhastrikā and Kapālabhāti activate and invigorate the liver, spleen, pancreas and abdominal muscles. Thus digestion is improved, the sinuses are drained, the eyes feel cool and one has a general sense of exhilaration.

Caution

1. As a locomotive engine is stoked with coal to generate steam to pull the train, so Bhastrikā generates prāṇā to activate the entire body. Too much stoking burns out the boiler of the engine. So also too long a practice of Bhastrikā wears out the system as the breathing process is forceful.

2. Persons with a weak constitution and poor lung capacity should not attempt Bhastrikā or Kapālabhāti.

3. Those suffering from ear or eye complaints (pus in the ear, detachment of the retina or glaucoma) should not attempt them either.

4. Nor should persons with high or low blood pressure.

5. If the nose starts to bleed or the ears to throb and ache, immediately stop Bhastrikā or Kapālabhāti.

6. Do not practise either for some time.

208. *Bhamarī Prāṇāyāma*

Bhamarī means a large black bee.

Technique

The technique of Bhamarī Prāṇāyāma is the same as that of Ujjāyi. The difference is that in Bhamarī, during exhalation, a soft humming sound like the murmuring of bees is made. After completion lie down in Śavāsana. (Plate 592)

Effects

The humming sound in Bhamarī Prāṇāyāma is helpful in cases of insomnia.

209. *Śītalī Prāṇāyāma* (Plate 601)

Śītala means cool. This prāṇāyāma cools the system, hence the name.

Technique

1. Sit in Padmāsana (Plate 104), Siddhāsana (Plate 84) or Vīrāsana (Plate 89).

2. Keep the back erect and rigid and the head level. Perform the Jñāna Mudrā with the hands (see p. 433, para. 21). Here Jālandhara Bandha is not done during inhalation but later.

3. Open the mouth and form the lips into an 'O'.

4. The sides and tip of the tongue touching the teeth, from the molars to the front teeth, should be lifted and curled up. The shape of the tongue will resemble a fresh curled leaf about to open. (Plate 601)

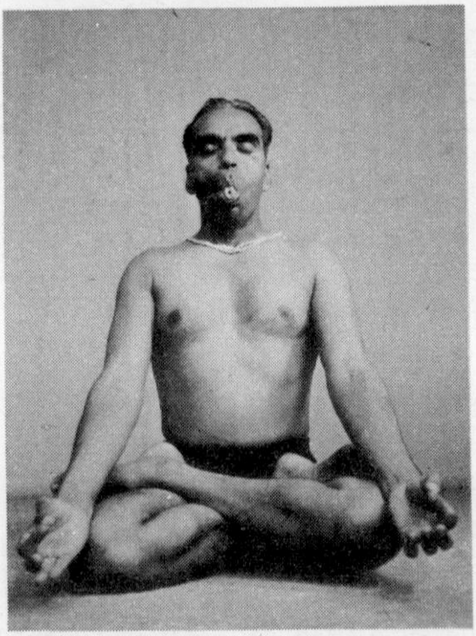

601

5. Protrude the curled tongue out of the lips. Draw in the air past the curled tongue with a sibilant sound (sssssssa) to fill the lungs completely. The air is drawn in as if through a pipette or a drinking straw. After full inhalation withdraw the tongue and close the mouth.

6. After full inhalation, lower the head, from the nape of the neck, to the trunk. The chin should rest in the notch between the collar-bones just above the breast-bone. The head is now in the Jālandhara Bandha position.

7. Now hold the breath (antara kumbhaka) for about 5 seconds, practising Mūla Bandha (see p. 437).

8. Exhale slowly with an aspirate sound (hhuuuuuuuum) through the nose as in Ujjāyī.

9. This completes one cycle of Śitalī Prāṇāyāma.

10. Lift the head and repeat the cycle for 5 to 10 minutes.

11. After completion lie down in Śavāsana. (Plate 592)

Effects

This cools the system and soothes the eyes and ears. It is beneficial in cases of low fever and biliousness. It activates the liver and the spleen, improves digestion and relieves thirst.

Caution

1. Persons suffering from high blood pressure should omit antara kumbhaka.

2. Those with heart trouble should not attempt Śitalī Prāṇāyāma in the beginning.

210. *Śitakārī Prāṇāyāma*

Śitakārī is that which causes cold. This is a variation of Śitalī Prāṇāyāma.

Technique

Here the tongue is not curled. The lips are kept slightly parted and only the tip of the tongue protrudes between the teeth. The tongue is kept flat as in its normal state. Follow the same technique as in Śitalī Prāṇāyāma.

Effects

The effects are the same as those mentioned for Śitalī Prāṇāyāma.

Caution

Persons with high blood pressure may find greater strain in Śitakārī than in Śītalī Prāṇāyāma.

211. *Sama Vṛtti Prāṇāyāma*

1. Sama means the same or identical, straight, entire, whole and complete: also similarly or in the same manner.

2. Vṛtti means action, movement, function or operation, a course of conduct or method.

3. In Sama Vṛtti Prāṇāyāma, therefore, an attempt is made to achieve uniformity in the duration of all the three processes of breathing, namely, puraka or inhalation, kumbhaka or retention, and rechaka or exhalation in any type of prāṇāyāma. If one lasts 5 seconds so do the others.

4. This uniformity of 5 seconds should be maintained throughout all the cycles of breathing in any type of Prāṇāyāma like Ujjāyī, Sūrya Bhedana, Nāḍī Śodhana, Śitalī and so on.

Caution

5. In the beginning Sama Vṛtti Prāṇāyāma should be confined only to inhalation (puraka) and exhalation (rechaka).

6. First, achieve uniformity of length of time in puraka and rechaka then only attempt antara kumbhaka (retention of breath after full inhalation).

7. Start the antara kumbhaka gradually. In the beginning, the ratio of time for pūraka, antara kumbhaka and rechaka should be kept at $1 : \frac{1}{4} : 1$. Very slowly increase the proportions to $1 : \frac{1}{2} : 1$. After this is firmly established attempt $1 : \frac{3}{4} : 1$. Only after mastering this, increase the proportion of antara kumbhaka so as to achieve the ratio of $1 : 1 : 1$.

8. Do not attempt bāhya kumbhaka (restraint of breath after full exhalation) until you have achieved the desired ratio of $1 : 1 : 1$ in pūraka, antara kumbhaka and rechaka.

9. If all air is expelled from the lungs, the vacuum inside and the atmospheric pressure outside will create a tremendous strain upon the lungs. Therefore, in the beginning, do not do both antara kumbhaka and bāhya kumbhaka together.

10. Practise antara kumbhaka and bāhya kumbhaka separately or alternately. It is beneficial to practise kumbhakas first by interspersing

them after two or three cycles of deep breathing with pūraka and rechaka alone. For example do two or three cycles of deep breathing and one cycle of antara kumbhaka. Then do two or three cycles of deep breathing followed by one cycle of bāhya kumbhaka. Start with 3 antara kumbhakas and 3 bāhya kumbhakas, and increase the number of kumbhakas very gradually.

212. *Viṣama Vṛtti Prāṇāyāma*

1. Viṣama means among many other things irregular and difficult.

2. Viṣama Vṛtti Prāṇāyāma is so called because the same length of time for inhalation, retention and exhalation is not maintained. This leads to interruption of rhythm and the difference in ratio creates difficulty and danger for the pupil.

3. In this type of prāṇāyāma if full inhalation takes 5 seconds, the breath is held (antara kumbhaka) for 20 seconds, and exhalation takes 10 seconds, the ratio being 1 : 4 : 2. At first the pupil will find it hard to maintain the rhythm during exhalation, but it all eases with practice.

4. Conversely, if inhalation is for 10 seconds, the breath is held for 20 seconds and exhalation takes 5 seconds, the ratio here being 2 : 4 : 1.

5. Again if the length of time can be so varied that if inhalation is for 20 seconds, retention is for 10 seconds and exhalation for 5, the ratio being 4 : 2 : 1.

6. In one cycle of prāṇāyāma, one can adopt the ratios 1 : 2 : 4, 2 : 4 : 1, and 4 : 1 : 2. Then these three ratios are counted as one cycle of prāṇāyāma.

7. If bāhya kumbhaka (restraint after full exhalation and before fresh inhalation) is also observed, the combination of ratios will be greater still.

8. If the different ratios are observed in the Viloma, Anuloma and Pratiloma methods of prāṇāyāma (described below) in the basic varieties of prāṇāyāmas like Ujjāyi, Sūrya Bhedana, Nāḍī Śodhana, Bhramari, Śitalī and Śitakāri, the number of combinations will be astronomical.

9. No mortal could perform all these different combinations in one lifetime.

10. The path of Viṣama Vṛtti Prāṇāyāma is fraught with danger. Do

not, therefore, dream of attempting to practise it on your own without the personal supervision of an experienced Guru or teacher.

11. Due to disharmony caused by these different time ratios for inhalation, retention and exhalation, all the systems of the body, especially the respiratory and nervous ones, are overtaxed and unduly strained.

12. The caution given on Sama Vṛtti Prāṇāyāma (see p. 453), regarding the practice of kumbhaka in paragraphs 5 to 10, applies with greater force in Viṣama Vṛtti Prāṇāyāma.

13. One now begins to realise the truth of Svātmārāma's statement in the second chapter of the *Haṭha Yoga Pradīpikā*: 'Prāṇa should be tamed more slowly and more gradually than lions, elephants and tigers (according to one's capacities and physical limitations); otherwise it will kill the practitioner.'

VILOMA, ANULOMA AND PRATILOMA PRĀṆĀYĀMAS

Sama Vṛtti and Viṣama Vṛtti Prāṇāyāma are concerned with the maintenance of a particular ratio of time taken in inhalation, retention and exhalation.

The Viloma, Anuloma and Pratiloma types of Prāṇāyāma are concerned with the methods and techniques of inhalation and exhalation. In Viloma, the inhalation or exhalation is not one continuous process, but is done gradually with several pauses. In Anuloma, inhalation is through both nostrils as in Ujjāyi and exhalation is alternate through either nostril as in Nāḍī Śodhana. In Pratiloma, all inhalation is alternate through either nostril while all exhalation is through both nostrils as in Ujjāyi.

213. *Viloma Prāṇāyāma*

Loma means hair. The particle vi is used to denote negation or privation. Viloma thus means against the hair, against the grain, against the natural order of things.

In Viloma Prāṇāyāma inhalation or exhalation is not one uninterrupted continuous process, but is interrupted by several pauses. For instance, if continuous inhalation to fill the lungs or continuous exhalation to expel the air were to take 15 seconds in each case, in Viloma there would be a pause of about 2 seconds after every third second of inhalation or of exhalation. The process of inhalation or of exhalation is thus lengthened to 25 seconds. The technique given below is in two stages, which are distinct.

Technique: Stage I

1. Viloma Prāṇāyāma can be done either in a sitting posture or while lying down.

2. If done when seated, keep the back erect, lower the head to the trunk so that the chin rests in the notch between the collar-bones on the top of the breast-bone. This is Jālandhara Bandha. Keep the hands in Jñāna Mudra (see p. 433, para. 21).

3. Inhale for 2 seconds, pause for 2 seconds holding the breath, again inhale for 2 seconds, again pause for 2 seconds holding the breath, and continue like this until the lungs are completely full.

4. Now hold the breath for 5 to 10 seconds (antara kumbhaka) according to capacity, practising Mūla Bandha (see p. 437).

5. During the pauses in the process of inhalation Mūla Bandha should be practised.

6. Exhale slowly and deeply as in Ujjāyi with an aspirate sound (huuuum). During exhalation relax the Mūla Bandha.

7. This completes one cycle of the first stage of Viloma Prāṇāyāma.

8. Repeat 10 to 15 cycles of this first stage at a stretch.

Stage II

9. Rest for a minute or two.

10. Then take a deep breath without any pauses as in Ujjāyi with a sibilant sound (sssssssa), keeping the chin on the top of the breast-bone. Fill the lungs completely.

11. Hold the breath from 5 to 10 seconds (antara kumbhaka), keeping the Mūla Bandha grip.

12. Exhale for 2 seconds and pause for 2 seconds. Again exhale for 2 seconds, pause for 2 seconds and continue like this until the lungs are completely emptied.

13. During the pauses maintain the Mūla Bandha grip.

14. This completes one cycle of the second stage of Viloma Prāṇāyāma.

15. Repeat the second stage of Viloma 10 to 15 times at a stretch.

16. This completes Viloma Prāṇāyāma.

17. Then lie down in Śavāsana. (Plate 592)

Effects

Viloma Prāṇāyāma in the first stage helps those suffering from low blood pressure. In the second stage it benefits persons suffering from high blood pressure.

Caution

1. The second stage of Viloma should only be done when lying down by persons suffering from high blood pressure.

2. Those suffering from heart complaints should not attempt it until they have mastered the Nāḍī Śodhana and Ujjāyi Prāṇāyāmas.

214. *Anuloma Prāṇāyāma*

Anu means with, along with or connected: also in an orderly succession. Anuloma, therefore, means in regular gradation, with the hair (loma = hair), along the grain or in natural order. In Anuloma Prāṇāyāma, inhalation is done through both nostrils and exhalation alternately through either nostril.

Technique

1. Sit in any comfortable position like Padmāsana (Plate 104), Siddhāsana (Plate 84) or Vīrāsana (Plate 89).

2. Keep the back erect and rigid. Lower the head to the trunk and rest the chin in the notch between the collar-bones just above the breast-bone. (This is the Jālandhara Bandha.)

3. Inhale deeply through both nostrils as in Ujjāyi until the lungs are fully filled.

4. Hold the breath after inhalation (antara kumbhaka) from 5 to 10 seconds according to capacity, maintaining Mūla Bandha (see p. 437).

5. Bring the right hand to the nose as described in Sūrya Bhedana Prāṇāyāma, relax the Mūla Bandha and exhale slowly from the partially opened right nostril, keeping the left one completely blocked. Completely empty the lungs and then lower the hand.

6. Inhale through both nostrils, until the lungs are filled as in para. 3.

7. Hold the breath after inhalation (antara kumbhaka) from 5 to 10 seconds according to capacity, maintaining Mūla Bandha. The retention of breath described in para. 4 and in this para. should be of equal length.

8. Again bring the right hand to the nose. Release the Mūla Bandha and close the right nostril completely. Now keep the left nostril

partially open, and exhale slowly and deeply to empty the lungs completely.

9. This completes one cycle of Anuloma Prāṇāyāma.

10. Do 5 to 8 cycles at a stretch.

11. Then lie down in Śavāsana. (Plate 592)

Effects

The effects are the same as those of Ujjāyi, Nāḍī Śodhana and Sūrya Bhedana.

Caution

1. In Anuloma Prāṇāyāma, the exhalation lasts longer than the inhalation. This leads to a variation in the rhythm of breathing. This is difficult and should therefore be done by advanced pupils only.

2. Persons suffering from blood pressure or heart ailments and nervous disorders should not attempt it as the results may be disastrous.

215. *Pratiloma Prāṇāyāma*

Prati means opposite. This type of Prāṇāyāma is the converse of Anuloma. In it inhalation is alternate through either nostril and then exhalation is through both nostrils as in Ujjāyi.

Technique

1. Sit in any comfortable position like Padmāsana (Plate 104), Siddhāsana (Plate 84) or Vīrāsana (Plate 89).

2. Keep the back erect and rigid. Lower the head to the trunk. Rest the chin in the notch between the collar-bones just above the breast-bone. This is the Jālandhara Bandha.

3. Stretch the left arm. Rest the back of the left wrist on the left knee. Perform the Jñāna Mudra with the left hand (see 203, 3).

4. Bend the right arm at the elbow, and the index and middle fingers towards the palm, keeping them passive. Bring the ring and little fingers towards the thumb. (Plate 598)

5. Place the right thumb on the right side of the nose just below the nasal bone and the ring and little fingers on the left side of the nose just below the nasal bone, just above the curve of the fatty tissue of the nostrils.

6. Press the ring and little fingers to block the left side of the nose completely.

7. With the right thumb, press the right side of the fatty tissue so as to make the outer edge of the nostril parallel to the lower edge of the cartilage of the septum.

8. The right thumb is bent at the top joint and the tip of the thumb is placed at a right angle to the septum. (Plate 599)

9. Now inhale slowly and deeply, controlling the aperture of the right nostril with the tip of the thumb nearer the nail. Fill the lungs to the brim (puraka).

10. Then block the right nostril so that both the nostrils are now blocked.

11. Hold the breath for about 5 to 10 seconds (antara kumbhaka) and stay in Mūla Bandha (see p. 437).

12. Lower the right hand. Release the Mūla Bandha grip. Exhale slowly and deeply as in Ujjāyi (203) until the lungs are completely empty.

13. Again raise the right hand to the nose. Inhale through the partially opened left nostril slowly and deeply, keeping the right nostril completely closed.

14. Fill the lungs to the brim.

15. Hold the breath with the Mūla Bandha grip from 5 to 10 seconds. The retention of breath (antara kumbhaka) after inhalation from either nostril should be of equal duration.

16. Lower the right hand, release the Mūla Bandha, exhale slowly and deeply, completely expelling all air from the lungs as in Ujjāyi.

17. This completes one cycle of Pratiloma Prāṇāyāma.

18. Do 5 to 8 cycles at a stretch.

19. Then lie down in Śavāsana. (Plate 592)

Effects

The effects are the same as those of Ujjāyi, Nāḍī Śodhana and Sūrya Bhedana Prāṇāyāma.

Caution

1. Here, as in Anuloma, there is variation in the breath rhythm as the inhalation is longer than the exhalation. This difficult type of prāṇāyāma should, therefore, only be done by advanced pupils.

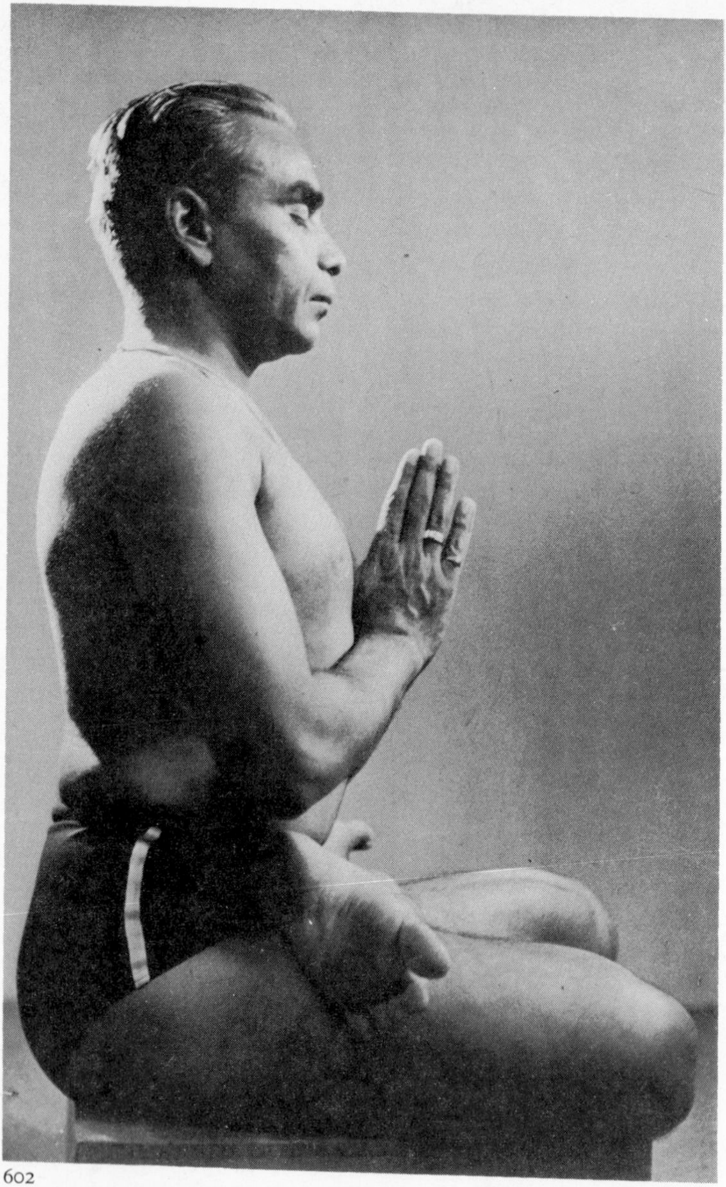

602

2. Persons suffering from blood pressure, heart ailments and nervous disorders should not attempt it, as the results will be disastrous.

216. *Sahita and Kevala Kumbhaka Prāṇāyāma*

Sahita means accompanied by, together with or associated with.

When prāṇāyāma practices are observed with the intentional aid and deliberate accompaniment of bāhya and antara kumbhaka, they are known as Sahita Kumbhaka Prāṇāyāmas.

Kevala means isolated, pure, absolute and perfect. When the practices of kumbhaka becomes *instinctive*, they are called Kevala Kumbhaka.

When the pupil has mastered Kevala Kumbhaka, he has isolated himself from the world and is in tune with the Infinite. He has obtained a measure of control over one of the most subtle and powerful of elements which can pervade the smallest crevice as well as the vast sky. His mind is completely absorbed with Prāṇa and becomes as free as Prāṇa itself.

As a wind drives smoke and impurities from the atmosphere, prāṇāyāma drives away the impurities of the body and the mind. Then, says Patañjali, the DIVINE FIRE within blazes forth in its full glory and the mind becomes fit for concentration (dhāraṇā) and meditation (dhyāna). (*Yoga Sutras*, chapter II, 52 and 53.) This takes a long time. By degrees is the darkness banished by the dawn.

Appendix I

Āsana Courses

I am dividing the āsanas into three groups; the primary, intermediate and advanced courses. I am giving the series of āsanas in a serial order for practice and the possible time it may take to gain control in all these three courses.

(The figures within the brackets after the āsanas denote the serial number of the illustrations.)

COURSE ONE

1st and 2nd week

Tāḍāsana (1); Vṛkṣāsana (2); Utthita Trikoṇāsana (4 and 5); Utthita Pārśvakoṇāsana (8 and 9); Vīrabhadrāsana I & II (14 and 15); Pārśvottānāsana (26); Sālamba Sarvāngāsana I (223); Halāsana (244); Śavāsana (592).

3rd and 4th week

Utthita Trikoṇāsana (4 and 5); Utthita Pārśvakoṇāsana (8 and 9); Vīrabhadrāsana I & II (14 and 15); Parivṛtta Trikoṇāsana (6 and 7); Pārśvottānāsana (26); Prasārita Pādottānāsana I (33 and 34); Sālamba Sarvāngāsana I (223); Halāsana (244); Śavāsana (592).

5th and 6th week

Utthita Trikoṇāsana (4 and 5); Utthita Pārśvakoṇāsana (8 and 9); Vīrabhadrāsana I & II (14 and 15); Parivṛtta Trikoṇāsana (6 and 7); Pārśvottānāsana (26); Prasārita Pādottānāsana I (33 and 34); Ūrdhva Prasārita Pādāsana (276 to 279); Paripoorṇa Nāvāsana (78); Ardha Nāvāsana (79); Sālamba Sarvāngāsana I (223); Halāsana (244); Ujjāyī Prāṇāyāma (Section 203) for five minutes in Śavāsana (592).

7th week

Consolidate the āsanas and increase the length of stay in all of them.

8th week

Utthita Trikoṇāsana (4 and 5); Utthita Pārśvakoṇāsana (8 and 9); Vīrabhadrāsana I, II & III (14, 15 and 17); Ardha Chandrāsana (19); Parivṛtta Trikoṇāsana (6 and 7); Pārśvottānāsana (26); Prasārita

Pādottānāsana I & II (33 and 34, 35 and 36); Ūrdhva Prasārita Pādāsana (276 to 279); Paripoorṇa Nāvāsana (78); Ardha Nāvāsana (79); Sālamba Sarvāngāsana (223); Halāsana (244); Ujjāyī Prāṇāyāma (Section 203) for five minutes in Śavāsana (592).

9th and 10th week

Utthita Trikoṇāsana (4 and 5); Utthita Pārśvakoṇāsana (8 and 9); Vīrabhadrāsana I, II and III (14, 15 and 17); Ardha Chandrāsana (19); Parivṛtta Trikoṇāsana (6 and 7); Parivṛtta Parśvakoṇāsana (10 and 11); Pārśvottānāsana (26); Prasārita Pādottānāsana I & II (33 and 34, 35 and 36); Parighāsana (39); Ūrdhva Prasārita Pādāsana (276 to 279); Paripoorṇa Nāvāsana (78); Ardha Nāvāsana (79); Sālamba Sarvangāsana I (223); Halāsana (244); Karṇapīdāsana (246); Ekapāda Sarvāngāsana (250); Jaṭara Parivartanāsana (274 and 275); Ujjāyī Prāṇāyāma with inhalation retention (Section 203) for five minutes in Śavāsana (592).

11th and 12th week

Utthita Trikoṇāsana (4 and 5); Parivṛtta Trikoṇāsana (6 and 7); Utthita Pārśvakoṇāsana (8 and 9); Parivṛtta Pārśvakoṇāsana (10 and 11); Vīrabhadrāsana I, II & III (14, 15 and 17); Ardha Chandrāsana (19); Pārśvottānāsana (26); Prasārita Pādottānāsana I & II (33 and 34, 35 and 36); Pādānguṣṭhāsana (44); Pādahastāsana (46); Uttānāsana (48); Parighāsana (39); Ūrdhva Prasārita Pādāsana (276 to 279); Paripoorṇa Nāvāsana (78); Ardha Nāvāsana (79); Sālamba Sarvāngāsana I (223); Halāsana (244); Karṇapīdāsana (246); Ekapāda Sarvāngāsana (250); Jaṭara Parivartanāsana (274 and 275); Ujjāyī Prāṇāyāma with inhalation retention (Section 203) in Śavāsana (592).

13th week

Repeat and become steady in your daily practices. Those who find it difficult to master all these āsanas within this period can continue with them for several more weeks.

14th and 15th week

Sālamba Śīrṣāsana I (184); Utthita and Parivṛtta Trikoṇāsana (4 and 5, 6 and 7); Utthita and Parivṛtta Pārśvakoṇāsana (8 and 9, 10 and 11); Vīrabhadrāsana I, II & III (14, 15 and 17); Ardha Chandrāsana (19); Pārśvottānāsana (26); Prasārita Pādottānāsana I & II (33, 34, 35 and 36) Pādānguṣṭhāsana (44); Pādahastāsana (46); Uttānāsana (48); Parighāsana (39); Śalabhāsana or Makarāsana (60 or 62); Dhanurāsana (63); Bhujangāsana I (73); Ūrdhva Prasārita Pādāsana (276 to 279); Paripoorṇa Nāvāsana (78); Ardha Nāvāsana (79); Sālamba Sarvāngāsana I (223);

Halāsana (244); Karṇapīḍāsana (246); Supta Koṇāsana (247); Pārśva Halāsana (249); Ekapāda Sarvāngāsana (250); Jaṭara Parivartanāsana (274 and 275); Mahāmudra (125); Januśīrṣāsana (127); Daṇḍāsana (77); Paschimottānāsana (160); Ujjāyī Prāṇāyāma with inhalation retention (Section 203) in Savāsana (592).

16th and 17th week (Observe the change in the order of the āsanas)

Sālamba Śīrṣāsana I (184); Utthita and Parivṛtta Trikoṇāsana (4, 5, 6 and 7); Utthita and Parivṛtta Pārśvakoṇāsana (8, 9, 10 and 11); Vīrabhadrāsana I, II & III (14, 15 and 17); Ardha Chandrāsana (19); Pārśvottānāsana (26); Prasārita Pādottānāsana I & II (33, 34, 35 and 36); Pādānguṣṭhāsana (44); Pādahastāsana (46); Uttānāsana (48); Ūrdhva Prasārita Ekapādāsana (49); Utkaṭāsana (42); Parighāsana (39); Uṣṭrāsana (41); Salabhāsana or Makarāsana (60 or 62); Dhanurāsana (63); Chaturanga Daṇḍāsana (67); Bhujangāsana I (73); Ūrdhva Mukha Śvānāsana (74); Adho Mukha Śvānāsana (75); Vīrāsana (86); Sālamba Sarvāngāsana I (223); Halāsana (244); Karṇapīḍāsana (246); Supta Koṇāsana (247); Pārśva Halāsana (249); Ekapāda Sarvāngāsana (250); Pārśvaikapāda Sarvāngāsana (251); Jaṭara Parivartanāsana (274 and 275); Ūrdhva Prasārita Pādāsana (276 to 279); Paripoorṇa Nāvāsana (78); Ardha Nāvāsana (79); Mahāmudrā (125); Jānuśīrṣāsana (127); Paschimottānāsana (160); Poorvottānāsana (171); Śavāsana (592); Siddhāsana (84). Do Ujjāyī Prāṇāyāma (without inhalation retention) (Section 203) in Siddhāsana.

18th week

Repeat.

If you now find all the standing āsanas are easy enough, you can do them on alternate days or twice a week.

19th to 21st week

Sālamba Śīrṣāsana I (184); Pārśva Śīrṣāsana (202 and 203); Ekapāda Śīrṣāsana (208 and 209); Sālamba Sarvāngāsana I (223); Sālamba Sarvāngāsana II (235); Nirālamba Sarvāngāsana I (236); Nirālamba Sarvāngāsana II (237); Halāsana (244); Karṇapīḍāsana (246); Supta Koṇāsana (247); Pārśva Halāsana (249); Ekapāda Sarvāngāsana (250); Pārśvaikapāda Sarvāngāsana (251); Ūrdhva Prasārita Pādasana (276 to 279); Jaṭara Parivartanāsana (275); Chakrāsana (280 to 283); Paripoorṇa Nāvāsana (78); Ardha Nāvāsana (79); Utkaṭāsana (42); Uṣṭrāsana (41); Vīrāsana (89); Śalabhāsana (60); Dhanurāsana (63); Chaturanga Daṇḍāsana (67); Bhujangāsana I (73); Urdhva Mukha Svānāsana (74); Adho Mukha Svānāsana (75); Mahāmudra (125); Jānuśīrṣāsana (127); Triangmukhaikapāda Paschimottānāsana (139); Ardha Baddha Padma Paschimottānāsana (135); Marīchyāsana I & II (144, 146 and 147); Ubhaya Pādānguṣṭhāsana (167); Ūrdhva Mukha Paschimottānāsana I (168); Paschimottānāsana (160); Poorvottānāsana (171); Bharadwājāsana I & II (297, 298, 299 and 300); Mālāsana II (322); Baddha Koṇāsana (102); Śavāsana (592); Ujjāyī Prāṇāyāma without Kumbhaka or retention (Section 203) in Siddhāsana (84).

22nd to 25th week

Follow the serial order up to Chakrāsana (280 to 283) as in the 19th week. Then: Śalabhāsana (60); Dhanurāsana (63); Chaturanga Daṇḍāsana (67); Bhujangāsana I (73); Ūrdhva Mukha Śvānāsana (74); Adho Mukha Śvānāsana (75); Jānuśīrṣāsana (127); Ardha Baddha Padma Paschimottānāsana (135); Triangmukhaikapāda Paschimottānāsana (139); Marīchyāsana I & II (144, 146 and 147); Paschimottānāsana (160); Ubhaya Pādānguṣṭhāsana (167); Ūrdhva Mukha Paschimottānāsana I (168); Lolāsana (83); Gomukhāsana (80); Simhāsana I (109); Padmāsana (104); Parvatāsana (107); Tolāsana (108); Vīrāsana (89); Supta Vīrāsana (96); Paryankāsana (97); Uṣṭrāsana (41); Utkaṭāsana (42); Uttānāsana (48); Bharadwājāsana I & II (297, 298, 299 and 300); Marīchyāsana III (303 and 304); Ardha Matsyendrāsana I (311 and 312); Mālāsana II (322); Baddha Koṇāsana (102); Śavāsana (592); Ujjāyī Prāṇāyāma without retention (Section 203) in Siddhāsana (84).

26th to 30th week

Sālamba Śīrṣāsana I (184); Pārśva Śīrṣāsana (202 and 203); Ekapāda Śīrṣāsana (208 and 209); Ūrdhva Padmāsana (211); Pinḍāsana in Śīrṣāsana (218); Sālamba Sarvāngāsana I & II (223 and 235); Nirālamba Sarvāngāsana I & II (236 and 237); Halāsana (244); Karṇapīḍāsana (246); Supta Koṇāsana (247); Pārśva Halāsana (249); Ekapāda Sarvāngāsana (250); Pārśvaikapāda Sarvāngāsana (251); Ūrdhva Padmāsana (261); Pinḍāsana in Sarvāngāsana (269); Jaṭara Parivartanāsana (275); Paripoorṇa Nāvāsana (78); Ardha Nāvāsana (79); Jānuśīrṣāsana (127); Ardha Baddha Padma Paschimottānāsana (135); Triangmukhaikapāda Paschimottānāsana (139); Marīchyāsana I (144); Paschimottānāsana (160); Ūrdhva Mukha Paschimottānāsana I (168); Gomukhāsana (80); Lolāsana (83); Simhāsana I (109); Padmāsana (104); Parvatāsana (107); Tolāsana (108); Matsyāsana (113); Vīrāsana (89); Supta Vīrāsana (96); Paryankāsana (97); Marīchyāsana III (303 and 304); Ardha Matsyendrāsana I (311 and 312); Baddha Koṇāsana (102); Adho Mukha Śvānāsana (75); Ūrdhva Mukha Śvānāsana (74); Chaturanga Daṇḍāsana (67); Śalabhāsana (60); Dhanurāsana (63); Uṣṭrāsana (41); Utkaṭāsana (42); Uttānāsana (48); Garuḍāsana (56); Śavāsana (592); Ujjāyī Prāṇāyāma with Antar Kumbhaka (inhalation retention) (Section 203) in Siddhāsana (84), or in Vīrāsana (89) or in Padmāsana (104).

When you do the standing positions, eliminate the various movements in Śīrṣāsana and Sarvāngāsana cycles and do the rest. If Padmāsana has not yet been mastered, try to do so by continuing the āsanas for several weeks. One can add more of them to the programme if one can do so without strain.

For those who are satisfied with this first course I will now give a short three-day course which whenever followed will benefit the body and bring harmony to the mind.

First day of the week

Sālamba Śīrṣāsana I (184) for 10 minutes; Sālamba Sarvāngāsana I (223) for 10 minutes; Halāsana (244) for 5 minutes; Jaṭara Parivartanāsana (275) half a minute on each side; Paripoorṇa Nāvāsana (78) for one minute; Ardha Nāvāsana (79) for 20 to 30 seconds; Paschimottānāsana (160) for 3 to 5 minutes; Marīchyāsana III (303 and 304) for 30 seconds each side; Ardha Matsyendrāsana I (311 and 312) for 30 seconds on each side. If Marīchyāsana III or Ardha Matsyendrāsana I is difficult to perform then do Bharadwājāsana I and II (297, 298, 299 and 300). Parvatāsana (107) for one minute; Matsyāsana (113) for 20 to 30 seconds; Śalabhāsana (60) for 20 to 30 seconds; Dhanurāsana (63) for 30 seconds; Ūrdhva Mukha Śvānāsana (74) for 20 to 30 seconds; Adho Mukha Śvānāsana (75) for one minute; Uttānāsana (48) for 1 to 2 minutes; Śavāsana (592) for 5 minutes and Nāḍī Śodhana Prāṇāyāma in Padmāsana (104) or in Vīrāsana (89) or in Siddhāsana (84) with inhalation retention for 10 minutes and 6 Uḍḍīyānas (Section 201) and again do Śavāsana (592).

Second day of the week

Sālamba Śīrṣāsana I (184) for 10 minutes; Pārṣva Śīrṣāsana (202 and 203) for 20 seconds each side; Ekapāda Śīrṣāsana (208 and 209) for 10 to 15 seconds on each side; Ūrdhva Padmāsana (211) for 20 seconds; Piṇḍāsana in Śīrṣāsana (218) for 30 seconds (do all these at one stretch). Sālamba Sarvāngāsana I (223) for 8 to 10 minutes; Sālamba Sarvāngāsana II (235) for 30 seconds; Nirālamba Sarvāngāsana I & II (236 and 237) for 30 seconds each; Halāsana (244) for 5 minutes; Karṇapīḍāsana (246) for 30 seconds; Supta Koṇāsana (247) for 20 seconds; Pārśva Halāsana (249) for 20 seconds on each side; Ekapāda Sarvāngāsana (250) for 15 seconds on each side; Pārsvaikapāda Sarvāngāsana (251) for 15 seconds on each side; Ūrdhva Padmāsana (261) for 20 seconds; Piṇḍāsana in Sarvāngāsana (269) for 20 seconds (all to be done at one stretch). Jaṭara Parivartanāsana (275) for 15 seconds on each side; Ūrdhva

Prasārita Pādāsana (276 to 279) for 15 seconds on each position; Mahāmudra (125) for 20 to 30 seconds on each side; Jānuśīrṣāsana (127), Ardha Baddha Padma Paschimottānāsana (135), Triangmukhaikapāda Paschimottānāsana (139), Marīchyāsana I & II (144, 146 and 147) for 20 seconds on each side in all these āsanas; Paschimottānāsana (160) for 3 minutes; Ūrdhva Mukha Paschimottānāsana I (168) for one minute; Marīchyāsana III (303 and 304) for half a minute on each side; Ardha Matsyendrāsana I (311 and 312) for half a minute on each side; Baddha Koṇāsana (102) for one minute; Uttānāsana (48) for 2 minutes; Śavāsana (592) for 5 minutes. Ujjāyī Prāṇāyāma (Section 203) or Nāḍī Śodhana Prāṇāyāma (Section 205) for 8 minutes in any comfortable āsana and then end with Śavāsana (592).

Third day of the week

Sālamba Śīrṣāsana I (184) for 10 minutes; Utthita Trikoṇāsana (4 and 5) for half a minute on each side; Parivṛtta Trikoṇāsana (6 and 7) for half a minute on each side; Utthita Pārśvakoṇāsana and Parivṛtta Pārśvakoṇāsana (8, 9, 10 and 11) for 20 seconds each side; Vīrabhadrāsana I, II & III (14, 15 and 17) for 15 seconds on each side; Ardhachandrāsana (19) for 20 seconds on each side; Pārśvottānāsana (26) for 30 seconds on each side; Prasārita Pādottānāsana I (33 and 34), Pādānguṣṭhāsana (44) for 30 seconds; Pādahastāsana (46) for 30 seconds; Uttānāsana (48) for one minute; Ūrdhva Prasārita Ekapādāsana (49) for 15 seconds on each side; Garuḍāsana (56) for 10 seconds on each side; Utkaṭāsana (42) for 15 seconds; Parighāsana (39) for 15 seconds on each side; Uṣṭrāsana (41) for 20 seconds; Bhujangāsana I (73) for 20 to 30 seconds; Vīrāsana (89), Supta Vīrāsana (96) and Paryankāsana (97) for 30 to 40 seconds in each āsana; Padmāsana (104), Parvatāsana (107), Tolāsana (108), Matsyāsana (113) for 30 seconds in each āsana; Gomukhāsana (80) 15 seconds on each side; Lolāsana (83) for 15 seconds; Simhāsana I (109) for 20 seconds; Paschimottānāsana (160) for 3 to 5 minutes; Ujjāyī Prāṇāyāma (Section 203) or Nāḍī Śodhana Prāṇāyāma (Section 205) without Kumbhaka or retention for 10 minutes; Śavāsana (592) for 5 minutes.

Again one can repeat in the same order on the following days resting on Sundays or doing only Śīrṣāsana I (184) for 10 minutes; Sālamba Sarvāngāsana I (223) for 10 minutes; Halāsana (244) for 5 minutes; Paschimottānāsana (160) for 5 minutes and Nāḍī Śodhana Prāṇāyāma (Section 205) for 15 minutes with inhalation retention and Śavāsana (592) for 5 minutes.

If one finds that the number of āsanas or the length of time they take has increased, one can adjust according to capacity and the time at one's disposal. Do Śavāsana (592) after Prāṇāyāma.

Do Antarkumbhaka (inhalation retention) only when you have mastered the art of deep inhalation and deep exhalation without any jerks.

Do not do the āsanas and Prāṇāyāma together. You may feel the strain and the fatigue.

If you do Prāṇāyāma in the mornings, then āsanas can be done in the evenings or half an hour after the āsanas.

Never do āsanas immediately after Prāṇāyāma, but one can practise Prāṇāyāma after āsanas if one is still fresh.

Those who wish to prostrate to the sun (sūryanamaskar) and to develop the arms and chest, can do the following āsanas in sequence at first for six rounds, increasing the number according to capacity.

Āsanas	*Method of breathing*
1. Tāḍāsana (1)	Inhalation
2. Uttānāsana (47 and 48) and jump to,	Exhalation, inhalation (Plate 47)
3. Chaturanga Daṇḍāsana (66 and 67)	Exhalation
4. Ūrdhva Mukha Śvānāsana (74) and go back to,	Inhalation
5. Chaturanga Daṇḍāsana (67)	Exhale, inhale
6. Adho Mukha Śvānāsana (75) and from here jump to,	Exhale
7. Uttānāsana (47 and 48) and then back to,	Inhalation
8. Tāḍāsana (1)	Exhalation

Important āsanas in Course 1

Utthita Trikoṇāsana (4 and 5); Parivṛtta Trikoṇāsana (6 and 7); Utthita Pārśvakoṇāsana (8 and 9); Parivṛtta Pārśvakoṇāsana (10 and 11); Vīrabhadrāsana I & III (14 and 17); Ardhachandrāsana (19); Pārśvottānāsana (26); Prasārita Pādottānāsana I (33 and 34); Ustrāsana (41); Uttanāsana (48); Śalabhāsana (60); Dhanurāsana (63); Adho Mukha Śvānāsana (75); Paripoorṇa Nāvāsana (78); Ardha Nāvāsana (79); Siddhāsana (84); Vīrāsana (89); Baddha Koṇāsana (102); Padmāsana (104); Matsyāsana (113); Jānuśīrṣāsana (127); Paschimottānāsana (160); Sālamba Śīrṣāsana I (184); Sālamba Sarvāngāsana I (223); Halāsana (244); Marīchyāsana III (303 and 304); Ardha Matsyendrāsana I (311 and 312); and Śavāsana (592).

If these āsanas are mastered then the others given in this course will come even without regular practice.

COURSE TWO

31st to 35th week

Sālamba Śīrṣāsana I (184); Ūrdhva Daṇḍāsana (188); Pārśva Śīrṣāsana (202 and 203); Parivṛttaika Pāda Śīrṣāsana (206 and 207); Ekapāda Śīrṣāsana (208 and 209); Pārśvaikapāda Śīrṣāsana (210); Ūrdhva Padmāsana (211); Pārśva Ūrdhva Padmāsana (215 and 216); Piṇḍāsana in Śīrṣāsana (218); Sālamba Sarvāngāsana I & II (223 and 235); Nirālamba Sarvāngāsana I & II (236 and 237); Halāsana (244); Karṇapīḍāsana (246); Supta Koṇāsana (247); Pārśva Halāsana (249); Ekapāda Sarvāngāsana (250); Pārśvaikapāda Sarvāngāsana (251); Ūrdhva Padmāsana (261); Piṇḍāsana in Sarvāngāsana (269); Pārśva Piṇḍāsana (270 and 271); Setubandha Sarvāngāsana (259); Ekapāda Setubandha Sarvāngāsana (260); Jaṭara Parivartanāsana (275); Supta Pādānguṣṭhāsana (285 to 287); Chakrāsana (280 to 283); Paripoorna Nāvāsana (78); Ardha Nāvāsana (79); Uṣṭrāsana (41); Vīrāsana (89); Supta Vīrāsana (96) Paryankāsana (97); Jānu Sīrṣāsana (127); Ardha Baddha Padma Paschimottānāsana (135); Triang Mukhaikapāda Paschimottānāsana (139); Krouchāsana (141 and 142); Marīchyāsana I (144); Paschimottānāsana (160); Baddha Padmāsana (118); Yoga Mudrāsana (120); Parvatāsana (107); Kukkuṭāsana (115); Garbha Piṇḍāsana (116) (all the Padmāsana Cycle can be done at one stretch). Upaviṣṭa Koṇāsana (151); Ākarṇa Dhanurāsana (173 and 175); Baddha Koṇāsana (102); Marīchyāsana III (303 and 304); Ardha Matsyendrāsana I (311 and 312); Śalabhāsana (60); Dhanurāsana (63); Pārśva Dhanurāsana (64 and 65); Uttānāsana (48); Nāḍī Śodhana Prāṇāyāma (Section 205) without inhalation retention for 10 minutes and Ujjāyī Prāṇāyāma (Section 203) in Śavāsana (592).

36th to 40th week

Follow the above order in Sālamba Śīrṣāsana and cycle and Sālamba Sarvāngāsana and cycle up to Supta Pādānguṣṭhāsana (285 to 287); Utthita and Parivṛtta Trikoṇāsana (4 and 5, 6 and 7); Utthita and Parivṛtta Pārsvakoṇāsana (8 and 9, 10 and 11); Vīrabhadrāsana I & III (14 and 17); Ardha Chandrāsana (19); Pārśvottānāsana (26); Pādānguṣṭhāsana (44); Pāda Hastāsana (46); Uttānāsana (48); Utthita Hasta Pādānguṣṭhāsana (23); Ardha Baddha Padmottānāsana (52); Vātāyanāsana (58); Jānu-Śīrṣāsana (127); Parivṛtta Jānu-Śīrṣāsana (132); Ardha Baddha Padma Paschimottānāsana (135); Krounchāsana (141 and 142); Marīchyāsana I (144); Paschimottānāsana (160); Ūrdhvamukha Paschimottānāsana I (168); Ūrdhvamukha Paschimottānāsana II (170); Baddha Padmāsana (118); Yoga Mudrāsana (120); Kukkuṭāsana (115);

Garbha Piṇḍāsana (116); Simhāsana II (110); Matsyāsana (113); Baddha-koṇāsana (102); Upaviṣṭa Koṇāsana (151); Ākarṇa Dhanurāsana (173 and 175); Marīchyāsana III (303 and 304); Ardha Matsyendrasana I (311 and 312); Uttānapādāsana (292); Śalabhāsana (60); Dhanurāsana (63); Pārśva Dhanurāṣana (64 and 65); Ūrdhva Dhanurāsana I (482); Śavāsana (592); Nāḍī Śodhana Prāṇāyāma (Section 205) for 5 minutes; Sūryabhedana Prāṇāyāma (Section 204) for 5 minutes with inhalation retention; Uḍḍīyāna (Section 201) for 8 times.

40th to 44th week

Consolidate all the positions concentrating on the āsanas which were left out in Course I.

45th to 50th week

Sālamba Śīrṣāsana I (184); Sālamba Śīrṣāsana II (192); Sālamba Śīrṣāsana III (194 and 195); Baddha Hasta Śīrṣāsana (198); Mukta Hasta Śīrṣāsana (200 and 201); Pārśva Śīrṣāsana (202 and 203); Parivṛttaikapāda Śīrṣāsana (206 and 207); Ekapāda Śīrṣāsana (208 and 209); Pārśvaikapāda Śīrṣāsana (210); Ūrdhva Padmāsana (211); Pārśva Ūrdhva Padmāsana (215 and 216); Piṇḍāsana in Śīrṣāsana (218); Sālamba Sarvāngāsana I & II (223 and 235); Nirālamba Sarvāngāsana I & II (236 and 237); Halāsana (244); Karṇapīḍāsana (246); Supta Koṇāsana (247); Pārśva Halāsana (249); Ekapāda Sarvāngāsana (250); Pārśvaikapāda Sarvāngāsana (251); Pārśva Sarvāngāsana (254); Setubandha Sarvāngāsana (259); Ekapāda Setubandha Sarvāngāsana (260); Ūrdhva Padmāsana (261); Pārśva Ūrdhva Padmāsana (264 and 265); Piṇḍāsana in Sarvāngāsana (269); Pārśva Piṇḍāsana (270 and 271); Supta Pādānguṣṭhāsana (285 to 287); Anantāsana (290); Paschimottānāsana (160); Parivṛtta Paschimottānāsana (165); Jānu-Śīrṣāsana (127); Parivṛtta Jānu-Śīrṣāsana (132); Krounchāsana (141 and 142); Ākarṇa Dhanurāsana (173 and 175); Baddha Padmāsana (118); Yoga Mudrāsana (120); Kukkuṭāsana (115); Garbha Piṇḍāsana (116); Gorakṣāsana (117); Simhāsana II (110); Matsyāsana (113); Supta Vīrāsana (96); Bhekāsana (100); Baddha Koṇāsana (102); Ardha Matsyendrāsana I (311 and 312); Marīchyāsana III (303 and 304); Marīchyāsana IV (305); Mālāsana I (321); Uttānapādāsana (292); Ūrdhva Dhanurāsana I (482) 6 times and Śavāsana (592).

(All the Śīrṣāsana cycle can be done at one stretch staying 10 to 15 seconds on each side, except Sīrṣāsana I (184) where you have to stay for 5 minutes. Also stay for 5 minutes in Sālamba Sarvāngāsana I (234) and Halāsana (244) for 5 minutes each, and the rest for 15 seconds on each side. Do Paschimottānāsana (160) for 3 to 5 minutes and the rest of the āsanas from 15 to 20 seconds.)

Do Nāḍī Sodhana (Section 205) with Antara Kumbhaka or inhalation retention for 10 minutes, Bhastrika (Section 206) for 3 minutes and Uḍḍīyāna (Plates 593, 594) 8 times.

51st to 54th week

Do the important āsanas of Course I and perfect the poses in Course II. Some will be mastered quickly, but others will take longer. Adjust, therefore, to your own convenience.

55th to 60th week

Śīrṣāsana and cycle (184 to 218); Sarvāṅgāsana and cycle (234 to 271 except 267); Jatara Parivartanāsana (275); Supta Pādāngusthāsana (285 to 287); Anantāsana (290); Ūrdhva Prasārita Pādāsana (276 to 279); Paschimottānāsana (160); Parivṛtta Paschimottānāsana (165); Urdhva Mukha Paschimottānāsana I (168); Ākarṇa Dhanurāsana (173 and 175); Bhujapīdāsana (348); Kūrmāsana (363 and 364); Supta Kūrmāsana (368); Ekapāda Śīrṣāsana (371); Padmāsana cycle (104 to 120) and Supta Vajrāsana (124); Bhekāsana (100); Baddha Koṇāsana (102); Marīchyāsana III (303 and 304); Ardha Matsyendrāsana I (311 and 312); Mālāsana I (321); Pāśāsana (328 and 329); Uttānapādāsana (292); Setubandhāsana (296); Ūrdhva Dhanurāsana II (486) twelve times following the technique 11 in the section on the āsana; Uttānāsana (48); Śavāsana (592); Prāṇāyāma as mentioned above and start meditation in Siddhāsana (84), Vīrāsana (89), Baddha Koṇāsana (103) or Padmāsana (104).

61st to 65th week

Śīrṣāsana and cycle (184 to 218). If the Sālamba Śīrṣāsana II & III (192, 194 and 195), Baddha Hasta Śīrṣāsana (198) and Mukta Hasta Śīrṣāsana (200 and 201) are mastered, they can be dropped as daily practices but should be done once in a while so that the balance is not lost. Sarvāṅgāsana and cycle (234 to 271 except 267); Jaṭara Parivartanāsana (275); Supta Pādanguṣṭhāsana (285 to 287); Anantāsana (290); Paschimottānāsana (160); Parivṛtta Paschimottānāsana (165); Ākarṇa Dhanurāsana (173 and 175); Kūrmāsana (363 and 364); Supta Kūrmāsana (368); Ekapada Śīrṣāsana (371); Skandāsana (372); Bhujapīdāsana (348); Aṣṭāvakrāsana (342 and 343); Ekahasta Bhujāsana (344); Dwihasta Bhujāsana (345); Adhomukha Vṛkṣāsana (359 – against the wall); Padmāsana cycle (104 to 124); Marīchyāsana III (303 and 304); Ardha Matsyendrāsana I (311 and 312); Pāśāsana (328 and 329); Uttānāpādāsana (292); Setubandhāsana (296); Ūrdhva Dhanurāsana for 12 to 15 times as stated in the 55th week; Uttānāsana (48); Śavāsana (592). Follow the Prāṇāyāma as stated previously and increase the length of inhalation, inhalation retention, exhalation and also the cycles and finish with meditation in the āsanas as stated above.

66th to 70th week

Śīrṣāsana I and cycle (184 to 218 except 192, 194, 195, 198 and 200–1); Adhomukha Vṛkṣāsana (359); Mayūrāsana (354); Padma Mayūrāsana (355); Nakrāsana (68 to 71); Sālamba Sarvāngāsana and cycle (234 to 271 except 267); Jaṭara Parivartanāsana (275); Supta Padanguṣṭhāsana (285 to 287); Anantāsana (290); Uttānapādāsana (292); Setubandhāsana (296); Ūrdhva Dhanurāsana (486); from Vṛkṣāsana (359) for 12 times and arch up to Tāḍāsana (1); Marīchyāsana III (303 and 304); Ardha Matsyendrāsana I (311 and 312); Pāśāsana (328 and 329); Bhujapīḍāsana (348); Aṣṭavakrāsana (342 and 343); Bakāsana (406); Paschimottānāsana (160); Parivṛtta Paschimottānāsana (165); Upaviṣṭa Koṇāsana (151); Ākarṇa Dhanurāsana (173 and 175); Padmāsana cycle (104 to 124); Kūrmāsana (363 and 364); Supta Kūrmāsana (368); Ekapāda Śīrṣāsana (371); Skandāsana (372); Baddha Koṇāsana (102); Bhekāsana (100); Supta Vīrāsana (96); Śavāsana (592).

71st to 73rd week

Do as explained in the 66th week but at the time of performing Ūrdhva Dhanurāsana (486) add Ekapada Ūrdhva Dhanurāsana (501 and 502) and proceed with Marīchyāsana III (303 and 304) and do the rest. Do Prāṇāyāma as stated above and after Uddiyāṇa, add Nauli (Section 202) 6 to 8 times and finish with meditation.

74th to 78th week

Repeat all the āsanas of Course One and Course Two.

Important āsanas in Course Two

Utthita Hasta Pādānguṣṭhāsana (23); Vātāyanāsana (58); Nakrāsana (68 to 71); Bhekāsana (100); Simhāsana II (110); Garbha Piṇḍāsana (116); Yoga Mudrāsana (120); Supta Vajrāsana (124); Parivṛtta Jānu-Śīrṣāsana (132); Krounchāsana (141 and 142); Upaviṣṭa Koṇāsana (151); Parivṛtta Paschimottānāsana (165); Ākarṇa Dhanurāsana (173 and 175); Ūrdhva Daṇḍāsana (188); Śīrṣāsana and Sarvāngāsana cycles; Supta Pādānguṣṭhāsana (285 to 287); Anantāsana (290); Setubandhāsana (296); Pāśāsana (328 and 329); Aṣṭāvakrāsana (342 and 343); Bhujapīḍāsana (348); Mayūrāsana (354); Ādhomukha Vṛkṣāsana (359); Kūrmāsana (363 and 364); Supta Kūrmāsana (368); Ekapāda Śīrṣāsana (371); Skandāsana (372); Bakāsana (406); and Ūrdhva Dhanurāsana (486).

For those who like to do the āsanas from Course One and Two, I now give the method of practice in a week's course.

First day of the week

Śīrṣāsana and cycle (184 to 218 except 192, 194–5, 198, 200–1); Sarvāngāsana and cycle (234 to 271 except 267); Supta Pādānguṣṭhāsana (285 to 287); Anantāsana (290); Paschimottānāsana (160); Utthita and Parivṛtta Trikoṇāsana (4 and 5, 6 and 7); Utthita and Parivṛtta Pārśva Koṇāsana (8 and 9, 10 and 11); Virabhadrāsana I, II and III (14, 15 and 17); Ardha Chandrāsana (19); Utthita Hasta Pādānguṣṭhāsana (23); Pārśvottānāsana (26); Prasārita Pādottānāsana I and II (33 and 34, 35 and 36); Ardha Baddha Padmottānāsana (52); Pādānguṣṭhāsana (44); Pādahastāsana (46); Uttānāsana (48); Marīchyāsana II, III and IV (144–6, 303–4, 305); Ardha Matsyendrāsana I (311 and 312); Mālāsana I & II (321 and 322); Pāśāsana (328 and 329); Ūrdhva Dhanurāsana (486) for 12 times; Śavāsana (592). Nāḍī Śodhana Prāṇāyāma (Section 205) for 15 minutes and meditation for 5 minutes.

Second day of the week

Śīrṣāsana and cycle (184 to 218); Adhomukha Vṛkṣāsana (359); Mayūrāsana (354); Padma Mayūrāsana (355); Nakrāsana (68 to 71); Salabhāsana or Makarāsana (60 or 62); Dhanurāsana (63); Pārśva Dhanurāsana (64 and 65); Chaturanga Daṇḍāsana (67); Bhujangāsana I (73); Ūrdhva Mukha Śvānāsana (74); Adhomukha Śvānāsana (75); Sālamba Sarvāngāsana cycle (234 to 271 except 267); Jaṭara Parivartanāsana (275); Supta Pādānguṣṭhāsana (285 to 287); Ūrdhva Prasārita Pādottānāsana (276 to 279); Chakrāsana (280 to 283); Paripoorṇa Nāvāsana (78); Ardha Nāvāsana (79); Utkaṭāsana (42); Uṣṭrāsana (41); Parighāsana (39); Garuḍāsana (56); Vātāyanāsana (58); Marīchyāsana III (303 and 304); Ardha Matsyendrāsana I (311 and 312); Pāśāsana (328 and 329); Paschimottānāsana (160); Kūrmāsana and Supta Kūrmāsana (363–4 and 368); Ekapāda Śīrṣāsana and Skandāsana (371 and 372); Ūrdhva Dhanurāsana (486) for 15 times and Śavāsana (592); Uḍḍīyāna (Section 201) and Nauli (Section 202) for 8 times each. Ujjāyi Prāṇāyāma (Section 203) with inhalation retention for 10 minutes and meditation for 5 minutes.

Third day of the week

Sālamba Śīrṣāsana (184) 10 minutes; Sarvāngāsana I (234) 10 minutes; Halāsana (244) 5 minutes; Supta Pādānguṣṭhāsana (285 to 287); Ūrdhva Prasārita Pādāsana (276 to 279); Paripoorṇa Nāvāsana (78); Ardha Nāvāsana (79); Jānu-Śīrṣāsana (127); Parivṛtta Jānu-Śīrṣāsana (132); Ardha Baddha Padma Paschimottānāsana (135); Triang Mukhaikapāda

Paschimottānāsana (139); Krounchāsana (141 and 142); Marīchyāsana I (144); Paschimottānāsana (160); Ūrdhva Mukha Paschimottānāsana I & II (168 and 170); Parivṛtta Paschimottānāsana (165); Ākarṇa Dhanurāsana (173 and 175); Kūrmāsana and Supta Kūrmāsana (363–4 and 368); Ekapāda Sīrsāsana and Skandāsana (371 and 372); Ūrdhva Dhanurāsana (486) for 15 times and Ekapāda Urdhva Dhanurāsana once (501 and 502); Uttānāsana (48) and Savāsana (592). Sūryabhedana Prāṇāyāma (Section 204) for 10 minutes; Ujjāyi (Section 203) for 5 minutes; Bhastrika (Section 206) for 3 minutes and meditation for 5 minutes.

Fourth day of the week

Sālamba Śīrṣāsana and cycle (184 to 218 except 192, 194–5, 198, 200 and 201); Sālamba Sarvāngāsana and cycle (234 to 271 except 267); Jaṭara Parivartanāsana (275); Supta Pādānguṣṭhāsana (285 to 287); Paschimottānāsana (160) for 5 minutes; Padmāsana and cycle (104 to 124); Vīrāsana (89); Supta Vīrāsana (96); Paryankāsana (97); Upaviṣṭa Koṇāsana (151); Baddha Koṇāsana (102); Kūrmāsana (363 and 364) for one minute each; Supta Kūrmāsana (368) for 3 minutes; Ekapāda Śīrṣāsana (371) one minute on each side; Skandāsana (372) for 30 seconds on each side; Marīchyāsana III (303 and 304); Ardha Matsyendrāsana I (311 and 312); Pāśāsana (328 and 329); Uttānapādāsana (292); Setubandhāsana (296); Ūrdhva Dhanurāsana (486) for 12 times staying 20 seconds each time; Śavāsana (592). Nāḍī Śodhana Prāṇāyāma (with inhalation retention) (Section 205) for 15 minutes and meditation to capacity in any āsana as stated earlier.

Fifth day of the week

Sālamba Śīrṣāsana and cycle (184 to 218); Sālamba Sarvāngāsana and cycle (234 to 271 except 267); Supta Pādānguṣṭhāsana (285 to 287); Paschimottānāsana (160); Parivṛtta Paschimottānāsana (165); Kūrmāsana (363 and 364); Supta Kūrmāsana (368); Bhujapīdāsana (348); Aṣṭāvakrāsana (342 and 343); Mayūrāsana and Padma Mayūrāsana (354 and 355); Ūrdhva and Mukha Svānāsana (74); Bakāsana (406); Lolāsāna (83); Adho Mukha Vṛkṣāsana (359); Adho Mukha Svānāsana (75); Chaturanga Daṇḍāsana (67); Nakrāsana (68 to 71); Ūrdhva Dhanurāsana for 15 to 20 times (486); Savāsana (592). Prāṇāyāma and meditation as in the 3rd day.

Sixth day of the week

Sālamba Śīrṣāsana I (184) for 15 minutes. Ūrdhva Daṇḍāsana (188) for 1 minute; Sālamba Sarvāngāsana I (234) for 10 minutes; Halāsana (244) for 5 minutes; Paschimottānāsana (160) for 5 minutes; Ūrdhva Mukha

Paschimottānāsana I (168) for 1 minute; Paripoorṇa Nāvāsana (78) for 1 minute; Ardha Nāvāsana (79) for 30 seconds; Supta Vīrāsana (96) for 3 to 5 minutes; Krounchāsana (141 and 142) for 20 seconds each side; Kūrmāsana and Supta Kūrmāsana (363–4 and 368) for 1 minute each; Ardha Matsyendrāsana I (311 and 312) for 30 seconds each side; Pāśāsana (328 and 329) for 1 minute on each side; Adhomukha Vṛkṣāsana (359) for 1 minute; Mayūrāsana (354) for 1 minute; Ūrdhva Dhanurāsana (486) for 6 times, each time staying for 20 to 30 seconds; Śavāsana (592) for 10 to 15 minutes.

(Wherever the time is not given, it should be done according to one's capacity and the time at one's disposal.)

Seventh day of the week

You can rest or do only Prāṇāyāma of all types. Uḍḍīyāna (Section 201) and Nauli (Section 202) for 8 times each.

COURSE THREE

This course is mainly for those who like to persevere further and who have sufficient devotion for the Science.

79th to 84th week

Śīrṣāsana and cycle (184 to 218 except 192, 194–5, 198, 200–1); Sarvāngāsana and cycle (234 to 271 except 267); Paschimottānāsana (160); Kūrmāsana and Supta Kūrmāsana (363–4 and 368); Ekapāda Śīrṣāsana (371); Skandāsana (372); Bhairavāsana (375); Yoganidrāsana (391); Bhujapīdāsana (348); Bakāsana (406); Aṣṭāvakrāsana (342 and 343); Adhomukha Vṛkṣāsana (359); Pincha Mayūrāsana (357); Mayūrāsana (354); Marīchyāsana III (303 and 304); Ardha Matsyendrāsana I (311 and 312); Pāśāsana (328 and 329); Ardha Matsyendrāsana II (330 and 331); Setubandhāsana (296); Ūrdhva Dhanurāsana (486) for 8 times; Dwipāda Viparīta Daṇḍāsana (516); Ekapāda Ūrdhva Dhanurāsana (501 and 502); Uttanāsana (48); Śavāsana (592). Nāḍī Śodhana Prāṇāyāma (Section 205) for 10 minutes and meditation for 5 minutes in Siddhāsana (84) or Vīrāsana (89) or Padmāsana (104) or Baddha Koṇāsana (102).

85th to 90th week

Śīrṣāsana and cycle (184 to 218); Sarvāngāsana and cycle (234 to 271 except 267); Jaṭara Parivartanāsana (275); Ūrdhva Prasārita Pādāsana (276 to 270); Supta Pādānguṣṭhāsana (285 to 287); Anantāsana (290); Jānu-Śīrṣāsana (127); Parivṛtta Jānu-Śīrṣāsana (132); Ardha Baddha Padma Paschimottānāsana (135); Triang Mukhaikapāda Paschimottānāsana (139); Krounchāsana (141 and 142); Marīchyāsana I (144); Paschimottānāsana (160); Parivṛtta Paschimottānāsana (165); Upaviṣṭa Koṇāsana (151); Baddha Koṇāsana (102); Baddha Padmāsana (118); Yoga Mudrāsana (120); Kukkuṭāsana (115); Garbha Piṇḍāsana (116); Siṃhāsana II (110); Gorakṣāsana (117); Matsyāsana or Supta Vajrāsana (113 or 124); Vīrāsana (89); Supta Vīrāsana (96); Paryankāsana (97); Bhekāsana (100); Kūrmāsana and Supta Kūrmāsana (363–4 and 368); Yoganidrāsana (391); Ekapāda Śīrṣāsana (371); Bhairavāsana (375); Skandāsana (372); Chakorāsana (379 and 380); Bhujapīdāsana (348); Bakāsana (406); Pincha Mayūrāsana (357); Adhomukha Vṛkṣāsana (359); Mayūrāsana (354); Ardha Matsyendrāsana I & II (311–12 and 330–1); Mālāsana I & II (321 and 322); Pāśāsana (328 and 329); Dwipada Viparīta Daṇḍāsana (516); Ūrdhva Dhanurāsana (486) for 8 times and Śāvāsana (592). Follow the Prāṇāyāma as in 79th week.

91st to 94th week

Do the important āsanas in Course One and Two as well as all the āsanas which have been added so far in Course Three including the Śīrṣāsana and Sarvāngāsana cycles.

95th to 100th week

Śīrṣāsana and cycle (184 to 218); Sarvāngāsana and cycle (234 to 271 except 267); Supta Pādānguṣṭhāsana (285 to 287); Paschimottānāsana (160); Kūrmāsana and Supta Kūrmāsana (363–4 and 368); Yoganidrāsana (391); Ekapāda Śīrṣāsana (371); Bhairavāsana (375); Skandāsana (372); Chakorāsana (379 and 380); Pincha Mayūrāsana (357); Śayanāsana (358); Mayūrāsana (354); Haṃsāsana (356); Bhujapīdāsana (348); Bakāsana (406); Adhomukha Vṛkṣāsana (359); Vasiṣṭhāsana (398); Viśvāmitrāsana (403); Ūrdhva Dhanurāsana (486) for 8 times, stretching the legs and arms out straight after each time (487) to relieve stiffness in the back; Dwipāda Viparīta Daṇḍāsana (516) for 1 minute; Kapotāsana (507); Ardha Matsyendrāsana I & II (311–12 and 330–1); Pāśāsana (328 and 329); Uttānāsana (48); Śavāsana (592). Prāṇāyāma as before.

101st to 108th week

As the 95th week but do Viparīta Daṇḍāsana (516) from Sālamba Śīrṣāsana I (184) and again swing back to Śīrṣāsana I. For many this period is too short for acquiring control of Viparīta Daṇḍāsana. Concentrate then on this and shorten the time spent on the other āsanas.

109th to 125th week

Follow the 95th week course, add Viparīta Daṇḍāsana (516) as above and learn Viparīta Chakrāsana (488 to 499) by doing it 15 times daily at a stretch. It is a difficult āsana and it needs perseverance to perfect it. If you cannot do so in this period, do not lose heart but continue with it for several more weeks.

126th to 130th week

Śīrṣāsana and cycle (184 to 218); Ūrdhva Kukkuṭāsana (419); Bakāsana (410) from Śīrṣāsana II (192); Adhomukha Vṛkṣāsana (359); Pincha Mayūrāsana (357) following these four āsanas with Ūrdhva Dhanurāsana (486); and Viparīta Chakrāsana (488 to 499); Bhuja Pīdāsana (348); Aṣṭāvakrāsana (342–3); Mayurāsana (354); Hamsāsana (356); Vasiṣṭhāsana (398); Kaśyapāsana (399–400); Visvāmitrāsana (403); Sālamba Sarvāngāsana and cycle (234 to 271 except 267); Supta Pādānguṣṭhāsana (285 to 287); Paschimottānāsana (160); Kūrmāsana (363–4); Supta Kūrmāsana (368); Yoganidrāsana (391); Ekapāda Śīrṣāsana

(371); Skandāsana (372); Bhairavāsana (375); Kālabhairavāsana (378); Chakorāsana (379–80); Dwipāda Viparīta Daṇḍāsana (516) from Śīrṣāsana (184); Kapotāsana (507); Viparīta Chakrāsana (488 to 499) 6 times; Ardha Matsyendrāsana I & II (311–12, 330–1); Pāśāsana (328–9); Uttānāsana (48); Śavāsana (592). Prāṇāyāma as before with meditation.

131st to 136th week

Go back to Courses One and Two and do Ūrdhva Kukkuṭāsana (419); Yoganidrāsana (391); Viparīta Chakrāsana (488 to 499) for 15 times; Dwipāda Viparīta Daṇḍāsana (516) and Kapotāsana (507).

Note – Viparīta Chakrāsana (488 to 499) is a strenuous āsana so that one may not be able to do Prāṇāyāma daily. In that event, do Prāṇāyāma on alternate days and the cycles of Śīrṣāsana and Sarvāngāsana on alternate days. Also, if the body is stiff and you cannot cope with the table as given above, then spread the āsanas and the weeks to your convenience. Unless you improve these back-bending postures you cannot proceed much with the other difficult āsanas. It is also possible that those over 35 will find it difficult to master Viparitā Chakrāsana in so short a time. I have instructed many people of different ages and some learn quicker than others. But there is no age limit for these āsanas.

137th to 142nd week

Śīrṣāsana and cycle (184 to 218); Ūrdhva Kukkuṭāsana (419); Bakāsana (410) from Śīrṣāsana II (192); Pārśva Bakāsana (412); Gālavāsana (427 and 428); Adhomukha Vṛkṣāsana (359); Pincha Mayūrāsana (357); Mayūrāsana (354); Vasiṣṭhāsana (398); Kaśyapāsana (399 and 400); Viśvāmitrāsana (403); Sālamba Sarvāngāsana and cycle (234 to 271 except 267); Supta Pādānguṣṭhāsana (285 to 287); Paschimottānāsana (160); Kūrmāsana and Supta Kūrmāsana (363–4 and 368); Yoganidrāsana (391); Ekapāda Śīrṣāsana (371); Skandāsana (372); Bhairavāsana (375); Kālabhairavāsana (378); Dūrvāsāsana (383); Ruchikāsana (384); Dwipāda Viparīta Daṇḍāsana (516) from Śīrṣāsana I (184) and back 3 times; Maṇḍalāsana (525 to 535); Kapotāsana (507); Viparīta Chakrāsana (488 to 499) for 12 times; Ardha Matsyendrāsana I & II (311–12 and 330–1); Pāśāsana (328 and 329); Uttānāsana (48); Savāsana (592); Prāṇāyāma as before with meditation.

143rd to 145th week

Repeat the 137th week course up to Ruchikāsana (384) and add Viranchyāsana I & II (386–7 and 388) and continue with Dwipāda Viparīta Daṇḍāsana (516) and the remaining exercises of that course.

If you can add the different methods of Prāṇāyāma explained in Part Three, do so. Then do early morning Prāṇāyāma; the difficult āsanas in the morning and only the Śīrṣāsana and Sarvāṅgāsana cycles in the evening. If you have not the time, do Prāṇāyāma in the morning and the āsanas in the evening.

146th to 155th week

Śīrṣāsana and cycle (184 to 218); Ūrdhva Kukkutāsana (419); Bakāsana (410); Pārśva Bakāsana (412); Gālavāsana (427 and 428); Ekapāda Gālavāsana (432 and 433); Adhomukha Vṛkṣāsana (359); Pincha Mayūrāsana (357); finishing these āsanas with Viparīta Chakrāsana (488 to 499); Vasiṣṭhāsana (398); Kaśyapāsana (399 and 400); Viśvamitrāsana (403); Sālamba Sarvāṅgāsana and cycle (234 to 271 inclusive) of Uttāna Padma Mayūrāsana (267); Supta Pādānguṣṭhāsana (285 to 287); Paschimottānāsana (160); Kūrmāsana and Supta Kūrmāsana (363–4 and 368); Ekapāda Śīrṣāsana (371); Skandāsana (372); Buddhāsana (373); Kapilāsana (374); Bhairavāsana (375); Kālabhairavāsana (378); Chakorāsana (379 and 380); Dūrvāsāsana (383); Ruchikāsana (384); Viranchyāsana I & II (386 and 388); Dwipāda Śīrṣāsana (393); Tittibhāsana (395); Ardha Matsyendrāsana I & II (311–12 and 330–1); Pāśāsana (328); Ardha Matsyendrāsana III (332 and 333); Dwipāda Viparīta Daṇḍāsana (516); Mandalāsana (525 to 535); Kapotāsana (512); Ekapāda Viparīta Daṇḍāsana (521); Chakrabandhāsana (524); Śavāsana (592). Prāṇāyāma of Ujjāyī (Section 203) or Sūryabhedana (Section 204) or Nāḍī Śodhana (Section 205) with inhalation retention (Antarkumbhaka); Uḍḍīyāna (Section 201) 8 times; Nauli (Section 202) 8 times and meditation for 5 to 10 minutes.

156th to 160th week

Repeat the important āsanas from Courses One and Two and then do the āsanas of Course Three so far learnt.

161st to 165th week

Śīrṣāsana and cycle (184 to 218); Ūrdhva Kukkutāsana (419); Bakāsana (410); Pārśva Bakāsana (412); Gālavāsana (427 and 428); Ekapāda Gālavāsana (432 and 433); Dwipāda Kouṇḍinyāsana (438); Ekapāda Kouṇḍinyāsana I (441); Adhomukha Vṛkṣāsana (359); Pincha Mayūrāsana (357) finishing each āsana with Viparīta Chakrāsana (488 to 499); Aṣṭāvakrāsana (342 and 343); Bhujapīdāsana (348); Vaśiṣṭhāsana (398); Viśvāmitrāsana (403); Sarvāṅgāsana and cycle (234 to 271); Paschimottānāsana (160); Kūrmāsana and Supta Kūrmāsana (363–4 and 368); Ekapāda Śīrṣāsana and cycle (371 to 384); Dwipāda Śīrṣāsana and Tittibhāsana (393 and 395); Yoganidrāsana (391); Ardha Matsyendrāsana I, II & III (311–12, 330–1, 332–3); Pāśāsana (328); Yogadaṇḍāsana (456); Supta Bhekāsana (458).

166th to 175th week

Sālamba Śīrṣāsana I (184) for 10 minutes; Sālamba Sarvāngāsana I (234) for 10 minutes; Halāsana (244) for 5 minutes; Jaṭara Parivartanāsana (275); Supta Pādānguṣṭhāsana (285 to 287); Ūrdhva Kukkuṭāsana (419); Bakāsana (410); Pārśva Bakāsana (412); Gālavāsana (427); Ekapāda Gālavāsana (432); Dwipāda Kouṇḍinyāsana (438); Ekapāda Koundinyāsana I & II (441 and 442); Ekapāda Bakāsana I & II (446 and 451); finishing each āsana with Viparīta Chakrāsana (488 to 499); Paschimottānāsana (160); Kūrmāsana and Supta Kūrmāsana (363–4 and 368); Ekapāda Śīrṣāsana and cycle (371 to 384); Dwipāda Śīrṣāsana (393); Yoganidrāsana (391); Yogadaṇḍāsana (456); Supta Bhekāsana (458); Mūlabandhāsana (462 and 463); Vāmadevāsana I & II (465 and 466); Dwipāda Viparīta Daṇḍāsana (516); Maṇḍalāsana (525 to 535); Ekapāda Viparīta Daṇḍāsana I & II (521 and 522); Chakrabandhāsana (524); Kapotāsana (512); Laghuvajrāsana (513); Ardha Matsyendrāsana I, II & III (311, 330 and 332); Pāśāsana (328); Śavāsana (592). Prāṇāyāma as before.

176th to 180th week

Repeat the 166th week's course, add Pārśva Kukkuṭāsana (424 and 425) after Ūrdhva Kukkuṭāsana (419) and Paripoorṇa Matsyendrāsana (336 and 339) after Pāśāsana (328).

Paripoorṇa Matsyendrāsana (336 and 339) may take a longer time to master than I have anticipated. One should try this āsana every day irrespective of failures. If one cannot master the āsanas of Course Three so far dealt with in the stipulated period, spread them out over several more weeks.

As the other āsanas take years to master, I shall try my best to give a résumé for each day's practice of all these āsanas.

First day of the week

Sālamba Śīrṣāsana I (184) for 8 to 10 minutes; Sālamba Sarvangāsana I (234) for 10 minutes; Halāsana (244) for 5 minutes; Jaṭara Parivartanāsana (274); Supta Pādānguṣṭhāsana (285 to 287); Bhujapīdāsana (348); Aṣṭāvakrāsana (342 and 343); Adhomukha Vṛkṣāsana (359); Pincha Mayūrāsana (357); Mayūrāsana (354); Haṃsāsana (356); Ūrdhva Kukkuṭāsana (419); Pārśva Kukkuṭāsana (424 and 425); Bakāsana (410); Pārśva Bakāsana (412); Dwipāda Kouṇḍinyāsana (438); Ekapāda Kouṇḍinyāsana I & II (441 and 442); Ekapāda Bakāsana I & II (446 and 451); Gālavāsana (427); Ekapāda Gālavāsana (432) and finish each of these āsanas with Viparīta Chakrāsana (488 to 499); Uttānāsana (48); Śavāsana (592). Nāḍī Śodhana Prāṇāyāma (Section 205) for 10 minutes, Uḍḍīyāna (Section 201) 8 times and Nauli 8 times (Section 202).

Second day of the week

Śīrṣāsana and cycle (184 to 218); Sarvāngāsana and cycle (234 to 271); Jaṭara Parivartanāsana (274); Supta Pādānguṣṭhāsana (285 to 287); Jānu-Śīrṣāsana (127); Parivṛtta Jānu-Śīrṣāsana (132); Ardha Baddha Padma Paschimottānāsana (135); Triang Mukhaikapāda Paschimottānāsana (139); Krounchāsana (141); Marichyāsana I & II (144 and 146); Upaviṣṭa Koṇāsana (151); Paschimottānāsana (160); Padmāsana and cycle (104 to 124); Baddha Koṇāsana (102); Vīrāsana (89); Vātāyanāsana (58); Paripoorṇa Nāvāsana (78); Ardha Nāvāsana (79); Gomukhāsana (80); Ūrdhva Mukha Paschimottānāsana I (168); Yoganidrāsana (391); Śavāsana (592). Prānāyāma as before with Bhastrikā (Section 206) and Śītali (Section 209).

Third day of the week

Śīrṣāsana and cycle (184 to 218); Sarvāngāsana and cycle (234 to 271); all the standing positions (4 to 36); Dhanurāsana (63); Salabhāsana (60); Chaturanga Daṇḍāsana (67); Ūrdhva Mukha Śvānāsana (74); Adho Mukha Śvānāsana (75); Paschimottānāsana (160); Parivṛtta Paschimottānāsana (165); Ākarṇa Dhanurāsana (173 and 175); Uttānapādāsana (292); Setubandhāsana (296); Marīchyāsana III & IV (303 and 305); Ardha Matsyendrāsana I (311); Pāśāsana (328); Mayūrāsana (354); Yoganidrāsana (391); Dwipāda Śīrṣāsana (393); Dwipāda Viparīta Daṇḍāsana (516); Maṇḍalāsana (525 to 535); Kapotāsana (512); Viparīta Chakrāsana (488 to 499) 8 times at a stretch; Uttānāsana (48); Śavāsana (592). Prāṇāyāma to capacity without strain.

Fourth day of the week

Śīrṣāsana and cycle (184 to 218); Sarvāngāsana and cycle (234 to 271); Adhomukha Vṛkṣāsana (359); Pincha Mayūrāsana (357); Śayanāsana (358); Mayūrāsana (354); Haṃsāsana (356); Paschimottānāsana (160); Kūrmāsana and Supta Kūrmāsana (363–4, 368); Ekapāda Śīrṣāsana and cycle (371 to 384); Virinchyāsana I & II (386 and 388); Yoganidrāsana (391); Dwipāda Viparīta Daṇḍāsana (516); Maṇḍalāsana (525 to 535); Ekapāda Viparīta Daṇḍāsana I & II (521 and 523); Chakrabandhāsana (524); Laghuvajrāsana (513); Kapotāsana (512); Uttānāsana (48); Śavāsana (592). Nāḍī Śodhana Prāṇāyāma without retention for 15 minutes and meditation in Siddhāsana (84) or in Padmāsana (104).

Fifth day of the week

Sālamba Śīrṣāsana I (184) for 10 minutes; Sālamba Sarvāngāsana I (234) for 10 minutes; Halāsana (244) for 5 minutes; Paschimottānāsana (160) for 5 minutes; Vasiṣṭhāsana (398); Kaśyapāsana (399); Viśvāmitrāsana

(403); Ūrdhva Kukkuṭāsana (429); Pārśva Kukkuṭāsana (424 and 425); Bakāsana (410); Pārśva Bakāsana (412); Dwipāda Kouṇḍinyāsana (438); Ekapāda Kouṇḍinyāsana I & II (441 and 442); Ekapāda Bakāsana I & II (446 and 451) (all these balancing āsanas at one stretch); Yogadaṇḍāsana (456); Mulabandhāsana (462); Vāmadevāsana I & II (465 and 466); Dwipāda Viparīta Daṇḍāsana (516); Maṇḍalāsana (525 to 535); Kapotāsana (512); Paschimottānāsana (160) for 5 minutes; Uttānāsana (48) for 3 minutes; Śavāsana (592) for 5 minutes; Ujjāyī Prāṇāyāma for 10 minutes.

Sixth day of the week

Śīrṣāsana and cycle (184 to 218); Sarvāngāsana and cycle (234 to 271); Paschimottānāsana (160) for 5 minutes; Yoganidrāsana (391) one minute on each way changing the legs; Dwipāda Śīrṣāsana (393) half a minute each way; Marichyāsana III (303); Ardha Matsyendrāsana I, II & III (311, 330 and 332); Mālāsana I & II (321 and 322); Pāśāsana (328); Paripoorṇa Matsyendrāsana (336 and 339); Dwipāda Viparīta Daṇḍāsana (516); Maṇḍalāsana (525 to 535); Ekapāda Viparīta Daṇḍāsana I & II (521 and 523); Kapotāsana (512); and 6 of Viparīta Chakrāsana (488 to 499); Śavāsana (592).

Seventh day of the week

Rest completely or do only Prāṇāyāma.

181st to 190th week

Śīrṣāsana and cycle (184 to 218); Sarvāngāsana and cycle (234 to 271); Ūrdhva Kukkuṭāsana (419); Pārśva Kukkuṭāsana (424); Bakāsana (410); Pārśva Bakāsana (412); Dwipāda Kouṇḍinyāsana (438); Ekapāda Kouṇḍinyāsana I & II (441 and 442); Ekapāda Bakāsana I & II (446 and 451); Vasiṣṭhāsana (398); Viśvāmitrāsana (403); Paschimottānāsana (160); Kūrmāsana and Supta Kūrmāsana (363–4 and 368); Ekapāda Śīrṣāsana and cycle (371 to 384); Yoganidrāsana (391); Dwipāda Śīrṣāsana and Tittibhāsana (393 and 395); Yogadaṇḍāsana (456); Mulabandhāsana (462); Ardha Matsyendrāsana I (311); Pāśāsana (328); Paripoorṇa Matsyendrāsana (326); Dwipāda Viparīta Daṇḍāsana (516); Maṇḍalāsana (525 to 535); Ekapāda Viparīta Daṇḍāsana I & II (521 and 523); Kapotāsana (512); Laghuvajrāsana (513); Ekapāda Rājakapotāsana I (542); Hanumānāsana (475 and 476); Uttānāsana (48); Śavāsana (592). Nāḍī Śodhana Prāṇāyāma (Section 205) for 20 minutes.

191st to 200th week

Śīrṣāsana (184); Sarvāngāsana (234); Halāsana (244); Ūrdhva Kukkuṭāsana (419); Pārśva Kukkuṭāsana (424); Bakāsana (410); Pārśva Bakāsana

(412); Dwipāda Kouṇḍinyāsana (438); Ekapāda Kouṇḍinyāsana I & II (441 and 442); Ekapāda Bakāsana I & II (446 and 451) finishing each āsana with Viparīta Chakrāsana (488 to 499); Dwipāda Viparīta Daṇḍāsana (516); Maṇḍalāsana (525 to 535); Ekapāda Viparīta Daṇḍāsana I & II (521 and 523); Chakrabandhāsana (524); Kapotāsana (512); Ekapāda Rājakapotāsana I (542); Hanumānāsana (475); Samakoṇāsana (477); Yogadaṇḍāsana (456); Mulabandhāsana (462); Vasiṣṭhāsana (398); Viśvāmitrāsana (403); Paschimottānāsana (160); Kūrmāsana and Supta Kūrmāsana (363–4 and 368); Yoganidrāsana (391); Ekapāda Śīrṣāsana and cycle (371 to 384); Dwipāda Śīrṣāsana (393); Ardha Matsyendrāsana I (311); Pāśāsana (328); Paripoorṇa Matsyendrāsana (336); Kandāsana (470); Śavāsana (592). Prāṇāyāma as above.

201st to 225th week

Follow the 191st week's course up to Ekapāda Rājakapotāsana I (542) and add Ekapāda Rājakapotāsana II (545); Pādānguṣṭha Dhanurāsana (555); Bhujangāsana II (550); Rājakapotāsana (551); Hanumānāsana (475); Samakoṇāsana (477); Supta Trivikramāsana (478); Yogadaṇḍāsana (456); Mūlabandhāsana (462); Kandāsana (470); Ardha Matsyendrāsana I (311); Pāśāsana (328); Paripoorṇa Matsyendrāsana (336); Yoganidrāsana (391); Dwipāda Śīrṣāsana (393); Paschimottānāsana (160); Śavāsana (592). Prāṇāyāma as before.

226th to 250th week

Follow the 200th week's course up to Rājakapotāsana (551); add Vṛschikāsana I & II (537 and 538); Gheruṇḍāsana I & II (561 and 564); Kapinjalāsana (567) and again follow from Hanumānāsana (475) of the 200th week.

251st to 275th week

Śīrṣāsana and cycle (184 to 218); Sarvāngāsana and cycle (234 to 271); Ūrdhva Kukkuṭāsana (419); Pārśva Kukkuṭāsana (424); Bakāsana (410); Pārśva Bakāsana (412); Dwipāda Kouṇḍinyāsana (438); Ekapāda Kouṇḍinyāsana I (441); Ekapāda Bakāsana I and Ekapāda Bakāsana II with Ekapāda Kouṇḍinyāsana II (446, 451 and 442) finishing each āsana with Viparīta Chakrāsana (488 to 499); Dwipāda Viparīta Daṇḍāsana, Maṇḍalāsana, Ekapāda Viparīta Daṇḍāsana I & II at one stretch (516, 525 to 535, 521 and 523); Kapotāsana (512); Vṛschikāsana I (537); Bhujangāsana II (550); Rājakapotāsana (551); Pādānguṣṭha Dhanurāsana (555); Gheruṇḍāsana I & II (561 and 564); Ekapāda Rājakapotāsana I, II, III & IV (542, 545, 546 and 547); Gaṇḍa-Bheruṇḍāsana (580); Natarājāsana (590 and 591) and then follow the 200th week course from Hanumānāsana (475) onwards.

276th to 300th week

Follow the 251st week's course up to Ekapāda Rājakapotāsana I (542); then do Vālakhilyāsana (544); Ekapāda Rājakapotāsana II, III and IV (545, 546 and 547); Sīrṣapādāsana (570); Gaṇḍa-Bheruṇḍāsana and Viparīta Śalabhāsana together (580, 581 and 584) at one stretch and go to Ūrdhva Dhanurāsana (486) to do Tiriang-Mukhottānāsana (586); Natarājāsana (590 and 591). Then follow the 200th week's course from Hanumānāsana (475) and Prāṇāyāma as before.

To start with many fail to advance further than the exercises given for the 166th week. But by tenacity and persistent practice one can master every āsana and prāṇāyāma recommended in this book. In my earlier years it took me four years of hard work in which optimism and pessimism were balanced equally. When you have achieved mastery of the 166th week of the course, I ask you in all sincerity to persevere in the work you have undertaken happy in what you have attained and never despairing at any temporary failure. Most people, however, take far longer than I have stipulated to master all these āsanas with comfort and ease. When you have perfected all those detailed in this third course, you can divide them up into a week's course as suggested below. Then by daily practice, learn to remain master of them all.

First day of the week

Śīrṣāsana and cycle (184 to 218); Sarvāngāsana and cycle (234 to 271); Bhujapīdāsana (348); Aṣṭāvakrāsana (342 and 343); Bakāsana (410); Pārśva Bakāsana (412); Ūrdhva Kukkuṭāsana (419); Pārśva Kukkuṭ-āsana (424); Dwipāda Kouṇḍinyāsana (438); Ekapāda Kouṇḍinyāsana I (441); Ekapāda Bakāsana I (446); Ekapāda Bakāsana II with Ekapāda Kouṇḍinyāsana II (451 with 442); Gālavāsana (427); Ekapāda Gālav-āsana (432); finishing each āsana with Viparīta Chakrāsana (488 to 499); Adhomukha Vṛkṣāsana (359); Pincha Mayūrāsana (357); Mayūrāsana (354); Paschimottānāsana (160) for 5 minutes; Śavāsana (592). Nāḍī Sodhana Prāṇāyāma for 15 minutes; Ujjāyī Prāṇāyāma with Antarkum-bhaka (inhalation retention) for 8 times; Meditation in Padmāsana (104) or Siddhāsana (84) for 5 minutes.

Second day of the week

Śīrṣāsana and cycle (184 to 218); Sarvāngāsana and cycle (234 to 271); Supta Pādānguṣṭhāsana (285 to 287); Jaṭara Parivartanāsana (274); Paschimottānāsana (160); Ākarṇa Dhanurāsana (173 and 175); Kūrm-āsana and Supta Kūrmāsana (363, 364 and 368); Ekapāda Śīrṣāsana and cycle (371 to 384); Viranchyāsana I & II (386 and 388); Dwipāda

Śīrṣāsana (393); Yoganidrāsana (391); Yogadaṇḍāsana (456); Mulabandhāsana (462); Vāmadevāsana I & II (465 and 466); Kandāsana (470); Hanumānāsana (475); Uttānāsana (48); Savāsana (592).

Prāṇāyāma as before with 8 times Uddiyāṇa and 8 times Nauli.

Third day of the week

Śīrṣāsana and cycle (184 to 218); Sarvāngāsana and cycle (234 to 271); Dwipāda Viparīta Daṇḍāsana (516); Maṇḍalāsana (525 to 535); Ekapāda Viparīta Daṇḍāsana I & II (521 and 523); Chakrabandhāsana (524); Kapotāsana (512); Laghu Vajrāsana (513); Vṛśchikāsana I (537); Bhujangāsana II (550); Rājakapotāsana (551); Pādānguṣṭha Dhanurāsana (555); Gheraṇḍāsana I & II (561 and 564); Ekapāda Rājakapotāsana I & II (542 and 545); Vālakhilyāsana (544); Sīrṣapādāsana (570) and Gaṇḍa Bheruṇḍāsana, Viparīta Śalabhāsana and Tiriang-Mukhottānāsana (580, 581, 584 and 586) all together; Paschimottānāsana (160); Marichyāsana III (303); Ardha Matsyendrāsana I (311); Pāśāsana (328); Paripoorṇa Matsyendrāsana (336); Śavāsana (592). Nāḍī Śodhana Prāṇāyāma without retention for 10 to 15 minutes.

Fourth day of the week

Śīrṣāsana and cycle (184 to 218); Sarvāngāsana and cycle (234 to 271); Paschimottānāsana (160); Yoganidrāsana (391); Marichyāsana III (303); Ardha Matsyendrāsana I (311); Pāśāsana (328); Paripoorṇa Matsyendrāsana (336); Yogadaṇḍāsana (456); Mūlabandhāsana (462); Kandāsana (470); Hanumanāsana (475); Samakoṇāsana (477); Supta Trivikramāsana (478); Ūrdhva Mukha Paschimottānāsana I & II (168 and 170); Śavāsana (592). Prāṇāyāma as on the first day of the week.

Fifth day of the week

Śīrṣāsana and cycle (184 to 218); Sarvāngāsana and cycle (234 to 271); Ūrdhva Kukkuṭāsana (419); Pārśva Kukkuṭāsana (424); Bakāsana (410); Pārśva Bakāsana (412); Dwipāda Kouṇḍinyāsana (438); Ekapāda Kouṇḍinyāsana I (441); Ekapāda Bakāsana I & II (446 and 451); Ekapāda Kouṇḍinyāsana II (442); Gālavāsana (427); Ekapāda Gālavāsana (432); all these āsanas at one stretch without going to Ūrdhva Dhanurāsana (486); Vasiṣṭhāsana (398); Kaśyapāsana (399); Visvamitrāsana (403); Maṇḍalāsana (525 to 535); Kapotāsana (512); Vṛṣchikāsana I (537); Rājakapotāsana (551); Pādānguṣṭha Dhanurāsana (555); Śīrṣapādāsana (570); Gaṇḍa Bheruṇḍāsana (580 and 581); Uttānāsana (48); Śavāsana (592). Nāḍī Śodhana Prāṇāyāma without retention for 15 minutes.

Sixth day of the week

Śīrṣāsana and cycle (184 to 218); Sarvāngāsana and cycle (234 to 271); Paschimottānāsana (160); Yoganidrāsana (391); Marichyāsana III (303); Ardha Matsyendrāsana I (311); Pāśāsana (328); Paripoorṇa Matsyendrāsana (336); Hanumānāsana (475); Samakoṇāsana (477); Supta Trivikramāsana (478); Mūlabandhāsana (462); Kandāsana (470); Maṇḍalāsana (525 to 535); Kapotāsana (512); Vṛśchikāsana I (537); Rājakapotāsana (551); Ekapāda Rajakapotāsana I (542); Vālakhilyāsana (544); Śīrsapādāsana (570); Gaṇḍa Bheruṇḍāsana (580 and 581); Uttānāsana (48); Śavāsana (592). Nāḍī Śodhana Prāṇāyāma, Ujjāyī Prāṇāyāma with inhalation retention and 8 times Uḍḍīyāna.

Seventh day of the week

Complete rest or only Śīrṣāsana I (184); Sālamba Sarvāngāsana I (234); Halāsana (244); Paschimottānāsana (160) and Nāḍī Śodhana Prāṇāyāma without retention for 30 minutes.

Appendix II

Curative Āsanas for Various Diseases

After working for 25 years as a teacher, I am giving groups of āsanas for different functional and organic ailments and diseases, based on experiences with my pupils.

I have listed a number of āsanas under each complaint, so it is advisable to seek the guidance of an experienced teacher and to adopt them according to one's ability, suppleness of body and constitution. When practising āsanas it is important to use common sense and to watch the reactions of your body, thereby judging the time that you stay in them.

Acidity

Utthita Trikoṇāsana (4 and 5); Parivṛtta Trikoṇāsana (6 and 7); Utthita Pārśvakoṇāsana (8 and 9); Parivṛtta Pārśvakoṇāsana (10 and 11); Vīrabhadrāsana I, II & III (14, 15 and 17); Ardha Chandrāsana (19); Pārśvottānāsana (26); Pādānguṣṭhāsana (44); Pāda Hastāsana (46); Uttānāsana (48); Sālamba Śīrṣāsana and cycle (184 to 218); Sālamba Sarvāngāsana and cycle (234 to 271); Jaṭara Parivartanāsana (275); Paripoorṇa Nāvāsana (78); Ardha Nāvāsana (79); Ūrdhva Prasārita Pādāsana (276 to 279); Jānu-Śīrṣāsana (127); Parivṛtta Jānu-Śīrṣāsana (132); Paschimottānāsana (160); Marīchyāsana I, II & III (144, 146 and 303); Ardha Matsyendrāsana I, II & III (311, 330 and 332); Pāśāsana (328); Paripoorṇa Matsyendrāsana (336); Yoganidrāsana (391); Śalabhāsana (60); Dhanurāsana (63); Bhujangāsana I (73); Mayūrāsana (354); Ūrdhva Dhanurāsana (486) and Uḍḍīyāna (Section 201).

Anaemia

Śīrṣāsana and cycle (184 to 218); Sarvāngāsana and cycle (234 to 271); Paschimottānāsana (160); Uttānāsana (48); Ujjāyī Prāṇāyāma; Nāḍī Śodhana Prāṇāyāma without Kumbhaka (retention) for 2 to 3 months. After 3 months do Antarkumbhaka (inhalation retention). Savāsana (592) whenever possible from 10 to 15 minutes at a stretch.

Ankles

Utthita and Parivṛtta Trikoṇāsana (4, 5, 6 and 7); Utthita and Parivṛtta

Pārśvakoṇāsana (8, 9, 10 and 11); Vīrabhadrāsana I, II and III (14, 15 and 17); Pārśvottānāsana (26); Prasārita Pādottānāsana (33); Adhomukha Śvānāsana (75); Gomukhāsana (80); Vīrāsana (89); Supta Vīrāsana (96); Bhekāsana (100); Baddha Padmāsana and cycle (104 to 124); Baddha-koṇāsana (102); Supta Pādāngusthāsana (285 to 287); Triang Mukhaikapāda Paschimottānāsana (139); Krounchāsana (141); Bharadwājāsana I & II (297 and 299); Ākarṇa Dhanurāsana (173 and 175); Śalabhāsana (60); Dhanurāsana (63); Uṣṭrāsana (41); Vātāyanāsana (58); Garuḍāsana (56); Supta Bhekāsana (458); Mālāsana I and II (321 and 322).

Appendicitis

Śīrṣāsana and cycle (184 to 218); Sarvāngāsana and cycle (234 to 271); Paschimottānāsana (160); Ūrdhvamukha Paschimottānāsana I & II (168 and 170); Poorvottānāsana (171); Mahā Mudra (125); Jānu-Śīrṣāsana (127); Ardha Matsyendrāsana I (311); Pāśāsana (328); Ūrdhva Dhanurāsana (468); Dwipāda Viparīta Daṇḍāsana (516); Uttānāsana (48). Nāḍī Śodhana Prāṇāyāma (Section 205) without retention for 2 months, then with retention after inhaling.

Arthritis of the lower back

Utthita and Parivṛtta Trikoṇāsana (4, 5, 6 and 7); Utthita and Parivṛtta Pārśvakoṇāsana (8, 9, 10 and 11); Vīrabhadrāsana I, II & III (14, 15 and 17); Ardhachandrāsana (19); Pādānguṣṭhāsana (44); Pāda Hastāsana (46); Uttānāsana (48); Śīrṣāsana and cycle (184 to 218); Sarvāngāsana and cycle (234 to 271); Marichyāsana I, II, III & IV (143, 145, 303 and 305); Bharadwājāsana I & II (297 and 299); Ardha Matsyendrāsana I (311); Pāśāsana (328); Parighāsana (39); Śalabhāsana (60); Dhanurāsana (63); Pārśva Dhanurāsana (64 and 65); Uttānapādāsana (292); Uṣṭrāsana (41); Setubandhāsana (296); Ūrdhva Dhanurāsana (486); Dwipāda Viparīta Daṇḍāsana (516); Adhomukha Vṛkṣāsana (359); Pincha Mayūrāsana (357).

Arthritis of the dorsal region

Padmāsana and cycle (104 to 124); Vīrāsana (91); Paryankāsana (97); Gomukhāsana (80); all standing positions (4 to 36); Parighāsana (39); Paschimottānāsana (160); Ūrdhva Mukha Paschimottānāsana I & II (168 and 170); Bhujangāsana I (73); Ūrdhva Mukha Śvānāsana (74); Adhomukha Śvānāsana (75); Pincha Mayūrāsana (357); Adhomukha Vṛkṣāsana (359); Śīrṣāsana and cycle (184 to 218); Sarvāngāsana and cycle (234 to 271); Bharadwājāsana I & II (297 and 299); Marīchyāsana I & III (143 and 303); Ardha Matsyendrāsana I & II (311 and 330); Pāśāsana (328); Uṣṭrāsana (41); Dhanurāsana (63); Urdhva Dhanurāsana (486 and 487); Ekapāda Ūrdhva Dhanurāsana (501); Dwipāda Viparīta Daṇḍāsana (516); Ekapāda Viparīta Daṇḍāsana I (521); Kapotāsana (512); Laghuvajrāsana (513).

Arthritis of the shoulder joints

Utthita and Parivṛtta Trikoṇāsana (4, 5, 6 and 7); Utthita and Parivṛtta Pārśvakoṇāsana (8, 9, 10 and 11); Vīrabhadrāsana I, II & III (14, 15 and 17); Ardhachandrāsana (19); Pārśvottānāsana (26); Sālamba Sīrṣāsana (184); Sālamba Sarvāngāsana I & II (234 and 235); Halāsana (244); Dhanurāsana (63); Ūrdhva Mukha Śvānāsana (74); Adhomukha Śvānāsana (75); Vīrāsana (89); Parvatāsana (107); Ardha Baddha Padmottānāsana (52); Ardha Baddha Padma Paschimottānāsana (135); Paschimottānāsana (160); Gomukhāsana (80); Baddha Padmāsana (118); Yogamudrāsana (120); Pincha Mayūrāsana (357); Adhomukha Vṛkṣāsana (359); Vasiṣṭhāsana (398); Kaśyapāsana (399); Viśvamitrāsana (403); Bhujapidāsana (348); Bakāsana (410); Marichyāsana I, II & III (144, 146 and 303); Ardha Matsyendrāsana I & II (311 and 330); Bharadwājāsana I & II (297 and 299); Pāśāsana (328); Paripoorṇa Matsyendrāsana (336); Uṣṭrāsana (41); Yogadaṇḍāsana (456); Ūrdhva Dhanurāsana (486); Kapotāsana (512); Maṇḍalāsana (525 to 535); Pādānguṣṭha Dhanurāsana (555).

Arms and abdominal organs

Chaturanga Daṇḍāsana (67); Nakrāsana (68 to 71); Ūrdhva Mukha Śvānāsana (74); Adhomukha Śvānāsana (75); Lolāsana (83); Tolāsana (108); Simhāsana II (110); Mayūrāsana (354); Padma Mayūrāsana (355); Haṃsāsana (356); Aṣṭāvakrāsana (342); Bhujapīdāsana (348); Pincha Mayūrāsana (357); Adhomukha Vṛkṣāsana (359); Bakāsana (410); Pārśva Bakāsana (412); Ekahasta Bhujāsana (344); Dwihasta Bhujāsana (345); Chakorāsana (379); Vasiṣṭhāsana (398); Viśvāmitrāsana (403); Tittibhāsana (395); Ūrdhva Kukkuṭāsana (419); Parśva Kukkuṭāsana (424); Dwipāda Kouṇḍinyāsana (438); Ekapāda Kouṇḍinyāsana I & II (441 and 442); Ekapāda Bakāsana I & II (446 and 451); Gālavāsana (427); Ekapāda Gālavāsana (432); Viparīta Chakrāsana (488 to 499).

Asthma

Śīrṣāsana and cycle (184 to 218); Sarvāngāsana and cycle (234 to 271); Mahāmudra (125); Jānu-Śīrṣāsana (127); Uttanāsana (48); Paschimottānāsana (160); Bhujangāsana I & II (73 and 550); Śalabhāsana (60); Dhanurāsana (63); Ūrdhva Mukha Śvānāsana (74); Adhomukha Śvānāsana (75); Vīrāsana (89); Supta Vīrāsana (96); Paryankāsana (97); Padmāsana and cycle (104 to 124); Uttānapādāsana (292); Setubandhāsana (296); Poorvottānāsana (171); Ardha Matsyendrāsana I & II (311 and 330); Pāśāsana (328); Uṣṭrāsana (41); Ūrdhva Dhanurāsana (486); Dwipāda Viparīta Daṇḍāsana (516). Ujjāyī Prāṇāyāma (Section 203) and Nāḍī Śodhana Prāṇāyāma (Section 205) without retention when there is an attack and at other times with inhalation retention and Uḍḍīyāna (Section 201).

Backache

Śīrṣāsana and cycle (184 to 218); Sarvāngāsana and cycle (234 to 271); all standing poses (4 to 36); Jaṭara Parivartanāsana (275); Supta Pādānguṣṭhāsana (285 to 287); Mahāmudra (125); Jānu-Śīrṣāsana (127); Parivṛtta Jānu-Śīrṣāsana (132); Paschimottānāsana (160); Ūrdhva Mukha Paschimottānāsana I and II (168 and 170); Parivṛtta Paschimottānāsana (165); Marichyāsana I & III (144 and 303); Ardha Matsyendrāsana I & II (311 and 330); Pāśāsana (328); Paripoorṇa Matsyendrāsana (336); Mālāsana I & II (321 and 322); Adhomukha Śvānāsana (75); Uṣṭrāsana (41); Śalabhāsana (60); Dhanurāsana (63); Pārśva Dhanurāsana (64 and 65); Ūrdhva Dhanurāsana (486); Viparīta Chakrāsana (488 to 499); Dwipāda Viparīta Daṇḍāsana (516); Maṇḍalāsana (525 to 535).

High blood pressure

Halāsana (244); Jānu-Śīrṣāsana (127); Ardha Baddha Padma Paschimottānāsana (135); Triang Mukhaikapāda Paschimottānāsana (139); Paschimottānāsana (160); Vīrāsana (89); Siddhāsana (84); Padmāsana (104); Śavāsana (592). Nāḍī Śodhana Prāṇāyāma (Section 205) without retention. Meditation with closed eyes. (If the blood pressure is very high, then it is better to do Ujjāyī Prāṇāyāma (Section 203) in the lying position without pillows first for 5 minutes and then to perform Nāḍī Śodhana Prāṇāyāma (Section 205) and immediately do Śavāsana (592) for 15 minutes.)

Low blood pressure

Sālamba Śīrṣāsana I (184); Sālamba Sarvāngāsana I (234); Halāsana (244); Karṇapīḍāsana (246); Paschimottānāsana (160); Vīrāsana (89); Siddhāsana (84); Padmāsana (104); Baddhakoṇāsana (102); Nāḍī Śodhana Prāṇāyāma (Section 205) without retention in the beginning and Śavāsana (592).

Brain

Śīrṣāsana and cycle (184 to 218); Sarvāngāsana and cycle (234 to 271); Adhomukha Śvānāsana (75); Paschimottānāsana (160); Uttānāsana (48); Kūrmāsana and Supta Kūrmāsana (363, 364 and 368); Yoganidrāsana (391); Ūrdhva Dhanurāsana (486); Viparīta Chakrāsana (488 to 499); Dwipāda Viparīta Daṇḍāsana (516); Ekapāda Viparīta Daṇḍāsana I & II (521 and 523); Vṛśchikāsana I & II (537 and 538); Śīrṣapādāsana (570); Gaṇḍa Bheruṇḍāsana (580 and 581); Viparīta Śalabhāsana (584); Nāḍī Śodhana (Section 205), Sūryabhedana (Section 204), Bhastrikā (Section 206) and Śītali Prāṇāyāmas (601); Śavāsana (592).

Loss of memory

Śīrṣāsana and cycle (184 to 218); Sarvāngāsana and cycle (234 to 271); Uttānāsana (48); Paschimottānāsana (160); Ūrdhva Mukha Paschimottānāsana I & II (168 and 170); Trāṭaka or gazing at the middle of the eyebrows or tip of the nostrils. Nāḍī Śodhana Prāṇāyāma (Section 205) with inhalation retention and Bhastrikā Prāṇāyāma (Section 206).

Breathlessness

Sālamba Śīrṣāsana I (184); Sālamba Sarvāngāsana I (234); Halāsana (244); Paschimottānāsana (160); Uttānāsana (48); Adhomukha Śvānāsana (75); Parvatāsana (107); Ūrdhva Dhanurāsana (486); Ūjjāyi Prāṇāyāma Nāḍī Śodhana Prāṇāyāma; Uḍḍīyāna; Śavāsana (592).

Bronchitis

All standing positions (4 to 39); Śīrṣāsana and if possible cycle (184 to 218); Sarvāngāsana and cycle (234 to 271 except 267); Paschimottānāsana (160); Jaṭara Parivartanāsana (275); Ūrdhva Mukha Paschimottānāsana I & II (168 and 170); Jānu-Śīrṣāsana (127); Mahāmudra (125); Bhujangāsana I (73); Adhomukha Śvānāsana (75); Gomukhāsana (80); Marīchyāsana I & III (144 and 303); Ardha Matsyendrāsana I (311); Mālāsana I & II (321 and 322); Pāśāsana (328); Vīrāsana (89); Supta Vīrāsana (96); Paryankāsana (97); Padmāsana and whatever possible in the cycle (104 to 124); Baddha Koṇāsana (102); Upaviṣṭha Koṇāsana (151); Ekapāda Śīrṣāsana and cycle (371 to 384); Yoganidrāsana (391); Dwipāda Śīrsāsana (393); Kūrmāsana and Supta Kūrmāsana (363, 364 and 368); Śalabhāsana (60); Dhanurāsana (63); Uṣṭrāsana (41); Urdhva Dhanurāsana (486); Kapotāsana (512); Dwipāda Viparīta Daṇḍāsana (516); Ujjāyī (Section 203), Nāḍī Sodhana (Section 205) and Sūrya Bhedana Prāṇāyāmas (Section 204) with inhalation retention.

Broncho-pneumonia

Sālamba Śīrṣāsana I (184); Sālamba Sarvāngāsana I (234); Halāsana (244); Paschimottānāsana (160); Uttānāsana (48); Mahā Mudra (125);

Adhomukha Śvānāsana (75); Vīrāsana (89); Siddhāsana (84); Padmāsana (104); Baddha Padmāsana (118); Baddha Koṇāsana (102); Ujjāyi, Nāḍī Sodhana and Sūrya-bhedana Prāṇāyāmas; Śavāsana (592).

Chest

All standing positions (1 to 48); Śīrṣāsana and cycle (184 to 218); Sarvāngāsana and cycle (234 to 271); Dhanurāsana (63); Chaturanga Daṇḍāsana (67); Bhujangāsana I & II (73 and 550); Ūrdhva-mukha Śvānāsana (74); Adhomukha Śvānāsana (75); Padmāsana and cycle (104 to 124); Paschimottānāsana (160); Ākarna Dhanurāsana (173 and 175); Ubhaya Pādānguṣṭhāsana (167); Ūrdhva Mukha Paschimottānāsana I & II (168 and 170); Baddha Koṇāsana (101); Bhujapīdāsana (348); Marīchyāsana III (303); Ardha Matsyendrāsana I, II & III (311, 330 and 332); Pāśāsana (328); Pincha Mayūrāsana (357); Adhomukha Vṛkṣāsana (359); Bakāsana (410); Pārśva Bakāsana (412); Dwipāda Kouṇḍinyāsana (348); Ekapāda Koundinyāsana I & II (441 and 442); Ekapāda Bakāsana I & II (446 and 451); Ūrdhva Kukkuṭāsana (419); Pārśva Kukkuṭāsana (424); Vāmadevāsana I & II (465 and 466); Ūrdhva Dhanurāsana (486); Viparīta Chakrāsana (488 to 499); Kapotāsana (512); Laghuvajrāsana (513); Dwipāda Viparīta Daṇḍāsana (516); Ekapāda Viparīta Daṇḍāsana I & II (521 and 523); Chakrabandhāsana (524); Maṇḍalāsana (525 to 535); Vṛischikāsana I (537); Rājakapotāsana (551); Ekapāda Rājakapotāsana I, II, III and IV (542, 545, 546 and 547); Vālakhilyāsana (544); Pādānguṣṭha Dhanurāsana (555); Gaṇḍa Bheruṇḍāsana (580 and 581); Viparīta Śalabhāsana (584); Tiriang Mukhottānāsana (586); Natarājāsana (590); Ujjāyi (Section 203) and Nāḍī Śodhana Prāṇāyāma (Section 205) with inhalation retention.

Chill

Śīrṣāsana and cycle (184 to 218); Sarvāngāsana and cycle (234 to 271); Uttānāsana (48); Paschimottānāsana (160); Ardha Matsyendrāsana I (311); Pāśāsana (328); Ūrdhva Dhanurāsana (486). Ujjāyi (Section 203), Bhastrikā (Section 206), Nāḍī Śodhana (Section 205) and Sūryabhedana (Section 204) Prāṇāyāmas.

Coccyx (Pain and displacement)

Vīrāsana (86); Supta Vīrāsana (96); Padmāsana and cycle (104 to 124); Śīrṣāsana I (184); Sarvāngāsana I (234); Setubandha Sarvāngāsana and Ekapāda Setubandha Sarvāngāsana (259 and 260); Śalabhāsana (60); Dhanurāsana (63); Pārśva Dhanurāsana (64 and 65); Bhujangāsana I & II (73 and 550); Adhomukha-Vṛkṣāsana (359); Pincha-Mayūrāsana (357); Ūrdhva Mukha Śvānāsana (74); Vātāyanāsana (58); Uṣṭrāsana (41); Ūrdhva Dhanurāsana (486 and 487); Dwipāda Viparīta Daṇḍāsana (516); Kapotāsana (512); Laghuvajrāsana (513); Vṛiśchikāsana I (537); Rājakapotāsana (551); Ekapāda Rājakapotāsana I, II, III & IV (542, 545, 546 and 547); Vālakhilyāsana (544); Gaṇḍa Bheruṇḍāsana (580 and 581); Viparīta Salabhāsana (584); Pādānguṣṭha Dhanurāsana (550); Tiriang Mukhottānāsana (586); Hanumānāsana (475); Mulabandhāsana (462).

Cold

Śīrṣāsana and cycle (184 to 218); Sarvāngāsana and cycle (234 to 271); Uttānāsana (48); Paschimottānāsana (160); Kūrmāsana and Supta Kūrmāsana (363, 364 and 368); Yoganidrāsana (391); Ujjāyi Prāṇāyāma (Section 203) with inhalation retention.

Cough

Śīrṣāsana and cycle (184 to 218); Sarvāngāsana and cycle (234 to 271); Uttānāsana (48); Paschimottānāsana (160); Ardha Matsyendrāsana I (311); Pāśāsana (328); Ūrdhva Dhanurāsana (486); Ujjāyi Prāṇāyāma (Section 203) with inhalation retention.

Colic

Śīrṣāsana and cycle (184 to 218); Sarvāngāsana and cycle (234 to 271); Uttānāsana (48); Jaṭara Parivartanāsana (275); Paripoorṇa Nāvāsana (78); Ardha Nāvāsana (79); Vīrāsana (89); Supta Vīrāsana (96); Mahāmudra (125); Uḍḍīyāna 6 to 8 times (Section 201).

Colitis

Śīrsāsana and cycle (184 to 218); Sarvāngāsana and cycle (234 to 271); Uttānāsana (48); Paschimottānāsana (160); Vīrāsana (89); Supta Vīrāsana (96); Jaṭara Parivartanāsana (275); Paripoorṇa Nāvāsana (78); Ardha Nāvāsana (79); Marīchyāsana III (303); Ardha Matsyendrāsana I (311); Pāśāsana (328); Mahāmudra (125); Adhomukha Śvānāsana (75); Jānu-Śīrṣāsana (127); Yoganidrāsana (391); Śalabhāsana (60); Dhanurāsana (63); Urdhva Dhanurāsana (486); Ujjāyī (Section 203) and Nāḍī Śodhaṇa Prāṇāyāma (Section 205).

Constipation

Śīrṣāsana and cycle (184 to 218); Sarvāngāsana and cycle (234 to 271); all the standing poses (4 to 36); Uttānāsana (48); Paschimottānāsana (160); Jaṭara Parivartanāsana (275). Nāḍī Śodhana Prāṇāyāma (Section 205).

Coronary thrombosis

Ujjāyī Prāṇāyāma (Section 203) in the lying position without retention.

(Even the deep breathing, this should be done without strain and preferably with the guidance of a competent teacher.) Śavāsana (592) for 15 minutes twice a day.

Deformity in legs

All the standing positions (4 to 48); Jānu-Śīrṣāsana (127); Ardha Baddha Padma Paschimottānāsana (135); Triangmukhaikapāda Paschimottānāsana (139); Krounchāsana (141); Upaviṣhṭa Koṇāsana (151); Ubhaya Pādānguṣṭhāsana (167); Ūrdhva Mukha Paschimottānāsana I & II (168 and 170); Halāsana (244); Jaṭara Parivartanāsana (275); Supta Pādānguṣṭhāsana (284 to 287); Anantāsana (290); Adhomukha Śvānāsana (75); Salabhāsana (60); Hanumānāsana (475); Samakoṇāsana (477); Supta Trivikramāsana (478).

Deformity in arms

All the standing poses (1 to 48); Parvatāsana (107); Halāsana (244); Ūrdhva Mukha Śvānāsana (74); Adhomukha Śvānāsana (75); Adhomukha Vṛkṣāsana (359); Gomukhāsana (80); Marīchyāsana I & III (144 and 303); Ardha Matsyendrāsana I (311); Baddha Padmāsana (118); Mālāsana I (321); Pāśāsana (328).

Diabetes

Śīrṣāsana and cycle (184 to 218); Sarvāngāsana and cycle (234 to 271); Mahāmudra (125); Jānu-Śīrṣāsana (127); Paschimottānāsana (160); Vīrāsana (89); Supta Vīrāsana (96); Ākarṇa Dhanurāsana (173 and 175); Śalabhāsana (60); Dhanurāsana (63); Paripoorṇa Nāvāsana (78); Ardha Nāvāsana (79); Jatara Parivartanāsana (275); Uttānāsana (48); Marīchyāsana I, II, III and IV (146, 303 and 305); Ardha Matsyendrāsana I, II and III (311, 330 and 332); Pāśāsana (328); Paripoorṇa Matsyendrāsana (336); Ūrdhva Dhanurāsana (486); Dwipāda Viparīta Daṇḍāsana (516); Mayūrāsana (354); Hamṣāsana (356); Bhujangāsana I and II (73 and 550); Uḍḍīyāna (Section 201), Nauli (Section 202), Nāḍī Śodhana Prāṇāyāma (Section 205) with inhalation retention; Śavāsana (592).

Diarrhoea

Sālamba Śīrṣāsana I (184); Sālamba Sarvāngāsana I (234); Nāḍī Śodhana Prāṇāyāma (Section 205) without retention.

Dilation of heart

Nāḍī Śodhana Prāṇāyāma (Section 205) without retention.

Displacement of uterus

Śīrṣāsana and cycle (184 to 218); Sarvāngāsana and cycle (234 to 271);

Uttānāsana (48); Pādāngusṭhāsana (44); Pāda-Hastāsana (46); Adho-mukha Śvānāsana (75); Daṇḍāsana (77); Parvatāsana (107); Matsyāsana (114); Baddha Koṇāsana (101); Upaviṣṭha Koṇāsana (151); Ujjāyi (Section 203) and Nāḍī Śodhana Prāṇāyāma (Section 205); Uḍḍīyāna (Section 201).

Displacement of the spinal discs

All the standing poses (4 to 19); Pādāngusṭhāsana (43); Pāda Hastāsana (45); Uttānāsana (47); Paschimottānāsana (160); Śalabhāsana (60 and 61); Makarāsana (62); Dhanurāsana (63); Uṣṭrāsana (41); Bhujangāsana I (73); Ūrdhva Mukha Śvānāsana (74); Uttānapādāsana (292); Setu-bandhāsana (296); Sarvāngāsana I (234); Setubandha Sarvāngāsana (259); Pincha Mayūrāsana (357); Adhomukha Vṛkṣāsana (359); Parvat-āsana (107); Matsyāsana (113); Supta Vīrāsana (96); Paryankāsana (97); Parighāsana (39); Ūrdhva Dhanurāsana (486 and 487); Dwipāda Viparīta Daṇḍasāna (516); Ujjāyi (Section 203) and Nāḍī Śodhana Prāṇāyāma (Section 205).

Dysentery

Śīrṣāsana and possible āsanas in the cycle (184 to 218); Sarvāngāsana and possible āsanas in the cycle (234 to 271); Mahāmudra (125); Jānu-Śīrṣāsana (127); Nāḍī Śodhana Prāṇāyāma (Section 205) without retention.

Dyspepsia

Follow the āsanas dealing with *Acidity*

Epilepsy

Sālamba Śīrṣāsana I (184); Sālamba Sarvāngāsana I (234); Halāsana (244); Mahāmudra (125); Paschimottānāsana (160); Ujjāyi Prāṇāyāma with inhalation retention and Nāḍī Śodhana Prāṇāyāma without retention; Śanmukhi Mudra (106) for 5 minutes; Śavāsana (592) for any length of time at disposal. Sītali Prāṇāyāma (601); Dhyāna or meditation.

Eyes

Śīrṣāsana and cycle (184 to 218); Sarvāngāsana and cycle (234 to 271); Uttānāsana (48); Paschimottānāsana (160); Trāṭaka or gazing with eyes closed at the tip of the nose for some time and in between the eyebrows for some time. Śanmukhi Mudra (106); Śītali (601) and Nāḍī Śodhana Prāṇāyāma (Section 205); Śavāsana (592).

Fatigue

Sālamba Śīrṣāsana I (184); Sālamba Sarvāngāsana I (234); Halāsana (244); Paschimottānāsana (160); Ūrdhva Mukha Paschimottānāsana II (170); Adhomukha Śvānāsana (75); Uttānāsana (48); Ardha Matsyendrāsana I (311); Pāśāsana (328); Mālāsana II (322); Dwipāda Viparīta Daṇḍāsana (516); Nāḍī Sodhana Prāṇāyāma (Section 205) without retention; Śavāsana (592).

Flat foot

All the standing positions (1 to 48); Śīrṣāsana I (184); Sarvāngāsana I (234); Vīrāsana (89); Supta Vīrāsana (96); Paryankāsana (97); Bhekāsana (100); Supta Bhekāsana (458); Triang Mukhaikapāda Paschimottānāsana (139); Krounchāsana (141); Baddha Padmāsana (118); Baddha Koṇāsana (102); Mūlabandhāsana (462); Supta Pādānguṣṭhāsana (284 to 287); Gomukhāsana (80); Yogadaṇḍāsana (456); Vāmadevāsana I & II (465 and 466); Gheraṇḍāsana I (561).

Flatulence

Śīrṣāsana and cycle (184 to 218); Sarvāngāsana and cycle (234 to 271); all the standing positions (1 to 36); Pādānguṣṭhāsana (44); Pāda Hastāsana (46); Uttānāsana (48); Mahāmudra (125); Jānu-Śīrṣāsana (127); Ardha Baddha Padma Paschimottānāsana (135); Triang Mukhaikapāda Paschimottānāsana (139); Krounchāsana (142); Marīchyāsana I (144); Paripoorṇa Nāvāsana (78); Ardha Nāvāsana (79); Marīchyāsana III (303); Ardha Matsyendrāsana I & III (311 and 332); Mālāsana II (322); Pāśāsana (328); Paripoorṇa Matsyendrāsana (336); Paschimottānāsana (160); Ūrdhva Mukha Paschimottānāsana I & II (168 and 170); Jaṭara Parivartanāsana (275); Ūrdhva Prasārita Pādāsana (276 to 279); Chakrāsana (280 to 283); Supta Vīrāsana (96); Yoga Mudrāsana (120); Ekapāda Śīrṣāsana and cycle (371 to 384); Kūrmāsana and Supta Kūrmāsana (363, 364 and 368); Yoganidrāsana (391); Dwipāda Śīrṣāsana (393); Śalabhāsana (60); Dhanurāsana (63); Mayūrāsana (354); Ūrdhva Dhanurāsana (486); Dwipāda Viparīta Daṇḍāsana (516); Maṇḍalāsana (525 to 535); Uḍḍīyāna (Section 201) and Nauli (Section 202).

Gall bladder and liver exercises

Follow the āsanas given under the headings *Acidity*, *Dyspepsia* and *Flatulence*.

Gastritis

Same as in *Flatulence*.

Giddiness

Sālamba Śīrṣāsana I (184); Sālamba Sarvāngāsana I (234); Halāsana (244); Paschimottānāsana (160); Śanmukhi Mudra (106); Nāḍī Śodhana Prāṇāyāma (Section 205) without retention; Śavāsana (592).

Gout

Śīrṣāsana and whatever possible in the cycle (184 to 218); Sarvāngāsana and whatever possible in the cycle (234 to 271); standing positions (4 to 36); if possible Padmāsana and cycle (104 to 124); Vīrāsana (89); Supta Vīrāsana (96); Paryankāsana (97); Parighāsana (39); Garuḍāsana (56); Gomukhāsana (80); Uttānāsana (48); Paschimottānāsana (160); Ubhaya Pādānguṣṭhāsana (167); Ākarṇa Dhanurāsana (173 and 175); Krounchāsana (142); Marīchyāsana III (303); Ardha Matsyendrāsana I (311); Mālāsana I & II (321 and 322); Pāśāsana (328); Yogadaṇḍāsana (456); Bhekāsana (100); Supta Bhekāsana (458); Mūlabandhāsana (462); Vāmadevāsana I & II (465 and 466); Kandāsana (470); Hanumānāsana (475).

Halitosis (Bad breath)

Śīrṣāsana and cycle (184 to 218); Sarvāngāsana and cycle (234 to 271); Uttānāsana (48); Jaṭara Parivartanāsana (275); Paschimottānāsana (160); Simhāsana I & II (109 and 110); Ujjāyi (Section 203), Nāḍī Śodhana (Section 205) and Śītali Prāṇāyāma (601); Uḍḍīyāna (Section 201).

(While doing āsanas and Prāṇāyāma, open the mouth, extend the tongue and curl it upwards so that the tip is pushed towards and brought close to the glottis throughout the practices. This not only removes the foul smell but also quenches the thirst. It is called Kāka Mudrā in Yoga. Kāka means a crow and mudrā a symbol.)

Hamstring muscles

All the standing positions (4 to 36); Sālamba Śīrṣāsana and whatever possible in the cycle (184 to 218); Sālamba Sarvāngāsana and whatever possible in the cycle (234 to 271); Jaṭara Parivartanāsana (275); Supta Pādānguṣṭhāsana (284 to 287); Anantāsana (290); Paschimottānāsana (160); Poorvottānāsana (171); Baddha Koṇāsana (101); Upaviṣṭha Koṇāsana (151); Ākarṇa Dhanurāsana (173 and 175); Kūrmāsana (363 and 364); Ustrāsana (41); Śalabhāsana (60); Dhanurāsana (63); Ūrdhva Dhanurāsana (486 and 487); Dwipāda Viparīta Daṇḍāsana (516); Maṇḍalāsana (525 to 535); Ardha Matsyendrāsana I (311); Mālāsana II (322); Pāśāsana (328); Hanumānāsana (475); Samakoṇāsana (477); Supta Trivikramāsana (478).

Headache

Sālamba Śīrṣāsana I (184) for 10 minutes; Sālamba Sarvāngāsana I (234) for 10 minutes; Halāsana (244) for 5 minutes and possible āsanās in Sarvāngāsana cycle; Paschimottānāsana (160) for 5 minutes; Uttānāsana (48) for 3 minutes; Nāḍī Śodhana Prāṇāyāma (Section 205) without retention for 10 to 15 minutes; Śavāsana (592) for 10 minutes.

Heart trouble

Ujjāyī (Section 203) or Nāḍī Śodhana Prāṇāyāma (Section 205) without retention and without strain. Meditation. Śavāsana (592).

Heartburn

Follow the exercises given under the headline *Acidity*.

Heels (Pain or spurs)

Śīrsāsana and cycle (184 to 218); Sarvāngāsana and cycle (234 to 271); Adhomukha Śvānāsana (75); Vīrāsana (89); Supta Vīrāsana (96); Paryankāsana (97); Bhekāsana (100); Supta Bhekāsana (458); Baddha Koṇāsana (101); Mulabandhāsana (462); Ardha Matsyendrāsana I (311); Mālāsana I & II (321 and 322); Pāśāsana (328); Paripoorṇa Matsyendrāsana (336); Ūrdhva Mukha Paschimottānāsana I & II (168 and 170); Gomukhāsana (80); Pincha Mayūrāsana (357); Adhomukha Vṛkṣāsana (359); Vāmadevāsana I & II (465 and 466); Yogadaṇḍāsana (456); Kandāsana (470).

Hernia (Umbilical)

Śīrṣāsana and cycle (184 to 218); Sarvāngāsana and cycle (234 to 271); Baddhakoṇāsana (103); Upavista Koṇāsana (151); Paschimottānāsana (160); Ūrdhva Mukha Paschimottānāsana I & II (168 and 170); Ākarṇa Dhanurāsana (173 and 175); Supta Pādānguṣṭhāsana (284 to 287); Mahāmudra (125); Adhomukha Śvānāsana (75); Pādānguṣṭhāsana (43); Pāda Hastāsana (45); Uttānāsana (57); Ūrdhva Dhanurāsana (486); Dwipāda Viparīta Daṇḍāsana (516); Kūrmāsana and Supta Kūrmāsana (363, 364 and 368); Ekapāda Śīrṣāsana and cycle (371 to 384); Yoganidrāsana (391); Dwipāda Śīrṣāsana (393); Paripoorṇa Nāvāsana (78); Ardha Nāvāsana (79); Uḍḍīyāna.

Hernia (Inguinal)

Śīrṣāsana and cycle (184 to 218); Sarvāngāsana and cycle (234 to 271); Ubhaya Pādānguṣṭhāsana (167); Ūrdhva Mukha Paschimottānāsana I & II (168 and 170); Krounchāsana (141); Ākarṇa Dhanurāsana (173 and 175); Supta Pādānguṣṭhāsana (284 to 287); Upaviṣṭa Koṇāsana

(151); Baddha-Koṇāsana (102); Hanumānāsana (475); Samakoṇāsana (477); Supta Trivikramāsana (478); Yogadaṇḍāsana (456); Mūlabandhāsana (462); Yoganidrāsana (391); Uḍḍīyāna (Section 201).

(It is advisable to do Baddha Koṇāsana (101) in the lying position while retiring. Do not immediately stand or move about after performing the āsana. Do Śavāsana after the above āsana.)

Hunch-back

All the standing positions (1 to 36); Chaturanga Daṇḍāsana (67); Śalabhāsana (60); Makarāsana (62); Dhanurāsana (63); Uṣṭrāsana (41); Pādānguṣṭhāsana (43); Pāda Hastāsana (45); Uttānāsana (47); Bhujangāsana I (73); Ūrdhva Mukha Śvānāsana (74); Adhomukha Śvānāsana (75); Mahāmudra (125); Jānu-Śīrṣasana (127); Upaviṣṭa Koṇāsana (151); Gomukhāsana (80); Parvatāsana (107); Bharadwājāsana I & II (297 and 299); Marīchyāsana I, II, III and IV (144, 146, 303 and 305); Baddha Padmāsana (118); Paryankāsana (97); Ardha Matsyendrāsana I & II (311 and 330); Jaṭara Parivartanāsana (275); Supta Pādānguṣṭhāsana (285 to 287); Ūrdhva Dhanurāsana (486); Pincha Mayurāsana (357); Adhomukha Vṛkṣāsana (359); Dwipāda Viparīta Daṇḍāsana (516).

Hydrocele

Śīrṣāsana and cycle (184 to 218); Sarvāngāsana and cycle (234 to 271); Padmāsana and cycle (104 to 124); Adhomukha Vṛkṣāsana (359); Pincha Mayūrāsana (357); Adhomukha Śvānāsana (75); Jaṭara Parivartanāsana (275); Supta Pādānguṣṭhāsana (285 to 287); Baddha Koṇāsana (101); Upaviṣṭa Koṇāsana (151); Paschimottānāsana (160); Yoganidrāsana (391); Yogadaṇḍāsana (456); Mulabandhāsana (462); Vāmadevāsana I & II (465 and 466); Kandāsana (470); Hanumānāsana (475); Samakoṇāsana (477); Uḍḍīyāna (Section 201) and Nauli (Section 202).

Impotency

Śīrṣāsana and cycle (184 to 218); Sarvāngāsana and cycle (234 to 271); Paschimottānāsana (160); Uttānāsana (48); Mahāmudra (125); Baddha Koṇāsana (101); Ardha Matsyendrāsana I (311); Pāśāsana (328); Mūlabandhāsana (462); Kandāsana (470); Hanumānāsana (475); Yoganidrāsana (391); Ūrdhva Dhanurāsana (486); Dwipāda Viparīta Daṇḍāsana (516); Uḍḍīyāna; Nāḍī Śodhana Prāṇāyāma (Section 205) with inhalation retention.

Indigestion

All the standing positions (4 to 48); Śīrṣāsana and cycle (184 to 218); Sarvāngāsana and cycle (234 to 271); Jaṭara Parivartanāsana (275); Ūrdhva Prasarīta Pādāsana (276 to 279); Paripoorṇa Nāvāsana (78);

Ardha Nāvāsana (79); Mahāmudra (125); Śalabhāsana (60); Dhanurāsana (63); Paschimottānāsana (160); Yoganidrāsana (391); Marīchyāsana III (303); Ardha Matsyendrāsana I (311); Pāśāsana (328); Paripoorṇa Matsyendrāsana (336); Supta Vīrāsana (96); Uḍḍīyāna (Section 201) and Nauli (Section 202), Bhastrika Prāṇāyāma (Section 206), Nāḍī Śodhana Prāṇāyāma (Section 205) with inhalation retention.

Insomnia

Śīrṣāsana and cycle (184 to 218); Sarvāngāsana and cycle (234 to 271); Paschimottānāsana (160); Uttānāsana (48); Bhastrika, Nāḍī Śodhana and Sūryabhedana Prāṇāyāma without retention, Śanmukhi Mudra (106) and Śavāsana (592).

Kidneys

Śīrṣāsana and cycle (184 to 218); Sarvāngāsana and cycle (234 to 271); all the standing positions (4 to 48); Ūrdhva Mukha Śvānāsana (74); Adhomukha Śvānāsana (75); Śalabhāsana (60); Dhanurāsana (63); Jānu-Śīrṣāsana (127); Parivṛtta Jānu-Śīrṣāsana (132); Paschimottānāsana (160); Parivṛtta Paschimottānāsana (165); Baddha Koṇāsana (103); Upaviṣṭa Koṇāsana (151); Jaṭara Parivartanāsana (275); Ardha Nāvāsana (79); Marīchyāsana III (303); Ardha Matsyendrāsana I, II and III (311, 330 and 332); Pasāśāna (328) Paripoorṇa Matsyendrāsana (336); Bhujangāsana I and II (73 and 550); Mulabandhāsana (462); Kandāsana (470); Hanumānāsana (475); Yoganidrāsana (391); Ūrdhva Dhanurāsana (486 and 487); Dwipāda Viparīta Daṇḍāsana (516); Maṇḍalāsana (525 to 535); Kapotāsana (512); Rājakapotāsana (551); Vṛiśchikāsana I or II (537 or 538); Pādānguṣṭha Dhanurāsana (555); Śīrṣapādāsana (570); Gaṇḍa Bheruṇḍāsana (580 and 581); Viparīta Śalabhāsana (584); Tiriang Mukhottānāsana (586); Natarājāsana (590); Uḍḍīyāna (Section 201) and Nāḍī Śodhana Prāṇāyāma (Section 205).

Knees

All the standing positions (1 to 48); Jānu-Śīrṣāsana (127); Parivṛtta Jānu-Śīrṣāsana (132); Ardha Baddha Padma Paschimottānāsana (135); Triangmukhaikapāda Paschimottānāsana (139); Krounchāsana (141); Marīchyāsana I, II, III & IV (144, 146, 303 and 305); Ākarṇa Dhanurāsana (173 and 175); Padmāsana and cycle (104 to 124); Vīrāsana (89); Supta Vīrāsana (96); Paryankāsana (97); Gomukhāsana (80); Siddhāsana (84); Baddha Koṇāsana (101); Bharadwājāsana I & II (297 and 299); Ardha Matsyendrāsana I (311); Mālāsana I & II (321 and 322); Pāśāsana (328); Kūrmāsana and Supta Kūrmāsana (363, 364 and 368); Yoganidrāsana (391); Yogadaṇḍāsana (456); Bhekāsana (100); Supta Bhekāsana (458); Mulabandhāsana (462); Vāmadevāsana I & II

(465 and 466); Kandāsana (470); Hanumānāsana (475); Gheraṇḍāsana I & II (561 and 564).

Labour pain

Vīrāsana (89); Baddha Koṇāsana (101 and 103); Upaviṣṭa Koṇāsana (148) but with or without holding the toes; Ujjāyi Prāṇāyāma (Section 201) with inhalation retention and Nāḍī Śodhana Prāṇāyāma (Section 203) without retention; Śavāsana (592).

Legs

All the standing positions (1 to 58); Śalabhāsana (60); Dhanurāsana (63); Bhujangāsana I & II (73 and 550); Chaturanga Daṇḍāsana (67); Ūrdhva-mukha Śvānāsana (74); Adhomukha Śvānāsana (75); Paripoorṇa Nāvāsana (78); Ardha Nāvāsana (79); Paschimottānāsana (160); Ūrdhva Mukha Paschimottānāsana I & II (168 and 170); Ākarṇa Dhanurāsana (173 and 175); Upaviṣṭa Koṇāsana (151); Jaṭara Parivartanāsana (275); Supta Pādānguṣṭhāsana (285 to 287); Krounchāsana (141); Sālamba Sīrṣāsana I (184); Sālamba Sarvāngāsana (234); Halāsana (244); Pincha Mayūrāsana (357); Adhomukha Vṛkṣāsana (359); Anantāsana (290); Ekapada Śīrṣāsana and cycle (371 to 384); Vasiṣṭhāsana (398); Viśvāmitrāsana (403); Hanumānāsana (475); Samakoṇāsana (477); Supta Trivikramāsana (478).

Liver, Spleen, Pancreas and Intestines

Follow the āsanas given under *Arms* and *Kidneys*.

Lumbago

All the standing positions (4 to 48); Śalabhāsana (60); Dhanurāsana (63); Bhujangāsana I (73); Poorvottānāsana (171); Mālāsana I & II (321 and 322); Bharadwājāsana I & II (297 and 299); Marīchyāsana III (303); Ardha Matsyendrāsana I (311); Pāśāsana (328); Ūrdhva Mukha Paschimottānāsana II (170); Jaṭara Parivartanāsana (275); Parvatāsana (107); Śīrṣāsana and cycle (184 to 218); Sarvāngāsana and cycle (234 to 271); Ūrdhva Dhanurāsana (486 and 487); Viparīta Chakrāsana (488 to 499); Dwipāda Viparīta Daṇḍāsana (516); Maṇḍalāsana (525 to 535).

Lungs

Śīrṣāsana and cycle (184 to 218); Sarvāngāsana and cycle (234 to 271); Padmāsana and cycle (104 to 124); Vīrāsana (89); Supta Vīrāsana (96); Paryankāsana (97); all the standing positions (4 to 36); Urdhva Dhanurāsana (486); Dwipāda Viparīta Daṇḍāsana (516); all the types of Prāṇāyāma with inhalation retention.

Menstrual disorders

Śīrṣāsana and cycle (184 to 218); Sarvāngāsana and cycle (234 to 271); Paschimottānāsana (160); Uttanāsana (48); Adhomukha Śvānāsana (75); Baddha Padmāsana (118); Yogamudrāsana (120); Parvatāsana (107); Matsyāsana (113); Kūrmāsana and Supta Kūrmāsana (363, 364 and 368); Vīrāsana (89); Supta Vīrāsana (96); Paryankāsana (97); Baddha Koṇāsana (102); Upaviṣṭa Koṇāsana (151); Ūrdhva Mukha Paschimottānāsana I & II (168 and 170); Yoganidrāsana (391); Marīchyāsana III (303); Ardha Matsyendrāsana I (311); Pāśāsana (328); Ūrdhva Dhanurāsana (486); Dwipāda Viparīta Daṇḍāsana (516); Śavāsana (592); Nāḍī Śodhana Prāṇāyāma with inhalation retention and Uḍḍīyāna (Section 201).

Migraine

Sālamba Śīrṣāsana (184); if possible cycle of Śīrṣāsana; Sarvāngāsana (and whatever possible in the cycle) (234 to 271); Paschimottānāsana (160); Uttānāsana (48); Nāḍī Śodhana Prāṇāyāma without retention; Śītali Prāṇāyāma; Śanmukhi Mudra (106); Meditation in Vīrāsana (89) or Siddhāsana (84) or Baddha Koṇāsana (103) or Padmāsana (104); Śavāsana (592).

Nasal catarrh

Śīrṣāsana and cycle (184 to 218); Sarvāngāsana and cycle (234 to 271); Paschimottānāsana (160); Uttānāsana (48); Adhomukha Śvānāsana (75); Ujjāyī (Section 203), Bhastrikā (Section 206), Sūryabhedana (Section 204) and Nāḍī Śodhana Prāṇāyāma (Section 205).

Nervous debility

Śīrṣāsana and cycle (184 to 218); Sarvāngāsana and cycle (234 to 271); Uttānāsana (48); Paschimottānāsana (160); Nāḍī Śodhana Prāṇāyāma without retention; Śanmukhi Mudra (106); Meditation and Śavāsana (592).

Obesity

Follow the āsanas under *Acidity*, *Dyspepsia* and *Gastritis*.

Ovaries

Follow the āsanas under *Menstrual disorders*.

Palpitation

Sālamba Śīrṣāsana I (184); Sālamba Sarvāngāsana I (234); Halāsana (244); Paschimottānāsana (160); Uttānāsana (48); Adhomukha

Śvānāsana (75); Dwipada Viparīta Daṇḍāsana (516); Vīrāsana (89), Supta Vīrāsana (96); Ujjāyī (Section 203) and Nāḍī Sodhana Prāṇāyāma (Section 205) without retention in the beginning. After 2 or 3 months start with 5 seconds of inhalation retention and increase the time gradually. Śavāsana (592).

Polio

All the standing positions (1 to 36). Śalabhāsana (60); Dhanurāsana (63) and so on. But with Polio in my experience direct guidance is essential so do not work from the book. The āsanas have to be adjusted to the individual needs and state of the patient.

Paralysis

Here also, guidance from a competent teacher is a necessity. All the standing positions (1 to 36); Pādāṅguṣṭhāsana (44); Pāda Hastāsana (46); Uttānāsana (48); Śalabhāsana (60 and 61); Makarāsana (62); Dhanurāsana (63); Bhujangāsana I (73); Sālamba Śīrṣāsana I (184); Sālamba Sarvāngāsana I (234); Halāsana (244); Ekapāda Sarvāngāsana (250); Pārśvaikapāda Sarvāngāsana (251); Pārśva Halāsana (249); Supta Koṇāsana (247); Supta Pādāṅguṣṭhāsana (284, 285 and 287); Ūrdhva Prasārita Pādāsana (276 to 279); Śavāsana (592); Ujjāyi (Section 203) and Nāḍī Śodhana Prāṇāyāma (Section 205).

Piles

Śīrṣāsana and cycle (184 to 218); Sarvāngāsana and cycle (234 to 271); Jaṭara Parivartanāsana (275); Supta Pādāṅguṣṭhāsana (285 to 287); Matsyāsana (114); Simhāsana II (110); Śalabhāsana (60); Dhanurāsana (63); Ūrdhva Dhanurāsana (486); Dwipāda Viparīta Daṇḍāsana (516); Ujjāyi (Section 203) and Nāḍī Śodhana Prāṇāyāma (Section 205) with retention and Śavāsana (592).

Pleurisy and pneumonia

(After medical treatment and rest, the patient can conveniently take to yoga practices to gain strength and lead a normal life in a shorter time.)

Sālamba Śīrṣāsana I (184); Sālamba Sarvāngāsana I (234); Halāsana (244); Paschimottānāsana (160); Uttānāsana (48); Vīrāsana (89); Parvatāsana (107); Matsyāsana (114); Ujjāyi (Section 203) and Nāḍī Śodhana Prāṇāyāma (Section 205) without retention, meditation and Śavāsana (592).

Prostates

Śīrṣāsana and cycle (184 to 218); Sarvāngāsana and cycle (234 to 271); Jaṭara Parivartanāsana (275); Uttānāsana (48); Śalabhāsana (60);

Dhanurāsana (63); Adhomukha Śvānāsana (75); Paripoorna Nāvāsana (78); Ardha Nāvāsana (79); Jānu-Śīrṣāsana (127); Vīrāsana (89); Supta Vīrāsana (96); Baddha Koṇāsana (102); Padmāsana and cycle (104 to 124); Kūrmāsana and Supta Kūrmāsana (363, 364 and 368); Ekapāda Śīrṣāsana and cycle (371 to 384); Yoganidrāsana (391); Ardha Matsyendrāsana I & II (311 and 320); Pāśāsana (328); Paripoorna Matsyendrāsana (336); Mūlabandhāsana (462); Kandāsana (470); Hanumānāsana (475); Samakoṇāsana (477); Ūrdhva Dhanurāsana (486); Viparīta Chakrāsana (488 to 499); Dwipāda Viparīta Daṇḍāsana (516); Maṇḍalāsana (525 to 535); Uḍḍīyāna (Section 201), Nāḍī Śodhana (Section 205) and Ujjāyi Prāṇāyāma (Section 203) with retention.

Rheumatic pains

Follow the āsanas given under *Arthritis* and *Lumbago.*

Sciatica

All standing positions (1 to 36); Śīrṣāsana and do whatever is possible in the cycle (184 to 218); Sarvāngāsana and possible āsanas in the cycle (234 to 271); Jaṭara Parivartanāsana (275); Supta Pādānguṣṭhāsana (284 to 287); Anantāsana (290); Uttānapādāsana (292); Setubandhāsana (296); Paschimottānāsana (160); Śalabhāsana (60); Dhanurāsana (63); Bhujangāsana I (73); Ūrdhva Mukha Śvānāsana (74); Adhomukha Śvānāsana (75); Ūrdhva Mukha Paschimottānāsana I & II (168 and 170); Poorvottānāsana (171); Kūrmāsana (363 and 364); Mūlabandhāsana (462); Bharadwājāsana I & II (297 and 299); Marīchyāsana III (303); Ardha Matsyendrāsana I (311); Mālāsana I & II (321 and 322); Pāśāsana (328); Hanumānāsana (475); Supta Trivikramāsana (478); Uṣṭrāsana (41); Dwipāda Viparīta Daṇḍāsana (516). If possible, Paripoorṇa Matsyendrāsana (336).

Spermatorrhoea

Śīrṣāsana and cycle (184 to 218); Sarvāngāsana and cycle (234 to 271); Paschimottānāsana (160); Baddha Koṇāsana (103); Mūlabandhāsana (462); Kandāsana (470); Ujjāyi (Section 203) and Nāḍī Śodhana Prāṇāyāma (Section 205) without retention for 2 to 3 months, then do them with inhalation retention.

Sterility

Follow the āsanas under *Spermatorrhoea.*

Thrombosis of the legs

Sālamba Sarvāngāsana I, if possible (234); Halāsana (244); Vīrāsana

(89); Siddhāsana (84); Baddha Koṇāsana (102); and any sitting āsanas without strain. Ujjāyi (Section 203) and Nāḍī Śodhana Prāṇāyāma (Section 205) and Śavāsana (592).

Tonsillitis

Śīrṣāsana and whatever āsana is possible in the cycle (184 to 218); Sarvāṅgāsana and possible āsanas in the cycle (234 to 271); Vīrāsana (89); Paryankāsana (97); Padmāsana and cycle (104 to 124); standing positions (1 to 36); Uṣṭrāsana (41); Dhanurāsana (63); Ūrdhva Mukha Śvānāsana (74); Marīchyāsana III (303); Ardha Matsyendrāsana I (311); Pāśāsana (328); Paripoorṇa Matsyendrāsana (336); Paschimottānāsana (160); Yoganidrāsana (391); Ūrdhva Dhanurāsana (486); Dwipāda Viparīta Daṇḍāsana (516); Ujjāyi (Section 203) and Nāḍī Śodhana Prāṇāyāma (Section 205); Bhastrikā (Section 206) and Uḍḍīyāna (Section 201).

Tuberculosis

It is advisable to get the guidance of a competent teacher after medical treatment.

Tumour of the stomach

(Only if the disease is in the beginning stage.)
Sālamba Śīrṣāsana I and possible āsanas in the cycle (184 to 218); Sālamba Sarvāṅgāsana I and possible āsanas in the cycle (234 to 271); standing positions (1 to 36); Uttānāsana (48); Mahāmudra (125); Jānu-Śīrṣāsana (127); Supta Vīrāsana (96); Matsyāsana (114); Parvatāsana (107); Paschimottānāsana (160); Uḍḍīyāna (Section 201) and Ujjāyī (Section 203) or Nāḍī Śodhana Prāṇāyāma (Section 205).

Ulcer (Gastric)

Follow the āsanas under *Acidity*, *Dyspepsia* and *Flatulence*.

Ulcer (Duodenal)

Śīrṣāsana and cycle (184 to 218); Sarvāṅgāsana and cycle (234 to 271); Mahāmudra (125); Jānu-Śīrṣāsana (127); Paschimottānāsana (160); Kūrmāsana and Supta Kūrmāsana (363, 364 and 368); Yoganidrāsana (391); Marīchyāsana III (303); Ardha Matsyendrāsana I (311); Pāśāsana (328); Dwipāda Viparīta Daṇḍāsana (516); Uḍḍīyāna (Section 201), Ujjāyī (Section 203) and Nāḍī Śodhana Prāṇāyāma (Section 205) with inhalation retention.

Urine (Dribbling or excessive)

Śīrṣāsana and what you can in the cycle (184 to 218); Sarvāṅgāsana and what you can in the cycle (234 to 271); Supta Vīrāsana (96); Matsyāsana (114); Siṃhāsana II (110); Mahāmudra (125); Baddha Koṇāsana (101); Uḍḍīyāna (594); Nāḍī Śodhana Prāṇāyāma (Section 205) with Antara Kumbhaka and Bāhya Kumbhaka.

Varicose veins

Śīrṣāsana and cycle (184 to 218); Sarvāṅgāsana and cycle (234 to 271); Vīrāsana (89); Supta Vīrāsana (96); Paryankāsana (97); Bhekāsana (100).

A Table to Correlate the Āsanas with the Plates that Illustrate them

Names of Āsanas, etc.	Intermediate Āsana Plate No.	Final Āsana Plate No.
1. Tāḍāsana	—	1
2. Vṛkṣāsana	—	2
3. Utthita Trikoṇāsana	3	4 and 5
4. Parivṛtta Trikoṇāsana	—	6 and 7
5. Utthita Pārśvakoṇāsana	—	8 and 9
6. Parivṛtta Pārśvakoṇāsana	—	10 and 11
7. Vīrabhadrāsana I	12 and 13	14
8. Vīrabhadrāsana II	—	15
9. Vīrabhadrāsana III	16	17
10. Ardha Chandrāsana	18	19
11. Utthita Hasta Pādānguṣṭhāsana	20 to 22	23
12. Pārśvōttānāsana	24 and 25	26, 27 and 28
13. Prasārita Pādottānāsana I	29 to 32	33 and 34
14. Prasārita Pādottānāsana II	—	35 and 36
15. Parighāsana	37 and 38	39
16. Uṣṭrāsana	40	41
17. Utkaṭāsana	—	42
18. Pādānguṣṭhāsana 44	43	44
19. Pāda Hastāsana	45	46
20. Uttānāsana	47	48
21. Ūrdhva Prasārita Ekapādāsana	—	49
22. Ardha Baddha Padmottānāsana	50 and 51	52, 53, 54 and 55
23. Garuḍāsana	—	56
24. Vātāyanāsana	57	58 and 59
25. Śalabhāsana	61	60
26. Makarāsana	—	62
27. Dhanurāsana	—	63
28. Pārśva Dhanurāsana	—	64 and 65
29. Chaturanga Daṇḍāsana	66	67
30. Nakrāsana	—	68 to 71
31. Bhujangāsana I	72	73
32. Ūrdhva Mukha Śvānāsana	—	74
33. Adho Mukha Śvānāsana	—	75 and 76
34. Daṇḍāsana	—	77
35. Paripūrṇa Nāvāsana	—	78

Names of Āsanas, etc.	Intermediate Āsana Plate No.	Final Āsana Plate No.
36. Ardha Nāvāsana	—	79
37. Gomukhāsana	—	80 and 81
38. Lolāsana	82	83
39. Siddhāsana	—	84
40. Vīrāsana	85 to 92	89
41. Supta Vīrāsana	93 to 95	96
42. Paryankāsana	—	97
43. Bhekāsana	98 and 99	100
44. Baddha Koṇāsana	101	102 and 103
45. Padmāsana	—	104 and 105
46. Ṣanmukhī Mudrā	—	106
47. Parvatāsana	—	107
48. Tolāsana	—	108
49. Siṃhāsana I	—	109
50. Siṃhāsana II	—	110 and 111
51. Matsyāsana	112 and 114	113
52. Kukkuṭāsana	—	115
53. Garbha Piṇḍāsana	—	116
54. Gorakṣāsana	—	117
55. Baddha Padmāsana	—	118 and 119
56. Yoga Mudrāsana	—	120, 121 and 122
57. Supta Vajrāsana	123	124
58. Mahā Mudrā	—	125
59. Jānu Śīrṣāsana	126	127, 128 and 129
60. Parivṛtta Jānu Śīrṣāsana	130 and 131	132
61. Ardha Baddha Padma Paschimottānāsana	133, 134 and 136	135 and 137
62. Triang Mukhaikapāda Paschimottānāsana	138	139
63. Krounchāsana	140	141 and 142
64. Marīchyāsana I	143	144
65. Marīchyāsana II	145	146 and 147
66. Upaviṣṭha Koṇāsana	148 to 150	151 and 152
67. Paschimottānāsana (or Ugrāsana or Brahmacharyāsana)	153 to 160	161 and 162
68. Parivṛtta Paschimottānāsana	163 and 164	165 and 166
69. Ubhaya Pādānguṣṭhāsana	—	167
70. Ūrdhva Mukha Paschimottānāsana I	—	168
71. Ūrdhva Mukha Paschimottānāsana II	169	170
72. Pūrvottānāsana	—	171
73. Ākarṇa Dhanurāsana	172 and 174	173 and 175
74. Sālamba Śīrṣāsana I	176 to 183 and 186 to 189, 191	184, 185 and 190

Names of Āsanas, etc.	*Intermediate Āsana Plate No.*	*Final Āsana Plate No.*
75. Ūrdhva Daṇḍāsana	—	188
76. Sālamba Śīrṣāsana II	—	192
77. Sālamba Śīrṣāsana III	193, 196 and 197	194 and 195
78. Baddha Hasta Śīrṣāsana	—	198
79. Mukta Hasta Śīrṣāsana	199	200 and 201
80. Pārśva Śīrṣāsana	—	202 and 203
81. Parivṛttaikapāda Śīrṣāsana	204	205, 206 and 207
82. Eka Pāda Śīrṣāsana	—	208 and 209
83. Pārśvaika Pāda Śīrṣāsana	—	210
84. Ūrdhva Padmāsana in Śīrṣāsana	—	211 and 212
85. Pārśva Ūrdhva Padmāsana in Śīrṣāsana	—	213 to 216
86. Piṇḍāsana in Śīrṣāsana	217	218
87. Sālamba Sarvāngāsana I	219 to 222 and 226 to 235	223 and 224, 225 and 234
88. Sālamba Sarvāngāsana II	—	235
89. Nirālamba Sarvāngāsana I	—	236
90. Nirālamba Sarvāngāsana II	—	237
91. Halāsana	238 to 243	244
92. Karṇapīḍāsana	245	246
93. Supta Koṇāsana	—	247 and 248
94. Pārśva Halāsana	—	249
95. Eka Pāda Sarvāngāsana	—	250
96. Pārśvaika Pāda Sarvāngāsana	—	251
97. Pārśva Sarvāngāsana	252 and 253	254 and 255
98. Setu Bandha Sarvāngāsana (or Uttana Mayūrāsana)	256 to 258	259
99. Eka Pāda Setu Bandha Sarvāngāsana (or Eka Pāda Uttāna Mayūrāsana)	—	260
100. Ūrdhva Padmāsana in Sarvāngāsana	—	261
101. Pārśva Ūrdhva Padmāsana in Sarvāngāsana	—	262 to 265
102. Uttāna Padma Mayūrāsana	266	267
103. Piṇḍāsana in Sarvāngāsana	268	269
104. Pārśva Piṇḍāsana in Sarvāngāsana	—	270 and 271
105. Jaṭhara Parivartanāsana	272 and 273	274 and 275
106. Ūrdhva Prasārita Pādāsana	—	276 to 279
107. Chakrāsana	—	280 to 283
108. Supta Pādānguṣṭhāsana	284	285 to 287
109. Anantāsana	288 and 289	290
110. Uttāna Pādāsana	291	292
111. Setu Bandhāsana	293 to 295	296

Names of Āsanas, etc.	*Intermediate Āsana Plate No.*	*Final Āsana Plate No.*
112. Bharadvājāsana I	—	297 and 298
113. Bharadvājāsana II	—	299 and 300
114. Marīchyāsana III	301 and 302	303 and 304
115. Marīchyāsana IV	—	305 and 306
116. Ardha Matsyendrāsana I	307 to 310 and 313 to 316	311 and 312
117. Mālāsana I	317 to 320	321
118. Mālāsana II	—	322
119. Pāśāsana	323 to 327	328 and 329
120. Ardha Matsyendrāsana II	—	330 and 331
121. Ardha Matsyendrāsana III	—	332 and 333
122. Paripūrṇa Matsyendrāsana	334 and 335, 337 and 338	336 and 339
123. Aṣṭāvakrāsana	340 and 341	342 and 343
124. Eka Hasta Bhujāsana	—	344
125. Dwi Hasta Bhujāsana	—	345
126. Bhujapidāsana	346 and 347, 349 and 350	348
127. Mayūrāsana	351 to 353	354
128. Padma Mayūrāsana	—	355
129. Haṃsāsana	—	356
130. Pīncha Mayūrāsana	—	357
131. Śayanāsana	—	358
132. Adho Mukha Vṛkṣāsana	—	359
133. Kūrmāsana	360 to 362	363 and 364
134. Supta Kūrmāsana	365 to 367	368
135. Eka Pāda Śīrṣāsana	369 and 370	371
136. Skandāsana	—	372
137. Buddhāsana	—	373
138. Kapilāsana	—	374
139. Bhairavāsana	—	375
140. Kāla Bhairavāsana	376 and 377	378
141. Chakorāsana	—	379 and 380
142. Dūrvāsāsana	381 and 382	383
143. Ruchikāsana	—	384 and 385
144. Viranchyāsana I	—	386 and 387
145. Viranchyāsana II	—	388
146. Yoganidrāsana	389 and 390	391
147. Dwi Pāda Śīrṣāsana	392	393 and 394
148. Tittibhāsana	—	395
149. Vasiṣṭhāsana	396 and 397	398
150. Kaśyapāsana	—	399 and 400
151. Viśvāmitrāsana	401 and 402	403
152. Bakāsana	404 and 405, 407 to 409	406 and 410
153. Pārśva Bakāsana	411	412

Names of Āsanas, etc.	*Intermediate Āsana Plate No.*	*Final Āsana Plate No.*
154. Ūrdhva Kukkuṭāsana	413 to 416	417 to 419
155. Pārśva Kukkuṭāsana	420 to 423	424 and 424a, 425 and 425a
156. Gālavāsana	426	427 and 428
157. Eka Pāda Gālavāsana	429, 430 and 432	431 and 433
158. Dwi Pāda Kouṇḍinyāsana	434 to 437	438
159. Eka Pāda Kouṇḍinyāsana I	439 and 440	441
160. Eka Pāda Kouṇḍinyāsana II	444	442 and 443
161. Eka Pāda Bakāsana I	445	446 and 447
162. Eka Pāda Bakāsana II	448 to 450	451 and 452
163. Yogadaṇḍāsana	453 to 455	456
164. Supta Bhekāsana	457	458
165. Mūlabhandāsana	459 to 461	462 and 463
166. Vāmadevāsana I	464	465
167. Vāmadevāsana II	—	466
168. Kandāsana	467 to 469	470 to 471b
169. Hanumānāsana	472 to 474	475 to 476a
170. Samakoṇāsana	—	477
171. Supta Trivikramāsana	—	478
172. Ūrdhva Dhanurāsana I	479 to 481	482
172a. Ūrdhva Dhanurāsana II	483 to 485	486 and 487
173. Viparīta Chakrāsana in Ū. Dh.	—	488 to 499
174. Eka Pāda Ūrdhva Dhanurāsana	500	501 and 502
175. Kapotāsana	503 to 506, 508 to 511	507 and 512
176. Laghuvajrāsana	—	513
177. Dwi Pāda Viparīta Daṇḍāsana	514 and 515, 517 to 520	516
178. Eka Pāda Viparīta Daṇḍāsana I	—	521
179. Eka Pāda Viparīta Daṇḍāsana II	522	523
180. Chakra Bandhāsana	—	524
181. Maṇḍalāsana	—	525 to 535
182. Vṛśchikāsana I	—	536 and 537
183. Vṛśchikāsana II	—	538
184. Eka Pāda Rājakapotāsana I	539 to 541	542
185. Vālakhilyāsana	543	544
186. Eka Pāda Rājakapotāsana II	—	545
187. Eka Pāda Rājakapotāsana III	—	546
188. Eka Pāda Rājakapotāsana IV	—	547
189. Bhujaṅgāsana II	548 and 549	550
190. Rājakapotāsana	552	551
191. Pādāṅguṣṭha Dhanurāsana	553 and 554, 556 and 557	555
192. Gheraṇḍāsana I	558 to 560	561 to 563

Names of Āsanas, etc.	*Intermediate Āsana Plate No.*	*Final Āsana*
193. Gheraṇḍāsana II	—	564 to 566
194. Kapiñjalāsana	—	567
195. Śīrṣa Pādāsana	568 and 569	570
196. Gaṇḍa Bheruṇḍāsana	571 to 579, 582 and 583	580 and 581
197. Viparīta Śalabhāsana	—	584
198. Tiriang Mukhottānāsana	585	586
199. Naṭarājāsana	587 to 589	590, 591 and 591a
200. Śavāsana (or Mṛtāsana)	—	592
201. Uḍḍtyāna Bandha	—	593 and 594
202. Nauli	—	595 and 596
Prāṇāyāma		
203. Ujjāyi	—	597
204. Sūrya Bhedana	598	599
— Bāhya Kumbhaka	—	600
205. Nāḍī Śodhana	—	—
206. Bhastrikā	—	—
207. Kapālabhāti	—	—
208. Bhamarī	—	—
209. Śitalī	—	601
210. Śitakārī	—	—
211. Sama Vṛtti	—	—
212. Viṣama Vṛtti	—	—
213. Viloma	—	—
214. Anuloma	—	—
215. Pratiloma	—	—
216. Sahita and Kevala	—	—
— Dhyāna	—	602

Glossary

A	Negative particle meaning 'non', as in non-violence.
Abhaya	Freedom from fear.
Abhiniveśa	Instinctive clinging to life and the fear that one may be cut off from all by death.
Abhyāsa	Constant and determined study or practice.
Adhaḥ	Down, lower.
Ādhāra	A support.
Adhimātra	Beyond measure, superior.
Adhimātratama	The supreme one, the highest.
Adho-mukha	Face downwards.
Ādīśvara	The primeval Lord; an epithet of Śiva.
Aditi	The mother of the gods, known as Ādityas.
Āditya	Son of Aditi or gods.
Advaita	Non-duality of the Universal Spirit with the individual soul.
Āgama	Testimony or proof of an acceptable authority when the source of knowledge has been checked and found trustworthy.
Ahaṁkāra	Ego or egotism; literally 'the I-Maker', the state that ascertains 'I know'.
Ahiṁsā	Non-violence. The word has not merely the negative and restrictive meaning of 'non-killing or non-violence', but the positive and comprehensive meaning of 'love embracing all creation'.
Ajapa-mantra	Unconscious repetitive prayer. Every living creature unconsciously breathes the prayer 'So'ham' (Saḥ = He (the Universal Spirit), aham = am I) with each inward breath, and with each outgoing breath prays 'Haṁsaḥ' (Aham = I am, Saḥ = He (the Universal Spirit)).
Ājñā-chakra	The nervous plexus situated between the eyebrows, the seat of command.
Ākarṇa	Near to the ear, towards the ear.
Akrodha	Freedom from anger.

Alabhdha-bhūmikatva	Failure to attain firm ground or continuity in practice, feeling that it is not possible to see reality.
Ālamba	Support.
Ālasya	Idleness, sloth, apathy.
Amanaska	The mind which is free from thoughts and desires.
Amṛta	Nectar of immortality.
Anāhata-chakra	The nervous plexus situated in the cardiac region.
Ananta	Infinite; a name of Viṣṇu as also of Viṣṇu's couch, the serpent Śeṣa.
Ananta-padmanābha	A name of Viṣṇu.
Anavasthitattva	Instability to continue the practices feeling that it is not necessary to continue as he thinks that he has reached the highest state of Samādhi.
Aṅga	The body; a limb or a part of the body; a constituent part.
Aṅgamejayatva	Unsteadiness or tremor of the body.
Aṅgula	A finger; the thumb.
Aṅguṣṭha	The big toe.
Añjanā	Name of the mother of Hanumān, a powerful monkey chief.
Antara	Within; interior.
Antara Kumbhaka	Suspension of breath after full inhalation.
Antaranga Sādhanā	The inward quest of the soul by Prāṇāyāma and Pratyāhāra whereby the mind is brought under control and the senses are emancipated from the thraldom of objects of desire.
Antarātmā	The Supreme Soul residing in the heart of man.
Antarātmā Sādhanā	The innermost quest of the soul by means of Dhāraṇā (concentration), Dhyāna (meditation) and Samādhi.
Anuloma	With the hair, with the grain, regular. In a natural order.
Anumāna	An inference.
Apāna	One of the vital airs which move in the sphere of the lower abdomen and control the function of elimination of urine and faeces.
Aparigraha	Freedom from hoarding or collecting.
Apuṇya	Vice or demerit.
Ardha	Half.
Arjuna	A Pāṇḍava prince, the mighty bowman and hero of the epic Mahābhārata.
Āsana	Posture. The third stage of yoga.

Asmitā	Egotism.
Aṣṭa	Eight.
Aṣṭāṅga Yoga	The eight limbs of Yoga described by Patañjāli.
Aṣṭāvakra	One whose body was crooked in eight places. Name of a sage, who, though born physically deformed, became the spiritual preceptor of King Janaka of Mithilā.
Asteya	Non-stealing.
Aśva	A horse.
Aśvinī-mudrā	The contraction of the anal sphincter muscles. It is so called because it brings to the mind the image of a horse excreting.
Ātmā or *Ātman*	The Supreme Soul or Brahman.
Ātma Ṣaṭkam	A group of six verses written by Śankarāchārya describing the soul in the state of Samadhi.
Ātmīyatā	The feeling of oneness, as a mother's feeling for her children.
Auṁ	Like the Latin word 'Omne', the Sanskrit word 'Auṁ' means 'all' and conveys concepts of 'Omniscience', 'Omnipresence' and 'Omnipotence'.
Avasthā	State or condition of the mind.
Avatāra	Descent, advent or incarnation of God. There are ten avatāras of Viṣṇu: Matsya (the Fish); Kūrma (the Tortoise); Varāha (the Boar); Narasiṁha (the Man-lion); Vāmana (the Dwarf); Paraśurāma; Rāma (hero of the epic Rāmāyaṇa); Krishna (hero of the epic Mahābhārata who related the Bhagavad Gītā); Balarāma and Kalki.
Avidyā	Ignorance.
Avirati	Sensuality.
Āyāma	Length, expansion, extension. It also conveys the idea of restraint, control and stopping.
Baddha	Bound, caught, restrained, firm.
Bahiraṅga Sādhanā	The outward quest of the soul for its Maker. The first three stages of Yoga, namely, Yama, Niyama and Āsana, are the outward quest and keep the seeker in harmony with his fellow men and nature.
Bāhya Kumbhaka	Suspension of breath after full exhalation when the lungs are completely empty.
Baka	A crane, a wading bird.
Bali	Name of a demon king.
Bandha	Bondage or fetter. It means a posture where certain

	organs or parts of the body are contracted and controlled.
Bhagavad Gītā	The Song Divine, the sacred dialogues between Krishna and Arjuna. It is one of the source books of Hindu philosophy, containing the essence of the Upanishads.
Bhagavān	Lord; venerable, holy.
Bhairava	Terrible, formidable; one of the forms of Śiva.
Bhakti	Worship, adoration.
Bhakti-mārga	The way or path to realisation through adoration of a personal god.
Bharadvāja	A sage.
Bhastrikā	A bellows used in a furnace. Bhastrikā is a type of prāṇāyāma where air is forcibly drawn in and out as in a blacksmith's bellows.
Bhaya	Fear.
Bhedana	Piercing, breaking through, passing through.
Bheka	A frog.
Bheruṇḍa	Terrible, frightful. It also means a species of bird.
Bhoga	Enjoyment; an object of pleasure.
Bhoktṛ	One who enjoys or experiences.
Bhramara	A large black bee.
Bhramarī	A type of prāṇāyāma where during exhalation a soft humming sound like the murmuring of a bee is made.
Bhrānti-darśana	Erroneous (bhrānti) vision or knowledge (darśana), delusion.
Bhu	Land.
Bhūdāna	The donation of land.
Bhuja	The arm or the shoulder.
Bhuja-pīdā	Pressure on the arm or shoulder.
Bhujaṅga	A serpent, a snake.
Bhūmikatva	Firm ground.
Bīja	Seed or germ.
Bīja-mantra	A mystical syllable with a sacred prayer repeated mentally during prāṇāyāma, and the seed thus planted in the mind germinates into one-pointedness.
Brahmā	The Supreme Being, the Creator. The first deity of the Hindu Trinity entrusted with the work of creation of the world.
Brahma-randhra	An aperture in the crown of the head through which the soul is said to leave the body on death.
Brahma-vidyā	The knowledge of the Supreme Spirit.
Brahmachāri	A religious student vowed to celibacy and abstinence.

	One who is constantly moving (chārin) in Brahman (the Supreme Spirit); one who sees divinity in all.
Brahmacharya	A life of celibacy, religious study and self-restraint.
Brahman	The Supreme Being, the cause of the universe, the all-pervading spirit of the universe.
Brahmāṇḍa-prāṇa	The cosmic breath.
Brahmarṣī	A Brahmin sage.
Buddhi	Intellect, reason, discrimination, judgement.
Chakra	Literally, a wheel or circle. Energy (prāṇa) is said to flow in the human body through three main channels (nāḍīs), namely, Suṣumṇā, Piṅgalā and Idā. Suṣumṇa is situated inside the spinal column. Piṅgalā and Idā start respectively from the right and left nostrils, move up to the crown of the head and course downwards to the base of the spine. These two nāḍīs intersect with each other and also the Suṣumṇā. These junctions of the nāḍīs are known as chakras or the fly-wheels which regulate the body mechanism. The important chakras are: (a) Mūlādhāra (mūla = root, source; ādhāra = support, vital part) situated in the pelvis above the anus; (b) Svādhiṣṭhāna (sva = vital force, soul; adhiṣṭhāna = seat or abode) situated above the organs of generation; (c) Maṇipūraka (maṇipūra = navel) situated in the navel; (d) Manas (mind) and (e) Sūrya (the Sun), which are situated in the region between the navel and the heart; (f) Anāhata (= unbeaten) situated in the cardiac area; (g) Viśuddha (= pure) situated in the pharyngeal region; (h) Ājñā (= command) situated between the eyebrows; (i) Sahasrāra (= thousand), which is called the thousand-petalled lotus in the cerebral cavity; and (j) Lalāta (= forehead) which is at the top of the forehead.
Chakra-bandha	The binding or sealing posture where all the chakras are exercised.
Chandra	The moon.
Chatur	The number four.
Chidambaram	A place of pilgrimage in South India. (Chit = consciousness, ambara = atmosphere or dress.) A name of God, who covers all with His consciousness.
Chitta	The mind in its total or collective sense, being composed of three categories: (a) Mind, having the faculty

	of attention, selection and rejection; (b) Reason, the decisive state which determines the distinction between things and (c) Ego, the I-maker.
Chitta-vikṣepa	Distraction, confusion, perplexity.
Chitta-vṛtti	Fluctuations of the mind. A course of behaviour, mode of being, condition or mental state.
Dadhīcha	A celebrated sage, who donated his bones to the gods. From these bones was fashioned the thunderbolt, with which Indra, the king of the gods, slew the demon Vṛtra.
Daitya	A son of Diti. A demon.
Dakṣa	A celebrated prajāpati, a lord of created beings.
Dakṣiṇa	The right side.
Damanī	A layer within a nāḍī or channel for the passage of energy.
Dānava	A demon.
Daṇḍa	A staff.
Daṇḍakā	The forest region in the Deccan between the rivers Narmāda and Godāvarī.
Daurmanasya	Despair, dejection.
Deva	A god.
Devadatta	One of the vital airs which provides for the intake of extra oxygen in a tired body by causing a yawn.
Dhanu	A bow.
Dhāraṇā	Concentration or complete attention. The sixth stage of Yoga mentioned by Patañjali.
Dhasañjaya	One of the vital airs which remains in the body even after death, and sometimes bloats up a corpse.
Dhenu	A cow.
Dhṛ	To hold, to support, to maintain.
Dhyāna	Meditation. The seventh stage of Yoga mentioned by Patañjali.
Diti	The mother of the demons called Daityas.
Droṇa	The preceptor of the Pāṇḍava and Kaurava princes in the arts of war, especially archery. He was the son of the sage Bharadvāja.
Duḥkha	Pain, sorrow, grief.
Durvāsā	A very irascible sage.
Dveṣa	Hate, dislike, repugnance.
Dwi	Two, both.
Dwi-hasta	Two hands.
Dwi-pāda	Two feet or legs.

Eka	One, single, alone, only.
Eka-pāda	One leg.
Eka-tattvābhyāsa	The study of the single element, the Supreme Spirit that pervades the innermost self of all beings.
Ekāgra	(Eka = one; agra = foremost.) Fixed on one object or point only; closely attentive, where the mental faculties are all focussed on a single object.
Ekāgratā	One-pointedness.
Gālava	A sage.
Gaṇa	A troop of demigods, who were Śiva's attendants.
Gaṇḍa	The cheek, the whole side of the face including the temple.
Gaṇḍa-bheruṇḍa	A species of bird.
Gaṅgā	The river Ganges, the most sacred river in India.
Garbha-piṇḍa	Embryo in the womb.
Garuḍa	An eagle. Name of the king of birds. Garuḍa is represented as a vehicle of Viṣṇu and as having a white face, an aquiline beak, red wings and a golden body.
Gheraṇḍa	A sage, the author of Gheraṇḍa-Saṁhitā, a classical work on Haṭha-yoga.
Gheraṇḍa-Saṁhitā	*See* above.
Go	A cow.
Gomukha	Face resembling a cow. It is also a kind of musical instrument, narrow at one end and broad at the other like the face of a cow.
Gorakṣa	A cowherd. Name of a famous Yogi.
Gotra	A family, race, lineage.
Gu	First syllable in the word 'Guru', meaning darkness.
Gulma	The spleen.
Guṇa	A quality, an ingredient or constituent of nature.
Guṇātīta	One who is freed from and gone beyond or crossed the three guṇas of Sattva, Rajas and Tamas.
Guru	Spiritual preceptor, one who illumines the darkness of spiritual doubt.
Ha	First syllable of the word 'Haṭha', which is composed of the syllables 'ha' meaning the sun, and 'ṭha' meaning the moon. The object of Haṭha-yoga is to balance the flow of solar and lunar energy in the human system.

Hala	A plough.
Haṁsa	A swan.
'Haṁsaḥ'	'I am He, the Universal Spirit', the unconscious repetitive prayer that goes on with each exhalation within every living creature throughout life.
Hanumān	A powerful monkey chief of extraordinary strength and prowess, whose exploits are celebrated in the epic Rāmāyaṇa. He was the son of Añjana and Vāyu, the god of wind.
Hasta	The hand.
Haṭha	Force. The word 'haṭha' is used adverbially in the sense of 'forcibly' or 'against one's will'. Haṭha-yoga is so called because it prescribes rigorous discipline, in order to find union with the Supreme.
Haṭha-vidyā	The science of Haṭha-yoga.
Haṭha-yoga	The way towards realisation through rigorous discipline.
Haṭhā-yoga-pradīpikā	A celebrated textbook on Haṭha-yoga written by Svātmārāma.
Himālaya	The abode of ice and snow. Name of the mountain ranges on the northern borders of India.
Hiṁsā	Violence, killing.
Hiraṇya-kaśipu	A celebrated demon king, slain by Viṣṇu to save Prahlāda, his devotee.
Iḍā	A nāḍī, a channel of energy starting from the left nostril, then moving to the crown of the head and thence descending to the base of the spine. In its course it conveys lunar energy and so is called chandra nāḍī (channel of the lunar energy).
Indra	Chief of the gods. The god of thunder, lightning and rain.
Indriya	An organ of sense.
Indriya-jaya	Conquest, restraint or mastery of the senses by controlling desires.
Īśvara	The Supreme Being, God.
Īśvara-praṇidhāna	Dedication to the Lord of one's actions and one's will.
Jāgrata-avasthā	The complete awareness of the state of the mind.
Jālandhara-bandha	Jālandhara is a posture where the neck and throat are contracted and the chin is rested in the notch between the collar-bones at the top of the breast-bone.

Jamunā	A tributary of the Ganges.
Janaka	A famous philosopher king of Videha or Mithilā.
Jānu	The knee.
Japa	A repetitive prayer.
Jaṭhara	The abdomen, stomach.
Jaṭhara-parivartana	An āsana, in which the abdomen is made to move to and fro.
Jaya	Conquest, victory. It also means control, mastery.
Jīva	A living being, a creature.
Jīvana	Life.
Jīvana-mukta	A person who is emancipated during his lifetime by true knowledge of the Supreme Spirit.
Jīvana-mukti	The emancipated state.
Jīvātmā	The individual or personal soul.
Jñāna	Sacred knowledge derived from meditation on the higher truths of religion and philosophy, which teaches a man how to understand his own nature.
Jñāna-mārga	The path of knowledge by which man finds realisation.
Jñāna-mudrā	The gesture of the hand where the tip of the index finger is brought in contact with the tip of the thumb, while the remaining three fingers are kept extended. The gesture is a symbol of knowledge (jñāna). The index finger is the symbol of the individual soul, the thumb signifies the Supreme Universal Soul, and the union of these two symbolises true knowledge.
Jñānendriya	Hearing, touch, sight, taste and smell.
Kagola or *Kahola*	The father of the sage Aṣṭāvakra.
Kailāsa	A mountain peak in the Himālayas, considered as the abode of Śiva.
Kaivalya	Final emancipation.
Kaivalya-pāda	The fourth and last part of Patañjāli's Yoga Sūtra, dealing with Absolution.
Kāla-Bhairava	A name of Śiva.
Kālidāsa	The most renowned dramatist and poet in Sanskrit literature, whose work 'Śakuṅtalā' is universally respected.
Kāma	Desire, lust. Name of the god of Passion.
Kāma-dhenu	The heavenly cow yielding all desires.
Kāma-rūpa	The seat of the genitals, so named after Kāma, the god of passion.
Kaṅda	A bulbous root, a knot. The kaṅda is of a round shape of about four inches situated twelve inches above the

	anus and near the navel, where the three main nāḍīs – Suṣumṇā, Iḍā and Piṅgalā – unite and separate. It is covered as if with a soft white piece of cloth.
Kanyākubja	An ancient city and country situated on a tributary of the Ganges, now called Kanoja.
Kapālabhāti	Kapāla = skull; bhāti = light, lustre. A process of clearing the sinuses.
Kapila	A sage, the founder of the Sānkhya system, one of the six orthodox systems of Hindu philosophy.
Kapiñjala	The chātaka bird, which is supposed to drink only raindrops.
Kapota	A dove, pigeon.
Karma	Action.
Karma-mārga	The way of an active man towards realisation through action.
Karma-yoga	The achievement of union with the Supreme Universal Soul through action.
Karmendriya	Organs of excretion, generation, hands, feet and speech.
Karṇa	The ear, also one of the heroes in the Mahābhārata.
Karṇa-pīḍā	Pressure around the ear.
Kārtikeya	The god of war, also known as Kumāra, Ṣaṇmukha and Skanda. He is a son of Śiva and is so called because he was reared by the Kṛttikās, the Pleiades, each six of whom fed him at her breast (Ṣaṇ = six; mukha = mouth or face). The story of his birth is told by Kalidasa in his epic 'Kumāra-saṁbhava'.
Karuṇā	Compassion, pity, tenderness. It also implies devoted action to alleviate the suffering of the afflicted ones.
Kaśyapa	A sage, husband of Aditi and Diti. He is one of the lords or progenitors of living beings.
Kaṭhopaniṣad	One of the principal Upanishads in verse and in the form of a dialogue between the seeker Nachiketā and Yama, the god of Death.
Kauṇḍinya	A sage.
Kauravas	Descendants of Kuru, who fought the fratricidal Mahābhārata war with their cousins the Pāṇḍavas.
Kāyā	The body.
Kāyika	Relating to the body.
Kevala	Whole, entire, absolute, perfect, pure.
Kevala Kumbhaka	When the practices of Kumbhaka (respiratory processes) become so perfect that they are instinctive, they are known as Kevala Kumbhaka.

Kleśa	Pain, anguish, suffering.
Koṇa	An angle.
Krauncha	A bird like a heron, the name of a mountain.
Krishṇa	The most celebrated hero in Hindu mythology. The eighth incarnation of Viṣṇu.
Kriyā	An expiatory rite, a cleaning process.
Kṛkara	Name of one of the subsidiary vital airs, whose function is to prevent substances going up the nasal passages and throat by bringing on sneezes and coughing.
Kṛta	Name of first of the four ages of the world of men.
Kṣatriya	A member of the warrior class.
Kṣipta	Distracted, neglected.
Kukkuṭa	A cock.
Kumāra-saṁbhava	*See* Kārtikeya.
Kumbha	A water pot, a pitcher, a chalice.
Kumbhaka	Kumbhaka is the interval of time or retention of breath after full inhalation or after full exhalation.
Kuṇḍalinī	The Kuṇḍalinī (kuṇḍala = the coil of a rope; Kuṇḍalinī = a coiled female serpent) is the divine cosmic energy. This force or energy is symbolised as a coiled and sleeping serpent lying dormant in the lowest nerve centre at the base of the spinal column, the Mūlādhāra-chakra. This latent energy has to be aroused and made to ascend the main spinal channel, the Suṣumṇa piercing the chakras right up to the Sahasrāra, the thousand-petalled lotus in the head. Then the Yogi is in union with the Supreme Universal Soul.
Kūrma	A tortoise. It is also the name of one of the subsidiary vital airs whose function is to control the movements of the eyelids to prevent foreign matter or too bright a light going into the eyes.
Lac	100,000.
Laghu	Little, small. It also means handsome.
Lakṣmana	A brother of Rāma, hero of the epic Rāmāyaṇa.
Lakṣmī	The goddess of beauty and fortune, consort of Viṣṇu.
Lalāṭa	The forehead. It is also the name of a chakra.
Lankā	The kingdom of the demon king Rāvaṇa. It is identified with Ceylon.

Lauliki	The same as nauli, q.v.
Laya	Dissolution; absorption of the mind, devotion.
Laya-yoga	The achievement of union with the Supreme Universal Soul through adoration or devotion.
Lobha	Greed.
Lola	Tremulous, dangling, moving to and fro like a swing or a pendulum.
Loma	Hair.
Madhyama	Middling, average, mediocre.
Mahā	Great, mighty, powerful, lofty, noble.
Mahābhārata	The celebrated epic composed by Vyāsa. It includes the Bhagavad Gītā.
Maharṣi	A great sage.
Maitri	Friendliness coupled with a feeling of oneness.
Makara	A crocodile.
Mālā	A garland, wreath.
Man	To think.
Manas	The individual mind having the power and faculty of attention, selection and rejection. The ruler of the senses.
Manas-chakra	Nervous plexus situated between the navel and the heart.
Mānasika	Of the mind, mental.
Maṇḍala	A circle. It also means a collection, a division of the Ṛgveda.
Mandara	A mountain used by the gods and demons as a churning stick when they churned the cosmic ocean for nectar.
Maṇḍūka	A frog.
Maṇipūraka-chakra	The nervous plexus situated in the region of the navel.
Manomanī	The state of samādhi.
Mantra	A sacred thought or a prayer.
Manu	Name of the father of the human race.
Mārga	A way, road, path.
Marīchi	Name of one of the sons of Brahmā. He was a sage and the father of Kaśyapa, q.v.
Matsya	A fish.
Matsyendra	One of the founders of Haṭha-yoga.
Mayūra	A peacock.
Menakā	A nymph, the mother of Śakuntalā.
Meru-daṇḍa	The spinal column.

Mithilā	The capital of the kingdom of Videha, ruled by King Janaka.
Moha	Delusion, infatuation.
Mokṣa	Liberation, final emancipation of the soul from recurring births.
Mṛdu	Soft, gentle, mild.
Mṛta	Dead, a corpse.
Mūdha	Perplexed, confounded, foolish, dull, stupid.
Muditā	Joy, delight.
Mudrā	A seal: a sealing posture.
Mukha	Face, mouth.
Mukta	Liberated.
Mukti	Release, liberation, final absolution of the soul from the chain of birth and death.
Mūla	The root, base.
Mūla-bandha	A posture where the body from the anus to the navel is contracted and lifted up and towards the spine.
Mūlādhāra-chakra	Nervous plexus situated in the pelvis above the anus at the base or root of the spine, the main support of the body.
Muṇḍakopaniṣad	Name of an Upanishad dealing with the mystic syllable Auṁ.
Nachiketā	Name of the seeker and one of the principal characters in the Kaṭhopaniṣad. His father Vājaśravas wanted to give away all his possessions so as to acquire religious merit. Nachiketā felt puzzled and asked his father again and again: 'To whom will you give me?' His father said: 'I give you to Yama (the god of Death).' Nachiketā went down to the realm of Death and obtained three boons, the last of which was the knowledge of the secret of life after death. Yama tried to divert Nachiketā from obtaining his wish by offering the greatest earthly pleasures, but Nachiketā was not swayed from his purpose and ultimately Yama gave him the knowledge desired.
Nāda	Inner mystical sound.
Nāḍī	A tubular organ of the subtle body through which energy flows. It consists of three layers, one inside the other, like insulation of an electric wire. The innermost layer is called the 'sirā' and the middle layer 'damanī'. The entire organ as well as the outer layer is called 'nāḍī'.

Nāḍī-śodhana	The purification or cleansing of the nāḍīs.
Nāga	One of the subsidiary vital airs which relieves abdominal pressure, causing one to belch.
Nakra	A crocodile.
Nara	A man.
Narasiṁha	The man-lion, Visnu in his fourth incarnation.
Naṭarāja	A name of Śiva, the lord of the dancers.
Nauli	A process in which the abdominal muscles and organs are made to move vertically and laterally in a surging motion.
Nāva	A boat.
'*Neti Neti*'	'Not this! Not this!' The experience of samādhi is not like other experiences, which can be described in words. About it the sages say 'It is not this! It is not this!', for speech fails to convey the feeling of joy and peace experienced in that state.
Nirālamba	Without support.
Niranjana	Unstained; free from falsehood, pure.
Nirodha	Restraint, suppression.
Niruddha	Restrained, checked, controlled.
Niyama	Self-purification by discipline. The second stage of yoga mentioned by Patañjāli.
Pāda	The foot or leg; also part of a book.
Pādāṅguṣṭha	The big toe.
Padma	A lotus.
Padmanābha	A name of Viṣṇu who is said to have a lotus growing out of his navel. From this lotus came forth Brahmā.
Pāṇḍava	Name of any of the five sons of Pāṇḍu, the heroes in the Mahābhārata.
Paramapāda	The highest step, the supreme state, final beatitude.
Paramātmā	The Supreme Spirit.
Parāṅgmukhi	Facing inwards.
Paraśurāma	The sixth incarnation of Viṣṇu, who destroyed the Kṣatriya or warrior class with his battle-axe (paraśu).
Parigha	A beam or a bar used for bolting or shutting a gate.
Parigraha	Hoarding.
Paripūrṇa	Entire, complete.
Parivartana	Turning round, revolving.
Parivṛtta	Turned around, revolved.
Parivṛttaika-pāda	With one leg turned around.
Pārśva	The side, flank; lateral.

Parśvaika-pāda	With one leg turned sideways.
Parvata	A mountain.
Pārvati	A goddess, consort of Śiva, daughter of Himālaya.
Paryanka	A bed, a couch.
Pāśa	A fetter, trap, noose.
Paśchima	West; the back of the whole body from head to heels.
Paśchimottana	Intense stretch of the back side of the body from the nape to the heels.
Pātāla	The nether region.
Patañjali	The propounder of Yoga philosophy. He was the author of the Yoga Sūtras, the Mahābhāśya (a classical treatise on grammar) and a treatise on medicine.
Pīḍā	Pain, suffering, pressure.
Pincha	The chin, a feather.
Piṇḍa	The foetus or embryo, the body.
Piṇḍa-prāṇa	The individual breath, as contrasted with the cosmic or Universal breath.
Piṅgalā	A nāḍī or channel of energy, starting from the right nostril, then moving to the crown of the head and thence downwards to the base of the spine. As the solar energy flows through it it is also called the sūrya-nāḍī. Piṅgalā means tawny or reddish.
Plīhā	The spleen.
Prahlāda	A great devotee of Viṣṇu. He was the son of the demon king Hiraṇya-kaśipu.
Prajāpati	The lord of created beings.
Prajñā	Intelligence, wisdom.
Prajñātmā	The intelligential self.
Prakṛti	Nature, the original source of the material world, consisting of three qualities, sattva, rajas and tamas.
Pramāda	Indifference, insensibility.
Pramāṇa	A standard or ideal; authority.
Prāṇa	Breath, respiration, life, vitality, wind, energy, strength. It also connotes the soul.
Prāṇa-vāyu	The vital air which pervades the entire human body. It moves in the region of the chest.
Praṇava	Another word for the sacred syllable Auṁ.
Prāṇāyāma	Rhythmic control of breath. The fourth stage of yoga.
Praṇidhāna	Dedication.
Prasārita	Spread out, stretched out.
Praśvāsa	Expiration.

Pratiloma	Against the hair, against the grain.
Pratyāhāra	Withdrawal and emancipation of the mind from the domination of the senses and sensual objects. The fifth stage of yoga.
Pratyakṣa	Direct evidence.
Puṇya	Virtue, merit, righteous, just, good.
Puraka	Inhalation.
Pūrṇatā	Fullness, perfection.
Pūrva	East. The front of the body.
Pūrvottana	The intense stretch of the front side of the body.
Rāga	Love, passion, anger.
Rāja	A king, a ruler.
Rāja-kapota	King pigeon.
Rāja-mārga	The royal road to self-realisation through the control of the mind.
Rāja-yoga	The achievement of union with the Supreme Universal Spirit, by becoming the ruler of one's own mind by defeating its enemies. The chief of these enemies are: Kāma (passion or lust), krodha (anger or wrath), lobha (greed), moha (delusion), mada (pride) and matsara (jealousy or envy). The eight-fold yoga of Patañjāli shows the royal road (rāja-mārga) for achieving this objective.
Rāja-yogī	One who has complete mastery over his mind and self. One who has conquered himself.
Rājarṣi	A royal sage, a philosopher king.
Rajas	Mobility or activity; one of the three qualities or constituents of everything in nature.
Rajo-guṇa	The quality of mobility or activity.
Rāma	The hero of the epic Rāmāyaṇa. The seventh incarnation of Viṣṇu.
Rāmāyaṇa	Name of the celebrated epic about the exploits of Rāma. It is the work of the sage Vālmīki.
Rāvaṇa	Name of the demon king of Lankā who abducted Sītā, wife of Rāma.
Rechaka	Exhalation, emptying of the lungs.
Retus	Semen.
Ṛṣi	An inspired sage.
Ṙu	The second syllable in the word 'guru', meaning light.
Ruchika	A sage.

Sādhaka	A seeker, an aspirant.
Sādhanā	Practice, quest.
Sādhana-pāda	The second part of Patañjāli's Yoga Sūtras, dealing with the means.
Sahajāvasthā	The natural state of the soul in samādhi.
Sahasrāra-chakra	The thousand-petalled lotus in the cerebral cavity.
Sahita Kumbhaka	'Sahita' means 'accompanied' or 'attended by' or 'together with'. An intentional suspension of breath.
Śakuntalā	The daughter of the sage Viśvāmitra and the nymph Menakā. She is the heroine of Kālidāsa's play bearing her name.
Śalabha	A locust.
Sālamba	With support.
Sama	Same, equal, even, upright.
Sama-sthiti	Standing still and straight.
Sama-vṛtti	Of equal movement in inhalation, exhalation and suspension of breath in Prāṇāyāma.
Samādhi	A state in which the aspirant is one with the object of his meditation, the Supreme Spirit pervading the universe, where there is a feeling of unutterable joy and peace.
Samādhi-pāda	The first part of Patañjāli's Yoga Sūtras, dealing with the state of samādhi.
Samāna	One of the vital airs, whose function is to aid digestion.
Sambhava	Birth.
Śāmbhava or *Śāmbhavī*	Belonging to Śambhu or Śiva.
Śambhu	A name of Śiva.
Saṁśaya	Doubt.
Saṁskāra	Mental impression of the past.
Ṣaṇ	Six.
Sanjīvani	A kind of elixir or medicinal plant, said to restore the dead to life.
Śankarāchārya	A celebrated teacher of the doctrine of Advaita.
Ṣaṇmukha	Literally with six mouths. Another name of Kārtikeya, the god of war.
Ṣaṇmukhī-mudrā	A sealing posture where the apertures in the head are closed and the mind is directed inwards to train it for meditation.
Santoṣa	Contentment.
Saraswatī	A tributary of the Ganges. Also the name of the

goddess of speech and learning, the consort of Brahmā.

Sarva All, whole.

Sarvāṅga The whole body.

Satī The daughter of Dakṣa Prajāpati. She immolated herself for the insult offered to her husband Śiva by her father, and was then reborn as the daughter of Himālaya and again won Siva as her husband. She was the mother of Kārtikeya (the god of war) and of Ganapati (the god of learning, wisdom and good luck).

Sattva The illuminating, pure and good quality of everything in nature.

Sattva-guṇa The quality of goodness and purity.

Śaucha Purity, cleanliness.

Śava A corpse, a dead body.

Śayana A bed, a couch.

Śeṣa A celebrated serpent, said to have a thousand heads. Śeṣa is represented as the couch of Viṣṇu, floating on the cosmic ocean, or as supporting the world on his hoods. Other names of Śeṣa are Ananta and Vāsuki.

Setu A bridge.

Setu-bandha The construction of a bridge. Name of an āsana in which the body is arched.

Siddha A sage, seer or prophet; also a semi-divine being of great purity and holiness.

Siṁha A lion.

Sirā A tubular organ in the body. *See* nāḍī.

Śirṣa The head.

Śiṣya A pupil, a disciple.

Sītā Name of the wife of Rāma, the heroine of the epic Rāmāyaṇa.

Śita Cool, cold.

Sitakārī and *Śitalī* Types of prāṇāyāma which cool the system.

Śiva Name of the third god of the Hindu Trinity, who is entrusted with the task of destruction.

Śiva-saṁhitā A classical textbook on Haṭha-yoga.

Skanda A name of Kārtikeya, the god of war.

Smrti Memory, a code of law.

Śodhana Purification, cleansing.

'*Soham*' 'He am I'; the unconscious repetitive prayer that

	goes on with every inhalation within every living creature throughout life.
Śoka	Anguish, distress, grief, sorrow.
Śraddhā	Faith, trust.
Steya	Theft, robbery.
Sthita-prajñā	One whose wisdom is firmly established and does not waver; one who is unmoved by the dualities of pleasure and pain, gain and loss, joy and sorrow, victory and defeat.
Sthiti	Stability.
Styāna	Languor, sloth.
Sugrīva	A monkey chief who assisted Rāma in his search and recovery of Sītā, who had been abducted by the demon king Rāvaṇa.
Sukha	Happiness, delight, joy, pleasure, comfort.
Sumanasya	Benevolence.
Śunyāśūnya	The mind is in a state of void (Śūnya) and yet a state that is not void (aśūnya).
Supta	Sleeping.
Sūrya	The sun.
Sūrya-bhedana	Piercing or passing through (bhedana) the sun. Here the inhalation is done through the right nostril, from where the Piṅgalā-nāḍī or Sūrya-nāḍī starts. Exhalation is done through the left nostril, from where the Iḍā-nāḍī or Chandra-nāḍī starts.
Sūrya-chakra	Nervous plexus situated between the navel and the heart.
Sūrya-nāḍī	The nāḍī of the sun. Another name for Piṅgalā-nāḍī.
Suṣumṇā	The main channel situated inside the spinal column.
Suṣupti-avasthā	The state of the mind in dreamless sleep.
Sva	One's own, innate, vital force, soul, self.
Svādhiṣṭhāna-chakra	The nervous plexus situated above the organs of generation.
Svādhyāya	Education of the self by study of divine literature.
Śvāna	A dog.
Svapnāvasthā	The state of the mind in a dream.
Śvāsa	Inspiration.
Śvāsa-praśvāsa	Heaving and sighing.
Svātmārāma	The author of the Haṭha-yoga-pradīpikā, a classical textbook on Haṭha-yoga.
Tāḍa	A mountain.

Tamas	Darkness or ignorance, one of the three qualities or constituents of everything in nature.
Tamo-guṇa	The quality of darkness or ignorance.
Tan or *Tān*	To stretch, extend, lengthen out.
Tāṇḍava	The violent dance of Śiva, symbolising the destruction of the universe.
Tap	To burn, to blaze, to shine, to suffer pain, to be consumed by heat.
Tapas	A burning effort which involves purification, self-discipline and austerity.
Tāraka	A demon slain by Kārtikeya, the god of war.
'Tat twam asi'	'That thou art.' The realisation of the real nature of man as being part of the divine, and of the divinity within himself, which liberates the human spirit from the confines of his body, mind, intellect and ego.
Tattva	The true or first principle, an element or primary substance. The real nature of the human soul or the material world and the Supreme Universal Spirit pervading the universe.
Tattva-jñāna	The knowledge of the true principle.
Tejas	Lustre, brilliance, majesty.
Ṭha	The second syllable of the word 'haṭha'. The first syllable 'ha' stands for the sun, while the second syllable 'ṭha' stands for the moon. The union of these two is Haṭha-yoga.
Tirieng	Horizontal, oblique, transverse, reverse and upside down.
Tittibha	A firefly.
Tola	A balance.
Tri	Three.
Triaṅga	Three limbs.
Trikoṇa	A triangle.
Trivikrama	Viṣṇu is his fifth incarnation, who with his three steps (krama) filled the earth, heaven and hell.
Tṛṣṇā	Thirst, longing, desire.
Turīyāvasthā	The fourth state of the soul, combining yet transcending the other three states of waking, dreaming and sleeping state – the state of samādhi.
Ubhaya	Both.
Udāna	One of the vital airs which pervades the human body, filling it with vital energy. It dwells in the thoracic cavity and controls the intake of air and food.

Uḍḍīyāna	A fetter or bondage. Here the diaphragm is lifted high up the thorax and the abdominal organs are pulled back towards the spine. Through the Uḍḍīyāna-bandha the great bird Prāṇa (life) is forced to fly up through the Suṣumṇā-nāḍī.
Ugra	Formidable, powerful, noble.
Ujjāyi	A type of prāṇāyāma in which the lungs are fully expanded and the chest is puffed out.
Ullola	A large wave or surge.
Umā	Another name of the goddess Pārvati, consort of Śiva.
Unmanī	The state of samādhi.
Upaniṣad	The word is derived from the prefixes 'upa' (near) and 'ni' (down), added to the root 'sad' (to sit). It means sitting down near a Guru to receive spiritual instruction. The Upanishads are the philosophical portion of the Vedas, the most ancient sacred literature of the Hindus, dealing with the nature of man and the universe and the union of the individual soul or self with the Universal Soul.
Upaviṣṭha	Seated.
Upekṣā	Disregard. Upekṣā is not only a feeling of disdain for a person who has fallen into vice or a feeling of indifference or superiority towards him. It is also a self-examination to find out how one would have behaved in like circumstances and also how far he is responsible for the state of the fallen one and to help him on to the right path.
Ūrdhva	Raised, elevated, tending upwards.
Ūrdhva-mukha	Face upwards.
Ūrdhva-retus	(Ūrdhva = upwards, retus = semen.) One who lives in perpetual celibacy and abstains from sexual intercourse. One who has sublimated sexual desire.
Uṣṭra	A camel.
Ut	A particle, denoting intensity.
Utkaṭa	Powerful, fierce.
Uttāna	An intense stretch.
Utthita	Raised up, extended, stretched.
Vāchā	Speech.
Vāchika	Relating to speech, oral.
Vaikuṇṭha	An epithet of Viṣṇu.
Vairāgya	Absence of worldly desires.

Vajra	A thunderbolt, the weapon of Indra.
Vakra	Crooked.
Vālakhilya	A class of divine personages of the size of a thumb, produced from the Creator's body, and said to precede the chariot of the sun.
Valli	A chapter of the Upanishads.
Vāma	The left side.
Vāmadeva	A sage.
Vāmana	Viṣṇu in his fifth incarnation, when he was born as a dwarf to humble the demon king Bali.
Vaṇḍi	A court scholar at the court of king Janaka.
Vāsanā	Desire, inclination, longing.
Vasanta	The season of spring personified as a deity. A companion of Kāma, the god of love and passion.
Vasiṣṭha	A celebrated sage, author of several Vedic hymns.
Vāsuki	Another name of Śeṣa, q.v.
Vātāyana	A horse.
Vāyu	The wind, the vital airs.
Veda	The sacred scriptures of the Hindus, revealed by the Supreme Being.
Vibhūti	Might, power, greatness.
Vibhūti-pāda	The third part of the Yoga Sūtras of Patañjāli, dealing with the powers that the yogi comes across in his quest.
Vidyā	Knowledge, learning, lore, science.
Vikalpa	Fancy, resting merely on verbal expression, without any factual basis.
Vikṣepa	Distraction, confusion, perplexity.
Vikṣipta	Agitated state of the mind.
Viloma	Against the hair, against the order of things. The particle 'vi' denotes negation or privation.
Viparīta	Inverted, reversed.
Viparyaya	A mistaken view, which is later observed to be such, after study.
Vīra	A hero, brave.
Vīrabhadra	A powerful hero created out of Śiva's matted hair.
Virancha or *Viranchi*	A name of Brahma.
Virochana	A demon prince, who was the son of Prahlāda and the father of Bali.
Vīrya	Vigour, strength, virility, enthusiasm.
Viṣama-vṛtti	Uneven or vehement movement while breathing.

Viṣṇu	The second deity of the Hindu trinity, entrusted with the preservation of the world.
Viśuddha-chakra	The nervous plexus in the pharyngeal region.
Viśvāmitra	A celebrated sage.
Vitasti	A span.
Vṛkṣa	A tree.
Vṛśchika	A scorpion.
Vṛt	To turn, to revolve, to roll on.
Vṛtti	A course of action, behaviour, mode of being, condition or mental state.
Vyādhi	Sickness, disease, illness.
Vyāna	One of the vital airs, which pervades the entire body and circulates the energy derived from food and breathing all over the body.
Yama	The god of death. Yama is also the first of the eight limbs or means of attaining yoga. Yamas are universal moral commandments or ethical disciplines transcending creeds, countries, age and time. The five mentioned by Patañjali are: non-violence, truth, non-stealing, continence and non-coveting.
Yoga	Union, communion. The word 'yoga' is derived from the root 'yuj' meaning to join, to yoke, to concentrate one's attention on. It is the union of our will to the will of God, a poise of the soul which enables one to look evenly at life in all its aspects. The chief aim of yoga is to teach the means by which the human soul may be completely united with the Supreme Spirit pervading the universe and thus secure absolution.
Yoga-mudrā	A posture.
Yoga-nidrā	The sleep of yoga, where the body is at rest as if in sleep while the mind remains fully conscious, though all its movements are stilled. Yoga-nidrā is also the name of an āsana.
Yoga Sūtra	The classical work on yoga by Patañjali. It consists of 185 terse aphorisms on yoga and it is divided into four parts dealing respectively with samādhi, the means by which yoga is attained, the powers the seeker comes across in his quest and the state of absolution.
Yogi or *Yogin*	One who follows the path of yoga.
Yoni-mudrā	Yoni means the womb or source and mudrā a seal.

	Yoni-mudrā is a sealing posture where the apertures of the head are closed and the aspirant's senses are directed within to enable him to find out the source of his being.
Yuga	An age.
Yuj	To join, to yoke, to use, to concentrate one's attention on.
Yukta	One who has attained communion with the Supreme Spirit pervading the universe.

Index